Breastfeeding the Newborn

CLINICAL STRATEGIES FOR NURSES

Breastfeeding the Newborn

CLINICAL STRATEGIES FOR NURSES

Marie Biancuzzo, RN, MS, IBCLC
Perinatal Clinical Nurse Specialist
Herndon, Virginia

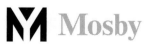

St. Louis   Baltimore   Boston   Carlsbad   Chicago   Minneapolis   New York   Philadelphia   Portland
London   Milan   Sydney   Tokyo   Toronto

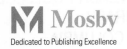

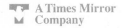

Mosby
Dedicated to Publishing Excellence

A Times Mirror
Company

Publisher: Nancy L. Coon
Editor: Michael Ledbetter
Developmental Editor: Nancy L. O'Brien
Project Manager: John Rogers
Production Editor: Helen Hudlin
Designer: Lee Goldstein, Kathy Gosche
Manufacturing Manager: Karen Lewis

A Note To The Reader:
The author and publisher have made every attempt to check dosages and nursing content for accuracy. Because the science of pharmacology is continually advancing, our knowledge base continues to expand. Therefore we recommend that the reader always check product information for changes in dosage or administration before administering any medication. This is particularly important with new or rarely used drugs.

Composition by Clarinda Company
Printing/binding by R.R. Donnelley & Sons Company

Mosby, Inc.
11830 Westline Industrial Drive
St. Louis, Missouri 63146

International Standard Book Number 0-8151-2453-8

99 00 01 02 03 / 9 8 7 6 5 4 3 2 1

CONTRIBUTOR

Daniel J. Cobaugh, Pharm.D.
Finger Lakes Regional Poison Center and
Department of Emergency Medicine
University of Rochester Medical Center
Rochester, New York

R E V I E W E R S

Lois D. W. Arnold, MPH, IBCLC
Executive Director
Human Milk Banking Association of
North America, Inc.
Sandwich, Massachusetts

Debi Leslie Bocar, RN, MS, MEd, IBCLC
Nurse Lactation Consultant
Mercy Health Center
Oklahoma City, Oklahoma

Charlotte Breithaupt, RN, MN, IBCLC
Lecturer and Clinical Faculty
Baylor University School of Nursing
Dallas, Texas

Karin Cadwell, RN, PhD, IBCLC
Faculty
Healthy Children 2000
Sandwich, Massachusetts

Dorothy Sholes Crowder, RN, BS, MS, CCE
Associate Professor Emeritus
Medical College of Virginia School of
Nursing
Virginia Commonwealth University
Richmond, Virginia

Kathy Della Porta, RN, MS
NICU Discharge Planning Coordinator
University of Rochester Medical Center
Rochester, New York

Donna A. Dowling, RN, PhD
Assistant Professor of Nursing
Frances Payne Bolton School of Nursing
Case Western Reserve University
Cleveland, Ohio

Nancy Hurst, RN, MSN, IBCLC
Director
Lactation Program and Milk Bank
Texas Children's Hospital
Houston, Texas

Jill Janke, RN, MN, DNSc
Professor
University of Alaska—Anchorage
Anchorage, Alaska

Susan K. Krug, MS, RD, CSP
Clinical Research Coordinator
Department of Pediatric Gastroenterology
and Nutrition
Children's Hospital Medical Center
Cincinnati, Ohio

Ruth A. Lawrence, MD
Professor of Pediatrics and Ob/Gyn
School of Medicine
University of Rochester
Rochester, New York

Mary L. Overfield, RN, MN, IBCLC
Lactation Consultant at Wake Medical
International Board Certified Lactation
Consultant
Raleigh, North Carolina

Toni Ross, RNC, PNP, PhD
Infectious Diseases Consultant
Glen Cove, New York

Sharleen H. Simpson, BSN, MSN, MA, PhD
Associate Professor, College of Nursing
University of Florida
Gainesville, Florida

Amy Kathryn Spangler, BSN, MN, IBCLC
Education Coordinator
Marietta OB/GYN Affiliates
Atlanta, Georgia

June D. Thompson, RN, MSN, DrPH
Director, Research, Education, and
Standards
University of New Mexico Health
Sciences Center
Albuquerque, New Mexico

Susan M. Tucker, RN, MSN, PhN, CNAA
Healthcare Consultant
Roseville, California

**Beverley Walker, M.Bioeth, B.App.Sc.,
IBCLC, RM, RN**
Consultant
Breastfeeding Education Victoria
Victoria, Australia

To my parents, who provided education and support for all of my endeavors
To my husband, David, who gives me unconditional love
And for the greater glory of God

PREFACE

The idea for this book was conceived in a corridor of the Georgetown University Levey Conference Center. At the time, I was a clinical nurse specialist at the University of Rochester Medical Center and had flown to Washington, DC to give a lecture. After the lecture, Karen Rechnitzer, RN, IBCLC (who later became my colleague at Georgetown University Hospital), said to me: "I've been doing this for years and I learned a lot from your presentation. All of that good information should be in one handy place. You should write a book!" I was amused by the idea but had no intention of writing a book. On the return flight, however, I found myself creating one more handout for a class, writing one more policy for the department, and later scurrying to the library for one more article that might help to solve our latest clinical crisis. It took a few years before I realized that I had several drawers full of articles, handouts, and related materials that could be assembled into a book.

This book was born out of necessity. From my earliest days as a staff nurse, I needed a book that told me how to manage breastfeeding, similar to the dozens of books that told me how to provide nursing care for the laboring patient. My early years in clinical practice were fraught with many frustrations; hospital policies and protocols that restricted breastfeeding made little sense to me. I soon began reading articles in medical journals but found them difficult to comprehend. I wanted a book on my shelf that would help me with my everyday role and responsibility as a staff nurse. My role changed over the years, and my need for knowledge increased. As the breastfeeding coordinator at the University of Rochester Medical Center, I found myself giving direct patient care, writing policies and procedures, and coordinating interdisciplinary efforts on a topic that I needed to know more about—breastfeeding! I wanted a book for nurses that would give clinical strategies based on an understanding of physiology and scholarly research.

This book reflects my own philosophy about the nurse's role and responsibility. I believe the staff nurse must use all of her knowledge, skills, and resources to meet the patient's physical, emotional, and spiritual needs as completely as possible. She cannot pick and chose which needs to meet based on her current knowledge or personal biases. Whether the nurse assumes care for the breastfeeding newborn or for the adult with a lung transplant, regardless of the patient's needs, she uses the same four components of the nursing process: assessment, planning, implementation, and evaluation. This book shows how to use interviewing, physical assessment, and other data-gathering mechanisms to make assessments about the mother's or the newborn's biological, psychological, and sociocultural needs in relation to breastfeeding. The proposed plan of care establishes goals to promote wellness but respects the mother's choices for how to achieve those goals. In each chapter there are concrete examples of how to implement care for the breastfeeding dyad: collaborating with members of the interdisciplinary team, becoming an advocate for the mother and newborn, facilitating informed consent, administering medications, prioritizing care, and enabling the mother to become confident and independent in breastfeeding her newborn. The book also gives specific ideas for how to evaluate the effectiveness of interventions. Within these pages the nurse will learn how to assess, plan, implement, and evaluate care for most of the clients she will encounter. I hope that this book will become a starting point for advanced practice nurses who function in the expanded role. When advanced practice nurses assume care for women and infants who are breastfeeding under difficult circumstances, they need to gain the same level of specialization and expertise as they would when working with groups of patients having other complex needs—for example, those with diabetes or those undergoing renal dialysis. It is my hope that the advanced practice nurse would gain sufficient knowledge about breastfeeding to become a clinical expert for individual patients, as well as a change agent within her health care setting and an advocate for national policy.

The basic organization of the book promotes breastfeeding at the personal, interpersonal, and system level, delivering evidence-based care across the health-illness continuum. Section 1 describes the basic sociocultural, psychological, and biological factors that influence breastfeeding. Section 2 describes the how-to of client education and clinical management of the well mother and newborn. Section 3 explains the underlying pathophysiology that can interfere with breastfeeding. Section 4 explores strategies to enhance the breastfeeding relationship when the mother and infant must be separated from each other. The book assumes that if the nurse adequately supports mothers and neonates (newborns from birth to 28 days old), the continuation of breastfeeding is likely.

There are three special boxed features in the book. **Clinical Scenarios** describe real people, although names have been changed. Most of the clinical scenarios are designed to help nurses think critically about how to solve a problem while a few help the reader to reflect on the philosophy or approach that was used in the scenario. **Historical Highlights** include perspectives and wisdom contributed to the art and science of breastfeeding before most of us were in practice.

Research Highlights discuss studies that have not yet been fully applied to the clinical area, or that refute a commonly-held myth. Boxes designated as *Priorities for Care* were designed to help the busy nurse prioritize when she is holding the book open with one hand and eating lunch with the other.

This book will be enlightening to some and unsettling to others. Although I have tried to provide clear directives in some cases, I have also tried to avoid giving the impression that there is only one right answer or strategy. Readers are encouraged to use clinical judgment. Furthermore, I presume that readers are like me, continually generating questions and seeking further clarity. Therefore I encourage readers to send their questions and comments to me at

bookcomments@wmc-worldwide.com.

My struggle to become both scholar and clinical expert becomes evident in these pages. Yet, after many years as a staff nurse, clinical nurse specialist, and university instructor, I wrote this book not to help the nurse *know* more, but to help her *do* something that will effect better patient outcomes. I like to imagine myself standing next to the reader, showing techniques, suggesting strategies, and asking provocative questions about cases that require a decision but have no easy answers. At the same time, I want to inspire the reader to yearn for the library and spend hours there reading about breastfeeding. Relatively few of us need to *generate* new research. All of us need to *apply* the existing research to clinical practice in order to achieve better clinical outcomes.

I labored through this book during two of the most exciting and difficult years of my life. The first four chapters were written amid paint fumes and nail-pounding that occurred during the extensive repair of our storm-damaged home. Just after I completed Chapter 8, my father died and it became very difficult for me to write. Knowing that my father didn't have much respect for people who waste time, however, I pressed on. The text was written on planes and trains while I was criss-crossing the country from Virginia to California. I wrote in hotel rooms in Alaska and next to swimming pools in Florida. Mothers, nurses, and colleagues continually inspired me to write a book that went straight to the heart of clinical matters.

This book was nurtured by numerous people. Two of my former students at Georgetown University School of Nursing helped immensely. Megan McGratty, RN, copied dozens of articles and always had a word of encouragement for the project. Cathy Zilinskas, RN, carried the heaviest load for the most laborious and boring tasks of finding, copying, collating, and organizing hundreds of articles and filing them with the hundreds of others I had been collecting for nearly 20 years. She performed numerous other tasks with efficiency and cheerfulness and helped me to never lose heart. My sister-in-law, Barbara Savins, verified the titles, cost, and availability of the patient education materials and contact information listed in the appendices; an awesome task. My friend, Mary Beauchamp, helped me through the last difficult miles of the book. Without her superb organizational skills, attention to detail, and ability to stay calm in my chaotic and cluttered office, this book may never have existed.

Karin Cadwell, RN, PhD, graciously responded to multiple phone calls when I have felt confused and uninformed. I am completely indebted to Sarah Coulter Danner, whose expertise and publications about breastfeeding the infant with cleft or neurological defects have greatly influenced my clinical approach. Sarah has graciously tutored me through many pages of this book. Debi Bocar, RN, MS, IBCLC, has reviewed more than half of the chapters in the book and has made numerous constructive suggestions. Moreover, Debi's creativity appears throughout these pages; her photographs and other materials have greatly enhanced the quality of this book.

Numerous colleagues at the University of Rochester Medical Center have helped me, including Kathy Della Porta who has reviewed various portions of this book and responded to several panicked, last-minute phone calls. My friend and former colleague, Ruth Lawrence, MD, was a tremendous influence on me during my years at University of Rochester Medical Center and continues to mentor me. She has graciously loaned articles and responded to the multiple e-mail, fax, and phone queries I sent on a weekly or daily basis since starting the book. I am enormously indebted to her not only for her expertise but for her ongoing support of my endeavors to provide direct care for patients and continuing education for nurses. I could never begin to thank her for all she has done for me throughout the years.

At Mosby, my editor, Michael Ledbetter, recognized the need for a new book on breastfeeding for nurses and had confidence in the potential of a first-time book author. My developmental editor, Nancy O'Brien, encouraged me with her consistently positive attitude and ability to put up with my numerous quirks. Her incredible gift for recognizing the fine line between pushing me and challenging me has been a true blessing.

My parents have been a tremendous source of inspiration. My mother went against the grain, breastfeeding her children in the 1940s and 1950s when bottle feeding was the social norm. She was often horrified by my tales of how we restrict breastfeeding in the hospital and wholeheartedly supported my efforts to reduce barriers to breastfeeding within the hospital and on the national front. Without her insistence that every woman can breastfeed, I would have undoubtedly believed that it was reserved for the chosen few. My father always insisted that education was cheaper than ignorance. If this book educates just one nurse, I will never count the cost of the time, energy, and money that went into creating it.

My husband, David Vaklyes, has been a pillar of strength for me. Beyond his daily reminder of "you can do this, dear," he took many evenings, weekends, and vacation days to give hands-on support for the project. I shudder to think how many small errors might have gone unnoticed if he had not carefully reviewed the calculations and graphs within these pages. Many times he made the 380-mile trip with me to the Miner Library at the University of Rochester Medical Center or accompanied me to the Dahlgren Library at Georgetown University Medical Center here in Washington, DC. He has also spent hours on the Internet identifying pertinent web sites, finding e-mail addresses for authors of articles, and downloading citations from MedLine. He also plowed through newspapers finding everything from articles about breastfeeding legislation to cartoons about authors, editors, and breastfeeding mothers. (The cartoons helped me to keep my sense of humor.) Without his help and encouragement, I would still be complaining about the need for the book, rather than writing the book.

C O N T E N T S

Section 3

Breastfeeding Under Difficult Circumstances

Section 4

Choices: Sources of Nutrition and Delivery Techniques

1

Factors Influencing Successful Breastfeeding

1

Social/Cultural Factors

SOCIETAL INFLUENCES

Infants have been breastfed for thousands of years. During the late nineteenth and early twentieth centuries, however, breastfeeding rates began to decline as other options became readily available. Nestlé had manufactured and distributed its Milk Food for Infants in the 1870s throughout the United States and Europe and in other areas. Shortly after the turn of the century, American medical researchers were also involved in creating artificial milk for infants.[1] Thereafter, breastfeeding was no longer the norm in American society; infants could be either breastfed or bottle fed.

Several social changes occurred in the 1930s. More and more women began delivering in hospitals with central nurseries, and the ease of sterilization processes made bottle feeding possible there and at home. Furthermore, physicians and commercial companies throughout the world were making more and more precise "formulas" for infants. Formula, meaning artificial milk or human milk substitute, soon became widely available. Even the word *formula* connoted a scientific method, and these milk substitutes gained favor as the scientific way of feeding. Eventually, the mother was able to make the "formula" because the directions for mixing were simply printed on the container. Physicians, worried that their influence on infant feeding would be usurped by "commercial men," began to have talks with artificial milk companies about advertising. Between 1929 and 1932 the American Medical Association exerted pressure on the formula industry to advertise only to physicians. This understanding between the professional and corporate worlds continued for nearly 50 years.

In the 1940s the dairy industry exploded, resulting in an abundance of leftover whey. Rather than let it go to waste, the industry used the whey to create a huge industry for artificial milk. As a result of effective marketing strategies, artificial milk and bottles became a status symbol for those who could afford them. Americans hailed the scientific advances of artificial milk, considering it equal to or better than human milk. With virtually no studies on human milk and an emphasis on "science-based" artificial milk, breastfeeding management was soon based more on myth than on science; hence, inaccurate information from health care providers and changing social norms later led to a decline in breastfeeding. Several key influences became either facilitators for or barriers to breastfeeding.

Facilitators for Breastfeeding

Events of the 1940s, 1950s, and 1960s

In the late 1940s a great facilitator of breastfeeding was related to consumer demand for rooming-in. One woman, anticipating a delivery at Yale New Haven Hospital, requested rooming-in for herself and her infant. Although her request was denied, ironically, she had a communicable disease when she was admitted to the hospital, and "rooming-in" was initiated as an infection control measure. This woman's initial request served as the impetus for the Yale New Haven Rooming-In Project, which was enthusiastically received by mothers and improved breastfeeding efforts.[2] Few hospitals adopted this model, however, and central nurseries and bottle feeding predominated; in 1957 only 21% of infants discharged from the hospitals were exclusively breastfed.[1] Artificial feeding, which predominated throughout the 1950s, 1960s, and 1970s, was often viewed as superior, or at least equal, to breastfeeding. One physician, a breastfeeding advocate, noted that the decline in breastfeeding was caused by perception: "Formula feeding has become so simple, safe and uniformly successful that breastfeeding no longer seems worth the bother."[3]

Events of the 1970s

In the late 1970s and 1980s, attitudes and practices related to childbearing began to undergo dramatic changes. The movement toward home birth and birthing centers in the San Francisco Bay area fueled the fires to promote natural methods as desirable and superior to the overmedicalized styles of perinatal management. Furthermore, providers of perinatal health care began to change. Certified nurse-midwives were more frequently involved in perinatal care, nurse practitioners were beginning to perform well-baby assessments, and the number of female obstetricians and pediatricians was increasing. These changes in the general philosophy and the gender of health care providers bolstered efforts to focus on the woman's capabilities and needs rather than the medical management of natural processes.

In 1978 the United States began to recognize the centrality of breastfeeding to the health and nutrition of the nation. The Carter administration appointed a committee to develop the first "Goals for The Nation"; one of these goals was increasing breastfeeding incidence and duration. The committee set a goal that, by 1990, breastfeeding would be initiated for 75% of infants and that 35% of those infants would still be breastfeeding at age 6 months.[4] These goals were revised in 1988, but the general intention was to promote breastfeeding as a way to achieve optimal health and nutrition. See Box 1-1.

In 1978 a similar movement began internationally. The Thirty-first World Health Assembly identified the prevention of infant malnutrition as a priority, and breastfeeding as one way to overcome it. In the latter part of 1978, the World Health Organization (WHO) and the United Nations Children's Fund (UNICEF) convened a meeting of 150 representatives of governments, the United Nations system and other intergovernmental bodies, nongovernmental organizations, the infant-food industry, and experts in related disciplines. Of the five main themes related

Box 1-1
Goals for the Nation

In 1978 goals were set that stated that by the year 1990:

- 75% of women would initiate breastfeeding
- 35% of women would continue breastfeeding for at least 6 months[4]

In 1988 goals were set that stated that by the year 2000:

- 75% of women would initiate breastfeeding
- 50% of women would continue breastfeeding for at least 6 months[12]

to breastfeeding undertaken by participants, perhaps the most important was the marketing and distribution of breast-milk substitutes. Several recommendations emerged from this joint WHO/UNICEF meeting.

Events of the 1980s

In 1980 the Thirty-third World Health Assembly endorsed the statements and recommendations of the joint WHO/UNICEF meeting of late 1978. The assembly specified that an international code for marketing infant formula and other products used as breast-milk substitutes should be developed. This code, to be prepared by the director general of WHO, was to be drafted in consultation with all other parties concerned. Several drafts were sent out for comment. In 1981 the WHO endorsed the fourth draft of the code and recommended to the Thirty-fourth World Health Assembly that the code be accepted as a recommendation rather than a regulation.

In May 1981 the World Health Assembly adopted the International Code for Marketing of Breast-Milk Substitutes, with 118 votes in favor, 1 against, and 3 abstentions. (The single vote against the code was from the United States.) The aim of the code was "to contribute to the provision of safe and adequate nutrition for infants, by the protection and promotion of breast-feeding, and by ensuring the proper use of breast-milk substitutes, when these are necessary, on the basis of adequate information and through appropriate marketing and distribution."[5] The main points from the code are found in Appendix D. (The United States did not officially endorse the code until 1994.)

In the 1980s several significant events in the United States increased breastfeeding incidence and continuation. In 1982 the American Academy of Pediatrics (AAP) issued a policy statement entitled "The Promotion of Breast-feeding" that strongly favored breastfeeding.[6] It followed an earlier statement, entitled "Encouraging Breast-Feeding," which was somewhat less directive; the earlier statement drew general conclusions, whereas the later statement made four clear recommendations. Later, the AAP reaffirmed its statement in conjunction with the American College of Obstetricians.[7,8] Most recently, the AAP has strengthened its original statement; the title, "Breastfeeding and the Use of Human Milk"[9] emphasizes the use of human milk even when breastfeeding is not possible, and the statement itself delivers a strong assertion that artificial milk is clearly inferior in all cases.

In 1984 the Maternal and Child Health Bureau (MCHB) of the U.S. Department of Health and Human Services (DHHS) convened the Surgeon General's Workshop. The purpose of the workshop was to assess the current status of breastfeeding in the United States and to develop strategies to facilitate reaching the 1990 breastfeeding objective for the nation. Work groups were formed to identify and prioritize issues related to breastfeeding and lactation and to develop recommendations that would remove the barriers to breastfeeding and better enable the United States to meet breastfeeding goals. This workshop was the first formal attempt to facilitate breastfeeding at the national level through a multidisciplinary group. A report summarizing the themes and recommendations[10] was generated at the conclusion of the meeting, and two follow-up reports were written in subsequent years.

In 1987 the Institute of Medicine Subcommittee on Nutrition During Lactation convened and generated several recommendations,[11] as well as an official statement that endorsed breastfeeding under ordinary circumstances.

In a follow-up to the 1978 effort, the Bush administration in 1988 appointed a committee to develop goals for the nation for the year 2000. A goal was established to increase to 75% the number of mothers who breastfeed their newborns on discharge from the hospital and to 50% those who continue breastfeeding for the first 6 months of life.[12] (Currently, the goals for the year 2010 are being developed.) Despite such promotion throughout the 1980s and 1990s, however, American women have fallen short of this goal as shown in Figure 1-1.

In 1989 the WHO/UNICEF put forth their statement, *Protecting, Promoting, and Supporting Breast-Feeding: The Special Role of Maternity Services*.[13] This statement, which outlined univer-

sally relevant principles and action steps, was intended as a summary of what needed to be done to improve perinatal breastfeeding efforts throughout the world. The Ten Steps to Successful Breastfeeding contained in that document were intended as an executive summary. The Ten Steps, shown in Box 1-2 became the cornerstone for the Baby-Friendly™ Hospital Initiative (BFHI) in 1991. This document also contained

Box 1-2
The Ten Steps to Successful Breastfeeding

The Baby-Friendly™ Hospital Initiative promotes, protects and supports breastfeeding through The Ten Steps to Successful Breastfeeding for Hospitals as outlined by UNICEF and WHO. The steps for the United States are:

1. Have a written breastfeeding policy that is routinely communicated to all health care staff.
2. Train all health care staff in skills necessary to implement this policy.
3. Inform all pregnant women about the benefits and management of breastfeeding.
4. Help mothers initiate breastfeeding within an hour of birth.*
5. Show mothers how to breastfeed and how to maintain lactation even if they should be separated from their infants.
6. Give newborn infants no food or drink other than breastmilk, unless medically indicated.
7. Practice "rooming-in" by allowing mothers and infants to remain together 24 hours a day.
8. Encourage breastfeeding on demand.
9. Give no artificial teats, pacifiers, dummies, or soothers to breastfeeding infants.
10. Foster the establishment of breastfeeding support groups and refer mothers to them on discharge from the hospital or birthing center.

*When written in 1989, this step required breastfeeding initiation within the first *half* hour. Research in the 1990s showed that the natural sequence of behavior is for suckling to occur within the first hour. Therefore, this step was modified for United States hospitals by BFHI.

From WHO and UNICEF. *Protecting, Promoting, and Supporting Breastfeeding. The Special Role of Maternity Services.* Geneva: World Health Organization; 1989.

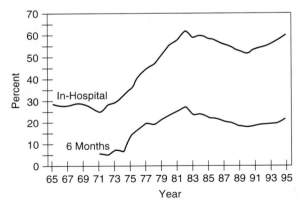

Fig. 1-1 U.S. breastfeeding rates: 1965 through 1995. *(From Ryan AS: The resurgence of breastfeeding in the United States.* Pediatrics *[www.pediatrics.org/cgi/content/full/99/4/e12] 1997;99:2.)*

the Checklist for Evaluating the Adequacy of Support for Breastfeeding. This very important document served as the backbone and impetus for breastfeeding promotion in the 1990s.

Events of the 1990s

Breastfeeding promotion was especially visible in the early 1990s. In the United States in August of 1990, a survey[14] was conducted as a follow-up to the 1984 Surgeon General's Workshop; the intent of this national survey was to identify breastfeeding promotion activities that were related to but happening after the completion of the 1984 workshop. The survey, discussed later in this chapter, provided valuable data about breastfeeding promotion activities throughout the country.

Meanwhile, on the international front, from July 30 to August 1, 1990, a WHO/UNICEF policy makers' meeting was held in Florence, Italy. From this meeting, "Breastfeeding in the 1990s: A Global Initiative," came the WHO/UNICEF joint statement, the "Innocenti Declaration," which described the current state of breastfeeding promotion worldwide and outlined goals to be reached by 1995. One of the goals was for government to ensure "that every facility providing maternity services fully practices all ten of the Ten Steps to Successful Breastfeeding set out in the joint WHO/UNICEF statement *Protecting, Promoting, and Supporting Breast Feeding: The Special Role of Maternity Services.*" Thus the "Innocenti Declaration" became the forerunner of the BFHI.

In 1991 UNICEF and the WHO launched the Baby-Friendly™ Hospital Initiative (BFHI), which sought to overcome some of the general barriers that hospitals imposed on women throughout the world. At the heart of the BFHI were the ten steps listed in the WHO/UNICEF statement. Subsequently, more than 13,000 hospitals throughout the world attained Baby-Friendly™ status. In the United States, the movement was spearheaded by the U.S. Committee for UNICEF (which provided the funding for the project) and Wellstart

International (which provided the technical expertise). Although the United States signed the "Innocenti Declaration," efforts to implement the ten steps were delayed. Currently, only 14 hospitals in the United States have achieved the Baby-Friendly™ award. Baby-Friendly U.S.A. is the official organization for the BFHI program in the United States (see Appendix D) for granting the award. Those hospitals that did change protocols to reflect the BFHI have had excellent results; initiation of breastfeeding, artificial milk supplementation, and support from hospital staff improved markedly in one southwestern hospital.[15]

Barriers to Breastfeeding

At the 1984 workshop, the U.S. Surgeon General, C. Everett Koop, said, "We must identify and reduce the barriers which keep women from beginning or continuing to breastfeed their infants."[10] In 1990, however, the National Center for Education in Maternal and Child Health, in consultation with Maternal and Child Health Bureau staff, conducted a pilot study to gather descriptive data on breastfeeding promotion. While the study identified some promotion activities, many barriers were also revealed in the following categories: (1) professional education, (2) public education, (3) support in the health care system, (4) support services in the community, (5) support in the workplace, and (6) research.

Nearly a decade later, multiple barriers continue to exist around these themes, although there have been some improvements in some areas. The following section describes some data from the national survey and presents observations about how or if the barriers have been removed.

Professional Education

Education for professionals—or, rather, the lack of it—has been and continues to be a barrier to breastfeeding. The national survey identified barriers to consumers that have their origins in professional education. When professionals fail to provide support, give poor advice, or are lacking in knowledge about breastfeeding and lactation management, or when knowledgable, skilled clinicians are inaccessible, barriers to initiating or continuing breastfeeding continue.[14]

Lack of Support

Breastfeeding, perhaps more than other topics in health care, is strongly affected by the personal attitudes, beliefs, and values of the health care provider. Lack of support or encouragement from physicians, nurses, hospital staff, or other health professionals may be related to the difficulty professionals have with setting aside their own attitudes, beliefs, and values. A factor that is consistently associated with promotion of breastfeeding is having had personal experience breastfeeding, or having a spouse who has breastfed.[16-19] One study found that female pediatric house staff were more likely to agree that pediatricians should encourage breastfeeding; male pediatric house staff were more likely to see breastfeeding as "instinctive."[20] This is just one of many examples of how beliefs can interfere with support for breastfeeding.

Nurses who have been practicing for over 20 years have often felt the sting of public perception that nurses are not supportive of breastfeeding. Unfortunately, there is some evidence to substantiate this perception. In one study, nutritionists and physicians had more positive beliefs about breastfeeding than nurses.[19] Furthermore, formal programs to educate nurses are only beginning to appear.

Poor Advice

Despite efforts to improve breastfeeding management, health care professionals, including nurses, continue to give poor advice about breastfeeding management. Poor advice has taken different forms. Sometimes it actually has been no advice. When the person being asked for advice has no answer for the problem, he or she typically recommends switching to artificial feeding. Sometimes it has been inconsistent advice; consumers are very confused when one professional says one thing while another says something to the contrary. Other times it has been inaccurate, incomplete, or inappropriate advice for the circumstances. Such poor advice may be related to the professional's attitude or to the health care provider's inadequate education.

Inadequate Education

A general lack of education among health professionals about breastfeeding and lactation management has been an ongoing barrier during the past few decades. Several studies have shown that formal education about breastfeeding has been sadly lacking in nursing school curricula. The majority of nurses have obtained most of their information about breastfeeding through clinical experience.[21] It is not only optimal but possible to successfully integrate lactation management into health care curricula,[22] and those who have done so have found it tremendously rewarding. Approximately half of the nurses in one study identified nursing school as their main source of information about breastfeeding, yet they were unable to give accurate information on such basic matters as the "letdown" reflex. Admittedly, this is an old study,[23] but those who attended nursing school during the time of the study are likely to be practicing today. Another study showed that entry-level nursing education correlated negatively with nurses' knowledge of breastfeeding[24] or did not correlate with their total score on the researcher's questionnaire.[21] Limited knowledge continues to be a problem.[21,25]

Improving nursing education about breastfeeding management is an ongoing effort. Fortunately, the national registered nurse licensure examination now includes questions about breastfeeding; this was a giant step forward in advancing nurses' awareness and competence in basic breastfeeding management. Today's textbooks have more (and more accurate) information about lactation and breastfeeding management than did textbooks a decade ago, but colleges of nursing have been slow to incorporate lectures on breastfeeding into student curricula at either the undergraduate or the graduate level.

Limited Access to Professional Support

Women have often lacked access to health professionals trained in lactation management. Therefore, even if health care providers are knowledgeable or supportive, they might not be available or accessible. It is also interesting to note that when mothers do seek advice, it is frequently not from health care providers.[26] Rather, women tend to rely on their friends and family for support.[27]

Public Education

In a national questionnaire, 44% of respondents identified public education—specifically, women's attitudes and societal attitudes—as a barrier to breastfeeding. Women's attitudes about modesty, embarrassment, loss of independence, lack of confidence, concern that their milk supply is inadequate, lack of motivation, concern with figure, problems breastfeeding a previous infant, and negative misconceptions were identified as barriers to breastfeeding (see Chapter 4). Several of these individual barriers may interfere with initiating and continuing breastfeeding and are likely to result from lack of accurate information.

The questionnaire noted only one societal attitude that became a barrier: "Breastfeeding is not accepted as the norm; general lack of societal support for breastfeeding." Many years after the survey, this attitude persists. Breastfeeding experts consider human milk as the standard, but others compare human milk or the breastfeeding experience to what they know about artificial feeding as though artificial feeding was the "standard." Mulford[28] shows how a bottle-feeding knowledge base can lead to inaccurate assumptions about breastfeeding. For example, mothers know that artificial milk can spoil if it is unrefrigerated for too

long; this mentality may be the basis for assuming that a breastfeeding mother's illness or ingestion of a particular food may spoil the milk and bother the infant. This bottle-feeding knowledge base may be what causes women to wonder whether their milk is "bad" following such an event.

While public education about breastfeeding has lagged in educational and health care settings, public education about bottle feeding has flourished. Commercial advertising is one form of public "education." Mothers learn about artificial feeding during the antepartum period. One survey showed that 65% of mothers recalled receiving offers for free formula antepartally; 90% cited their primary caregiver as the source of their samples, and 93% of the offers were from companies that market only to hospitals and physicians.[29] Thus physicians have become unintentional advertisers of artificial milk.[30]

It is widely acknowledged that the mass media are highly influential in American culture. Unfortunately, however, they have not always had a positive effect. It is common to see women bottle feeding on television, but breastfeeding is rarely depicted. Furthermore, the bottle has become a common symbol for the baby. Even educational material that is meant to support breastfeeding has not always been useful; frequently it is written at a literacy level that many women cannot comprehend.

Health Care System

Barriers in the health care system have been greatly reduced since they were first formally identified in the Surgeon General's Workshop and in the later survey. These barriers, as well as efforts to eliminate them, have been noted at the national, state, and local level.

National Level
POLICIES AND REGULATORY MECHANISMS
The "Innocenti Declaration" clearly stated, "All governments should develop national breastfeeding policies and set appropriate national targets

for the 1990s."[31] The "Goals for the Nation" were the first step toward setting national targets, but these targets have not been attained. Although there have been several efforts to form a national policy on breastfeeding, to date, none exists.

Progress may occur soon, however. The United States National Breastfeeding Committee was formed in January 1998, with representatives from many organizations, including the Association of Women's Health, Obstetrical and Neonatal Nurses (AWHONN) and the American College of Nurse-Midwives (ACNM). One of the committee's goals is to facilitate a national breastfeeding policy. Until a national policy exists, there will never be a unified and consistent statement to health care providers and consumers that supports breastfeeding, and barriers will continue to exist for the initiation and continuation of breastfeeding.

On a smaller scale, however, policies are beginning to appear. At the original Surgeon General's Workshop, participating organizations were directed to establish position statements on breastfeeding. Many position statements by various organizations have since been written; they are listed in Appendix D. When organizations create such statements and endorse breastfeeding, support for individual mothers is strengthened.

WIC

The Special Supplemental Nutrition Program for Women, Infants and Children (WIC) was legislated by Congress as a pilot program in 1972 and authorized as a permanent program in 1975. WIC was initiated for pregnant, lactating, or postpartum women and their infants and children up to 5 years of age. The goal of this federally funded program is to improve birth outcomes and early childhood development by providing nutrient-dense supplemental foods, nutrition education, and health care referrals. Women and their children are eligible for WIC benefits when their gross family income is below 185% of the poverty level and a nutritionally related medical condition and/or nutritional risk exists. The program has benefited from numerous legislative and regulatory acts over the years. An excellent history of WIC and its effects on women and their children is found elsewhere.[32]

For women, infants, and children, WIC provides supplemental foods that are high in protein, iron, vitamins A and C, and calcium. Because WIC serves over 40% of all infants born in the United States, it is a major purchaser of artificial milk. In the early years, WIC paid the full retail price for artificial milk; later it bid for contracts and then received rebates. This change strengthened the program's ability to serve additional participants; in fact, today this cost-saving measure supports about a quarter of WIC's 7.4 million participants. In addition, WIC's nutrition education and counseling efforts, particularly related to breastfeeding promotion and support, have shown significant improvement. Breastfeeding rates are growing faster among WIC participants than among the general population.[33]

Unlike other organizations and circumstances that perpetuated the barriers, WIC has actively facilitated breastfeeding. In 1989 the United States Department of Agriculture (USDA) set aside $8 million each year, which WIC state agencies were required to spend on breastfeeding promotion and support. Furthermore, each state WIC agency is required to designate a breastfeeding coordinator (see Appendix D). Breastfeeding women have a higher priority for enrollment in the WIC program, their benefits are more varied (more supplemental food benefits), and they have a longer participation period (1 year as opposed to 6 months) than those who choose artificial feeding. Furthermore, mothers receive an expanded food package if they exclusively breastfeed and do not receive any artificial milk from WIC.

In the late 1990s WIC stepped up efforts to provide education and support for breastfeeding. In 1994, Public Law 103-448, the Healthy Meals for Healthy Americans Act, revised the formula for determining the amount of funds to be spent for WIC breastfeeding promotion and support. The act replaced the $8 million target level with a national maximum for breastfeeding promotion and supported expenditures of $21 per year for each pregnant and breastfeeding woman. This amount is adjusted annually based on inflation.

WIC state agencies require staff training to assist mothers through all phases of breastfeeding from prenatal decision making to weaning. Furthermore, WIC has endeavored to be seen as a referral center and resource within the community. In August 1997 the USDA launched the WIC National Breastfeeding Promotion Campaign together with Best Start (a social marketing organization). This campaign includes television and radio spots, billboards, and pamphlets that advertise breastfeeding. The campaign's motto, "Loving support makes breastfeeding work," is designed to send a positive message not only to breastfeeding mothers but also to families and friends who support them.

State

Historically, state health departments have been involved in many matters related to health but minimally involved in breastfeeding promotion. Now, many years after the directives from the Surgeon General's conference, most states have done little to remove the barriers to breastfeeding at the state level. New York state, however, has been a leader. Some of the most serious barriers to breastfeeding in the hospital have been overcome in New York because the state health code incorporated specific directives about breastfeeding (see Appendix D). Because hospitals are required to comply with all aspects of the state health code, these directives were taken seriously by hospital personnel, and many improvements to breastfeeding management followed. Furthermore, the New York State Department of Health has sponsored training programs for health care professionals and has included information about breastfeeding in grade school curricula. These

state-mandated directives have done much to bring about social change.

A task force on breastfeeding has been established in some states, providing an opportunity for health care providers to interact with policy makers to identify barriers to breastfeeding and ways to overcome those barriers. Much work needs to be done, however. States that do not have an active task force on breastfeeding should consider establishing one, and existing task forces should focus on addressing the critical issues. Ideally, members of the task force should include those who are in clinical practice and should aim to identify ways to heighten awareness of other practicing clinicians. Publishing a newsletter that provides highlights of the state's legislation related to breastfeeding matters or WIC activities can serve as a practical tool in promoting breastfeeding management from the state level.

CONTINUUM OF POSTPARTUM CARE
The lack of postpartum services continues to be a barrier to breastfeeding, perhaps more so now than when the Surgeon General's Workshop identified this as a possible barrier. Shortened maternity stays appear to be a trend that will continue. However, a short hospital stay is not necessarily a deterrent to breastfeeding. One recent study found no difference in duration of breastfeeding between mothers who had a 48-hour hospital stay and those who had a 24-hour stay.[34]

There are no well-controlled studies that show the consequences of early discharge.[35,36] Also, studies typically measure mortality, morbidity, and hospital readmission. Any inference that early discharge causes these problems, or that breastfeeding is the culprit, is entirely unsubstantiated.

Postpartum follow-up is essential, but the specifics of how, how long, and by whom such services should be provided is less clear.[37] The follow-up differs markedly in the published studies, tending to be one of three types: (1) no follow-up, (2) telephone follow-up only, or (3) office or clinic follow-up. Unfortunately, no well-controlled studies have addressed breastfeeding specifically, but in general, outcomes for perinatal patients are best when early discharge is followed by an in-person visit rather than a telephone follow-up; providing no follow-up is undesirable.

Local

BREASTFEEDING COORDINATORS

The New York State health code mandates that a breastfeeding coordinator exist in every hospital and every WIC agency. Although this directive has done much to strengthen breastfeeding efforts, a barrier that continues, however, is that the qualifications and exact role of the hospital breastfeeding coordinator have never been spelled out.

Having spent much of my career as a breastfeeding coordinator at a major medical center, I am confident that the breastfeeding coordinator can have an overwhelming influence on hospital practices related to breastfeeding. The coordinator must be competent not only in breastfeeding management but also in program development and management, and should be expert at implementing change within the system. To overcome barriers within the system, the coordinator must be prepared to lead multiple interdisciplinary efforts that ultimately result in changes in breastfeeding not only for individuals but also for the system.

MATERIALS AND EQUIPMENT

Materials and equipment to support breastfeeding should be minimal. However, in situations where either the mother or infant is ill, the lack of materials and equipment has sometimes been a barrier. Furthermore, lack of reimbursement from third-party payers continues to be problematic, although some improvements are under way. A list of resources for locating materials and equipment related to breastfeeding is found in Appendices A and C.

Services in the Community

The national survey conducted prior to the 1984 Surgeon General's Workshop showed factors that influence breastfeeding initiation and continuation rates include lack of support from family and friends, lack of knowledge, lack of postpartum support services, and a lack of role models who breastfeed. Lack of support from family and friends is closely related to a lack of role models. Most women who are of childbearing age today were born in the 1960s and 1970s, when their mothers and mothers-in-law gave birth in a culture that strongly supported bottle feeding. There is also a strong correlation between the way a woman was fed and the way she chooses to feed her newborn; women who were breastfed are more likely to choose breastfeeding for their own children.

Lack of postpartum support services has been a problem, but many mechanisms to promote postpartum services have been initiated or strengthened since the 1980s. Hospitals now offer postpartum support groups, telephone hot lines, and other ongoing services. Physicians have employed certified nurse-midwives or nurse-practitioners to assist individuals with breastfeeding efforts and to establish and present group classes. A number of other postpartum support strategies have emerged.

La Leche League was begun in 1957 by a group of women attending a church picnic. Recognizing a need to support one another, they realized that all women could benefit from a mother-to-mother support network. La Leche League (meaning "the milk") soon grew; now La Leche League International, headquartered in Schaumburg, Illinois, extends to many countries throughout the world. La Leche League International provides many goods and services for breastfeeding mothers and professionals. Among other services, the national office has a library, sponsors conferences, and maintains a toll-free number for mothers to obtain quick advice or referrals to chapters in their area. The organization also produces a catalog of breastfeeding products, books, and other materials. At the local level, leaders hold regular meetings to support antepartum mothers in their choice to breastfeed and postpartum mothers in their efforts to continue. Health care professionals have finally become more at ease with referring mothers to the local chapter of La Leche League International. (To find a local chapter, contact headquarters; see Appendix A.)

Workplace Factors

Respondents in the Surgeon General's national survey cited the woman's return to work or school as the most frequent barrier to breastfeeding initiation and continuation. This is an interesting perception but one that appears to differ from reality. Published statistics, as well as more recent unpublished data from the Ross Mother's Survey, show that about the same number of employed women initiate breastfeeding, but breastfeeding continues longer when the mother is employed part-time rather than full-time.[38] Employment per se is probably not the barrier to breastfeeding. Employed mothers face a host of problems that are experienced by all breastfeeding mothers, but these problems tend to be magnified in the workplace. Lack of support, embarrassment, the stresses of the transition to parenthood, lack of practical information about how to maintain breastfeeding while separated from the infant, and other factors that are more intense for employed mothers are probably more reflective of the true barriers than employment alone (see Chapter 10).

Hospitals

The Surgeon General's Workshop did not single out hospitals as a barrier to breastfeeding. Because it is assumed, however, that most readers will be working in hospitals or working with women who have delivered in hospitals, it is important to understand how the hospital environment has been a barrier to breastfeeding and to recognize positive changes that are on the horizon.

During the last several decades, practices such as routine supplementation, separation of mothers and newborns through central nurseries, and rigid feeding schedules have been barriers to breastfeeding initiation and continuation. Some of these practices persist, but many hospitals, trying to improve consumer satisfaction, have done much to improve the environment to foster breastfeeding efforts. The BFHI criteria, mentioned earlier, have done much to abolish "routine" practices that have been barriers to breastfeeding.

It is notable that in 1988, the year the "Goals for the Nation" were drafted (but not yet published), companies that manufactured artificial milk broke their pact with the medical community and marketed directly to consumers, a move the AAP swiftly and staunchly opposed. The profession simply refused to accept money from the companies. Ironically, artificial milk companies had provided the medical profession with large sums of money to conduct breastfeeding studies. Because the vast majority of breastfeeding studies were carried out in the 1980s and were funded by artificial milk companies, the studies, along with the funding, diminished substantially.[39]

Advertising by artificial milk companies has been a continuing concern for breastfeeding advocates. It is important to recognize that advertisements by artificial milk companies *work;* if the company did not realize greater profits, it would discontinue its marketing strategies. The artificial milk business generates well over a billion U.S. dollars each year. One marketing strategy is to advertise during the antepartum period; another involves distributing free formula to hospitals.

Free Hospital "Formula"
The Surgeon General's questionnaire did not identify artificial milk or advertising by artificial

milk companies as a barrier to breastfeeding. Furthermore, little, if any, research shows a cause-and-effect relationship; we cannot say, for example, that advertising artificial milk to pregnant mothers causes them to choose artificial feeding rather than breastfeeding. What is known, however, is that practices designed to promote artificial milk have frequently undermined mothers' breastfeeding efforts.

Traditionally, hospitals have accepted free samples of artificial milk from manufacturers. A well-known marketing technique is getting a product's name out there where consumers can see it and try it. Consequently, hospitalized mothers receive artificial milk supplement—and videos, pamphlets, or infant items from artificial milk companies—in the hope that they will later purchase the brand with which they are most familiar. When mothers are not offered artificial milk, either as a supplement or as a gift pack, they are much less likely to recognize the "house brand."[40] Furthermore, supplementation is usually not necessary, but when artificial milk is readily available it is likely to be used, and using unnecessary supplements is a marker for breastfeeding failure.

Discharge Packs
Over the last several decades, artificial milk companies have routinely provided hospitals with "discharge packs" that may contain artificial milk, infant items, or coupons. In the past, these packs have been routinely and indiscriminately distributed in hospitals for breastfeeding mothers, sometimes with the approval of the physician.[41] Except where it is prohibited by state law, this practice continues, even though its effects have been deleterious to breastfeeding efforts[42] and the continuation of breastfeeding.[43]

Breastfeeding advocates have frequently implied that artificial milk and advertising by artificial milk companies is the "problem" with breastfeeding. Certainly, the availability of artificial milk and strong advertising for it have been deterrents to breastfeeding for some women. However, no single factor can be "blamed" for problems with breastfeeding.

CULTURAL ASSESSMENT OF INDIVIDUALS AND FAMILIES

Perhaps no two topics are more rooted in culture than food and sex. In the United States, breasts are thought of primarily as sexual objects, not as nourishing organs. And everyone readily agrees that breastfeeding provides food. However, the lactating woman is involved in something much more than simply producing food; breastfeeding has a significant emotional impact for mother and child. Feeding is the first and perhaps most enduring function of the mothering role.

Breastfeeding can be an emotionally and culturally charged topic. Providing culturally sensitive care can present a true challenge because we are all products of our own culture and therefore tend to project our values, beliefs, norms, and practices onto others who may not embrace our culture. Perhaps the first step in providing culturally sensitive care is to become aware of our own cultural biases here in the United States. Furthermore, it is difficult to delineate sociocultural matters from those that are psychological or biological. Giger and Davidhizar[44] define culture as:

> A patterned behavioral response that develops over time as a result of imprinting the mind through social and religious structures and intellectual and artistic manifestations. Culture is also the result of acquired mechanisms that may have innate influences but are primarily affected by internal and external environmental stimuli. Culture is shaped by values, beliefs, norms and practices that are shared by members of the same cultural group. Culture guides our thinking, doing and being and becomes patterned expressions of who we are. These patterned expressions are passed down from one generation to the next.

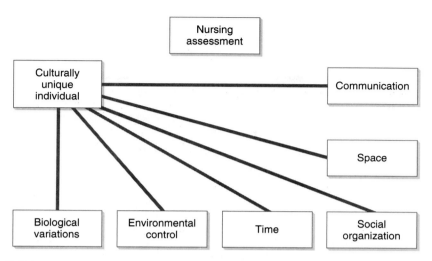

Fig. 1-2 Giger and Davidhizar's transcultural assessment model. *(From Giger JN, Davidhizar RE: Transcultural Nursing. 2nd ed. St. Louis: Mosby; 1995.)*

Culture provides implicit and explicit codes of behavior. In the United States, members of the dominant culture tend to be white, educated, and of the middle socioeconomic class; this is clearly the group in which breastfeeding has been most popular in recent decades. By contrast, ethnic groups are distinct from the dominant culture. In the United States, there are well over 100 ethnic groups, and breastfeeding typically is less popular among these groups than among the dominant culture. It is not possible here to address the needs of cultural groups throughout the world, nor is it possible to describe every nuance of the culture. Rather, the aim of this chapter is to examine the concept of culture as it relates to breastfeeding in America.

Giger and Davidhizar[44] recognize the overlap of culture, ethnicity, and religion and suggest a model for cultural assessment of the client, shown in Figure 1-2. The components of their model include (1) a culturally unique individual, (2) communication, (3) space, (4) social organization, (5) time, (6) environmental control, and (7) biological variations. These components identify several important concepts to be addressed for the breastfeeding mother.

Culturally Unique Individual

Certain cultural norms drive practices related to feeding in general and to breastfeeding in particular. From a clinical standpoint, it is useful to identify norms but not to rely on stereotypes. Knowing that a certain ethnic group embraces a particular norm (e.g., Italians serve wine with their meal) is helpful when anticipating someone's possible needs and preferences. This knowledge, however, must be tempered with the recognition that not all members of the ethnic group will embrace that norm or practice (e.g., my mother never serves wine with the meal). Furthermore, those who have been acculturated into the American way of life may not exhibit the norm at all. Thus, norm recognition is important but should not replace respect for individual variation and choice. Some cultural behaviors related to childbirth and breastfeeding are described in Table 1-1.

TABLE 1-1
CULTURAL BEHAVIORS RELATED TO ASSESSMENT OF CHILDBIRTH AND BREASTFEEDING

Nations of Origin	Important Cultural Considerations	Clinical Strategy
Native American (170 Native American tribes, Aleuts, Eskimos)	Extremely family-oriented and likely to value traditional healing methods.	Capitalize on the family as a support for breastfeeding.
Asian (China, Hawaii, Philippines, Korea, Japan) Southeast Asia (Laos, Cambodia, Vietnam)	Earlier generations more likely to breastfeed, but second-generation Asian-Americans may not. May delay breastfeeding or do "breast and bottle." Belief in yin and yang.	Determine if delay in breastfeeding is practiced because it is a part of strong belief system, or if the woman would be receptive to knowing the benefits of early breastfeeding.
African	African-American women in today's America are products of mothers who gave birth at a time when bottle-feeding was viewed as a status symbol; often friends or grandmothers provide primary support. Breastfeeding is popular among African-Americans in the southern United States, but not in the northern states.	Involve close friend or family member in discussions about breastfeeding. Be aware of media that frequently do not depict African-American women who breastfeed.
Hispanic (Spain, Cuba, Mexico, Central and South America)	Primary belief that breastfeeding is good. Woman's mother or mother-in-law is frequently the primary support person if modern-day mother must return to work. Belief in the hot and cold theory.	Involve mother or mother-in-law or female relatives in discussions about breastfeeding. Show respect for belief in hot and cold theory and facilitate woman's consumption of appropriate foods during pregnancy and lactation.

New immigrants may perceive bottle feeding as the cultural norm and may be eager to assimilate practices of their new culture in the United States. Immigrants may perceive that formula is superior to human milk because they see it used so frequently. Similarly, they may equate the cost of the product with its superiority. (If it costs a lot of money, it must be desirable.) Furthermore, they may draw conclusions about American products that have no basis in reality. A colleague described one Asian woman who said she wanted to use artificial milk "so the baby will grow tall like Americans."

Communication

Communication includes verbal exchange, nonverbal communication, and the use of silence. In a much broader sense, however, it is an outward manifestation of inner values and beliefs. For example, in some cultures it would be inappropriate to outwardly disagree with a nurse or other health care professional, so the client may respond affirmatively or be silent, implying agreement. Words that have one meaning for one culture may have a very different meaning for another. For example, African-Americans may describe the newborn's eating behavior as "greedy"; because the word *greedy* may have a negative connotation for the Anglo-American nurse, she may misinterpret the mother's meaning. Actually, the mother's description of the baby's "greedy" behavior at the breast should be understood as "eager" or "vigorous."

Eye contact is part of communication in general, and some specific norms about eye contact pertain to infant care. For example, in some cultures it is inappropriate for a nurse or other health care professional to make eye contact with an infant without touching him. Some Hispanics, for instance, believe that such a practice results in a curse known as *mal de ojo*. Those who hold this belief also think that the curse can be cured by having the person touch the infant.

Another aspect of communication is touch, and, along with it, modesty. In American culture, for example, it is considered immodest to breastfeed in public, even though little or no breast tissue may be visible. In other cultures, women may wear long sleeves to cover their arms and veils to cover their faces, yet at the same time partially expose their breasts while suckling an infant.

Space

The amount of personal space considered appropriate varies from culture to culture. The most general example pertains to the distance we maintain during a conversation. For the breastfeeding mother, some specific examples come into play. For example, the mother whose infant is in the neonatal intensive care unit may have difficulty breastfeeding her infant if she knows that other people are just on the other side of a flimsy curtain. This may be more than a matter of modesty; the sights and sounds of the environment may inhibit her as well.

Social Organization and Orientation

A basic structure of social organization is the family, and the social support of family becomes especially important during the childbearing period. A shift from an extended to a nuclear family gradually took place as the United States became more urban. The effect of this trend on breastfeeding can only be inferred, but fewer women have breastfed since this change has occurred. Nowadays, it is entirely possible that a woman has never seen a sister or a cousin or any other woman breastfeeding. Furthermore, how a woman was fed may influence her decision for how to feed her own child[45] and whether or not she is successful.[46]

Social support can be provided by one's family or friends. Baranowski's study differentiates between social support and social influence. Quoting Caplan et al, he asserts, "Social support is defined as any input directly provided by another person (or group) which moves the receiving person towards goals which the receiver desires."[47] He implies that social support is primarily a process, whereas social influence is the result—to choose or not choose breastfeeding. While social influence may result in the decision to breastfeed, social support of family and friends is as likely to sustain the breastfeeding mother's efforts later on.[27] It is helpful to identify the primary support person for the breastfeeding mother. This person tends to differ from culture to culture. African-American mothers generally identify a close friend as the primary support person for breastfeeding, whereas Mexican-Americans are more likely to turn to their mothers for breastfeeding support. Anglo-Americans are most likely to seek support from their male partners.[47]

One aspect of social organization in the United States is the presence of women in the workforce. The majority of American women with children younger than school age are now employed, and hence day care has become widespread. The long-term effects of this separation on child rearing in general are not well understood, but the effects on breastfeeding in particular deserve special mention. (See Chapter 10 for a discussion of breastfeeding and employment.) Employment outside the home does not preclude breastfeeding. Women who are employed full-time can and do continue to breastfeed their children, but more women who are employed part-time are doing so.[38]

Time

Time is influential in every culture, and the importance of the clock in American culture is discussed in the section on values. However, two central ideas that vary tremendously from culture to culture are the time of initiation of breastfeeding and the time of weaning.

Time of Initiation

In some cultures breastfeeding is not initiated until around the time the milk "comes in." For example, Mexican-American women, who believe that colostrum is dirty or bad, do not begin breastfeeding at the time of birth. If this cultural norm is not understood, there can be miscommunication between the newly delivered mother and the nurse. Do not presume that the woman has chosen to bottle feed if she folds her arms over her chest and announces, *"No leche."* She is not saying, "I don't want to breastfeed." She is giving a message that she is not going to breastfeed at this point, but she may and usually does go home and begin to breastfeed after her milk comes in. Similarly, Asian women often delay the initiation of breastfeeding.

Time of Weaning

In other parts of the world, children are typically weaned when they are around 3 to 4 years old, but in the United States infants are typically weaned before 6 months of age. An extensive review of weaning practices has been provided by Hervada and Newman.[48] Weaning is perhaps the most culturally charged issue related to breastfeeding in America today. Nearly half of mothers reported there is "no negative aspect" to breastfeeding at 6 months, but only about one quarter say there is no negative aspect to breastfeeding a 1-year-old. About 25% cite "social stigma" (i.e., negative attitudes of others) as a negative aspect of breastfeeding at 6 months, and about 40% cite it as a negative aspect of breastfeeding past 1 year.[49]

Environmental Control

Environmental control includes values and beliefs about health and illness, as well as about how to overcome adverse situations related to the conditions one is experiencing.

Beliefs

Perhaps the most basic belief is about life and health. Those who believe they can influence their own health by good health care practices—such as breastfeeding—are likely to embrace healthy practices. Some cultures have specific beliefs about human milk and breastfeeding. Very often, the younger members of the cultures—those of childbearing age—are not as likely to be as entrenched in the belief as their elders. If there is a strong cultural belief that breastfeeding is intrinsically good, however, the woman is likely to initiate and continue breastfeeding.

Some Americans believe that artificial feeding is truly equivalent to human milk (the product) or may believe that colostrum is "bad" but mature milk is "good." They may believe many myths about breastfeeding (the process) related to the appearance of the breasts; these myths and others will be explored in Chapter 4. Other beliefs may never be voiced but may underlie our decisions. For example, our bottle-feeding mindset may lead us to believe that when the bottle is empty, the feeding is over. The uninformed may believe the same is true for breastfeeding, which it is not. The breast is never truly empty. In addition, it is important to realize that infants (or older children) often come to the breast for comfort as much as nutrition, and breastfeeding mothers experience a pleasure that is not attainable through bottle feeding.

Values

The general values within a society are reflected in specific values about health and health care, and hence about breastfeeding. Leininger[50] identifies seven cultural values that influence American health care (presumably for either consumers or providers). Taking her work one step further, we can see how breastfeeding may be influenced by values.

1. Americans value optimal health as a human right and a civil right. We have often tried to convince women that "breast is best," based on the idea that breastfeeding promotes optimal health. Curiously, however, bottle feeding mothers tend to choose bottle feeding for reasons other than achieving optimal health.[45] Similarly, Americans have made breastfeeding a civil right, with a good deal of publicity and legislation surrounding the idea of whether or not women may breastfeed in public (see Appendix D).

More Americans have recently come to value natural foods, good nutrition, and safer environments, so it logical that the decision to breastfeed should follow. For example, women who bake their own whole-grain bread and recycle their newspapers have already demonstrated that they value high-quality nutrition and saving resources. It would be wonderful if society could see how breastfeeding epitomizes "health food" and preserving the environment.

2. The value of democracy implies majority-driven decisions and equality-driven treatment. This majority-wins mentality may influence women to make feeding decisions based on what they see the majority of women doing. (While a slim majority *do* breastfeed, few are *seen* breastfeeding.) This equality-driven value comes across in communication by health care providers who sometimes ask, "Are you going to breastfeed or bottle feed?"—with the implication that those two "treatments" are equal.

3. American culture values individualism, that is, the individual is more highly respected and valued than the group. In the case of breastfeeding, this seems to play out as an emphasis on a woman's breasts as sexual objects. In our culture, it is acceptable for the individual to expose her breasts—so long as the nipples and areolas are covered—when advertising a commercial product, sunbathing at the beach, or trying to attract male attention at a party. It is not acceptable, however, to breastfeed in public, even though the nipples and areola would indeed be covered by

the baby, and probably less breast tissue would be exposed than on the beach. When the breasts are used for individual gain, the culture approves, but using them to nourish another person is not favored in American culture these days.

Historically and in other cultures, this sex-object value has not necessarily been relevant. For example, women in Mali are bemused or horrified that men would be aroused by women's breasts, or that women would find "breast to mouth" contact pleasurable.[51] It is difficult to imagine anyone today admiring a celebrity and exclaiming, as in Luke 11:27, "Happy the womb that bore you and the breasts that nursed you!" When a contemporary researcher asked a Scottish woman how she felt about breastfeeding, the reply was "Euch, those are for your husband."[52] (*Euch* is a Scottish word that expresses disgust beyond that conveyed by the American word *yuk*.)

Women are more likely to breastfeed in cultures where the group is valued and where groups of women publicly breastfeed. This notion of the influence of the group on the individual's breastfeeding decision is one aspect of social support. For example, La Leche League International has provided one mechanism for helping women to see the value that a group attaches to breastfeeding.

4. Americans value achieving and doing. Women often say they are going to "try" breastfeeding, with the implication that they consider failure entirely possible, or even likely. Oftentimes, terminology used by professionals throughout the childbearing cycle has had negative connotations. Phrases such as "incompetent cervix," "trial labor," "failed induction," "failure to progress," and "lactation failure" have reinforced this pass-fail mentality. The literature is replete with the term "lactation failure" in reference to the lactating woman when it would often be more accurate to refer to the health care professional's failure to provide adequate education and support for the woman. (In this text, the phrase "lactation failure" is reserved for those rare situations in

which the woman's physiological functions interfere with milk production, much as "renal failure" refers to physiological dysfunctions of urine production.)

5. Our value of "cleanliness" being next to godliness may have had detrimental effects on breastfeeding. Americans have been indoctrinated into believing that artificial nipples should be sterilized, that artificial milk will spoil if it is unrefrigerated, and that anything disposable (e.g., disposable bottles or milk bags) is therefore cleaner than reusable. This value makes some erroneous advice seem plausible. For example, women have been instructed or have inferred that they should wash their nipples with sterile water, that they should discontinue breastfeeding if they are sick or have cracked nipples, and that certain foods taint human milk. Perhaps a better focus for this "cleanliness" value would be the environmental waste created by the use of artificial milk, bottles, and related paraphernalia.

6. American culture values time and time schedules, whereas other cultures place little importance on time; in fact, some cultures have no clocks or calendars whatsoever. "Scheduled" feedings, limited-time feedings, delayed feedings—however detrimental these may be to breastfeeding—have until recently been easily accepted in this culture. A review of the literature clearly shows that pediatric textbooks used the clock as the primary frame of reference for clinical management for over 100 years.[53] However, health care providers seldom mention that breastfeeding requires no time to prepare or reheat milk or to store leftovers. Similarly, with breastfeeding there are no bottles to buy, wash, and dry, and no cans to recycle. Our culture has valued convenience foods but has often overlooked breast milk, the original "fast food."

7. Americans value technology and automation. This is perhaps the most important value that has contributed to our preferences for bottle feeding. Artificial milk is a product of improved technology and automation. It is mass-produced

and shipped to consumers. Bottles, too, are the result of technology, and it is easy to be persuaded that this technology must be intrinsically good.

Practices

Some ethnic groups have specific beliefs about the consumption of hot and cold foods to improve health conditions. The theory of hot and cold is based on the four bodily humors (blood, phlegm, black bile, and yellow bile), which manifest themselves in dry, wet, hot, and cold. The basic premise is that the elements must be balanced, and the food that is ingested helps to balance the condition. Over the years, the wet and dry components of the theory have become insignificant, but the hot and cold components remain important in some cultures which believe that a "cold" condition would require a person to eat only "hot" foods, and vice versa. The "hot" or "cold" designation has nothing to do with the actual temperature or spiciness of the food; it is an arbitrary designation. Asians and Hispanics fre-

Box 1-3
Hot and Cold Food Classifications Among Puerto Ricans

Frio (cold)	*Caliente (hot)*
Milk	Alcoholic beverages
Avocado	Chili peppers
Coconut	Chocolate
Lima beans	Coffee
Sugarcane	Corn meal
White beans	Evaporated milk
Barley water	Kidney beans
Chicken	Onions
Fruits	Peas
Honey	Tobacco
Raisins	
Salt cod	
Watercress	

Box 1-4

Hot and Cold Food Classifications Among Chinese

Yin (cold)	Yang (hot)
Watercress	Soups
Water chestnuts	Herbs
Bamboo shoots	Broccoli
Mustard greens	Liver
Bok choy	Mushrooms
Chrysanthemum tea	Peanuts
Fruits	Peppers
Vegetables	Ginger
Seaweed	Chicken
Soybean	Meat
Sprouts	Pig's feet
Cola drinks	Broth
Rice milk	Nuts
Juices	Fried food
Milk	Coffee
Beer	Spices
	Infant formula

quently espouse the hot and cold theory. Hispanics refer to conditions or foods as *frio* or *fresco* (cold) and *caliente* (hot); examples are shown in Box 1-3. Similarly, Asians refer to the *yin* (cold) and *yang* (hot); examples are shown in Box 1-4.

Belief in the hot and cold theory influences dietary practices during the childbearing cycle. Pregnancy is viewed as a "hot" condition requiring "cold" foods. Once delivered, both mother and newborn are considered to be in a cold state for about 100 days and should consume hot foods for at least 30 days.[54] Human milk is thought to be neutral, because ideally the woman is in a state of balance. An important consideration cannot be overlooked, however; some women are actually relieved to be in the United States, far away from elders who may hold these beliefs about the bodily humors. They may not wish to abstain from certain foods, and so it is important to rec-

ognize that the hot and cold theory may or may not be part of their belief system.

In clinical practice we react to information that mothers give us about their cultural beliefs and practices. Before reacting, it is best to determine if the outcome of the cultural practice is efficacious, neutral, dysfunctional, or uncertain.[44] For example, if the woman believes that eating a hot fish stew will improve her milk supply, encourage this practice; doing so shows respect for her culture, and the outcome will be efficacious from a nutritional standpoint (she needs the fluid, high protein, and minerals that the stew provides). It becomes more difficult to react to practices that are dysfunctional. For example, the clinical scenario on p. 22 describes a mother who is not eating, which obviously is an undesirable behavior. The aim of the interaction is to remain respectful but to discourage the dysfunctional practice.

Biological Variations

Sometimes it is difficult to delineate sociocultural factors from psychological and biological factors because they are highly interrelated. This discussion will focus on how cultural patterns repress the natural motives that ensure survival of the species, as Benedek's model emphasizes.[55]

Lactose intolerance is a health variation that may affect the lactating mother. Asians, Africans, and Hispanics are all likely to be lactose intolerant. Drinking milk or consuming dairy products is not necessary for lactation, but those who abstain from consuming dairy products will need to obtain calcium from alternative sources.

The relationship between the incidence of diabetes mellitus and race is more clearly understood than the relationship between diabetes and infant feeding practices. Typically, those of European descent—especially Spanish descent—are more likely to have diabetes than those of African descent.

CLINICAL SCENARIO

Situation A

You are the nurse on the postpartum unit. Your patient, Ms. S., is a breastfeeding mother of Asian descent. She appears to have eaten little. On her lunch tray you see an apple, a ham sandwich, a crisp garden salad, and a carton of low-fat milk. The nurse on the shift ahead of you said that she tried to tell Ms. S. how important it is for lactating mothers to eat and drink, but to no avail. What would you do?

Situation B

You are the clinical instructor in the newborn nursery. One of your undergraduate students is caring for Mrs. C., a 39-year-old white, middle-class multipara. The student tells you that she can't possibly teach Mrs. C. anything about breastfeeding because the woman "'nursed her other baby." You caution the student that sometimes women nurse for only a couple of weeks but report that they have "nursed before," so you recommend that the student find out a little more about Mrs. C.'s past breastfeeding experience. The student comes back and reports to you that she is convinced that Mrs. C. nursed "for a fair chunk of time." You ask when Mrs. C. weaned her last baby, and the student responds, "I couldn't get that out of her." What do you think is going on? What would you recommend that the student do next?

Answers

The scenarios above describe real-life situations. There is seldom only one "right" answer to a clinical situation. The following answers are provided to give the reader guidance, with the full recognition that other answers may be appropriate.

SITUATION A

The fruit, vegetables, and milk are "cold" foods that are typically avoided by traditional Chinese postpartum women because the postpartum period is considered a "cold" condition. One strategy is to simply observe what has happened and talk with the woman about it. An example might be, "Ms. S., I notice you haven't eaten much on your lunch tray. I would be happy to order a different lunch for you. What kind of food would you prefer?" If she declines, encourage her to have family members bring in soup or other food from home. If she does not elaborate on her preferences, call the dietary department and ask for a meal that contains many of the "hot" foods.

SITUATION B

The woman was reluctant to answer because she was still breastfeeding a toddler at home. She felt that the student nurse might think this was "weird" and did not wish to reveal the real situation. There are several options for how to handle this. Students, who are always allowed to be in the learning role, have a wonderful opportunity to put the woman at ease by saying simply, "Mrs. C., you never really told me when you had weaned your last child. I'm wondering if you are still nursing her. If so, maybe you can tell me a little about how you've been able to be so successful." This is a good lead-in because it shows approval for the behavior and helps the woman to share her experience.

Nutritional Deficiencies and Preferences

It is difficult to separate the idea of food preferences from the beliefs one holds about certain foods' impact on health in general or on lactation specifically. Some cultures have specific beliefs about foods that are helpful or harmful to the mother's milk. The most notable example is the hot and cold theory that influences dietary choices during the childbearing cycle, as discussed earlier. Other examples are common in the dominant American culture. Health care professionals and women themselves have developed long lists of foods that are presumably bothersome to infants, but few foods have as much effect on the milk as they are presumed to have (see Chapter 4 for a discussion). For example, in American culture chocolate is thought to be "bad" for the mother's milk, while in other cultures it is thought to enhance the milk supply.

Another important belief is related to galactogogues, which are food and drink that are thought to increase milk supply.[56] Box 1-5 lists several common galactogogues. Somewhat surprisingly, foods that are presumed to be "bad" in some cultures may be considered galactogogues in others. One new mother reported that her mother-in-law, who lived in northern Mexico, gave her a hot drink made with chocolate, *masa* (cornmeal), cinnamon, sugar, and condensed milk in order to help her milk supply.

Psychological Characteristics and Coping

People in different cultures have different psychological characteristics and ways of coping. For example, in some cultures it is not appropriate for laboring women to make any noise that expresses the pain they feel during labor; in other cultures laboring women are quite vocal. Similarly, some breastfeeding mothers are unlikely to ask questions or report pain during the breastfeeding interaction. More subtle situations often occur, however. The woman who feels she has been belittled by a health care provider may not return for another appointment; the woman who is overwhelmed with messages about breastfeeding may "shut down" and not absorb further information. How women and their families cope with situations varies from culture to culture and from individual to individual.

In many cases, the differences among members within a group are greater than the differences between groups. Therefore, when interacting with an individual mother, it is best to use the three-step process developed by Best Start (Appendix C). This process has been successful for over two decades with women of many ethnic backgrounds, including those who are socioeconomically disadvantaged:

Step 1: Ask open-ended questions. Use the interviewing techniques suggested in Chapter 4 to elicit ideas, concerns, questions, and social norms.

Step 2: Affirm feelings. This step is the most difficult to master, particularly when the cultural feelings or biases are different from those of the interviewer.

Step 3: Educate. Education should be based on targeting the concerns uncovered in step 1, giving positive feedback, and providing small bits of information at a time. Chapter 4, which addresses maternal education, outlines in more detail how to educate and support women in positive ways.

SUMMARY

Multiple individual, family, and societal influences during the late nineteenth century and continuing into the twentieth century led to the decline of breastfeeding in the United States. Especially during the 1980s, multiple efforts at the national level were undertaken to increase breastfeeding initiation and continuation. Most of these efforts have had some degree of success and are continuing as we approach the new millennium. However, breastfeeding is more than just a biological matter of fact; individual, family, and social values and beliefs also influence practice. The United States has still not met the goal of having 75% of women choosing to breastfeed and 50% continuing until the infant is 6 months old.

Much work still must be done to convert the nation from a primarily artificial-feeding culture to a breastfeeding culture.

Apologizing for a personal anecdote, I feel compelled to mention my own mother, who is a good example of how the extended family influenced breastfeeding success, and how she, in turn, has influenced my values, beliefs, and practices related to breastfeeding. My mother was born in Italy in 1918. She came to the United States around 1928. Unlike the majority of women living in the United States in the 1940s and 1950s, she breastfed her children because bottle feeding "didn't make sense" to her. She grew up in an extended family, seeing her older sister and other family members and friends suckle their children. She is frequently taken aback at the notion of "teaching" women to breastfeed; to her breastfeeding seems like something "all women just know how to do." She appears to have been completely unencumbered by the rules and dictas given to American mothers, and it simply never occurred to her that she might not succeed. She considers a baby at the breast, a pot of sauce simmering on the stove, a loaf of bread in the oven, and a kiss on the cheek essential gifts a mother provides for her family.

References

1. Apple RD. *Mothers and Medicine: A Social History of Infant Feeding.* Madison, Wis: University of Wisconsin Press; 1987.
2. Jackson EB, Olmsted RW, Foord A, Thoms H, Hyder K. A hospital rooming-in unit for four newborn infants and their mothers: descriptive account of background, development and procedures with a few preliminary observations. *Pediatrics* 1948;1:28-43.
3. Hill LF. A salute to La Leche League International. *J Pediatr* 1968;73:161-162.
4. United States Department of Health and Human Services. *Healthy People: The Surgeon General's Report on Health Promotion and Disease Prevention.* Washington, DC: Government Printing Office; 1979.
5. World Health Organization. *International Code of Marketing of Breast-milk Substitutes.* Geneva: World Health Organization; 1981.
6. American Academy of Pediatrics. The promotion of breast-feeding: policy statement based on task force report. *Pediatrics* 1982;69:654-661.
7. American Academy of Pediatrics and the American College of Obstetricians and Gynecologists. *Guidelines for Perinatal Care.* 3rd ed. Elk Grove Village, Ill: American Academy of Pediatrics; 1992.
8. American Academy of Pediatrics and the American College of Obstetricians and Gynecologists. *Guidelines for Perinatal Care.* 4th ed. Elk Grove Village, Ill: American Academy of Pediatrics; 1997.
9. American Academy of Pediatrics Work Group on Breastfeeding. Breastfeeding and the use of human milk. *Pediatrics* 1997;100:1035-1039.
10. United States Department of Health and Human Services. *Report of the Surgeon General's Workshop on Breastfeeding and Human Lactation.* Rockville, Md: Health Resources and Services Administration; 1984.
11. Institute of Medicine. *Nutrition During Lactation.* Washington, DC: National Academy Press; 1991.
12. United States Department of Health and Human Services. *Healthy People 2000: National Health Promotion and Disease Prevention Objectives.* Washington, DC: Government Printing Office; 1991.
13. WHO and UNICEF. *Protecting, Promoting, and Supporting Breast-feeding: The Special Role of Maternity Services.* Geneva: World Health Organization; 1989.
14. Spisak S, Gross SS. *Second Followup Report: The Surgeon General's Workshop on Breastfeeding and Human Lactation.* Washington, DC: National Center for Education in Maternal and Child Health; 1991.

15. Wright A, Rice S, Wells S. Changing hospital practices to increase the duration of breastfeeding. *Pediatrics* 1996;97:669-675.

16. Freed GL, Clark SJ, Sorenson J, Lohr JA, Cefalo R, Curtis P. National assessment of physicians' breast-feeding knowledge, attitudes, training, and experience. *JAMA* 1995;273:472-476.

17. Freed GL, Clark SJ, Lohr JA, Sorenson JR. Pediatrician involvement in breast-feeding promotion: a national study of residents and practitioners. *Pediatrics* 1995;96(pt 1):490-494.

18. Freed GL, Clark SJ, Cefalo RC, Sorenson JR. Breast-feeding education of obstetrics-gynecology residents and practitioners. *Am J Obstet Gynecol* 1995;173:1607-1613.

19. Barnett E, Sienkiewicz M, Roholt S. Beliefs about breastfeeding: a statewide survey of health professionals. *Birth* 1995;22:15-20.

20. Williams EL, Hammer LD. Breastfeeding attitudes and knowledge of pediatricians-in-training. *Am J Prev Med* 1995;11:26-33.

21. Anderson E, Geden E. Nurses' knowledge of breastfeeding. *J Obstet Gynecol Neonatal Nurs* 1991;20:58-64.

22. Naylor AJ, Creer AE, Woodward-Lopez G, Dixon S. Lactation management education for physicians. *Semin Perinatol* 1994;18:525-531.

23. Hayes B. Inconsistencies among nurses in breastfeeding knowledge and counseling. *JOGN Nursing* 1981;10:430-433.

24. Crowder DS. Maternity nurses' knowledge of factors promoting successful breastfeeding: a survey at two hospitals. *JOGN Nursing* 1981;10:28-30.

25. Lewinski CA. Nurses' knowledge of breastfeeding in a clinical setting. *J Hum Lact* 1992;8:143-148.

26. Ferris AM, McCabe LT, Allen LH, Pelto GH. Biological and sociocultural determinants of successful lactation among women in eastern Connecticut. *J Am Diet Assoc* 1987;87:316-321.

27. Bryant CA. The impact of kin, friend and neighbor networks on infant feeding practices: Cuban, Puerto Rican and Anglo families in Florida. *Soc Sci Med* 1982;16:1757-1765.

28. Mulford C. Swimming upstream: breastfeeding care in a nonbreastfeeding culture. *J Obstet Gynecol Neonatal Nurs* 1995;24:464-474.

29. Howard CR, Howard FM, Weitzman ML. Infant formula distribution and advertising in pregnancy: a hospital survey. *Birth* 1994;21:14-19.

30. Howard FM, Howard CR, Weitzman M. The physician as advertiser: the unintentional discouragement of breast-feeding. *Obstet Gynecol* 1993;81:1048-1051.

31. WHO and UNICEF. *Innocenti Declaration: 30 July to 1 Aug, 1990, Florence Italy.* Geneva: WHO and UNICEF; 1990.

32. Owen AL, Owen GM. Twenty years of WIC: a review of some effects of the program. *J Am Diet Assoc* 1997;97:777-782.

33. Ryan A. The resurgence of breastfeeding in the United States. *Pediatrics* (www.pediatrics.org/cgi/content/full/99/4/e12) 1997;99:1-5.

34. Quinn AO, Koepsell D, Haller S. Breastfeeding incidence after early discharge and factors influencing breastfeeding cessation. *J Obstet Gynecol Neonatal Nurs* 1997;26:289-294.

35. Britton JR, Britton HL, Beebe SA. Early discharge and the term newborn: a continued dilemma. *Pediatrics* 1994;94:291-295.

36. Braveman P, Egerter S, Perl M, Marchi K, Miller C. Problems associated with early discharge of newborn infants. Early discharge of newborns and mothers: a critical review of the literature. *Pediatrics* 1995;96:716-726.

37. Brooten D. Perinatal care across the continuum: early discharge and nursing home follow-up. *J Perinat Neonatal Nurs* 1995;9:38-44.

38. Ryan AS, Martinez GA. Breast-feeding and the working mother: a profile. *Pediatrics* 1989;83:524-531.

39. Greer FR, Apple RD. Physicians, formula companies, and advertising: a historical perspective. *Am J Dis Child* 1991;145:282-286.

40. Reiff MI, Essock-Vitale SM. Hospital influences on early infant-feeding practices. *Pediatrics* 1985;76:872-879.

41. Hayden GF, Nowacek GA, Koch W, Kattwinkel J. Providing free samples of baby items to newly delivered parents: an unintentional endorsement? *Clin Pediatr (Phila)* 1987;26:111-115.

42. Perez-Escamilla R, Segura-Millan S, Pollitt E, Dewey KG. Effect of the maternity ward system on the lactation success of low-income urban Mexican women. *Early Hum Dev* 1992;31:25-40.

43. Lindenberg CS, Cabrera Artola R, Jimenez V. The effect of early post-partum mother-infant contact and breast-feeding promotion on the incidence and continuation of breast-feeding. *Int J Nurs Stud* 1990;27:179-186.

44. Giger JN, Davidhizar RE. *Transcultural Nursing.* 2nd ed. St. Louis: Mosby; 1995.

45. Lawrence RA. *Breastfeeding: A Guide for the Medical Profession.* 2nd ed. St. Louis: Mosby; 1985.

46. Sloper K, McKean L, Baum JD. Factors influencing breast feeding. *Arch Dis Child* 1975;50:165-170.

47. Baranowski T, Bee DE, Rassin DK et al. Social support, social influence, ethnicity and the breast-feeding decision. *Soc Sci Med* 1983;17:1599-1611.

48. Hervada AR, Newman DR. Weaning: historical perspectives, practical recommendations, and current controversies. *Curr Probl Pediatr* 1992;22:223-240.

49. Reamer SB, Sugarman M. Breast feeding beyond six months: mothers' perceptions of the positive- and negative consequences. *J Trop Pediatr* 1987;33:93-97.

50. Leininger M. The significance of cultural concepts in nursing. *J Transcul Nurs* 1990;2:52-59.

51. Dettwyler KA. Beauty and the breast: the cultural context of breastfeeding in the United States. In: Stuart-Macadam P, Dettwyler KA, eds. *Breastfeeding: Biocultural Perspectives.* New York: Aldine De Gruyter; 1995:167-215.

52. Morse JM. "Euch, those are for your husband": examination of cultural values and assumptions associated with breast-feeding. *Health Care Women Int* 1989;11:223-232.

53. Millard AV. The place of the clock in pediatric advice: rationales, cultural themes, and impediments to breastfeeding. *Soc Sci Med* 1990;31:211-221.

54. Fishman C, Evans R, Jenks E. Warm bodies, cool milk: conflicts in post partum food choice for Indochinese women in California. *Soc Sci Med* 1988;26:1125-1132.

55. Benedek T. Psychobiological aspects of mothering. *Am J Orthopsychiatry* 1956;26:272-278.

56. Lawrence RA. *Breastfeeding: A Guide for the Medical Profession,* 4th ed. St. Louis: Mosby, 1994.

2

$\mathcal{P}$sychological Factors

$\mathcal{T}$he anatomy, physiology, and biochemistry discussed in Chapter 3 show how breastfeeding is a biological process. Indeed, the breast is a nourishing organ, but breastfeeding is more than a matter of milk production and synthesis for infant consumption; it also is a matter of nurturing and mothering. Factors that impact on motherhood, maternal role attainment, symbolic interaction of the families, and the transition to parenthood are relevant theoretical concepts to breastfeeding.

MOTHERHOOD AND SYMBIOSIS

In her classic article psychiatrist Dr. Therese Benedek says, "Mothering, the suckling, feeding, succoring of the young, is a complex behavior pattern; its motivation is 'innate' and regulated by hormones. The pattern of maternal behavior is rigidly set and characteristic of the species throughout the animal kingdom."[1] She maintains that growth, neurophysiological maturation, and psychosexual development are interwoven, and that cultural patterns repress the natural motives that ensure survival of the species. Furthermore, she says, "The psychodynamic tendencies which motivate maternal behavior—the wish to feed, to succor the infant—originate in the alimentary (symbiotic) relationship which the mother-individual has experienced with her own mother. . . . The term symbiosis signifies a *continual reciprocal interaction* between mother and child."[1] Indeed the breastfeeding relationship is reciprocal, with both mother and infant enjoying its psychophysiological benefits, as described in the Historical Highlight.

Benedek has articulated a biological basis for the psychological maturation of the mother as an individual and the maturation of the mother-infant relationship. This biological basis (rooted in hormones associated with pregnancy and lac-

Historical Highlight

Breast or Bottle: Not Psychologically Equivalent

Few would dispute the psychological benefit of breast-feeding over bottle feeding. However, few have articulated these benefits as clearly as the late Niles Newton, a professor of psychiatry and behavioral sciences. Newton states, "It is a common assumption in our society today that the bottle-fed baby held in his mother's arms is receiving an experience equivalent to that of breastfeeding" (p. 993). She further clarifies that common restrictions placed on breastfeeding—limiting the number of feedings, length of feeding, duration of feedings, interval between feedings, limiting maternal contact—limit the psychological benefits of breastfeeding and mimic the bottle feeding experience. These practices still exist, and Newton's paper, a review of the existent literature nearly three decades ago, still holds implications for caregivers in today's society. Newton enumerates several points that differ psychologically for both mother and infant. She describes psychological benefits for the mother in terms of the initial experience, psychophysiological reactions during breastfeeding, long-term psychophysiological reactions, maternal in-terests and behavior, sexual behavior and attitude toward men, personality and adjustment, and social variations. She describes psychological benefits for the infant in terms of initial experience, assuagement of hunger, mother-baby interaction, oral gratification and anal sensation, activity and learning, and personality adjustment. She expounds upon each of these benefits. Perhaps the most compelling benefit she describes is the mother-baby interaction. She emphasizes how the mother interprets and meets her infant's need and that the infant's toes curl and feet move in rhythm during a satisfying breastfeeding interaction. She says, "Comfort sucking and feeding are regularly presented along with the mother as one united total experience" (p. 998), and goes on to say that "in restricted breastfeeding, nourishment and comfort sucking are split." Clearly, breast and bottle are not equivalent, and the mother who restricts breastfeeding provides food but not comfort or pleasure. Have you ever seen a newborn curl his toes or move his feet in rhythm while bottle feeding?

From Newton N. The uniqueness of human milk: psychological differences between breast and bottle feeding. *Am J Clin Nutr* 1971;24:993-1004.

tation) and the continual reciprocal interaction between mother and child are critical. Benedek wrote her article over four decades ago, when the great majority of women were artificially feeding their infants, which makes her message even more compelling. She defines mothering as "the suckling, feeding, succoring of the young." Like breastfeeding experts who look to the animal kingdom for information about components of milk, imprinting, and other data about lactating mammals, Benedek looks beyond the Homo sapiens species to the entire animal kingdom to explain how this suckling behavior *is* mothering.

Her words "continual reciprocal interaction between mother and child" are more perfectly fulfilled in breastfeeding than in any other context. In essence, Benedek explains that hormones are the basis for taking on the mothering role and that such hormones predispose the woman to assume the caregiver role.

FAMILIES AND SYMBOLIC INTERACTION

Although Benedek would not have considered herself an interactionist, she emphasizes that suckling, the act, is intrinsically bound to mothering, the role. An understanding of role is inherent in the theory of symbolic interactionism and its relationship to the breastfeeding experience.

The theory of symbolic interaction assumes that all interactions are purposeful and meaningful and that each person's action or relationship is dependent on the other. For example, if you are learning something from the words (symbols) on this page, you consider me to be a teacher; hence I become a teacher by virtue of the fact that you are a learner. If you are not learning, I am not teaching. Symbols may include words, actions, voice inflection, and touch. Burr and colleagues, who have illuminated the concept of symbolic interaction as it relates to the family, assert that "humans decide what to do and not to do primarily on the basis of the symbols they have learned in interaction with others and their beliefs about the importance of these meanings."[2] The symbols that we receive drive actions and reactions. If we were in a classroom, for example, I would interpret the scowl on your face as a symbol of confusion or the nodding of your head as a symbol that you understand; from that information I would decide what to do next. A scowl would cue me to clarify my explanation; I might even feel bad that I was unsuccessful in explaining the material. Conversely, if I saw you nodding I would be likely to continue with my next point and would feel successful in my role as teacher. This mutual giving and receiving of symbols and subsequent actions and reactions are what the relationship is all about.

Perhaps no relationship is more dependent on symbolism than the breastfeeding relationship, for behaviors (and later, words) are especially symbolic in this intimate, reciprocal relationship. The mother who correctly interprets her infant's hunger cues puts him to the breast. Similarly, her behaviors hold meaning for the infant. When she readily offers the breast, the infant assigns meaning to it; he learns that here he can find warmth, comfort, and nourishment. Early on, the mother will assign meaning to the behaviors of the infant; for example, she will learn to recognize cues of satiety. (Later on, when the child can talk, they will have a word, such as "ma" or "tah-tah," which represents breastfeeding, and each of them will know what this means.) Most of us have seen

mothers who show signs that they feel contented, gratified, and successful when the infant peacefully falls asleep at the end of feeding. Conversely, a mother may appear uneasy and full of self-doubts when the infant awakens and exhibits hunger cues again in two hours. It is important to recognize that her reaction is not related to breastfeeding per se but her interpretation that she has "failed" to adequately meet the infant's needs. The mother who understands how breastfeeding works is likely to interpret this behavior as a matter-of-fact message; the baby is hungry. A mother who has seen older infants or artificially fed newborns sleep for a longer duration has already assigned a different meaning to this wakefulness. She is likely to interpret this as a reflection of her inability to adequately meet the infant's needs.

Imogene King[3] discusses not only interaction but also interaction as it relates to goal attainment. Her main premise is that all interaction is meaningful, and that the nurse's responsibility is to help the client to achieve her (the client's) goal. For example, in the case of the lactating mother, the nurse's role is to provide information and support in order to set and achieve a goal by helping the mother understand the cues and communication from her infant in relation to the breastfeeding experience.

TRANSITION TO PARENTHOOD

Alice Rossi's classic article takes Benedek's premise a bit further. She asserts that the real transition in life is not from being single to being married but from being childless to being a parent.[4] This is an important point as one interacts with a breastfeeding primipara. Much of what may sometimes be labeled as a "breastfeeding problem" is often more a reflection of the transition to parenthood. Rossi states, "The birth of a child is not followed by any gradual taking on of responsibility, as in the case of a professional work role. It is as if the woman shifted from graduate student to full professor with little intervening apprenticeship experience of slowly increasing responsibility. The new mother starts out immediately on 24-hour duty, with responsibility for a fragile and mysterious infant totally dependent on her care."[4]

Rossi acknowledges Benedek's idea that the infant's need for dependence is absolute, whereas the woman's need to mother is relative. Rossi goes on, however, to say that lack of mothering can be compensated for by the extended family, but in our culture women are typically isolated from extended families at the time the infant is most dependent on mothering. This observation assumes that the newborn is completely dependent on someone to meet his needs, including feeding, diapering, and cuddling. If a woman is breastfeeding, all of these needs, except feeding, can be met by the extended family or other caregivers. In American culture, a strange paradox appears: feeding is viewed as the central caregiving activity, and everyone wants to participate. A woman who chooses artificial feeding, however, gives up her rights to this central caregiving activity.

Understanding this idea of transition to parenthood is critical when assisting the breastfeeding mother, because it enables one to accurately identify nonbreastfeeding problems. As a clinical nurse specialist, I have often been asked to solve a "breastfeeding problem" only to find that the real problem was a new mother struggling with the transition to parenthood. The mother may voice her feelings couched in breastfeeding language, but the real problem is likely to relate to the transition to parenthood and attaining the maternal role.

Maternal Role Attainment

Reva Rubin, author of several classic articles, describes maternal role attainment. For decades,

Rubin's works have been revered as insightful and practical by nurses who wish to gain a better understanding of the maternity experience. Recently, her work has suffered some criticism.[5] This is unfortunate, since Rubin has clearly delineated phases relative to maternity, and these phases can be easily observed in today's breastfeeding mother.

Rubin[6] used the terms *taking-in* and *taking-hold* to describe the mother during the first few days after birth. These terms have some similarity to the bonding and attachment definitions, but with a clearer description of how this significant time in the woman's life affects not only how she relates to the infant but also how she relates to others.

Rubin asserts that "taking-in" lasts for two to three days; during this period the woman is focused on food—her own hunger and her infant's intake. She frequently relives and retells the details of her labor. Rubin says that during this taking-in period, the mother exhibits passive and dependent behavior. (Benedek would say that this is biologically induced through hormones.) "She is a receiver at this point. She accepts what she is given, tries to do what she is told, awaits the actions of others and initiates very little herself."[6] Taking-in is a time when the mother herself needs to be "mothered." This is significant for the breastfeeding mother because she is frequently still in this taking-in period when she is cut off from the nurturing behaviors of the hospital nurse and is instead expected to "take hold," that is, assume full responsibility for the infant.

The taking-in phase is in contrast to the taking-hold phase, where the mother becomes the initiator, the producer. The taking-hold phase, which is marked by rapid and frequent mood swings, lasts about 10 days. Rubin says that during this period a woman needs to get on with things, to give up passivity for an active role. During the taking-hold phase, she is especially concerned with having control of her own body. It is at this time that she is able to take hold of the tasks of mothering. Rubin's observations about the woman's behaviors parallel Benedek's assertion that the mother needs to be a caregiver. Interestingly, the time line that she suggests for the taking-in phase is roughly equivalent to the time when the mother has colostrum, and the taking-hold phase begins at approximately when transitional milk appears.

Parenthood and the Family

Communication between individuals is frequently referred to as engrossment, bonding, and attachment. The term *engrossment* refers to the relationship between the father and his newborn.[7] In the past, the word *bonding* has been used to refer to the maternal aspect of the relationship.[8] The early literature used the word *attachment* to refer to the infant aspect of the relationship between mother and newborn, with the opposite of attachment being loss. Bowlby[9] and Ainsworth[10] are most frequently recognized for their early contributions to the concept of attachment, but this literature was derived in part from studies of maternally deprived infants; hence attachment was viewed as the opposite of loss. More recent literature has used the word *attachment* when referring to *either* the infant or the maternal aspect of the relationship. All sources seem to agree, however, that bonding is unique in that there is a sensitive period immediately after birth when this relationship is influenced. (Note that this is a sensitive period, not a critical period; a critical period implies that irreparable harm may occur if the interaction is not achieved during that time.) Attachment, on the other hand, is thought of as being more linear; it starts prenatally and continues throughout life. Attachment behaviors include eye-to-eye contact (enface position), physical contact of holding, touching, cuddling, or stroking, talking to the infant, and initiating care for the baby. Except for talking to the baby, all of these behaviors are inherent in the breastfeeding process.

The forerunner of our understanding of attachment was *imprinting* (or "stamping" as it was called in the 1930s), which focused on the infant aspect of the relationship. This concept suggests that the young animal finds an object of a particular shape. In mammals the mouth is the most sensitive organ, and the object that is first recognized is the maternal nipple. (The symbolic interactionists would explain this as a symbol that the infant assigned meaning to.) Hence, infants who are first introduced to the artificial nipple rather than the mother's nipple may be more apt to "recognize" it early and favor it.

MARKERS FOR SUCCESS

Maternal Personal Characteristics

Several factors may impact the breastfeeding experience. These include age, birth experience, commitment, confidence, self-esteem, stress and anxiety, embarrassment and guilt, and postpartum depression.

Age

Biologically, the mother is capable of lactation, regardless of her age. Her willingness to breastfeed, however, is likely to be a reflection of her maturation in chronological years as well as her social maturation. According to Erikson,[11] adolescents are grappling with the task of identity versus role confusion. Therefore, the teenage mother may be more focused on herself, and it may be difficult for her to simultaneously focus her energies on a dependent infant. Additionally, adolescents are much more focused on their body image and their emerging sexuality than are older mothers. They are likely to view breastfeeding as having a sexual connotation, and are probably more vulnerable to the body image myths surrounding breastfeeding.

Birth Experience

Bentovim[12] identifies several variables that affect breastfeeding. One variable is related to factors surrounding delivery. These include length of delivery, need for anesthesia, sleepiness of the mother and infant, joyfulness of response to infant, prolongation of state of excitation, management of first mother-infant contact, emotional contact and regressive experiences, prematurity, separation, and malformation. Clinical experience shows that, indeed, those mothers who antepartally decided to breastfeed can sometimes change their minds if adverse circumstances happen during the intrapartum experience.

Commitment, Confidence, and Self-Esteem

The concepts of commitment, confidence, and self-esteem are closely related, and all have received relatively little attention with respect to breastfeeding in the professional literature. At present, there are few studies on how these affect the initiation and continuation of breastfeeding. Mothers with low confidence are more likely to wean early.[13,14] Mothers who are more committed to breastfeeding as the best method of feeding are more likely to continue when problems or concerns arise.[15] Over many years of clinical practice, however, it has become apparent that bolstering the mother's confidence is a critical element in breastfeeding success.

Stress and Anxiety

The most frequent cause for inadequate milk ejection is stress,[16] and increased stress may result in decreased milk production. The milk ejection reflex is inhibited when mothers experience distractions. The distracters used in one experiment[17]—feet in ice water and other physical and psychological distracters—may provide some insight into the real-life distracters experienced in clinical settings. Breast or nipple pain and incisional pain after cesarean section are common real-life distracters. The milk ejection reflex can be impaired by anxiety; mothers may become anxious with irritable infants whose crying seems to be a constant distracter. When mothers can relax, they are more able to have an ample milk supply.[17]

Some women report feeling tense and overwhelmed by breastfeeding,[18] and mothers have many stressful internal and external pressures. Internal pressures might include maintaining high standards for housekeeping or entertaining at home. External stress might be related to paying the bills, marital discord, or sandblasting the house next door. Instead of expressing disappointment at not being able to feed the baby, the helpful father is the one who offers to relieve the mother of some of the tasks of ordinary life, thereby reducing her stress.

Good interviewing skills, as discussed in Chapter 4, and astute observation provide clues to stressful situations. Mothers frequently minimize stressful situations when asked, as a few anecdotes demonstrate. One legally blind mother who told me of her perceived low milk supply denied that there was any stress in her life. This woman, however, boarded a city bus every day to visit her 27-week gestation infant at a hospital on the other side of town. Another mother reported that she was unable to get any milk into the collection container attached to a hospital-grade pump. Her breasts were obviously full, so it was apparent that something was interfering with her milk-ejection reflex. She was in a private room adjacent to the intensive care nursery, so privacy was not a problem, but in talking with her it soon became evident that she was anxious about the uncertainty that surrounded her infant's well-being. Warm compresses and hand massage helped a little, but she was still unable to release her milk. Finally, with a locked door and her husband massaging her breasts, she had an enormous milk ejection reflex, and enough milk to feed several newborns!

Embarrassment and Guilt

Embarrassment is similar to stress. A woman may find it difficult to let her milk flow when bedside curtains between her and her roommate are not pulled, or when there is no screen or only an inadequate screen in the special care nursery to enhance privacy if she must breastfeed there. A woman might be embarrassed to breastfeed in front of her father-in-law or her younger children. In these cases the milk-ejection reflex may indeed be inhibited.

Some women who breastfeed toddlers have reported feeling guilty because they have experienced pleasurable feelings during breastfeeding. This guilt is largely a result of cultural norms that portray breasts as sexual objects rather than nutritional organs. From the beginning, therefore, it is helpful to explain to the woman that oxytocin is the "great sensation" hormone; these feelings are normal. In fact, the pleasure associated with oxytocin—and therefore with coitus and breastfeeding—ensures survival of the species.

Postpartum Depression

Lactating women are not immune to postpartum depression, but symptoms of depression may not be evident until after the infant is weaned. This is a result of hormonal influence. Is there a correlation between postpartum depression and breastfeeding? To date, there is little research on this topic. It appears that breastfeeding offers neither a risk nor a protective influence for mothers. Nurses bear a responsibility to recognize signs of postpartum depression and to refer mothers to support groups. Postpartum Support Interna-

tional, headquartered in California, can be reached at 805-967-7636 (927 N. Kellogg Avenue, Santa Barbara, CA 93111). Depression After Delivery, a nonprofit organization headquartered in Morrisville, Pennsylvania, can be reached at 800-944-4773.

Family Influence

Partner's Beliefs and Attitudes

Like women, men's attitudes about breastfeeding are culturally driven. Fathers who show a positive attitude about breastfeeding may focus on the physiological and psychological advantages for the mother and infant; fathers who have negative attitudes about breastfeeding focus on the misconception that breastfeeding will make the woman's breasts ugly.[19] However, a woman may be unable to accurately predict her partner's reactions to breastfeeding.[20] Fathers' influence in decision making is described in Chapter 4.

Fathers can, however, have an important role in breastfeeding. William Sears, a noted pediatrician, asserts that the role of the father is twofold: (1) to develop comforting skills to calm the infant, and (2) to support the new mother, relieving her of many household tasks that drain her energy.[21] Sears gives some practical strategies that help fathers to function more fully in that role, and that benefit the mother and infant as well.

Domestic Violence and Abuse

Recently, nurses and other health care professionals have become more concerned about the effects of physical and sexual abuse on all women, but particularly on the obstetrical patient. Typically, battering begins or escalates when a woman is pregnant, but at the present time no research describes the effect on the woman's ability to produce or eject milk for her infant. One study

ed a decrease in the incidence of domestic
e among breastfeeding families.[22] Anecdotally, colleagues have reported that abused women might willingly suckle a female infant but not a male infant; one could assume that the sexual partner's jealousy of an infant having access to the woman's breasts might be a deterrent for deciding to breastfeed. Once again we see how breastfeeding is related to breasts as sexual objects in American culture. It would be unwise to generalize the findings from one small study, but some preliminary evidence suggests that the majority of fathers do not mind if their partner breastfeeds in front of friends or relatives, but they do not like them to feed in front of strangers or in a public place.[23]

SUMMARY

Breastfeeding is a continual, reciprocal relationship. The mother learns to interpret cues and meet the needs of her infant and the infant learns that the mother's breasts provide warmth and nourishment. The process of attachment is perfectly fulfilled in the act of breastfeeding. Multiple factors can positively or negatively influence the breastfeeding relationship. The nurse's interactions with the mother can support the positive influences and counteract the negative influences.

References

1. Benedek T. Psychobiological aspects of mothering. *Am J Orthopsychiatry* 1956;26:272-278.

2. Burr WR, Leigh GK, Day RD, Constantine J. Symbolic interaction and the family. In: Burr WR, Hill R, Nye FI, Reiss IL, eds. *Contemporary Theories About the Family*. Vol. 3. New York: Free Press; 1979.

3. King I. *A Theory for Nursing: Systems, Concepts and Process*. New York: Wiley; 1981.

4. Rossi A. Transition to parenthood. *J Marriage Fam* 1968;30:26-40.

5. Gay JT, Edgil AE. Douglass AB. Reva Rubin revisited. *J Obstet Gynecol Neonatal Nurs* 1988;17:394-399.

6. Rubin R. Puerperal change. *Nurs Outlook* 1961; 9:753-755.

7. Greenberg M, Morris N. Engrossment: The newborn's impact upon the father. *Am J Orthopsychiatry* 1974;44:520-531.

8. Klaus MH, Kennell JH. *Parent-Infant Bonding*. 2nd ed. St. Louis: Mosby; 1982.

9. Bowlby J. *Attachment*. Vol. 1. New York: Basic Books; 1969.

10. Ainsworth MDS. Object relations, dependency and attachment: a theoretical review of the infant-mother relationship. *Child Development* 1969; 40:969-1026.

11. Erikson EH. Eight ages of man. In *Childhood and Society*. New York: Norton; 1969:247-274.

12. Bentovim A. Shame and other anxieties associated with breast-feeding: a systems theory and psychodynamic approach. *Ciba Found Symp* 1976; 45:159-178.

13. Coreil J, Murphy J. Maternal commitment, lactation practices, and breastfeeding duration. *J Obstet Gynecol Neonatal Nurs* 1988;17:273-278.

14. Loughlin HH, Clapp-Channing NE, Gehlbach SH, Pollard JC, McCutchen TM. Early termination of breast-feeding: identifying those at risk. *Pediatrics* 1985;75:508-513.

15. Hewat RJ, Ellis DJ. Breastfeeding as a maternal-child team effort: women's perceptions. *Health Care Women Int* 1984;5:437-452.

16. Lawrence RA. *Breastfeeding: A Guide for the Medical Profession*. 4th ed. St. Louis: Mosby; 1994.

17. Newton M, Newton NR. The let-down reflex in human lactation. *J Pediatr* 1948;33:698-704.

18. Graef P, McGhee K, Rozycki J, Fescina Jones D, Clark JA, Thompson J, Brooten D. Postpartum concerns of breastfeeding mothers. *J Nurse Midwifery* 1988;33:62-66.

19. Freed GL, Fraley JK, Schanler RJ. Attitudes of expectant fathers regarding breast-feeding. *Pediatrics* 1992;90(2, pt 1):224-227.

20. Freed GL, Fraley JK, Schanler RJ. Accuracy of expectant mothers' predictions of fathers' attitudes regarding breast-feeding. *J Fam Pract* 1993;37:148-152.

21. Sears W. The father's role in breastfeeding. *NAACOGS Clin Issu Perinat Womens Health Nurs* 1992;3:713-716.

22. Acheson L. Family violence and breast-feeding. *Arch Fam Med* 1995;4:650-652.

23. Voss S, Finnis L, Manners J. Fathers and breastfeeding: a pilot observational study. *J R Soc Health* 1993;113:176-180.

24. Newton N. The uniqueness of human milk: psychological differences between breast and bottle feeding. *Am J Clin Nutr* 1971;24:993-1004.

3

Biological Factors

MAKING HUMAN MILK: THE PROCESS

Breastfeeding: A Bio-Psycho-Sociocultural Process

Breastfeeding can be defined simply as the infant's suckling milk at the breast; *lactation* is the maternal process of making milk. Both are bio-psycho-sociocultural processes. The breast is the site where breastfeeding takes place, but multiple sites are involved in the process of lactation, most notably the pituitary gland. While the proper functioning of endocrine glands is important, the woman's emotional response directly impacts on the biological processes; like all mothering acts, breastfeeding and lactation happen within a cultural context. The following pages aim to provide an understanding of anatomy and physiology that will support clinical management strategies.

Structure of the Mammary Gland (Breast)

The breasts—paired mammary glands—are actually modified exocrine glands, having a ductule system for secreting outwardly to the surface of the organ.[1] The glands are anchored to the overlying skin and to the pectoral muscles by the suspensory ligaments of Cooper as shown in Figure 3-1. The three major structures of the breast are the skin, the subcutaneous tissue, and the body of the breast.

Skin

The general skin, nipple, and areola are visible externally. (Chapter 8 describes features that the examiner should note when inspecting the external anatomy of the breast.) The areola, or areola mammae, is a pigmented area that surrounds the nipple. In the areola are Montgomery's glands,

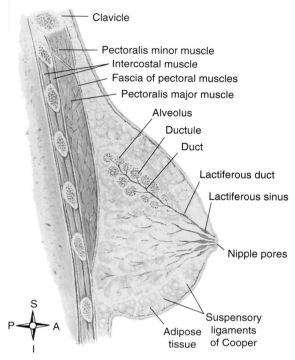

Fig. 3-1 Sagittal section of a lactating breast. *(From Thibodeau GA, Patton KT. Anatomy and Physiology. 3rd ed. St. Louis: Mosby; 1996.)*

which appear as raised projections. These are actually sebaceous glands that provide secretions to protect the areola and nipple.

The nipple (papilla mammae) is a raised projection in the center of the areola. Because the breast is an exocrine gland, the nipple is the external opening where the milk comes out. The nipple contains smooth muscle fibers and sensory nerve endings that cause it to become erect when stimulated.

Subcutaneous Tissue

The gland as well as fat and connective tissue are contained within the subcutaneous tissue. The size of a woman's breasts reflects the amount of fat

and connective tissue, not glandular tissue. Hence, the size of the breast has little or nothing to do with the functionality.

Body of the Breast (Corpus Mammae)

The corpus mammae from the Latin *corpus* "body" and *mammae* from the Latin *mamma,* meaning "breast," is the glandular organ. Like most organs, the breast is made up of two parts, the glandular tissue (parenchyma) and the supporting tissue (stroma).

Glandular Tissue (Parenchyma)

The parenchyma of the breast consists of the lobular, ductular, and alveolar structures. The breast has 15 to 25 *lobi* (singular, *lobus*). Like lobi in other parts of the body, each lobus is separated from neighboring lobi; in the breast it is separated by connective tissue. The duct from a lobus goes to the nipple. Lobi are subdivided into *lobuli* (about 20 to 40 lobuli in the breast), and each lobulus is again subdivided into 10 to 100 *alveoli.* Figure 3-2 shows the ductal system within the gland.

The *alveolus* (plural, *alveoli*) is the smallest functioning unit in the mammary gland. There are two types of cells in the alveolus as shown in Figure 3-3: the *secretory epithelial cells,* which synthesize fat and protein into milk, and the *myoepithelial cells,* which surround the secretory epithelial cells and are responsible for the milk ejection. The myoepithelial cells (*myo,* meaning "muscle") can be either at rest or contracted. When these myoepithelial cells contract, milk is ejected into the ductal system.

Milk flows through a ductular system that is embedded in the connective and fatty tissue. The ductular system is arranged in a treelike fashion, with larger "branches" and smaller "twigs" as shown in Figure 3-4. Ductules empty into ducts, which empty into the lactiferous sinuses, and eventually the milk is secreted through the nipple.

Stroma

The stroma contains the connective tissue, fat tissue, blood vessels, nerves, and lymphatics. The duct system of the breast is located within the connective tissue and fat.

CONNECTIVE TISSUE

Suspensory ligaments (Cooper's ligaments) help support the glandular and connective tissue and anchor them to the pectoral muscles, which are behind the breast.

BLOOD VESSELS

The lactating breast is a highly vascular organ. Not surprisingly, the internal mammary artery and the lateral thoracic artery provide most of the blood supply to the breast. Other arteries and veins are also involved in circulation to the breast.

NERVES

The breast is innervated primarily by branches from the fourth, fifth, and sixth intercostal nerves. However, the branch runs from deep to superficial, so the corpus mammae has less innervation than the areola or the nipple. The nipple/

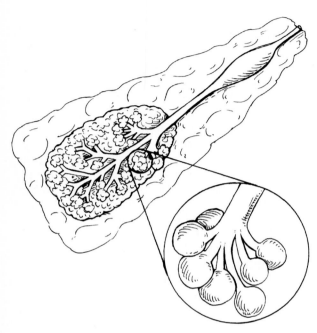

Fig. 3-2 Lobus (lobe) of the breast, with enlarged view of alveoli.

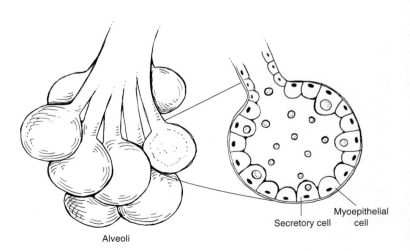

Fig. 3-3 Alveoli showing myoepithelial cells and secretory cells.

Alveoli

Secretory cell

Myoepithelial cell

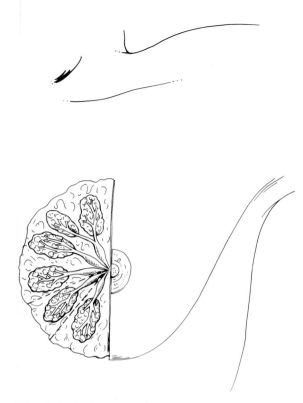

Fig. 3-4 Anterior view of the breast showing internal ductal structure.

areola complex is innervated by the lateral cutaneous branch of the fourth intercostal nerve. The nipple contains smooth muscle fibers, a rich blood supply, and multiple sensory nerve endings. Nerve endings in the nipple are receptive to *pain* and *pressure*. With stimulation, nerve endings send a message via the spinal cord to the brain; then the pituitary triggers the release of the hormones oxytocin and prolactin, and the nipple becomes erect. The nerve endings in the areola are sensitive to *pressure* and *suckling*. From the standpoint of breastfeeding management, this makes sense, because the infant should grasp and stimu-

late primarily the areola; he should not nipple suck (see Chapter 5).

LYMPHATICS

Lymph vessels carry a moving fluid (*lymph*) that is derived from blood and body fluid. Lymph is drained from the mammary gland and its surrounding tissues by two sets of lymphatic vessels. One set originates in and drains the skin over the breast, with the exception of the areola and nipple. The other set drains the corpus mammae as well as the skin of the areola and nipple. The lymphatic system in the breast is largely unrelated to lactation although lymphatic fluid accumulates during engorgement, contributing to visible distention.

The Process of Making Human Milk

Hormones Associated With Milk Production

Just as hormones govern birth, pubertal growth, conception, pregnancy, and delivery, they also govern lactation, which completes the reproductive cycle. Hormones associated with pregnancy and lactation are summarized in Table 3-1. During pregnancy, prolactin levels are very high, but estrogen and prolactin-inhibiting hormone (PIH; sometimes called prolactin-inhibiting factor) suppress the activity of prolactin at that time. Increased estrogen helps the gland to become sensitive to the effects of increased progesterone, which is responsible for proliferation of glandular tissue and ductule development during pregnancy; serum levels drop around the time of birth. Placental lactogen, human chorionic gonadotropin, and human chorionic somatomammotropin all contribute to mammary gland growth during pregnancy.

At birth, estrogen and progesterone levels drop. During lactation, growth hormone helps to

HORMONAL CONTRIBUTIONS TO BREAST DEVELOPMENT AND LACTATION

Hormone	Origin	Function Before and During Pregnancy	Function After Delivery
Prolactin	Anterior pituitary	Serum level rises, but estrogen suppresses its effect during pregnancy	Stimulates alveolar cells to produce milk; is probably of primary importance in initiating lactation but of secondary importance in maintaining lactation; may also cause lactation infertility by suppressing release of follicle-stimulating hormone and luteinizing hormone from pituitary or by causing ovaries to be unresponsive to gonadotropins; levels rise in response to various psychogenic factors, stress, anesthesia, surgery, high serum osmolality, exercise, nipple stimulation, and sexual intercourse
Prolactin-inhibiting factor (PIF)	Hypothalamus	Suppresses release of prolactin into blood; release stimulated by dopaminergic impulses (i.e., catecholamines)	Suppresses release of prolactin from anterior pituitary; agents that increase prolactin by decreasing catecholamines and thus PIF include phenothiazides and reserpine
Oxytocin	Posterior pituitary	Generally no effect on mammary function; sensitivity of myoepithelial cells to oxytocin increases during pregnancy	Causes myoepithelial cells to contract, leading to "milk ejection"; release is inhibited by stresses such as fear, anxiety, embarrassment, and distraction; also causes uterine contraction and postpartum involution of the uterus
Estrogen	Ovary and placenta	Stimulates proliferation of glandular tissue and ducts in breast; probably stimulates pituitary to secrete prolactin but inhibits prolactin effects at the mammary cell level	Blood level drops at parturition, which aids in initiating lactation; not important to lactation thereafter
Progesterone	Ovary and placenta	With estrogen, stimulates proliferation of glandular tissue and ducts in breast; inhibits milk secretion	Blood level drops at parturition, which aids in initiating lactation; probably unimportant to lactation thereafter
Growth hormone	Anterior pituitary		May act with prolactin in initiating lactation but appears to be most important in maintaining established lactation
ACTH	Anterior pituitary	Gradually increases in blood during pregnancy; stimulates adrenals to release corticosteroids	High level is believed necessary for maintenance of lactation
Placental lactogen	Placenta	Like growth hormone in structure; stimulates mammary growth; associated with mobilization of free fatty acids and inhibition of peripheral glucose utilization and lactogenic action	
Human chorionic gonadotropin	Placenta	Contributes to mammary gland growth during pregnancy	
Placental lactogen	Placenta	Contributes to mammary gland growth during pregnancy	
Human chorionic somatomammotropin	Placenta	Contributes to mammary gland growth during pregnancy	
Thyroxine	Thyroid	Normally no direct effect on lactation	Appears to be important in maintaining lactation either through some direct effect on the mammary glands or by control of metabolism
Thyrotropin-releasing hormone	Hypothalamus	Normally no effect on lactation	Stimulates release of prolactin; can be used to maintain established lactation

From Worthington-Roberts B, Williams SR. *Nutrition in Pregnancy and Lactation.* 6th ed. New York: McGraw-Hill; 1996.

maintain established lactation. A recent study suggests that it may be particularly helpful in maintaining lactation for mothers whose infants are not suckling vigorously at the breast.[2] Thyroxine appears to have some impact on maintaining lactation, and thyrotropin-releasing hormone stimulates the release of prolactin. The two main hormones associated with lactation, however, are oxytocin and prolactin.

Oxytocin

Oxytocin causes myoepithelial cells to contract—in the uterus during labor, in the genitals during orgasm, and in the ductule system of the lactating breast. Oxytocin is the primary hormone responsible for the milk-ejection reflex, or "let-down." This sensation—described as a "tingling" or "sensual" feeling by some mothers—varies in intensity from woman to woman and from day to day, just like labor contractions and orgasms. These sensations are completely normal, and relaxation helps milk ejection just the way it helps contractions and orgasms. Conversely, fatigue, stress, or a sense of fear or shame inhibits the milk ejection reflex. In the lactating mother, oxytocin release is both pulsatile and variable, and occurs before suckling.[3] Levels of oxytocin rise significantly during the first 45 minutes after delivery when compared with the 15 minutes prior to delivery.[4]

Prolactin

Perhaps prolactin could be described as the "great sensation" hormone. Prolactin (*pro* meaning "for" and *lactin* meaning "milk") can help a woman to feel relaxed or even euphoric. Prolactin levels rise during pregnancy and drop for a brief time prior to birth, then rise again a few hours after birth, or as soon as the neonate is suckled.[3] Prolactin levels should be around 150 to 200 ng/ml at term. Suckling, not the mere presence of an infant, causes higher prolactin levels; baseline serum prolactin levels during lactation gradually decrease over time after delivery until the infant is ulti-

mately weaned. During a breastfeeding episode, however, prolactin levels generally double. Prolactin release can be blocked, however, by prolactin-inhibiting factor. For a comparison of oxytocin and prolactin, see Table 3-2.

Stages of Mammary Function

There are four basic stages of mammary function: mammogenesis, lactogenesis, lactation, and involution.

Mammogenesis

Like all organs that undergo organogenesis, the breast undergoes mammogenesis (i.e., growth). Mammogenesis begins just prior to puberty and continues through puberty, the menstrual cycle, and pregnancy. The breast is never fully developed, however, until after it has produced milk.

Lactogenesis

Lactogenesis, that is, the gradual process of making milk, happens in three stages: lactogenesis I, II, and III. During these stages, human milk varies in components, appearance, and volume (supply).

LACTOGENESIS I

Lactogenesis I begins around 14 to 16 weeks gestation. The ductular and lobular proliferation occurs as a result of the influence of hormones when a colostrum-like substance is produced but not secreted in the gravida. (If the fetus is aborted at this time, however, these secretions can be observed clinically.) This stage continues until around the second trimester.

LACTOGENESIS II

Lactogenesis II begins around 28 weeks gestation. At this time the woman may become aware that she is leaking colostrum (especially if the breast is manipulated, which it should not be). Colostrum, the first "milk," is a thick substance that appears yellow because of its high carotene content. Colostrum is contained in the ducts during the sec-

T A B L E 3-2

COMPARISON OF OXYTOCIN AND PROLACTIN

	Oxytocin	Prolactin
Function	Essential for milk *ejection*	Essential for milk *production*
Secreted by	Posterior pituitary	Anterior pituitary
Release stimulated by	Hypothalamus	Hypothalamus
Release triggered by	(1) Can be stimulated by visual or auditory stimuli, but strongest release is triggered by suckling; after lactation is established, initial release is within 1 minute of suckling; release continues in a spurtlike fashion. (2) Visual or auditory stimuli also trigger release, but not as strongly as suckling	(1) Delivery of placenta, which removes prolactin-inhibiting hormone (PIH), triggers low estrogen and high prolactin level (2) Only tactile stimuli (suckling of the breast) triggers release; suckling provides a continuous stimulation for prolactin release
Relationship to milk volume	Levels of oxytocin not related to milk volume at given feeding	Actual level probably not related to milk volume Stimulating both breasts simultaneously increases prolactin level approximately 30%, thereby producing greater volume
Clinical implications	Peak and plateau is about every 6-10 minutes during a feeding Average pituitary contains 1000 mU of oxytocin. Only about 0.5 mU are required for the milk ejection reflex	Baseline levels rise during sleep: this correlates to the fact that infant suckling is greatest in the morning

Modified from Biancuzzo M. *Breastfeeding the Healthy Newborn: A Nursing Perspective.* White Plains, NY: March of Dimes Foundation; 1994. Used with permission.

ond trimester of pregnancy and is secreted the first few days postpartum.

The hormonal changes that occur during lactogenesis II involve primarily placental lactogen, progesterone, estrogen, and prolactin. After the placenta is delivered, a major source of *estrogen* is lost, and hence levels of this hormone drop abruptly. Incomplete delivery of the placenta delays lactogenesis if sufficient PIH is secreted to block mammary response.[5] *Progesterone* levels also fall but do not reach the levels seen in nonpregnant women for several days. *Prolactin* levels remain high. Levels of estradiol (the most potent naturally occurring estrogen), progesterone, and prolactin are shown in Figure 3-5.[6]

Colostrum is especially important for the newborn; it is rich in immunoglobulins and has a laxative effect on the gut, aiding with the passage of newborn meconium. Compared with mature milk, colostrum is higher in protein, lower in fat, and lower in carbohydrate. Colostrum is lower in energy than mature milk, containing about 67 kcal/100 ml (about 20 calories per ounce), whereas mature milk has about 75 kcal/100 ml (22.5 calories per ounce).[7]

Lactogenesis II continues only if the breast is adequately stimulated. With stimulation, colostrum is gradually replaced by transitional milk (consisting of colostrum and mature milk). When milk "comes in" (i.e., a sufficient volume of milk can be perceived by the mother and observed), this is transitional milk. Transitional milk is present from around 3 to 10 days postpartum[7]; in most cases the onset of transitional milk occurs before 5 days, depending on how early and how frequently the infant goes to breast. The woman experiences dramatic hormonal changes at this time; thus, about the time that the transitional milk comes in, so do the tears. Also around this time, her core temperature will rise due to engorgement of the breasts. After about 10 days of suckling, transitional milk is gradually replaced by mature milk.

LACTOGENESIS III

Lactogenesis III—once called *galatopoiesis*—begins around 10 days after birth. This is the establishment of a mature milk supply. Mature human milk contains about 22.5 calories per ounce, and *foremilk*—the milk that is produced and stored between feeding and released at the beginning of the next feeding—has an appearance similar to skimmed milk, with a characteristic blue tinge. *Hindmilk*—milk that is produced during and released at the end of a feeding—looks much richer. Sometimes human milk is a bit discolored. If the milk contains a little blood, it will have a pink tinge; if the mother has eaten an extraordinary amount of green vegetables, it will have a green tinge. This is usually harmless. Lawrence[8] has a more thorough discussion of colored milk.

Lactation

Lactation is the continuing production of milk. Established lactation is regulated primarily by prolactin and oxytocin, and throughout lactation these two hormones are secreted in response to suckling, as shown in Figure 3-6. Typically, lactation is said to have been "established" by around 4 weeks.[1]

Involution

Lactation can continue indefinitely, as long as the breast is suckled. Worldwide, the average time for complete cessation of breastfeeding may not occur until around 4 years. In some cultures, women long past menopause continue to suckle infants—often more than one infant or child—and will continue to lactate; cultural aspects of weaning are discussed in Chapter 1. The focus of this text is on the newborn, however, so the reader is referred to other professional[1] and consumer[9] sources for a more complete discussion of weaning.

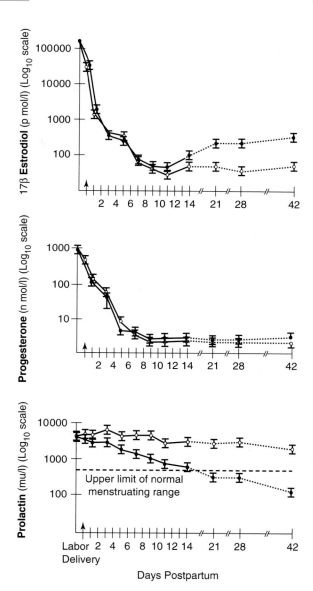

Fig. 3-5 Maternal hormone levels after birth in breastfeeding and nonbreastfeeding women. Breastfeeding subjects *(open circles)* and nonbreastfeeding subjects *(filled circles)*; *$p < 0.01$. (From Martin RH et al. Human alpha-lactalbumin and hormonal factors in pregnancy and lactation. Clin Endocrinol *1980;13:223-230.)*

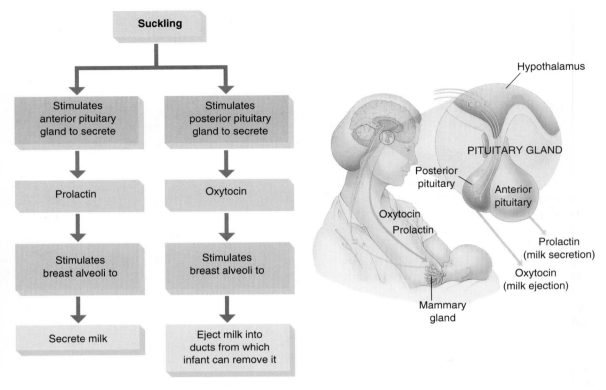

Fig. 3-6 Lactation: The illustration and accompanying flow chart summarize the mechanisms that control secretion and ejection of milk. *(From Thibodeau GA, Patton KT:* Anatomy and Physiology. *3rd ed. St. Louis: Mosby; 1996.)*

Ideally, weaning is initiated based on the infant's nutritional needs and developmental milestones, and it then progresses gradually. Whenever weaning does occur, however, the breast begins a postinvolution much as the uterus involutes after it has performed its intended function. During weaning the mother's milk changes in terms of its volume, nutritional components, and immunologic properties, whether weaning is gradual[10] or abrupt.[11] When the infant suckles less frequently, prolactin levels decrease, and when the breast is not emptied it becomes engorged; blood vessels are compressed, resulting in diminished oxytocin to the myoepithelium. Gradually, the alveoli col-

lapse, although even after the gland has returned to the resting state, the alveoli do not fully involute.

PROVIDING HUMAN MILK: THE PRODUCT

For a moment, ponder what human milk really is. What would you think if you saw the following newspaper headline: "Miracle Fluid Prevents Illness and Cures Disease"? Would you recognize this miracle fluid as human milk? As Palmer so eloquently writes,

If a multinational company developed a product that was a nutritionally balanced and delicious food, a wonder drug that both prevented and treated disease, cost almost nothing to produce and could be delivered in quantities controlled by the consumers' needs, the very announcement of their find would send their shares rocketing to the top of the stock market. The scientists who developed the product would win prizes and the wealth and influence of everyone involved would increase dramatically. Women have been producing such a miraculous substance, human milk, since the beginning of human existence, yet they form the half of the world's people who are the least wealthy and the least powerful.[12(p1)]

The word *product* may seem too commercialized to describe *breast milk*, but the term is used here to distinguish it from *breastfeeding*, the process. Those who heartily endorse breastfeeding sometimes forget that even if an infant is unable to perform breastfeeding the *process*, he should reap the benefits of human milk the *product*. Furthermore, it is useful to use the term *human milk* rather than *breast milk* because human milk comes only from a breast, so referring to it as *human milk* helps focus on its being species-specific. Because human milk is designed for humans, it has many biological, psychological, and sociocultural advantages.

Volume of Milk

Defining and Measuring Milk Volume

Studies about milk "volume" can be confusing or misleading without a thorough understanding of the terminology used and the physiology of milk production and transfer. This text uses Daly and Hartmann's terminology. *Milk production* refers to "the volume of milk removed from the breast," and *milk synthesis* refers to "the accumulation of milk within the breast."[13] Assuming that milk is removed by and transferred to the infant (as opposed to a pump), the volume of *infant intake* is considered to be the same as *milk production*. Milk *synthesis*, however, is not necessarily related to infant intake. This is an important distinction, because it explains many clinical phenomena. Milk may indeed be accumulating within the breast (i. e., the breast is synthesizing milk), but because the infant self-regulates his intake, the milk may simply be stored. Larger breasts may indeed have more storage capacity. Even when storage capacity is low, high production is still possible.[14]

Currently, studies that report maternal volume of milk are accomplished by test-weighing the infant on an electronic scale. Balance scales, which were used before the advent of electronic scales, were inaccurate, but test-weighing is now considered the most acceptable method. Intake is usually reported in grams because infants are weighed in grams. (Weighing the infant in pounds and ounces is less precise.) The density of human milk is approximately 1.03 g/ml.[15]

Normal Range of Milk Intake and Production

American mothers produce about 500 to 600 ml per day during the first 2 weeks and 700 to 800 ml per day thereafter, up to 6 months.[16-18] In the United States, where infants are frequently given solids after 4 to 6 months, milk volume decreases. Milk volume averages 769 g/day at 6 months, 637 g/day at 9 months, and 445 g/day at 12 months.[19]

Influences on Milk Production and Transfer

Infant Factors
During early lactation, volume (supply) of milk is indeed related to demand (i.e., removal of milk); frequency of feedings correlates with increased maternal milk volume.[20] The same is not true in later lactation. After breastfeeding has been well

established, increasing frequency does not result in increased volume.[18]

Maternal Factors

Age and parity of the mother appear to have little or no effect on the volume of milk produced. Despite early concerns of "disuse atrophy" after age 24, studies have shown no correlation between advancing maternal age and milk consumption.[21] At the other end of the spectrum, teenage mothers apparently produce enough milk to satisfy their infants.[22] Some evidence indicates that multiparous women may produce a greater supply of milk on the fourth postpartum day[23] but not after lactation is well established; there is no significant correlation between parity and infant intake in well-nourished populations.[17,24,25] Some culturally determined eating habits may explain the discrepancies.

Milk volume varies diurnally, with greater volume in the morning; milk volume peaks between 8:00 AM and 12:00 noon.[26] Milk volume can be significantly greater in one breast than in the other.[27] Other factors related to maternal health and health habits, especially smoking, can also influence milk production (see Chapter 4).

Composition of Human Milk

About 87% of human milk is water, and all other components are suspended in the water, as shown in Figure 3-7. Other components include fats, proteins, and carbohydrates, along with nonnitrogen compounds, and water-soluble and fat-soluble vitamins, cells, minerals, and trace elements. Furthermore, human milk is isotonic with plasma, so substances can readily cross the alveolar membrane either by diffusion or by active transport. Calcium, amino acids, glucose, magnesium, and sodium cross the membrane by active transport, whereas water, electrolytes, and water-soluble compounds move via diffusion.

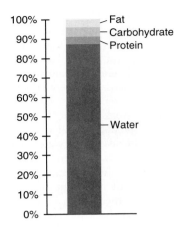

Fig. 3-7 Water and nutrients in human milk.

Primary Components of Human Milk

Components of milk either are synthesized in the secretory cells of the alveoli or are transferred from maternal plasma. The secretory cells synthesize the *macronutrients*: protein, fat, and carbohydrate (lactose). Maternal plasma transfers the macronutrients plus the *macronutrient elements*: vitamins and minerals.[28]

Fats

Fat is needed in human milk because it is (1) a vehicle for fat-soluble vitamins; (2) necessary for brain development; (3) a precursor of prostaglandin and hormones; and (4) an essential constituent of all cell membranes.[29] About 40% to 50% of the total calories in human milk are from fat.[30,31]

Human milk fat is composed mostly of triglycerides; cholesterol also is present and clinically important. Although cholesterol is known to have adverse effects on adult cardiovascular function, it has not been shown to have any negative effects on the infant, even though serum levels are higher in breastfed than artificially fed infants. To the contrary, higher levels of cholesterol are desirable because cholesterol is essential for brain

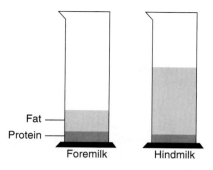

Fig. 3-8 Variation in composition of human milk. Note the greater amount of fat in hindmilk in comparison with foremilk. *(From the National Center for Education in Maternal and Child Health. The Art and Science of Breastfeeding. Arlington, VA: National Center for Education in Maternal and Child Health; 1986.)*

growth in infants. Artificial milk has about the same amount of its calories from fat, but it relies solely on vegetable fat, whereas human milk has cholesterol.

Fat is the most variable component of human milk from a variety of standpoints. Fat content is higher in mature milk than in colostrum, accounting for about 2% of all components of colostrum and about 3.6% of mature milk. Fat content is highest in the afternoon and evening (4:00 PM to 8:00 PM) and lowest between 4:00 AM to 8:00 AM.[26,32] Fat content is four to five times higher in hindmilk than in foremilk.[33,34] Figure 3-8 shows the fat in foremilk in comparison to the fat in hindmilk.

Although it does not influence other components of human milk, maternal diet can significantly influence fat in human milk. While the *amount* of fat is about the same and adequately meets the infant's needs, the *constituents* of fat differ when the mother is extremely malnourished or consumes mostly vegetable rather than animal fat. For example, if the mother consumes lower amounts of polyunsaturated fats, her milk will have a lower fatty acid content. Other factors, including length of gestation and parity, also seem to affect the fat amount.[29]

Proteins

The benefits of human milk and the risks of artificial milk can be best explained by understanding all of the components, but particularly the protein components, of human milk. Protein is synthesized from amino acids in the secretory cells or transferred from the maternal plasma. Amino acids are the "building blocks" of protein. While the terms *essential amino acids* and *nonessential amino acids* are frequently used, by definition they apply to adult needs and not to newborns. However, human milk contains all amino acids necessary for the nursling, as shown in Box 3-1. Protein levels are most concentrated in colostrum during the first few days after birth.[35] After milk volume increases, however, the "dose" continues to be about the same while the concentration decreases; protein accounts for about 2.3% of colostrum but only about 0.9% of mature milk.

Human milk contains two types of proteins: casein (curd) and whey (lactalbumins). Cow's milk contains these two proteins also, but the ratio of casein to whey can be significantly different. Human milk is made up of 60% whey and 40% casein, whereas cow's milk can be 20% whey and 80% casein. Human milk is easily and quickly digested and this greater proportion of whey produces softer stools. If artificial milk has a greater percentage of casein it is more difficult to digest and results in a more rubbery curd, and hence more rubbery stools.

WHEY PROTEINS

Whey proteins are synthesized in the mammary gland. The primary whey protein in human milk is a α-lactalbumin. Lactalbumin, together with the other key proteins lactoferrin and secretory immunoglobulin A, make up 60 to 80% of human milk protein. Other proteins (serum albumin, β-lactoglobulins, other immunoglobulins, and various glycoproteins) are also present.

Lactoferrin is also a whey protein that has several infection-protection properties. Present in higher concentrations in colostrum than in mature milk, lactoferrin inhibits the growth of iron-

Box 3-1

Amino Acids Present in Human Milk[28]

- Alanine
- Arginine
- Aspartic acid
- Cystine
- Glutamic acid
- Glycine
- Histidine
- Isoleucine
- Leucine
- Lysine
- Methionine
- Phenylalanine
- Proline
- Serine
- Taurine
- Threonine
- Tryptophan
- Tyrosine
- Valine

When compared with cow's milk, human milk is richer in cystine, which is needed for central nervous system development.

When compared with cow's milk, human milk is lower in phenylalanine and tyrosine. Higher amounts of phenylalanine and tyrosine may lead to central nervous system damage, especially in preterm infants.

Human milk is rich in taurine; newborns cannot synthesize taurine, and cow's milk does not contain any taurine. Taurine is essential for neurological development.

Secretory immunoglobulin A (sIgA), a whey protein, is the most abundant immunoglobulin in human milk. Without the secretory component, this immunoglobulin would be digested by proteolysis in the gastrointestinal tract. Furthermore, sIgA is enhanced by protein *complement*—a group of proteins found in human milk. The primary function of sIgA in human milk is to protect the infant against respiratory and enteric bacterial and viral organisms; it also may protect against allergies. Infants are less likely to have allergies to human milk not because of what it contains but because of the absence of food antigens.

Lysozyme is an enzyme that destroys Enterobacteriaceae and gram-positive bacteria. It also enhances the growth of intestinal flora, namely, lactobacilli, and has antiinflammatory functions. It is higher in human milk than in cow's milk, and concentrations increase as the course of lactation progresses.

CASEIN PROTEIN

Casein is a curd protein. Human milk caseins are predominately the beta type, while bovine casein is about 50% alpha-casein. The high alpha-casein ratio in bovine milk decreases iron absorption. Because iron is so poorly absorbed, relatively large amounts of it need to be added to artificial milk in order for infants to absorb the amount they need. The high beta-casein ratio in human milk allows about 80% of iron to be absorbed. This is important because iron is bound to lactoferrin, which inhibits the growth of iron-dependent bacteria in the gastrointestinal tract.

OTHER PROTEINS

Other proteins are also present in human milk, including serum albumin, β-lactoglobulins. β-Lactoglobulin makes use of some of the protein and some of the globulins. Cow's milk, where β-lactoglobulin predominates over α-lactalbumin, can cause insult to the pancreas and predispose the body to diabetes. Immunoglobulins IgG and IgM, which the fetus received via the placenta, are present in small amounts in hu-

dependent bacteria in the gastrointestinal tract. Therefore, organisms that require iron, such as coliforms and yeast, are inhibited by lactoferrin. It also acts synergistically with secretory immunoglobulin A to enhance antibacterial activity against *Escherichia coli*, but its effect diminishes when the infant is supplemented with cow's milk–based artificial milk. Lactoferrin also acts on microorganisms by blocking carbohydrate metabolism, attacking the cell wall, and binding calcium and magnesium.[36]

man milk, along with various glycoproteins and other substances. Complement proteins are a group of proteins found in human milk. The two that are most important in lactation are C3 and C4. Bifidus factor, which is also present in human milk, supports the growth of lactobacillus.

Carbohydrates

The main carbohydrate in human milk is lactose. Lactose (*lact* meaning "milk" and *ose* meaning "sugar") is a disaccharide, consisting of two monosaccharides, galactose, and glucose. It is synthesized in the secretory cells from circulating maternal blood glucose and galactose. About 4.8% of human milk is lactose, which represents about 40% of the total calories provided by human milk.[1] Nearly all of the carbohydrate in human milk is lactose, but trace amounts of other carbohydrates—glucose, galactose, glucosamines, and other nitrogen-containing oligosaccharides—are also present. Although there is a greater *amount* of carbohydrate in human milk, most of the total *calories* are from fat because carbohydrate yields approximately 4 kilocalories per gram, and fat yields 9 calories per gram.

Colostrum is lower in lactose (about 5.3g/100 ml), while mature milk is significantly higher (about 6.8 g/100 ml). Unlike fat, the amount of lactose varies little throughout the day. Lactose is unique in that it seems to regulate the volume of milk; that is, when less lactose is synthesized, the mother has a smaller total volume of milk and when more is synthesized, the mother has a larger total volume of milk. Therefore, the *concentration* of lactose in human milk is always about the same. Furthermore, lactose dramatically increases from day 4 to day 120,[37] and therefore milk production increases as well.

The percentage of lactose in human milk differs significantly from that in cow's milk. Whereas lactose accounts for about 6.8 g/100 ml of human milk, cow's milk contains only 0.3 g/100 ml. This is important because the higher amount of lactose creates a more acid environment for the gut, thus decreasing the amount of undesirable bacteria

there and improving the absorption of calcium, phosphorus, magnesium, and other elements. Lactose assists in the synthesis of the B vitamins and promotes the growth of lactobacilli, which are gram-positive normal flora of the gut that produce lactic acid from carbohydrate.

Vitamins

The vitamin content of human milk is influenced by maternal vitamin status. In general, chronically low maternal vitamin status results in low concentration of that vitamin in her milk. The Institute of Medicine Subcommittee on Nutrition[28] has carefully described the role of vitamins in human milk, so a summary will be reviewed briefly here.

FAT-SOLUBLE VITAMINS

Fat-soluble vitamins include vitamins A, D, E, and K, all of which are present in human milk. These vitamins vary significantly across the course of lactation. Vitamins A, E, and K all decrease over the course of lactation. Beta-carotene, a precursor of vitamin A, gives colostrum its characteristic yellow color. Colostrum is approximately twice as high in vitamin K concentration as mature milk.[38] Concentrations of tocopherols, the main component of vitamin E, are highest in colostrum and lower in mature milk.

WATER-SOLUBLE VITAMINS

Water-soluble vitamins include vitamin C, thiamin, riboflavin, niacin, vitamin B_6, folate, vitamin B_{12}, biotin, and panthothenic acid. The levels of water-soluble vitamins decrease over the course of lactation, with the exception of folacin,[39] but the volume increases, so total intake remains sufficient.

Minerals

Minerals regulate body function. The major minerals present in human milk include calcium, phosphorus, and magnesium. Maternal ingestion of these minerals has no strong impact on the concentrations found in milk. Most of the calcium, phosphorous, and magnesium is bound to casein.

ELECTROLYTES

Like the major minerals, potassium, sodium, and chloride are largely unaffected by maternal nutritional status. The amount of electrolytes is, however, related to the infant's health status. When infants fail to suckle well, the mammary glands involute; lactose concentration (and therefore milk volume) is reduced, while electrolytes are elevated.[11]

TRACE ELEMENTS

Trace elements in human milk include iodine, iron, copper, zinc, manganese, selenium, chromium, and cobalt. Iron, copper, and zinc levels are highest in human milk immediately after birth. Concentrations of copper decline between birth and 5 months and then stabilize, whereas zinc levels continue to decline throughout lactation.[40] Maternal levels of zinc[41] appear to have no influence on concentrations in milk.

Variations in Composition of Milk

Human milk is dynamic; it is literally a living and life-giving substance that contains thousands of living cells per milliliter, as shown in Figure 3-9. During the early postpartum period, most of the cells are leukocytes in the form of polymorphonuclear cells, macrophages, and lymphocytes[42]; after the first month the predominant cell type is no longer leukocytes but sloughed epithelial cells.[43] In contrast, artificial milk has no cells, as seen under the microscope in Figure 3-10, because the cells in unpasteurized fresh bovine milk have been destroyed by heat and other processes.

From a broad perspective, the composition of human milk is fairly similar among mothers. That is, milk is similar from one group of mothers (e.g., women who are 8 weeks postpartum) to another, and the same components are present in adequate amounts to meet the infant's needs, regardless of other factors. From a narrower perspective, however, milk varies tremendously in terms of both individual and time-related factors.

Individual Factors

Gestation at time of delivery, volume of milk secreted, time of day, age of infant, and the mother's age, parity, and general health status and habits influence the configuration of her milk components. Note, however, that maternal nutrition has very little to do with the makeup of milk. The mother's intake of vitamins and fatty acid content may alter her milk somewhat, but in general nature provides nutrients to the infant at the mother's expense. For this reason, severely undernourished women have been known to provide adequate milk to their infants. Most important, milk composition changes as the infant grows

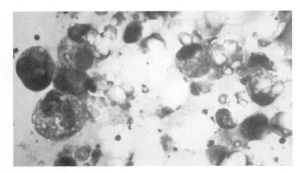

Fig. 3-9 Stain of human milk under the microscope. *(Courtesy Becky Baer.)*

Fig. 3-10 Stain of artificial milk under the microscope. *(Courtesy Becky Baer.)*

older, so that it more perfectly meets his nutritional needs. (Components of milk in relation to the preterm infant's needs will be discussed in later chapters.)

Components

HORMONES

Hormones in human milk include hypothalamic-hypophyseal hormones (prolactin, oxytocin, somatostatin, melatonin, growth hormone releasing factor, gonadotropin-releasing factor, thyrotropin-releasing factor, and thyroid-stimulating hormone), thyroid gland hormones (T3, T4, and calcitonin), adrenal gland hormones, sex hormones (estrogen and various others), insulin, epidermal growth factor, and other hormones and hormone-like substances.

CELLS

There are many white blood cells (WBCs) in human milk. When classified according to structure, granulocytes—having granules in the cytoplasm—include neutrophils, eosinophils, and basophils; agranulocytes include lymphocytes and monocytes. Neutrophils, lymphocytes, and monocytic macrophages (a phagocytic type of monocyte) are all present in human milk. Neutrophils are highest in colostrum, while monocytic macrophages are highest later in lactation.

OTHER

Human milk also contains other components, most notably nonprotein nitrogen components. These include urea, creatine, creatinine, uric acid, glucosamine, α-amino nitrogen, nucleic acids, nucleotides, and polyamines.

Advantages of Breastfeeding, Risks of Artificial Feeding

No one questions the critical role of the placenta, which is specially designed to nourish the fetus before delivery, yet the breast—specially designed to take over the job of nourishing the newborn after the placenta has been expelled—is frequently seen as optional and as equivalent to artificial feeding. In the adult world, artificial means are seen as poor seconds to the natural forms of eating and drinking whole, natural, unprocessed foods. Would we suggest intravenous fluids as an equivalent to quenching one's thirst with a tall glass of fruit juice? Would we claim that total parenteral nutrition is either superior in nutrient content or more appetizing than a Thanksgiving dinner? Why, then, would we promulgate the use of artificial methods of feeding for newborns? The mammary gland was designed to provide a superior food for the newborn, and the newborn's natural desire to suckle the sweet-tasting milk from his mother's warm breast is a far superior method to any artificial fluid or teat that can be produced by modern technology. An extensive review of the last decade's research studies shows that the advantages of human milk are indisputable,[44] and research from this decade continues to reinforce and expand upon these benefits.

The "Innocenti Declaration"[45] describes breastfeeding as a unique process that:

- Provides ideal *nutrition* for infants and contributes to their healthy growth and development
- Reduces incidence and severity of infectious *diseases*, thereby lowering infant morbidity and mortality
- Contributes to *women's health* by reducing the risk of breast and ovarian cancer, and by increasing the spacing between pregnancies
- Provides *social and economic* benefits to the family and the nation
- Provides women with a sense of *satisfaction* when successfully carried out.

Each of these statements was based on current research available when the "Innocenti Declaration" (see Appendix D) was written, and each has been reinforced by subsequent research. Following is a brief summary of these benefits.

Ideal Nutrition

Human milk is intended for human offspring; cow's milk is intended for cows' offspring. The human newborn's body is not designed to overcome the difficulties associated with digesting, absorbing, and utilizing nonhuman milk. It has been well documented that general morbidity among infants fed human milk is far less than among those fed artificial milk.[44,46] More specifically, differences in episodes of otitis media, lower respiratory illness, diarrhea, vomiting, and hospital admission are significant.[46]

Allergy
Breastfeeding appears to reduce the likelihood of allergy, but this relationship is not well understood. Numerous studies of the relationship between atopic eczema, asthma, allergic rhinitis, cow's milk allergy, and other food allergy have been reviewed, and few have been sufficiently controlled to provide definitive conclusions.[47] A recent study was particularly noteworthy, however, because it has the longest follow-up to date. The authors followed the subjects until they were 17 years old and concluded that breastfeeding in the first year of life protected subjects against food allergy, eczema, and respiratory allergies.[48]

Digestion
It is important to remember that digestion begins in the mouth. For the infant, the muscles of the lips, tongue, and jaw are better developed through breastfeeding. This provides long-term benefits, such as fewer orthodontic problems in later life. Infants who are exclusively breastfed are less likely to have (dental) malocclusions than their bottle-feeding cohorts,[49] and duration of breastfeeding lessened the likelihood of malocclusions in over 9000 cases.[50]

Human milk is easier for the infant to digest and absorb. It has long been recognized that breastfed infants have less diarrhea. Gastroesophageal reflux occurs significantly less often in breastfed than artificially fed infants, and median pH values are lower during episodes of reflux[51] when it does occur. Human milk has *half* the renal solute load as artificial milk because of lower levels of protein, calcium, sodium, potassium, and other ions.[39] The relatively low levels of these ions require less water for excretion, and hence lower levels of water are lost when the infant consumes human milk. This water conservation results in a more stable body temperature because water is a factor in thermoregulation.

Growth
Until recently, it has often been assumed that the optimal amount and rate of weight gain for breastfed infants is roughly equivalent to that of their artificially fed cohorts. Calorie and protein intakes are significantly higher for artificially fed infants than for breastfed infants at 3, 6, and 9 months.[52] However, to date, no studies exist to substantiate the generally accepted guidelines for weight gain during the first 28 days of life. A further discussion of clinical guidelines for weight gain is found in Chapter 5.

Immunologic Protection
The immunologic benefits of human milk can be best understood in the context of how the immune system works, and what immunoglobulins really are. First, the body can have either *nonspecific* immunity or *specific* immunity. Nonspecific immunity means that resistance occurs toward threatening pathogens, but the cells exhibit a sort of "shotgun approach" by simply responding to anything that is foreign. Specific immunity means that the immune response is focused; it goes about attacking a certain pathogen in a certain way.

The human body has three lines of defense. The first two lines are *nonspecific*. The first line of defense consists of mechanical or chemical barriers (e.g., skin and mucosa, or secretions). The second line of defense is an inflammatory response (blocking off the pathogens while a large number of immune cells arrive on the scene of the invader) or phagocytosis (ingesting and destroying the invading cells). The third line of defense involves both specific and nonspecific immunity. Nonspecific immunity includes natural killer cells (NK cells). NK cells are a group of nonspecific lymphocytes that take a "shotgun" approach to killing pathogens using direct means to lyse, or break apart, the invading cells. Interferon is a nonspecific protein. Complement is a group of about 20 enzymes that can exhibit specific or nonspecific immune responses. NK cells, interferon, and complement are all present in human milk.

Specific immunity is part of the body's third line of defense. The two major classes of cells that are important are the *B lymphocytes* and *T lymphocytes* (sometimes called *B cells* and *T cells*). B cells do not attack pathogens directly but instead produce *antibodies* to be the direct attackers (antibody-mediated immunity). T cells, however, attack pathogens directly (cell-mediated immunity). Antibodies are plasma proteins of the class called *immunoglobulins*. The major immunoglobulins (abbreviated Ig) include IgA, IgG, IgM, IgD, and IgE. In serum, the most abundant immunoglobulin is IgG, but in human milk the predominant immunoglobulin is secretory IgA. The mother produces secretory IgA in response to a specfic organism and passes it along through her milk. Thus the newborn gradually builds immunities towards most pathogens in his immediate environment.

Colostrum is really the first "inoculation." Secretory IgA antibodies are produced locally in the breast, and these antibodies amount to about 0.5 to 1 gram per day throughout the course of lactation. They are directed against food proteins and microorganisms often present in the intestine.[53]

Respiratory/Ear

Multiple studies have substantiated that breastfeeding decreases the risk of otitis media. In one study the type of day care, the sex of the infant, and the duration of breastfeeding were controlled. Significant associations were found between the occurrence of acute otitis media and breastfeeding.[54] Exclusive breastfeeding for 4 or more months appears to reduce single as well as recurrent episodes of otitis media.[55]

It also appears that breastfeeding provides protection against lower respiratory infections. While exclusive breastfeeding for four months marginally reduces the risk of pneumonia in some cultures,[56] early introduction of artificial milk may increase the risk for pneumonia.[57] Infants who have been breastfed may be at less risk for respiratory synctial virus–related lower respiratory infections, although many variables seem to contribute to morbidity.[58] Breastfed infants have reduced morbidity and are rarely hospitalized; they rarely require ventilation if respiratory difficulties do occur. Furthermore, the benefits of human milk may extend well beyond infancy, as described in the Research Highlight.

This text has endeavored to show the risks of artificial feeding in contrast to the benefits of breastfeeding, with the idea that health care providers and parents should become more focused on breastfeeding as the standard rather than on the threats of the alternative. However, a well-referenced and intriguing discussion of the hazards of artificial feeding is well worth reading.[59] The benefits of breastfeeding are clear when compared to the risks of infant formula, as shown in Box 3-2.

Women's Health

The act of suckling at the breast is advantageous to both the newborn and the mother. Even if artificial milk could be manufactured to exactly match the properties of human milk, and even if an artificial teat could exactly mimic the human

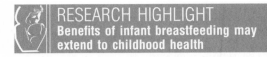

RESEARCH HIGHLIGHT
Benefits of infant breastfeeding may extend to childhood health

Citation: Wilson AC, Forsyth SF, Greene SA, Irvine L, Hau C, Howie PW. Relation of infant diet to childhood health: seven year follow up of cohort of children in Dundee infant feeding study. *Br Med J* 1998;316:21-25.

Focus: The current descriptive study was a follow-up to a study conducted in the United Kingdom between 1983 and 1986. The original prospective study showed multiple health benefits during infancy. These same subjects, whose mean age was 7.3 years for this study, were studied for respiratory illness, body composition (weight, height, body mass index, percentage of body fat), and blood pressure in relation to duration of breastfeeding and timing of introduction of solids.

Results: Exclusive breastfeeding was associated with a significant reduction in childhood respiratory illness. About 17% of the infants who were exclusively breastfed for at least 15 weeks had later respiratory illness, while about 30% and 32% of those who were partially or exclusively fed artificial milk experienced respiratory illness. Early introduction of solid food was associated with increased body fat and weight in childhood, and exclusive bottle feeding was associated with higher systolic blood pressure in childhood.

Strengths, limitations of the study: 545 (81%) of the original 674 subjects were available for the follow-up study. Possible confounding factors, including socioeconomic status, family history, and sex of the child were adjusted for using logistic regression analysis to ensure accurate results.

Clinical application: This study substantiates other studies that have shown that breastfeeding is associated with multiple health benefits. Parents should understand that the health, social, and economic impact of respiratory illness is not limited to infancy, and multiple other benefits of breastfeeding may extend far into childhood.

nipple/areola complex, advantages would still remain for the mother.

Sexuality and Fertility

Newton and Newton point out that "the survival of the human race, long before the concept of 'duty' evolved, depended upon the satisfactions gained from the two voluntary acts of reproduction—coitus and breastfeeding. These had to be sufficiently pleasurable to ensure their frequent occurrence."[60] Multiple physical and psychological responses that occur during lactation also occur during coitus.[60] Furthermore, multiple physical and psychological responses experienced during sexual excitement have similarities to those that occur during the act of giving birth.[61] These responses can be explained by the fact that the same hormones—including estrogen, progesterone, oxytocin, and prolactin—are involved in the menstrual cycle, sexual intercourse, pregnancy, birth, and lactation.

Few well-controlled studies address the impact of breastfeeding on sexual desire and behavior. Masters and Johnson, however, found that women who breastfeed are generally more interested in an early return to sexual activity.[62] However, the woman may have excessive vaginal dryness, due to the hormones associated with lactation, and may spray milk during orgasm. Some simple strategies—using lubricating jelly and feeding the infant before intercourse—minimize these effects.

Breastfeeding significantly suppresses fertility and contributes to limiting populations.[63] It is well-documented that mothers who breastfeed have longer intervals between births.[64] The elevated prolactin levels that occur during lactation suppress ovulation and the reproductive cycle. The time it takes for a woman's menses to return depends in large part on the frequency with which she suckles her infant. This amenorrhea, therefore, can last for weeks, months, or years. This difference has important teaching implications for child-spacing.

The World Health Organization has deemed that breastfeeding "has been the most effective contraceptive world-wide."[45] Yet the contraceptive value of natural family planning methods, including breastfeeding, has been ignored or inaccurately presented in the United States. Many of us have been educated in fine university programs that have scoffed at any type of birth control—

Box 3-2

Breast Milk: The Gold Standard Compared With the Risks of Infant Formula

Breastfeeding is the natural and normal way to provide optimal nutritional, immunologic, and emotional nurturing for the growth and development of infants. No artificial baby milk (formula) is the same as breast milk in terms of nutrients, enzymes, growth factors, hormones, or immunologic and antiinflammatory properties, or in infant growth and developmental outcomes. Therefore, breast milk doesn't just add benefits, but sets the standard for infant feeding.

The Standard of Health Outcomes

Artificially fed infants have

- Increased rates of respiratory disease[1]
- Increased rates of otitis media[2]
- Increased rates of gastroenteritis[3]
- Increased risk of sudden infant death syndrome (SIDS)[4]
- Increased incidence of allergies[5]
- Increased risk of childhood cancers[6]
- Increased risk of insulin-dependent diabetes mellitus (IDDM) in susceptible children[7]
- Increased risk of ulcerative colitis[8]
- Increased incidence of Crohn's disease[9]
- Increased possibility of improperly stimulated immune system[10]
- Increased risk for less favorable response to vaccines, with low antibody levels leaving some artifically fed babies underimmunized[11]

The Standard of Cognitive Outcomes

Artifically fed infants have

- A different brain composition than breastfed babies[12]
- A lower neurodevelopmental response at 4 months of age[13]
- Lower mental development scores at 18 months of age[14]
- Lower cognitive scores at 3 years of age[15]
- Twice the rate of minor neurological dysfunction at 9 years of age[16]
- Lower IQs at ages 11 to 16 years[17]

The Standard of Composition

Artificial baby milk does *not* contain[18]

- Secretory IgA
- Lysozyme
- Macrophages
- Hormones
- Enzymes
- Growth factors
- Long-chain polyunsaturated fatty acids (DHA and AA)

Artificial baby milk (formula) cannot meet these standards. The only food that meets them is breast milk—a living fluid and the gold standard.

References

1. Wright AL et al. *Br Med J,* 299, 1989
2. Duncan B et al. *Pediatr,* 91, 1993
3. Howie PW et al. *Br Med J,* 300, 1990
4. Frederickson DD et al. *Am J Dis Child,* 147, 1993
5. Saarinen UM et al. *Lancet,* 346, 1995
6. Davis MK et al. *Lancet,* 8/13, 1988
7. Mayer EJ et al. *Diabetes,* 37, 1988
8. Whorwell PJ et al. *Br Med J,* 1:382, 1979
9. Koletzko S et al. *Br Med J,* 298, 1989
10. Newman J. *Scientific American,* 12:76, 1995
11. Hahn-Zoric M et al. *Acta Paediatr Scand,* 79, 1990
12. Uauy R. *J Pediatr Gastroenterol Nutr,* 11, 1990
13. Agostoni C et al. *Pediatr Res,* 38, 1995
14. Florey CD, et al. *Int J Epidemiol,* 24 (suppl), 1995
15. Bauer G et al. *Psych Reports,* 68, 1991
16. Lanting CI et al. *Lancet,* 344, 1994
17. Greene LC et al. *Biochem Soc Trans,* 23, 1995
18. See labels on formula cans in your area

Courtesy of Barbara Heiser, RN, BSN, IBCLC, and Marsha Walker, RN, IBCLC, National Alliance for Breastfeeding Advocacy (NABA), Ellicott City, Maryland.

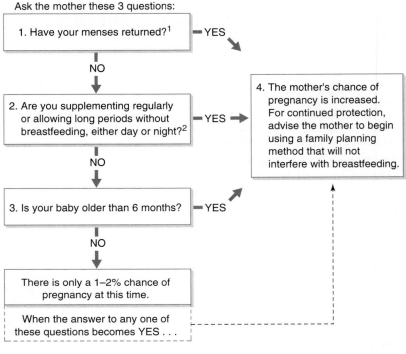

Ask the mother these 3 questions:

1. Have your menses returned?[1] ➤ YES

NO

2. Are you supplementing regularly or allowing long periods without breastfeeding, either day or night?[2] ➤ YES ➤

NO

3. Is your baby older than 6 months? ➤ YES

NO

4. The mother's chance of pregnancy is increased. For continued protection, advise the mother to begin using a family planning method that will not interfere with breastfeeding.

There is only a 1–2% chance of pregnancy at this time.

When the answer to any one of these questions becomes YES . . .

Fig. 3-11 The lactational amenorrhea method (LAM). *(From* The Lactational Amenorrhea Method: Are You Offering Your Clients All the Options? *Institute for Reproductive Health. Washington, DC: IRH; 1996.)*

[1] Spotting or bleeding during the first 56 days postpartum is not considered a menstrual bleed.
[2] Intervals between breastfeeds should not exceed 4 hours during the day, or 6 hours at night. Supplemental foods and liquids should not replace a breastfeed.

unless it is commercially produced. It is not at all uncommon for students in the health care professions to read a textbook or patient education materials about birth-spacing with no mention of breastfeeding. Excellent maternal and child nursing textbooks give few positive messages about natural family planning methods. Indeed, Pilliteri's discussion of natural family planning methods lumps calendar rhythm with symptothermal methods, with no mention of breastfeeding as a way to achieve child-spacing.[65] Some physicians seem convinced of the effectiveness of lactation on child-spacing,[66] while others, despite the evidence, seem skeptical.[67]

The lactational amenorrhea method (LAM) relies on the increased prolactin levels during lactation to avoid the occurrence of a pregnancy. Figure 3-11 shows that if menses has not returned, and if the mother is fully or almost fully breastfeeding the infant, pregnancy is highly unlikely to occur. Rigorous studies have shown that the pregnancy rate was less than 1% under these circumstances.[64,68] Breastfeeding can be a low-risk strategy to avoiding pregnancy under certain circumstances, and it provides an explanation for the woman who may be unsuccessfully trying to achieve a pregnancy while breastfeeding.

It is important to emphasize that American women, who frequently supplement their infants or restrict breastfeeding, rob themselves of the child-spacing benefits that can occur during lactation. However, a woman should not consider herself to be infertile simply because she is breastfeeding; breastfeeding is not a contraceptive.

Cancer

Breastfeeding's role in minimizing the risk of breast cancer has not been confirmed, although there is mounting evidence that breastfeeding contributes to lowered premenopausal breast cancer.[69-72] Current studies show little hope that breastfeeding protects against postmenopausal cancer. There is little conclusive evidence about the relationship of breastfeeding and ovarian cancer, but some studies suggest that reduced menstrual cycles may be a protective factor.[73,74]

Diabetes

Most of us can remember the days when diabetic women were blatantly discouraged from breastfeeding. Studies have shown, however, that breastfeeding is beneficial for both insulin-dependent mothers (IDDM) and gestational diabetic mothers (see Chapter 8).

Osteoporosis

Some studies have shown no clear benefits of breastfeeding on the development of osteoporosis,[75-78] but evidence is accumulating to support the idea that breastfeeding does have a protective effect against this common problem in women. Bone density may decrease transiently during lactation, but bone loss during lactation is regained after weaning.[79] Furthermore, bones recover to prelactation levels even with extended lactation and subsequent pregnancies.[80] The decreased urinary excretion of calcium and increased bone absorption during lactation may help to explain beneficial effects.[81] Epidemiological studies consistently demonstrate protection with breastfeeding.[44]

Other Benefits

Data are accumulating to suggest various other benefits of breastfeeding for women and their families. Breastfeeding may have a protective effect against rheumatoid arthritis[82] and against maternal urinary tract infections.[83] Breastfeeding mothers appear to lose weight more rapidly than nonlactating women between 3 and 6 months postpartum.[84] The existing and growing body of literature about breastfeeding suggests that more benefits of breastfeeding for both mother and child are yet to be discovered.

Social and Economic Advantages

Artificial milk costs are significant, depending on where it is purchased and how much the newborn or growing child consumes. Assuming for a moment that a newborn consumes an average of 2 ounces of artificial milk and takes 8 feedings a day during the first week, the parent would spend about $20 that week to buy artificial milk. Over and above the amount the infant consumes is the amount the parent wastes. (Typically, parents prepare a little more than they anticipate the infant will consume, resulting in waste.) Of course, as the infant grows, the amount consumed will increase substantially, as will the cost. Mother's milk, of course, is free, so the cost savings increases as the infant grows. Worse still, increased cost for artificial feeding goes beyond the price of buying the product. The paraphernalia associated with bottle feeding (nipples, bottles, bottle brushes, etc.) certainly adds to the cost of artificial feeding. The biggest expense, however, lies in increased health care costs due to infant illness.

Some people may argue that mother's milk is not really free because of the additional cost of feeding the mother. This rationale, however, has little to do with economics. First, a lactating mother's diet should be self-selected, and no "special" food is required. While the mother does need to consume more calories than a nonlactating mother, this requirement can be met by eating a peanut butter sandwich and a glass of milk in addition to her usual daily consumption. The milk that comes from her breasts is free, but artificial milk from the store is anything except economical.

It is difficult to imagine how artificial milk might be more "convenient" than human milk, although some women give this as a reason for not breastfeeding. Shopping for the product, putting it away at home, mixing, warming, and recycling the containers are chores that most of us would rather avoid. This is to say nothing of shopping for, assembling, cleaning, and sterilizing bottles, nipples, and related paraphernalia. Ironically, however, mothers often state that breastfeeding is "not convenient." There appears to be no research that interprets the meaning of this comment, but it certainly contradicts what is known about the tasks associated with artificial feeding. It is possible that "not convenient" is really a euphemism for "my boyfriend doesn't want me to" or "it will tie me down."

Sense of Satisfaction

During the past 50 years or so, some skeptics have challenged the benefits of breastfeeding. Historically, however, breastfeeding advocates and opponents have agreed that the bonding associated with breastfeeding is beneficial. Bonding, however, is only one aspect of the psychological experience, which was discussed in Chapter 2.

SUMMARY

The mammary gland, formed when the mother herself was only an embryo, undergoes structural changes during pregnancy that enable her to produce and provide milk after giving birth. The components of human milk vary to best accommodate the needs of the infant. Breastfeeding (the act of suckling the infant) and lactation (the process of making milk) provide advantages for infant nutrition, the woman's health, social and economic conservation, and a sense of satisfaction for the mother. It is no wonder, then, that human milk and breastfeeding truly constitute the "gold standard" by which other methods are measured.

References

1. Lawrence RA. *Breastfeeding: A Guide for the Medical Profession.* 4th ed. St. Louis: Mosby; 1994.
2. Gunn AJ, Gunn TR, Rabone DL, Breier BH, Blum WF, Gluckman PD. Growth hormone increases breast milk volumes in mothers of preterm infants. *Pediatrics* 1996;98(2, pt 1):279-282.
3. McNeilly AS, Robinson IC, Houston MJ, Howie PW. Release of oxytocin and prolactin in response to suckling. *Br Med J* 1983;286:257-259.
4. Nissen E, Lilja G, Widstrom AM, Uvnas-Moberg K. Elevation of oxytocin levels early post partum in women. *Acta Obstet Gynecol Scand* 1995; 74:530-533.
5. Neifert MR, McDonough SL, Neville MC. Failure of lactogenesis associated with placental retention. *Am J Obstet Gynecol* 1981;140:477-478.
6. Martin, RH, Glass MR, Chapman C, Wilson GD, Woods KL. Human alpha-lactalbumin and hormonal factors in pregnancy and lactation. *Clin Endocrinol (Oxf)* 1980;13:223-230.
7. Neville MC, Neifert MR, eds. *Lactation: Physiology, Nutrition and Breast-feeding.* New York: Plenum Press; 1983.
8. Lawrence RA. *Breastfeeding: A Guide for the Medical Profession.* 4th ed. St. Louis: Mosby; 1994.
9. Huggins K, Ziedrich L. *The Nursing Mother's Guide to Weaning.* Boston: Harvard Common Press; 1994.
10. Garza C, Johnson CA, Smith EO, Nichols BL. Changes in the nutrient composition of human milk during gradual weaning. *Am J Clin Nutr* 1983;37:61-65.

11. Hartmann PE, Kulski JK. Changes in the composition of the mammary secretion of women after abrupt termination of breast feeding. *J Physiol (Lond)* 1978;275:1-11.

12. Palmer G. *The Politics of Breastfeeding*. London: Pandora; 1988.

13. Daly, SE, Hartmann PE. Infant demand and milk supply. Part 2: The short-term control of milk synthesis in lactating women. *J Hum Lact* 1995;11:27-37.

14. Newton M, Newton NR. The normal course and management of lactation. *Clin Obstet Gynecol* 1962;5:44-46.

15. Neville MC, Keller R, Seacat J, et al. Studies in human lactation: milk volumes in lactating women during the onset of lactation and full lactation. *Am J Clin Nutr* 1988;48:1375-1386.

16. Lonnerdal B, Forsum E, Hambraeus L. A longitudinal study of the protein, nitrogen, and lactose contents of human milk from Swedish well-nourished mothers. *Am J Clin Nutr* 1976;29:1127-1133.

17. Butte NF, Garza C, Stuff JE, Smith EO, Nichols BL. Effect of maternal diet and body composition on lactational performance. *Am J Clin Nutr* 1984;39:296-306.

18. DeCarvalho M, Robertson S, Merkatz R, Klaus M. Milk intake and frequency of feeding in breast fed infants. *Early Hum Dev* 1982;7:155-163.

19. Dewey KG, Heinig MJ, Nommsen LA, Lonnerdal B. Maternal versus infant factors related to breast milk intake and residual milk volume: the DARLING study. *Pediatrics* 1991;87:829-837.

20. DeCarvalho M, Robertson S, Friedman A, Klaus M. Effect of frequent breast-feeding on early milk production and infant weight gain. *Pediatrics* 1983;72:307-311.

21. Butte NF, Garza C, Smith EO, Nichols BL. Human milk intake and growth in exclusively breast-fed infants. *J Pediatr* 1984;104:187-195.

22. Lipsman S, Dewey KG, Lonnerdal B. Breast-feeding among teenage mothers: milk composition, infant growth, and maternal dietary intake. *J Pediatr Gastroenterol Nutr* 1985;4:426-434.

23. Zuppa AA, Tornesello A, Papacci P, et al. Relationship between maternal parity, basal prolactin levels and neonatal breast milk intake. *Biol Neonate* 1988;53:144-147.

24. Dewey KG, Lonnerdal B. Infant self-regulation of breast milk intake. *Acta Paediatr Scand* 1986;75:893-898.

25. Rattigan S, Ghisalberti AV, Hartmann PE, Breastmilk production in Australian women. *Br J Nutr* 1981;45:243-249.

26. Stafford J, Villalpando S, Urquieta Aguila B. Circadian variation and changes after a meal in volume and lipid production of human milk from rural Mexican women. *Ann Nutr Metab* 1994;38:232-237.

27. Daly SE, Owens RA, Hartmann PE. The short-term synthesis and infant-regulated removal of milk in lactating women. *Exp Physiol* 1993;78:209-220.

28. Institute of Medicine. *Nutrition During Lactation*. Washington, DC: National Academy Press; 1991.

29. Hamosh M, Bitman J. Human milk in disease: lipid composition. *Lipids* 1992;27:848-857.

30. Jensen RG, Jensen GL. Specialty lipids for infant nutrition, I: milks and formulas. *J Pediatr Gastroenterol Nutr* 1992;15:232-245.

31. Hamosh M. Lipid metabolism in premature infants. *Biol Neonate* 1987;52(suppl 1):50-64.

32. Jackson DA, Imong SM, Silprasert A, et al. Circadian variation in fat concentration of breast-milk in a rural northern Thai population. *Br J Nutr* 1988;59:349-363.

33. Hall B. Uniformity of human milk. *Am J Clin Nutr* 1979;32:304-312.

34. Dorea JG, Horner MR, Bezerra VL, Campanate ML. Variation in major constituents of fore- and hindmilk of Brazilian women. *J Trop Pediatr* 1982;28:303-305.

35. Saint L, Smith M, Hartmann PE. The yield and nutrient content of colostrum and milk of women from giving birth to 1 month post-partum. *Br J Nutr* 1984;52:87-95.

36. Sanchez L, Calvo M, Brock JH. Biological role of lactoferrin. *Arch Dis Child* 1992;67:657-661.

37. Coppa GV, Gabrielli O, Pierani P, Catassi C, Carlucci A, Giorgi PL. Changes in carbohydrate composition in human milk over 4 months of lactation. *Pediatrics* 1993;91:637-641.

38. von Kries R, Shearer M, McCarthy PT, Haug M, Harzer G, Gobel U. Vitamin K_1 content of maternal milk: influence of the stage of lactation, lipid composition, and vitamin K_1 supplements given to the mother. *Pediatr Res* 1987;22:513-517.

39. Worthington-Roberts B, Williams SR. *Nutrition in Pregnancy and Lactation.* 5th ed. St. Louis: Mosby; 1993.

40. Casey CE, Neville MC, Hambidge KM. Studies in human lactation: secretion of zinc, copper, and manganese in human milk. *Am J Clin Nutr* 1989;49:773-785.

41. Feeley RM, Eitenmiller RR, Jones JB Jr, Barnhart H. Copper, iron, and zinc contents of human milk at early stages of lactation. *Am J Clin Nutr* 1983;37:443-448.

42. Ho FC, Wong RL, Lawton JW. Human colostral and breast milk cells: a light and electron microscopic study. *Acta Paediatr Scand* 1979;68:389-396.

43. Brooker BE. The epithelial cells and cell fragments in human milk. *Cell Tissue Res* 1980;210:321-332.

44. Cunningham AS, Jelliffe DB, Jelliffe EF. Breast-feeding and health in the 1980s: a global epidemiologic review. *J Pediatr* 1991;118:659-666.

45. WHO and UNICEF. *Protecting, Promoting, and Supporting Breast-feeding: The Special Role of Maternity Services.* Geneva: World Health Organization; 1989.

46. Cunningham AS. Morbidity in breast-fed and artificially fed infants. *J Pediatr* 1979;95(5, pt 1):685-689.

47. Kramer MS. Does breast feeding help protect against atopic disease? biology, methodology, and a golden jubilee of controversy. *J Pediatr* 1988; 112:181-190.

48. Saarinen UM, Kajosaari M. Breastfeeding as prophylaxis against atopic diease: prospective follow-up study until 17 years old. *Lancet* 1995;346:1065-1069.

49. Davis DW, Bell PA. Infant feeding practices and occlusal outcomes: a longitudinal study. *J Can Dent Assoc* 1991;57:593-594.

50. Labbok MH, Hendershot GE. Does breast-feeding protect against malocclusion? an analysis of the 1981 Child Health Supplement to the National Health Interview Survey. *Am J Prev Med* 1987;3:227-232.

51. Heacock HJ, Jeffery HE, Baker JL, Page M. Influence of breast versus formula milk on physiological gastroesophageal reflux in healthy, newborn infants. *J Pediatr Gastroenterol Nutr* 1992;14:41-46.

52. Heinig MJ, Nommsen LA, Peerson JM, Lonnerdal B, Dewey KG. Energy and protein intakes of breast-fed and formula-fed infants during the first year of life and their association with growth velocity: the DARLING Study. *Am J Clin Nutr* 1993;58:152-161.

53. Hanson LA, Ahlstedt S, Andersson B, et al. The immune response of the mammary gland and its significance for the neonate. *Ann Allergy* 1984; 53(6, pt 2):576-582.

54. Kero P, Piekkala P. Factors affecting the occurrence of acute otitis media during the first year of life. *Acta Paediatr Scand* 1987;76:618-623.

55. Duncan B, Ey J, Holberg CJ, Wright AL, Martinez FD, Taussig LM. Exclusive breast-feeding for at least 4 months protects against otitis media [see comments]. *Pediatrics* 1993;91:867-872.

56. Forman MR, Graubard BI, Hoffman HJ, Beren R, Harley EE, Bennett P. The Pima infant feeding study: breastfeeding and respiratory infections during the first year of life. *Int J Epidemiol* 1984;13:447-453.

57. Ford K, Labbok M. Breast-feeding and child health in the United States. *J Biosoc Sci* 1993;25:187-194.

58. Holberg CJ, Wright AL, Martinez FD, Ray CG, Taussig LM, Lebowitz MD. Risk factors for respiratory syncytial virus–associated lower respiratory illnesses in the first year of life. *Am J Epidemiol* 1991;133:1135-1151.

59. Walker M. A fresh look at the risks of artificial infant feeding. *JHL* 1993;9:97-107.

60. Newton N, Newton M. Psychologic aspects of lactation. *N Engl J Med* 1967;277:1179-1188.

61. Newton N. Trebly sensuous woman. *Psychology Today*. July 1971;98:68-71.

62. Masters WH, Johnson VE. *Human Sexual Response*. Boston: Little, Brown; 1966.

63. McNeilly AS. Lactational amenorrhea. *Endocrinol Metab Clin North Am* 1993;22:59-73.

64. Perez A, Labbok MH, Queenan JT. Clinical study of the lactational amenorrhoea method for family planning. *Lancet* 1992;339:968-970.

65. Pillitteri A. *Maternal and Child Health Nursing*. 2nd ed. Philadelphia: Lippincott; 1995.

66. Geerling JH. Natural family planning. *Am Fam Physician* 1995;52:1749-1756, 1759-1760.

67. Wang IY, Fraser IS. Reproductive function and contraception in the postpartum period. *Obstet Gynecol Surv* 1994;49:56-63.

68. Labbok MH, Stallings RY, Shah F, et al. Ovulation method use during breastfeeding: is there increased risk of unplanned pregnancy? *Am J Obstet Gynecol* 1991;165(6, pt 2):2031-2036.

69. Newcomb PA, Storer BE, Longnecker MP, et al. Lactation and a reduced risk of premenopausal breast cancer. *N Engl J Med* 1994;330:81-87.

70. United Kingdom National Case-Control Study Group. Breast feeding and risk of breast cancer in young women. *BMJ* 1993;307:17-20.

71. Yoo KY, Tajima K, Kuroishi T, et al. Independent protective effect of lactation against breast cancer: a case-control study in Japan. *Am J Epidemiol* 1992;135:726-733.

72. Katsouyanni K, Lipworth L, Trichopoulou A, Samoli E, Stuver S, Trichopoulos D. A case-control study of lactation and cancer of the breast. *Br J Cancer* 1996;73:814-818.

73. Rosenblatt KA, Thomas DB. Prolonged lactation and endometrial cancer: WHO Collaborative Study of Neoplasia and Steroid Contraceptives. *Int J Epidemiol* 1995;24:499-503.

74. Gwinn ML, Lee NC, Rhodes PH, Layde PM, Rubin GL. Pregnancy, breast feeding, and oral contraceptives and the risk of epithelial ovarian cancer. *J Clin Epidemiol* 1990;43:559-568.

75. Kritz-Silverstein D, Barrett-Connor E, Hollenbach KA. Pregnancy and lactation as determinants of bone mineral density in postmenopausal women. *Am J Epidemiol* 1992;136:1052-1059.

76. Melton LJ III, Bryant SC, Wahner HW, et al. Influence of breastfeeding and other reproductive factors on bone mass later in life. *Osteoporos Int* 1993;3:76-83.

77. Sowers M, Corton G, Shapiro B, et al. Changes in bone density with lactation *JAMA* 1993;269:3130-3135.

78. O'Neill TW, Silman AJ, Naves Diaz M, Cooper C, Kanis J, Felsenberg D. Influence of hormonal and reproductive factors on the risk of vertebral deformity in European women: European Vertebral Osteoporosis Study Group. *Osteoporos Int* 1997;7:72-78.

79. Kalkwarf HJ, Specker BL. Bone mineral loss during lactation and recovery after weaning. *Obstet Gynecol* 1995;86:26-32.

80. Sowers M, Randolph J, Shapiro B, Jannausch M. A prospective study of bone density and pregnancy after an extended period of lactation with bone loss. *Obstet Gynecol* 1995;85:285-289.

81. Specker BL, Vieira NE, O'Brien KO, et al. Calcium kinetics in lactating women with low and high calcium intakes. *Am J Clin Nutr* 1994;59:593-599.

82. Brun JG, Nilssen S, Kvale G. Breast feeding, other reproductive factors and rheumatoid arthritis: a prospective study. *Br J Rheumatol* 1995;34:542-546.

83. Coppa GV, Gabrielli O, Giorgi P, et al. Preliminary study of breastfeeding and bacterial adhesion to uroepithelial cells. *Lancet* 1990;335:569-571.

84. Dewey KG, Heinig MJ, Nommsen LA. Maternal weight-loss patterns during prolonged lactation. *Am J Clin Nutr* 1993;58:162-166.

Breastfeeding for Healthy Mothers and Newborns

4

Maternal Education and Support

ducation about infant feeding begins the first time feeding is observed. In the United States the first observation is often of bottle feeding; most American children grow up without ever having had the benefit of seeing an infant at the breast. Except in New York State, where breastfeeding education is part of the elementary school curriculum, education about breastfeeding as a feeding method is likely to begin when women hear about it from family and friends. Unfortunately, however, they frequently hear stories that describe negative breastfeeding experiences, which may affect their motivation to breastfeed and their attitude toward breastfeeding.

MOTIVATION AND ATTITUDE

Breastfeeding is a learned art, and the woman must be motivated to learn it. Six factors influence motivation to learn: attitudes, felt needs, stimulation, emotion, competence, and reinforcement.[1] These factors can impact either negatively or positively upon initiation and continuation of breastfeeding. For example, the mother may not be motivated to breastfeed if she feels there is no need to do so (artificial milk is equivalent to breastfeeding, or breastfeeding benefits only the infant but not the mother); the instructor does not stimulate her interest in breastfeeding; she has had previous negative emotional experiences related to breasts or breastfeeding; she perceives herself as unable to do it; or she does not receive adequate reinforcement for her efforts. The mother's attitude underlies all of these factors.

Breastfeeding is a behavior, but learning about breastfeeding can be enhanced or thwarted by attitudes. It is helpful, therefore, for breastfeeding educators and advocates to examine what an "attitude" is and how attitudes affect the teaching/ learning process.

Attitudes

Ellis[2] defines an attitude as a "combination of a perception with a judgment that often results in an emotion that influences behavior." This means that the learner takes in information through the senses, makes a judgment about whether it is negative or positive, and from that has some emotion attached; this negative or positive judgment influences her behavior.

Educators and psychologists have long recognized the ability of attitude to predict behavior. Health care professionals are beginning to recognize the impact of attitude on feeding choices. Reporting on numerous studies, Losch and colleagues[3] conclude that the ability of attitudes to predict behavior is strong, and that intentions prior to birth are very closely linked to actual feeding practices. Furthermore, the decision to breastfeed is often made before conception[4-6] and almost always by the end of gestation.[7] The link between intention and behavior once again becomes apparent, since those women who make the decision earlier (prior to or early in pregnancy) are more likely to continue breastfeeding longer,[8,9] and intention is a strong predictor of continuation past 6 weeks.[10]

The idea of attitudes as predictors of behavior has implications for those who educate pregnant women about breastfeeding. First, women who become pregnant with limited perceptions about breastfeeding will have fewer judgments and emotions, so the health care provider will likely have a greater influence on attitude. Second, those who come with a positive attitude about breastfeeding will require positive reinforcement. Third, those who come with negative attitudes are less likely to breastfeed. It is possible, however, to motivate these women to breastfeed by using two strategies that are effective with adult learners: (1) confront possible erroneous beliefs, expectations, and assumptions that may underlie learner attitude; and (2) reduce or remove components of the environment that result in failure or fear.[1]

Erroneous Beliefs, Expectations, Assumptions

Sometimes, women assume that their everyday health habits will need to be dramatically altered, or that less healthy habits preclude breastfeeding. These erroneous beliefs, such as those shown in Box 4-1, can be deterrents to either the initiation or the continuation of breastfeeding. Such beliefs should be replaced with science-based information, such as is provided in the following pages.

Box 4-1
Breastfeeding: Making an Informed Choice

Erroneous Beliefs About Breastfeeding Experience

Myth: Breastfeeding hurts.
Science: Sore nipples are not an expected consequence of breastfeeding. Nipples should not be sore when the infant is positioned correctly. Furthermore, breastfeeding is meant to be a pleasurable experience. If it were not, the human species might never have survived!

Myth: Breastfeeding will make my breasts sag.
Science: There is no support for the idea that breastfeeding will make a woman's breasts sag. Wearing a bra to support the ligaments of the breast, however, may be helpful.

Erroneous Beliefs About "Special" Requirements of Breastfeeding

Myth: I can't breastfeed because I didn't prepare my nipples
Science: There is no special preparation necessary.

Myth: I don't want to breastfeed because I don't like to drink milk.
Science: One does not need to drink milk to make milk.

Myth: I don't want to breastfeed because I don't want to give up [whatever food].
Science: Diet should be self-selected.

Confronting Possible Erroneous Beliefs, Expectations, and Assumptions

Erroneous beliefs, expectations, and assumptions about breastfeeding are common. The nurse needs to confront misunderstandings about food and nutrient needs, effects of food on the infant, maternal fluid requirements, and use of substances.

Nutritional and Fluid Requirements

Women do not need to eat any special foods while they are lactating. For the most part, lactating women should have a self-selected diet, choosing foods from the food pyramid shown in Figure 4-1. Groups that are particularly at risk for nutritional deficits, namely, those with restricted eating patterns (e.g., vegetarians, women who diet to lose weight, and those who avoid dairy products), adolescents, and low-

income women[11] may need special counseling. Suggest measures for improving nutrient intake for these women; Table 4-1 gives specific ideas. Refer a woman to a registered dietitian if her counseling needs appear to be extraordinary. Recommendations for calorie intake, weight loss, exercise, and use of caffeine, alcohol, and cigarettes are listed in Box 4-2.

Energy Requirements

The energy requirements of women who are lactating differ little from the requirements of those who are not. Nonpregnant adults need about 2200 kcal per day to maintain optimal nutrition. The pregnant woman needs about 2500 kcal per day, and the lactating woman needs about 2700 kcal per day. This need for 2700 kcal per day translates to about 500 kcal per day more than her prepregnant needs. Contrary to myths the woman may have heard, she does not need any

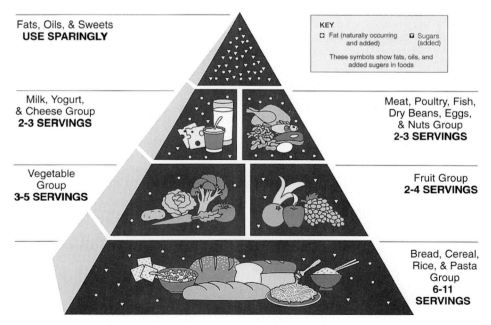

Fig. 4-1 Food guide pyramid. *(From U.S. Department of Agriculture.)*

special foods to meet this need. Recommend that she eat whatever nutritious food she would enjoy to obtain those extra 500 kcal. It can be a very simple food, such as a peanut butter sandwich and a glass of milk. For a thorough discussion of nutritional needs during pregnancy, see Worthington-Roberts and Williams[12] and the Institute of Medicine.[11]

Nutrient Requirements

Similarly, nutrient requirements for the lactating woman are nearly the same as for other women. The Institute of Medicine states, "Lactating women who meet the RDA (recommended daily allowance) for energy are likely to meet the RDA for all nutrients except calcium and zinc if the nutrient density of their diets is close to the average for young U.S. women. At energy levels less than 2700 kcal/day, the nutrients for which intake is most likely to be low, relative to need, include calcium, magnesium, zinc, vitamin B_6, and folate."[11] Therefore, encourage women who are at risk for low intake of these nutrients to eat the foods listed in Table 4-2.

Effects of Food on Infant

Mothers often talk among themselves about foods they believe to be bothersome to their infants. One example of such a food is garlic. However, whereas infants are apparently sensitive to the odor of garlic, they actually ingest more milk when the garlic odor is present.[13] One recent study suggested that cruciferous vegetables, including those listed in Box 4-3, and other "comon offenders" may be associated with fussy behavior.[14] This is not meant to be a list of "don'ts" but rather one that may be helpful as a mother keeps a log of foods she has ingested.

If a new mother asks about these or other foods that may affect her infant, acknowledge

---

T A B L E 4-1

SUGGESTED MEASURES FOR IMPROVING NUTRIENT INTAKE OF WOMEN WITH RESTRICTIVE EATING PATTERNS

Type of Restrictive Eating Pattern	Corrective Measures
Excessive restriction of food intake, i.e., ingestion of <1800 kcal of energy per day, which ordinarily leads to unsatisfactory intake of nutrients compared with the amounts needed by lactating women	Encourage increased intake of nutrient-rich foods to achieve an energy intake of at least 1800 kcal/day; if the mother insists on curbing food intake sharply, promote substitution of foods rich in vitamins, minerals, and protein for those lower in nutritive value; in individual cases, it may be advisable to recommend a balanced multivitamin-mineral supplement; discourage use of liquid weight loss diets and appetite suppressants
Complete vegetarianism i.e., avoidance of all animal foods, including meat, fish, dairy products, and eggs	Advise intake of a regular source of vitamin B_{12}, such as special vitamin B_{12} containing plant food products or a 2.6-μg vitamin B_{12} supplement daily
Avoidance of milk, cheese, or other calcium-rich dairy products	Encourage increased intake of other culturally appropriate dietary calcium sources, such as collard greens for blacks from the southeastern United States; provide information on the appropriate use of low-lactose dairy products if milk is being avoided because of lactose intolerance; if correction by diet cannot be achieved, it may be advisable to recommend 600 mg of elemental calcium per day taken with meals
Avoidance of vitamin D–fortified foods, such as fortified milk or cereal, combined with limited exposure to ultraviolet light	Recommend 10 μg of supplemental vitamin D per day

Reprinted with permission from *Nutrition During Lactation.* Copyright 1991 by the National Academy of Sciences. Courtesy the National Academy Press, Washington, DC.

that some foods may indeed bother some babies, but they may or may not have an effect on hers. Suggest that she avoid reportedly "bothersome" foods for the first week or so while she and the newborn are getting used to one another. This approach acknowledges that symptoms may appear but does not restrict the woman in her consumption of nutritious foods that she may enjoy. Advise her that the fussy behavior typically appears about 8 to 12 hours after she ingests the bothersome food and symptoms subside after 24 hours. Keeping a log is often helpful in identifying specific foods that cause problems.

Fluid Requirements

Contrary to popular myth, no arbitrary number of glasses of fluid is required to maintain lactation. Therefore, advise the mother to drink to satisfy thirst. For some, this might indeed be eight glasses of fluid, but for others it may be more or fewer. In the first few days postpartum, thirst may be intense; mothers who have had a long labor, multiple episodes of vomiting during labor, or a cesarean delivery may have some degree of dehydration, and hence a high degree of thirst.

As the postpartum course progresses, the lactating mother will indeed feel more thirsty than

---

Box 4-2
Recommendations for Intake During Lactation

Note: Nutritional status of lactating women in the United States has not been thoroughly or extensively studied; therefore, data are lacking on all aspects of this subject.

Normal weight loss: Advise women that the average rate of weight loss postpartum appears to be consistent with maintaining adequate milk volume. On average, lactating women who eat to appetite lose weight at the rate of 0.6 to 0.8 kg (1.3 to 1.6 lb) per month in the first 4 to 6 months of lactation, but there is wide variation in the weight loss experience of lactating women (some women gain weight during lactation). Those who continue breastfeeding beyond 4 to 6 months ordinarily continue to lose weight, but at a slower rate than during the first 4 to 6 months.

Reducing diets: If a lactating woman is overweight, a weight loss of up to 2 kg (~4.5 lb) per month is unlikely to adversely affect milk volume, but such women should be alert for any indications that the infant's appetite is not being satisfied. Rapid weight loss (>2 kg/month after the first month postpartum) is not advisable for breastfeeding women. Since the impact of curtailing maternal energy intake during the first 2 to 3 weeks postpartum is unknown, dieting during this period is not recommended.

Weight loss and milk volume: Advise women that the average rate of weight loss postpartum (0.5 to 1.0 kg, or 1 to 2 lb per month after the first month) appears to be consistent with maintaining adequate milk volume.

Nutritional assessments: Identify factors that predict whether women are at risk for adverse outcomes (such as

low socioeconomic status) or predict a beneficial effect (such as low weight for height). Obtaining measurements of skinfold thickness or conducting laboratory tests as part of the routine assessment of the nutritional status is not recommended because of difficulties with accuracy and expense for these assessments.

Energy intake and physical activity: Advise women about energy (calorie) intake based on a thorough understanding of their level of physical activity. Intakes below 1500 kcal/day are not recommended at any time during lactation, although brief fasts (lasting less than 1 day) are unlikely to decrease milk volume. Liquid diets and weight loss medications are not recommended.

Alcohol: If alcohol is used, advise the lactating woman to limit her intake to no more than 0.5 g of alcohol per kg of maternal body weight per day. Intake over this level may impair the milk-ejection reflex. For a 60-kg (132-lb) woman, 0.5 g of alcohol per kg of body weight corresponds to approximately 2 to 2.5 oz. of liquor, 8 oz. of table wine, or 2 cans of beer.

Cigarette smoking: Actively discourage cigarette smoking among lactating women, not only because it may reduce milk volume but also because of harmful effects on the mother and her infant.

Caffeine: Discourage intake of large quantities of coffee, other caffeine-containing beverages and medications, and decaffeinated coffee.

Condensed and modified from Institute of Medicine. *Nutrition During Lactation.* Washington, DC: National Academy Press; 1991:74, 104.

TABLE 4-2
FOODS CONTAINING NUTRIENTS NEEDED DURING LACTATION

Nutrient Needed	Foods Rich in This Nutrient
Calcium	Milk, cheese, yogurt, fish with edible bones, tofu processed with calcium sulfate, bok choy, broccoli, kale, collard, mustard, and turnip greens, breads made with milk
Zinc	Meat, poultry, seafood, eggs, seeds, legumes, yogurt, whole grains (bioavailability from this source is variable)
Magnesium	Nuts, seeds, legumes, whole grains, green vegetables, scallops, oysters (in general, this mineral is widely distributed in food rather than concentrated in a small number of foods)
Vitamin B_6	Bananas, poultry, meat, fish, potatoes, sweet potatoes, spinach, prunes, watermelon, some legumes, fortified cereals, and nuts
Thiamine	Pork, fish, whole grains, organ meats, legumes, corn, peas, seeds, nuts, fortified cereal grain (widely distributed in foods)
Folate	Leafy vegetables, fruit, liver, green beans, fortified cereals, legumes, and whole-grain cereals

Source: Institute of Medicine. *Nutrition During Lactation.* Washington, DC: National Academy Press; 1991:231.

Box 4-3
Foods that May Be Bothersome to Infants

- Broccoli
- Cabbage
- Cauliflower
- Chocolate
- Cow's milk
- Onion

These foods were identified as significantly affecting fussy behavior in infants less than 4 months old. The study did not specify what percentage of these infants were newborns, so whether or not the findings can be generalized to the newborn is uncertain. The authors caution that this study provides "initial evidence" that these foods are associated with fussy behavior.

This study also looked at other foods often assumed to be associated with fussy behavior, including green peppers, orange juice, brussel sprouts, and dried beans, but no significant associations were seen.

Source: Lust K, Brown J, Thomas W. Maternal intake of cruciferous vegetables and other foods in colic symptoms in exclusively breast-fed infants. *J Am Dietetic Assoc* 1996;96:47-48.

the nonlactating mother. This can be explained by the simple concept of intake and output; milk is output from her system just as perspiration or blood loss is output. The mother often puts her infant's needs ahead of her own, however, and may neglect to drink when she is thirsty. Therefore, suggest that she have a glass of liquid nearby when she breastfeeds, not because it is related to the act of breastfeeding but because this is a relaxing time for her to sip on a drink.

Women frequently hold the erroneous belief that increasing fluids will improve their milk supply. Health professionals who give this advice, which is not supported by research, do the woman a great disservice because the root of a supply problem, and hence the corrective strategy, may never be addressed. (See Chapter 8 for strategies to improve milk supply.) When women increase

their fluid intake by at least 25%, there is no change in milk volume, and no correlation between fluid intake and milk volume (see Figure 4-2).[15,16] When women increase their fluid intake by 50%, milk supply increases somewhat, but not significantly.[17]

Exercise and Weight Loss

Mothers frequently ask about how breastfeeding will affect their postpartum weight loss, and how exercise will affect their milk production and composition. To date, few studies have addressed these questions.

Typically, clinicians promise breastfeeding mothers that they will lose their pregnancy weight faster than their artificially feeding counterparts, based on the idea that breastfeeding burns about 500 kcal per day. However, there are conflicting study results about this question. An extensive review of the literature showed no evi-

A

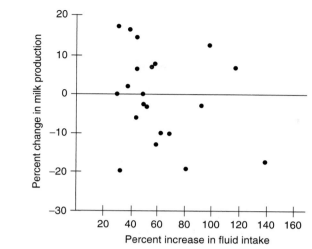

B

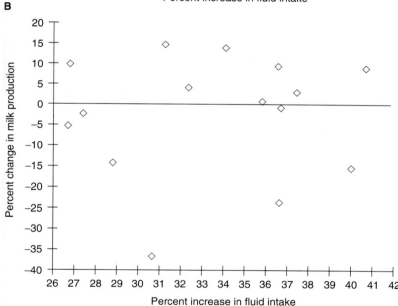

Fig. 4-2 These scattergrams show there is no significant relationship between percentage of fluid intake and percentage change in milk production over baseline. The studies were nearly identical, except that **A** shows percentages when mothers increased their fluid intake for 3 days, whereas **B** shows percentages when mothers increased their intake over a 7-day period. (**A,** *from Dusdieker et al. 1985. Effect of supplemental fluid on human milk production.* J Peds *1985;106:209.* **B,** *from Dusdieker et al. Prolonged maternal fluid supplementation in breast feeding.* Pediatrics *1990;86:739.)*

dence to support this notion,[18] and subsequent studies showed no correlation between maternal weight loss and infant feeding method.[19,20] However, a more recent study suggests that women who breastfeed have a greater weight loss than those who feed artificially.[21] Until further research is conducted, it may be unwise to promise mothers that they will lose weight faster if they breastfeed than if they feed artificially.

Postpartum exercise also does not seem to affect the rate of weight loss that breastfeeding mothers experience. Weight loss was not significantly different for breastfeeding mothers who exercised than for control subjects who did not.[22]

Recreational exercise, when compared with aerobic exercise, has not been associated with improved weight loss of exclusively breastfeeding women who are 6 to 8 weeks postpartum.[23]

Exclusively breastfeeding women with infants 9 to 24 weeks old had no difference in plasma hormones, milk energy, fat, protein, or lactose content when sedentary mothers were compared with those who performed aerobic exercise. Exercising subjects tended to have higher milk volume (839 vs. 776 g/day) and energy output in milk (538 vs. 494 kcal/day).[24] In another study there was no significant difference in milk volume, composition, or infant weight gain[22] for women 6 to 8 weeks postpartum. No adverse effects on milk production or composition occur when mothers exercise moderately four or five times a week.[25] Moderation seems to be the key, as strenuous exercise does have an adverse effect. Infants may be somewhat reluctant to take breast milk after the mother has exercised, presumably because of the high lactic acid concentration (and resulting sour taste) in the milk after strenuous exercise.[26,27]

Substance Use

Women who are pregnant or lactating need to understand the effects of substances on themselves and their fetuses or newborns. Women should also understand how cigarettes, alcohol, and illicit drugs affect lactation and the breastfeeding infant.

CIGARETTES

Mothers who smoke have a significantly decreased volume of milk.[28] It appears that smoking has an inhibitory effect on prolactin and oxytocin levels. Smoking simulates the release of epinephrine, which inhibits oxytocin release. Women who smoke have a 30% to 50% lower basal prolactin level on days 1 and 21, but when the infant suckles, the rise in prolactin level is not significantly different between smokers and nonsmokers. The smoking subjects, however, wean their infants sooner than nonsmokers.[29,30] Smoking has also been positively correlated with the incidence of colic.[31]

Women who smoke should be counseled to stop; smoking can decrease a mother's milk supply. If the woman is unable to stop, she should be counseled to at least decrease the number of cigarettes she smokes because the adverse effects vary directly with the number of cigarettes smoked. Quite apart from the issue of breastfeeding, mothers should be told that cigarette smoke is harmful to all in the household, especially to young children or infants.

ALCOHOL

Misunderstandings about the use of alcohol during lactation abound. Many women believe that drinking alcohol will aid in the milk ejection reflex. There is no research to support this idea, however. At the other end of the spectrum, some women believe that consuming any alcohol is prohibited during lactation, and health care providers have often reinforced this idea. However, it is important to remember that women in cultures outside of the United States have consumed small amounts of alcohol for centuries. Furthermore, the Institute of Medicine has clearly stated that lactating women may safely consume up to 8 oz of wine or 2 cans of beer per day. However, infants aged 25 days to 216 days apparently are sensitive to the odor in the milk after mothers have consumed ethanol, and they consume less milk despite more frequent suckling.[32] Breastfeeding is contraindicated when women are alcohol abusers.

ILLICIT DRUGS

Confirmation of the woman's current drug use is central to the question of whether the mother may or may not breastfeed. In cases where it is confirmed that the woman is using illicit drugs, she should be counseled to not breastfeed, in accordance with the American Academy of Pediatrics recommendations.[33] However, if the woman is only suspected of using illicit drugs, or if she has used them in the past, she may breastfeed.

Helping the Mother Develop Realistic Expectations

Concerns of breastfeeding mothers have been categorized as concerns about self (maternal concerns) or infant concerns, and subcategories of each have been identified.[34]

Concerns About Self

Throughout the literature, the worry of *not having enough milk* is the most frequently expressed concern.[7,35-42] This concern is so strong that women have reported it as the primary reason for terminating breastfeeding.[34,35,42,43] Effective counseling is critical. Before and after delivery, reassure mothers that they can easily achieve an adequate milk supply for a healthy newborn by establishing good latch-on (as described in Chapter 5) and that there are effective strategies to overcome an insufficient milk supply should it temporarily occur (see Chapter 8).

The second most frequently reported area of concern about self is *sore breasts* and/or *sore nipples*.[35,42,44] Unfortunately, the notion that pain is an expected consequence of breastfeeding is often a deterrent to choosing or continuing to breastfeed. Help women to understand that breastfeeding should not be painful; if it is, the pain can be alleviated with good latch-on, as described in Chapter 5.

Other commonly expressed concerns include fatigue and feelings of being tense and overwhelmed. If antepartum mothers express fears that they are "too nervous" to breastfeed, explain that the hormones associated with breastfeeding actually promote relaxation, as described in Chapter 3. When the postpartum woman says she is exhausted and overwhelmed, help her to understand that the transition to parenthood and/or the many responsibilities of providing care for a new infant, as discussed in Chapter 2, may cause one to feel tired and overwhelmed, and that artificial feedings will not necessarily alleviate the problem.

Concerns About Infants

Mothers raise many questions about care for the newborn. Most frequently, these include physical, feeding, and behavior concerns.

Physical Concerns

Physical concerns, including concerns about general wellness, growth, and development, have been reported. Some of the physical concerns—jaundice, stooling, and similar concerns—are related to breastfeeding. Mothers may be unaware of growth spurts, as described in Chapter 5, or may be unable to anticipate or recognize when they happen. These concerns are best addressed by anticipatory guidance and continuing support.

Feeding Concerns

"Feeding" is the most frequently cited infant concern, and mothers report it most often during the first and second week.[34] Concerns about feeding usually relate to the frequency of feeding, the need for supplementation, and techniques for feeding.

Frequency of feeding is a common concern for mothers.[42] Mothers may feel uneasy about feeding frequency because they do not understand how to read their newborn's signs of hunger and satiety, as described in Chapter 5, or because they expect a newborn to have longer intervals between feedings, as is characteristic of an older infant.

Mothers frequently ask whether they should supplement breastfeeding with artificial milk or water.[35] There is virtually no reason to give supplemental feedings to healthy newborns because this only upsets the natural symbiosis of supply and demand. There are few medical indications for supplementing (see Chapter 12).

Mothers frequently ask questions about the *technique for feeding*, usually about positioning and latch-on. Both positioning and latch-on require visual assessment and one-to-one teaching. While pamphlets or classes might be useful for other topics or questions, nothing can substitute for personal assistance with these questions. Focus teaching efforts on what the mother will *do*, not what she will *know*. This difference between doing and knowing is critical! Do not assume that a mother who *knows* can immediately *do* the technique unaided. See Chapter 5 for a discussion of feeding technique.

Behavioral Concerns

When the mother expresses worries about an insufficient milk supply, frequently she is asking a question about infant *satiety*. Mothers may have highly unrealistic expectations about how long newborns can wait before eating, and they may have difficulty determining whether the infant obtained milk or just sucked at the breast. Teach mothers to recognize signs of hunger, as well as signs of satiety (see Chapter 5).

Mothers are frequently concerned about infant *sleep* and *wakefulness*.[42,44] Concerns about sleep are frequently intertwined with questions and concerns about satiety. It is not realistic to think that newborns can sleep through the night. After about one month, if an infant has his last feeding around 11:00 PM and wakes for the next around 5:00 AM, the mother should consider this the longest sleeping interval she can hope for at that time.

From the beginning, parents need to be aware that infants are not simply awake or asleep. Rather, there are several different states of sleep and awake. Infant states of consciousness are more fully discussed in Chapter 6.

Rooming-In

Breastfeeding is most likely to be successful when obstacles that interfere with its success are removed or minimized. Separation of the mother and infant is one such obstacle, yet it is common practice in the United States to separate mothers from their infants.

The idea of "rooming-in," while it has gained much attention in this decade, is not a new concept. The first "rooming-in" project in the United States was begun in the 1940s,[45] as shown in the Historical Highlight. Today in the United States, rooming-in has become more popular with the advent of the Baby-Friendly™ Hospital Initiative program, but most hospitals have only daytime rooming-in and are struggling to implement 24-hour rooming-in as stated in the Baby-Friendly™ criteria. This limited contact is an obstacle to successful breastfeeding.

Rooming-in eliminates maternal and infant separation, which in general is unphysiological.[46] More specifically, infants who room in with their mothers breastfeed more frequently and show larger weight gains during the immediate postpartum period.[47] Anderson asserts that rooming-in provides a way for mothers and their newborns to be mutual caregivers.[46]

In this country, however, rooming-in is frequently perceived as more of a penalty than a privilege. It is not uncommon for a mother to request that the newborn go to the central nursery for the night so that she can "get her rest," and health care personnel not only support but often encourage this request. Worse still, well-intentioned health care providers frequently plant the seed for this request. The idea that a woman will get less sleep because of rooming-in, however, has not been documented in research studies. Mothers who roomed in at night reported that they slept 5.5 hours, while mothers with infants in the central nursery reported that they slept 5.35 hours, even after having taken sleeping pills.[48] Furthermore, newborns cried less when they were rooming-in with their mothers.[49]

Success?

It is often difficult to evaluate whether efforts to educate and support breastfeeding have been entirely successful. First, the definition of success can be rather subjectively defined. "Success" in breastfeeding is often discussed as though everyone agrees on the operational definition, which they do not. For example, success is sometimes

Historical Highlight

A Hospital Rooming-in Unit for Newborn Infants and Their Mothers

A brief survey conducted in 1937 at the New Haven Hospital showed that mothers did not feel adequately prepared to care for their infants after their discharge from the hospital. In response to this survey and the demands of mothers, a rooming-in arrangement, whereby the mother had her newborn in a crib by her bedside whenever she wished, was begun in New Haven, Connecticut, in 1946. Mothers who met the criteria (having a full-term, healthy newborn and similar criteria) were offered the opportunity to have rooming-in.

When breastfeeding women were offered this choice, their reactions in 1946 were similar to the responses of women today, but in different proportions than we might expect to see now. In those days, the majority of women considered rooming-in a privilege, and a typical response, quoted from the article, was, "Of course, after waiting so long, I would want to keep my baby with me!" A small minority declined the rooming-in arrangement, saying they believed they would get less rest in the rooming-in unit. Multiparas who participated in rooming-in, however, unanimously agreed that they felt they did not get less rest than during their previous hospitalizations, and said that their previous experience was more unsettling because they continually worried about what was happening to their babies in the nurseries.

After the rooming-in project was implemented, mothers who roomed in were almost unanimous in spontaneously expressing confidence in taking care of their newborns after discharge, while the mothers who were separated from their infants did not express this confidence.

It is noteworthy that the typical hospital stay was 8 days in 1946, and also that mothers were more likely to be in closer proximity to their own families. If these mothers lacked confidence, it is difficult to imagine how contemporary women, who are hospitalized for a much shorter time and often live hundreds of miles away from family members, can gain the skills and confidence they need to care for their newborns when they are separated from them.

---

defined as a subjective "report of success,"[50] or more objectively as breastfeeding at 4 to 6 weeks.[51] Perhaps a more pragmatic definition is "breastfeeding with less than 4 ounces of formula (supplementation) at 4 to 6 weeks postpartum."[52] This definition is useful in light of the fact that lactation is fairly well established by this time, and the use of artificial milk is the exception rather than the norm.

Further, it is entirely possible that a woman may receive inadequate education and support, yet breastfeed for three years. Conversely, it is possible that the woman who has received excellent instruction and support does not initiate breastfeeding, or discontinues breastfeeding early. Cessation of breastfeeding can occur at the end of a successful or unsuccessful experience. This text considers *weaning* to occur after a successful experience, and when the infant or mother has physically or psychologically "outgrown" breastfeeding, as opposed to breastfeeding attrition, which occurs when the woman is unable to overcome the obstacles that breastfeeding presents for her.

About one third of mothers who initiate breastfeeding in the hospital quit before 1 month. The reasons are many and varied, but many factors that occur during that time period can make the woman vulnerable to defeat. Sore nipples, lack of support, infant hospitalization, and the lack of a full milk supply are possible contributors to attrition at this time. Beyond these physiological factors, however, breastfeeding attrition has been linked to weak commitment[4,53-56] while continuation of breastfeeding has been associated with high motivation.[57,58] Although there are no studies beyond these that show lack of confidence as a primary factor in breastfeeding attrition, those who have worked with breastfeeding mothers over many years hear them state lack of confidence prior to giving up breastfeeding, and Jelliffe and Jelliffe call breastfeeding "a confidence game."[59]

Several factors have been shown to shorten the breastfeeding experience. Factors resulting in breastfeeding attrition were discussed in previous chapters, but, briefly include: (1) artificial milk products, either given in the hospital or supplied as discharge packs; (2) delayed initiation of breastfeeding; (3) supplementation with artificial milk or water; (4) perception of an insufficient milk supply; (5) lack of social support; and (6) factors related to birth (age of gestation and other factors). Most of these factors can be reduced when the mother has accurate information and the nurse uses a positive approach to learning.

POSITIVE LEARNING APPROACHES

Interactional Approaches

Teaching breastfeeding techniques is usually accomplished by a one-to-one situation or through group classes. Both methods are used, and both are effective.

Approaching Individuals: The Interview

One way to help the mother or parents overcome negative attitudes or let go of erroneous beliefs about breastfeeding is through the interview, which is a purposeful, therapeutic discussion between the nurse and the mother. A skilled interview may still be the best means to gather critical data from new mothers or mothers-to-be, despite superior physical assessment skills or modern technology. Establishing rapport, assuring privacy and confidentiality, explaining the process of the interview, giving the client the lead, and focusing the discussion are all essential to conducting a successful interview; other sources have covered these topics in more detail.[60] Two critical components of the interview—posing thoughtful questions and responding with active listening—will help the interviewer not only to understand women's choices but also to provide guidance in making those choices.

Closed-Ended Questions

Closed-ended questions are those that require a yes, no, or short-answer response. Closed-ended questions are useful for pertinent negatives (e.g., "Are you on any kind of medication?") or for obtaining specific information (e.g., "How many children do you have?"). For the lactating woman or one who is hoping to lactate, closed-ended questions such as these can be communication facilitators if they are not used too soon in the interview. For the most part, however, closed-ended questions are ineffective when one is interviewing the mother about breastfeeding. For example, do not ask, "Do you plan to breastfeed or bottle feed?" for that question implies that the choices are equal. Furthermore, the mother is likely to give a one-word answer to this closed-ended question, oftentimes, replying "Bottle." If she does, the interviewer is at a dead end; the interviewer is unable to explore the woman's reasons for the choice.

Open-Ended Questions

Use open-ended questions when interviewing mothers and teaching about breastfeeding. Open-ended questions provide the woman with a chance to give a broad response and give you the opportunity to listen. Ideally, incorporate the question into the context of the physical assessment or general antepartal teaching and ask, *"What do you know about breastfeeding?"* or *"What have you heard about breastfeeding?"* This approach invites the woman to explore her questions—and any myths she may have heard—and helps her come to a decision based on fact rather than myths.

T A B L E 4-3

COMMON MISTAKES IN ACTIVE LISTENING FEEDBACK

Example: "I'm sick and tired of getting up to breastfeed this baby twice each night."

Exaggerating	Overdoing your feedback of the feelings expressed	*Sounds like you're furious!*
Adding	Adding something or expanding the scope of what was said	*Nothing seems to be going well.*
Anticipating	Leading the speaker by saying what she may express next	*You're about ready to give up breastfeeding.*
Psychoanalyzing	Guessing about unexpressed underlying motives related to problems	*You're worried that your boyfriend will feel neglected in bed.*
Minimizing	Lessening the intensity of the expressed feeling	*You seem a little displeased with night feedings.*
Subtracting	Leaving out or missing the "kernel" of what was said	*You seem pretty unhappy.*
Backtracking	Feeding back something that was said earlier or not keeping up	*You said you hadn't had a good night's rest since the baby was born.*
Echoing	Repeating almost word for word what the speaker said	*You've had it with night feeds.*
Content	Reflecting content when speaker is really talking about feelings	*Your baby consistently wakes you up twice each night to breastfeed.*
Advising	Giving advice when speaker is venting feelings	*He's probably not eating frequently enough during the day. Let's talk about . . .*
Reassuring	Without acknowledging the feeling, telling speaker that this is okay	*Babies do that a lot at first; he'll settle down in a few weeks.*
Refocusing	Getting the focus off the speaker and onto someone or something else	*Oh yes, my baby did the same thing. He drove me crazy the first few weeks and I . . .*
Persuading	Assuming the speaker will take an action that you'd rather she didn't	*Yes, but you know, formula-fed babies can do that too.*

Better Responses:

When that happens night after night, you begin to wonder if there's a light at the end of the tunnel.

Waking up night after night can feel like a drag, huh?

My baby did that for the first few weeks. It gets pretty exhausting, doesn't it?

Active Listening

Listen *actively*. One way to do so is to make verbal or nonverbal responses that encourage the woman to keep talking. This might be nodding, maintaining silence, refocusing the interview, or probing. Although probing is usually used too soon, it can be effective in eliciting further information when it is done gently and at the right time. For example, "Tell me more about that" is a probing statement, but it is frequently successful in eliciting further information.

Reflective listening is a specific type of active listening that verifies content and acknowledges feelings. First, determine whether the woman is giving a message primarily about content (a play-by-play account of action) or feelings (deep-rooted feelings about how an action or event influenced her). Reflective listening requires a highly sophisticated interpretation of what has been said, followed by a response that accurately and succinctly captures the content, the feeling, or both. Reflective listening is not parroting. Common mistakes in active listening are listed in Table 4-3.

Teaching Groups: Prenatal and Postnatal Classes

Group classes have many advantages. First, they provide a time-efficient way to address common questions where the answers vary little or not at all from individual to individual. They also serve as a way to help mothers to interact with one another and establish a network of support from others who are also breastfeeding.

Group classes can be used any time throughout the perinatal period. Classes should be held at times that are convenient for parents and in a comfortable environment. The group setting has some distinct advantages. First, it encourages sharing of ideas and questions. The affective aspects of learning—discussing feelings and fears about breastfeeding—are often best accomplished in this environment, where other mothers may have the same thoughts and feelings, and frequently offer encouragement and support for difficulties or dilemmas that they have successfully resolved.

The group class also offers an advantage to the instructor. It is possible to cover material for several persons rather than for just one individual at a time. This works well for topics that have fairly straightforward answers that deviate little from individual to individual. For example, it would work well to describe ways to increase milk supply. However, specific questions about why a mother with a particular set of circumstances does not have enough milk require a one-to-one interaction.

Whether in a group or an individual setting, there are some specific challenges to teaching the *adolescent* mother as described in the Clinical Scenario. Young women at this stage in their lives are very conscious about their body image; they have scarcely outgrown their own childhood when they find themselves raising a child. Individual discussions often work well with teens because they need an individualized plan to help them succeed. On the other hand, they may do well with a group of their peers because they will relish the opportunity to talk about their decisions and circumstances. Teens are frequently reluctant to attend more generic group classes (i.e., women of all age groups, rather than teens only). Some priorities to keep in mind when counseling the adolescent mother are found in Box 4-4.

Resources

Consumer Education Materials

Media are useful for reinforcing the main points made in an interview or in a group class. The main criteria to consider when choosing media include the following:

1. Who is the audience? Will this material go primarily to antepartum women, adolescents, or parents who are not fluent in the English language? Can the audience understand the words?

2. What is the main need? Does the mother need motivation, how-to instruction for well infants, information about supplementation and separation, or information about special topics or complicated situations?

3. What is the cost for the media?

4. Is the material biased? Does it give subtle messages that only white, married, middle-class mothers can breastfeed? Does it give subtle messages that women will eventually need to use artificial milk?

5. Is the information accurate and up-to-date?

6. Are there strong positive messages about breastfeeding?

7. Are the graphics accurate?

Books, pamphlets, and videotapes are all helpful teaching aids. Appendix B lists multiple sources, and Appendix E lists how to contact the publisher or distributor. Appendix B also presents ways to summarize the content of the media and points for consideration when purchasing the materials.

Avoid promoting patient education material by corporations that want to advertise and promote a product. Some of these may have carefully targeted and often subtle messages about artificial feeding, and the information on breastfeeding is often inadequate or incomplete.

C L I N I C A L   S C E N A R I O

Adolescent Mother

Jody is 17 years old. She is unmarried, and gave birth to a healthy baby boy after a cesarean delivery about 36 hours ago. Her physician calls you on the postpartum unit to tell you that Jody "really wants to breastfeed but thinks she can't because her breasts are asymmetrical." You're an advocate of breastfeeding, but you're having some mixed feelings; this young woman has clearly told the nursing staff she wants to bottle feed, and the infant has been artificially fed since his birth. How can you respond to the physician, who insists that he has taken care of her since she became pregnant and "knows" she wants to breastfeed? How can you come to terms with yourself, trying to respect the patient's choice (rather than promote your own agenda)? And what, if anything, do you say to Jody?

Possible Strategies

Have faith in the physician's assessment that the mother "really wants" to breastfeed. Tell him that you will talk with Jody and explore her feelings about the method of feeding she has chosen, and her feelings about herself and her own body.

Ponder before you act. It is always difficult to know where to draw the fine line between supporting a patient's choice and providing more information for a truly informed choice. In Jody's case, it is likely that a 17-year-old who is grappling with her own identity and role is having difficulty integrating those concepts with her sexuality, mothering in general, and her chosen method of feeding in particular.

Establish rapport and talk with Jody about how *artificial* feeding is going. It is likely that she will have some questions or concerns. Use open-ended questions at first, then move to more closed-ended questions about any negative aspects of the feeding that she has noted. For example, "Jody, I have noticed that Danny has spit up quite a bit since the beginning of my shift.

Does he do this a lot?" This gives you a chance to segue into a discussion of the many inconveniences of artificial feeding for the *mother*. Focus on things that are important to her. Then ask in a nonjudgmental way about why she did not choose breastfeeding. She will probably tell you about the asymmetrical breasts. You will have the opportunity to help her explore her feelings, and she may agree to "try" breastfeeding.

Outcome

Jody put Danny to her breast after our conversation. Luckily, he latched on easily and suckled well. Five months after our interaction, I received a card from Jody. She said she had done everything wrong—that she had had a baby without being married and had had a cesarean delivery, which she saw as a failure. She went on to say that breastfeeding was the only thing she had done right. Danny was still breastfeeding almost exclusively, and she was soon going to return to high school.

Years elapsed, and I continued to work in perinatal nursing, although in different hospitals and different subspecialties. On one particularly busy shift, I volunteered to act as a preceptor for a new nurse because the regular preceptor was ill. The charge nurse quickly introduced me to the new nurse and assigned us to preterm twins. I was very focused on getting my assignment under way. Just as I was right in the middle of explaining how to place the EKG leads, I suddenly stopped short. My mind raced back nearly a decade and I said to the nurse, "Do you have a baby who isn't a baby any more?" The young woman grinned and said, "I wondered how long it would take you to recognize me, because I recognized you right away." The teenaged primipara with the asymmetrical breasts had married, had a second child, and eventually obtained a degree in nursing.

Box 4-4

Priorities for Care: Helping an Adolescent Mother Choose Breastfeeding

- Recognize that an adolescent mother makes decisions based on Erikson's stage of identity versus role confusion. Use strategies that help her achieve identity and minimize role confusion, for example:
  - Emphasize that she is the only one who can "mother" if she is breastfeeding.
  - Create a new paradigm: If she thinks breastfeeding will "tie her down," focus instead on how she is the "only one who can do it" and "her mother can't take over."
- Do more listening than talking and more teaching than preaching.
- Give practical suggestions to minimize embarrassment or exposure.
- Emphasize that breastfeeding is pleasurable.
- Set short-term and realistic goals; partial breastfeeding is better than no breastfeeding, and breastfeeding until she returns to school is better than not breastfeeding at all. Remind her that breastfeeding is not an all-or-nothing choice.
- Help her tune into Station WIIFM: "What's in it for me?"
- Present breastfeeding as "cool."
- Identify any issue the adolescent mother is committed to (e.g., saving the environment, empowering women) and show how breastfeeding promotes her stance on the issue.
- Enlist peer support/approval. Refer her to support groups for adolescent mothers who breastfeed.
- Focus on body image in a positive way; for example, tell her she is more likely to be able to zip up her jeans sooner if she breastfeeds.
- Encourage foods that are high in nutrition yet are also "social" foods.

Community Support

Ideally, women should start building a community support network early in pregnancy and continue this throughout the period of lactation. Help women to identify family and friends who have enjoyed breastfeeding, health care providers who are knowledgeable about breastfeeding, and mother-to-mother support groups.

A TEACHING PLAN THAT SUPPORTS EARLY HOSPITAL DISCHARGE

Discharge teaching has presented many challenges since 48-hour stays have become routine for uncomplicated obstetrical patients and their term infants. Sleepy infants, lack of maternal psychological readiness, and the lack of a full milk supply may frustrate efforts to teach breastfeeding during this limited time frame. The key is to develop a three-tiered teaching approach which includes affective, psychomotor, and cognitive learning during the antepartum, immediate postpartum, and long-term postpartum course.[63] A summary of priorities for teaching can be found in Box 4-5.

Antepartum: Anticipating Breastfeeding

Breastfeeding is not a topic separate from antepartum care. Antepartum care should encompass the woman's ability to support a healthy newborn; breastfeeding should be integrated into other prenatal assessments and the teaching plan. Assessment and teaching should include the psychological, physical, and sociocultural factors associated with the breasts and breastfeeding.

Assessment

The Decision to Breastfeed

While health care providers often recite a litany of advantages of breastfeeding and human milk, many other factors are likely to influence the mother's decision in choosing a method of feeding. Societal and cultural norms drive the

Box 4-5
Priorities for Teaching

Early Antepartum
- Explore feelings and ideas about infant feeding methods
- Identify questions and concerns
- Dispel commonly held myths, especially lifestyle restrictions
- Deliver carefully targeted positive messages; counter negative messages
- Explain benefits of breastfeeding for both mother and child
- Discuss negative impact of poor health habits, such as smoking, on the overall health of the pregnant or lactating mother and her fetus or infant
- Identify multiple sources of support
- Instill confidence in the mother
- Support any interest in breastfeeding

Later Antepartum
- Help mother develop realistic expectations about infant's needs and behavior
- Note maternal physical or psychological needs or poor health that require intervention; refer the woman for medical help as appropriate
- Explain that nipple preparation, creams, ointments, and so on are unnecessary and potentially harmful
- Anticipate postpartum clothing needs, including nursing bras and clothes for discrete nursing
- Emphasize advantages of rooming-in for families as well as infants

- Help mother to make a commitment to breastfeed based on informed choice (and then health care has to support it)

Immediate Postpartum
- Acknowledge feelings and respond to concerns
- Applaud mother's choice to initiate breastfeeding within first hour of life
- Demonstrate proper positioning and latch-on
- Verify audible swallowing; point this out to the mother
- Discourage supplements or restricted frequency or duration of feeding
- Discourage pacifiers
- Help mother to recognize her infant's behavioral cues
- Advocate for mother's right to have rooming-in
- Identify red flags that require follow-up
- Identify sources for professional and peer support after discharge

Continuing Postpartum
- Express confidence in the mother's ability to continue until she and infant decide to wean
- Reinforce need for periodic professional and peer support
- Establish collaborative systems that facilitate consistent information
- Follow up with red-flag situations

choices, fears, questions, and priorities of individuals. Family, friends, and neighbors have a significant impact on the woman's decision[61]; the nurse may have a relatively low influence. This text presumes that the nurse's role is to reduce the influence of the fears, anxieties, and myths that the woman has been exposed to and to help her reach an informed decision by providing answers to spoken and unspoken questions. In essence, the nurse's role is to help the woman to achieve her own goal through informed choice.

WHO INFLUENCES THE CHOICE?
We might like to believe that we exert a significant influence on mothers to make healthy choices for themselves and their infants. It appears, however, that women's choices are often more driven by their own attitudes, beliefs, and values than by advice from health care providers.

In a study at the University of Rochester[62] husbands were most influential as women made the decision to either breastfeed or bottle feed. The breastfeeding woman was more influenced by the obstetrician than was the bottle-feeding mother; similarly, obstetricians were more influential in the feeding choice than were pediatricians, presumably because women generally make their decision prior to giving birth.

Fathers can be very influential in the decision-making process. Middle-class mothers are more likely to choose breastfeeding when fathers approve (or if they are thought to approve) of breastfeeding than when they are indifferent about it[64] or negative.[65,66] Low-income women are also influenced by their partner's support.[67] Women do not accurately predict fathers' attitudes, however[64]; their predictions are little more accurate than guessing. Fathers are generally more favorable than mothers predict.

Unfortunately, fathers frequently have little knowledge of breastfeeding or how they can support their partner with breastfeeding; they harbor many misconceptions[68] but have more positive perceptions if they attend prenatal classes. There are several significant differences between fathers of breastfed and artificially fed infants. Fathers of breastfeeding infants have more positive perceptions of breastfeeding than fathers of artificially fed infants. Fathers of breastfed infants focus on benefits for the infants—better feeding, better bonding, protection from disease—and express a desire for the mother to breastfeed. Fathers of artificially fed infants focus on perceived negatives for themselves or the mother—less attractive, bad for breasts, makes breasts ugly, and interferes with sex. The perception that breastfeeding interferes with sex was very high among fathers whose infants were artificially fed.[69]

The clinical implication here is clear: it is important to involve both the mother and her partner in discussions about breastfeeding as soon as possible because the partner's attitude clearly influences the mother's decision.

Factors Influencing the Decision

Factors that influence the decision to breastfeed are many and varied. Lawrence[62] conducted a study soliciting women's reasons for choosing

---

TABLE 4-4

FACTORS THAT INFLUENCED DECISION TO BREASTFEED OR BOTTLE FEED

Factors	Bottle Feeding	Breastfeeding
Childbirth classes	44%	80%
"That's how my mother fed her babies"	40%	16%
"That's how my friends fed their babies"	30%	16%
"That's how I fed my other baby"	96% of all bottle feeding multiparas*	94% of all breastfeeding multiparas†
Other reasons	34%	68%

*60% of bottle feeding mothers were multiparas
†53% of breastfeeding mothers were multiparas
From Lawrence RA. *Breastfeeding: A Guide for the Medical Profession.* 2nd ed. St. Louis, Mosby; 1985.

---

their feeding method. Respondents were given four choices as reasons for why they decided to breast or bottle feed: (1) childbirth classes; (2) "that's how my mother fed her babies"; (3) "that's how my friends fed their babies"; (4) "that's how I fed my other baby"; (see Table 4-4). The questionnaire also provided space for the mother to write in "other" reasons. Lawrence observed that "other" reasons identified were perhaps the most interesting and significant part of the study. All of the mothers who chose bottle feeding were more focused on their own needs, and all of the mothers who chose breastfeeding focused on their infant's needs (see Table 4-5). Although these data are somewhat old, they have relevance for today's mother, and they mirror the previously mentioned studies about the father's focus. This has clinical implications for caregivers. First, the key is to help mothers inclined toward artificial feeding to realize that breastfeeding is best for *them.* It would be unethical to project a personal bias about feeding method on the woman, but unfair to assume that she has adequate resources to come to an informed decision unaided. Simi-

TABLE 4-5
REASONS VOLUNTEERED FOR THE CHOICE MADE

Bottle Feeding		Breastfeeding	
Breastfeeding did not appeal to me	3	Best for baby	8
Breastfeeding too annoying	1	More natural	8
Breastfeeding makes breasts sag	1	More nutritional	2
Breastfeeding ties me down	2	More beneficial	2
More convenient for me	3	Special immunities	2
No medical proof for breast milk	2	More satisfying	2
Infant won't sleep through night if breastfed	2	Prevent allergies	3
Best for me	3	Health reasons for infant	4
Want to take birth control pills	1	Wanted to	2
Want to go to work	1	Satisfying	3
Too nervous to breastfeed	2	More convenient	2
Total	21		38

From Lawrence RA. *Breastfeeding: A Guide for the Medical Profession.* 2nd ed. St. Louis, Mosby; 1985.

larly, avoid a list of "don'ts." Breastfeeding does not seem attractive to the woman who is told she can no longer eat this or do that. Present breastfeeding as a *positive* experience! Second, help the expectant couple discuss the infant feeding method, and try to dispel negative connotations about breastfeeding in relation to sexuality.

Physical Assessment

The aim of prenatal physical assessment is to establish that the pregnancy is progressing optimally and to identify any factors that might compromise the fetus or newborn. Because the breasts are designed to nourish the neonate, any prenatal assessment that excludes physical assessment of the breasts is negligent. The antenatal assessment of the breasts has an added benefit; it gives the mother confidence that she can breastfeed if the examiner says she can.[70] More specifically, the prenatal breast examination should focus on the adequacy of the breasts for breastfeeding. Physical assessment—inspection and palpation of the breasts—should be performed at least twice: once at the first prenatal visit and again during the third trimester. See Chapter 8 for a full discussion of performing physical assessments of the breasts and nipples; Box 4-6 is a summary of points that should be documented during the antepartum visit.

Breastfeeding is not a topic that is separate from other prenatal teaching. Present breastfeeding as the completion of the reproductive cycle. For example, while listening to the fetal heart tones, point out the sound of the placenta and explain its function in nourishing the fetus. This becomes an excellent segue for examining the breasts as the next part of the physical assessment. It is easy for the nurse to comment, "Oh, your breasts are enlarging. This is a good sign! Your breasts are getting ready to take over the job of nourishing the baby after he is born." In this way breastfeeding is presented as a normal, physiological process, which helps the woman to gain confidence that her body is already becoming capable of this task.

Planning and Implementation

During the antepartum period, the goal is to have the woman choose a feeding method. Women may ask "how-to" questions about breastfeeding or other mothering responsibilities, but the unvoiced question is really, "Am I capable of doing this?"

Responses and teaching during the antepartum period need to focus on affective learning to aid in decision making. In this way, the woman is likely to develop a stronger commitment. This affective dimension cannot be minimized, as early weaning is related to decreased professional and social support, the belief that breastfeeding is difficult, and the perception that there are more

Box 4-6
Antepartum Breastfeeding Assessment Form

Name _____ Age _____   Date of first visit _____

Term _____ Preterm _____ Abortion _____ Live _____   Re-examined _____

The Gravida

❏ Verbalizes feelings about breastfeeding, including prior breastfeeding experience, myths she has heard about breastfeeding, etc.

❏ Acknowledges benefits of breastfeeding for _____ self _____ infant

❏ Has not made decision about feeding method (date _____)

❏ Made decision to initiate _____ breastfeeding _____ artificial feeding

❏ Identified resources/support persons for feeding method chosen

Subjective and Objective Data

❏ Nipples well everted

❏ Flat or inverted nipples (circle one)

❏ Adequate nutritional intake

❏ Breast tenderness and enlargement

❏ Breasts symmetrical

❏ Cultural/dietary values _____

Recommendations

❏ Referred to breastfeeding class

❏ Received written materials

❏ Recommended breast shells

❏ Other

benefits to artificial feeding.[71] Without adequate teaching or positive reinforcement, women are likely to believe such myths.

During the early antepartum period, focus on positive and negative sides of choices. Dispel myths that the woman may have heard about breastfeeding. An easy way to do this is to say, "What have you heard about breastfeeding?" By using this approach, the interviewer can immediately go to the heart of the matter; the mother is unlikely to choose breastfeeding if she believes that it will make her nipples sore or her breasts sag. Giving the woman a litany of benefits for the infant—better digestion, fewer ear aches, and so on—is of limited value because mothers are more likely to choose artificial feeding because they perceive greater benefits for themselves.[62]

During the last decade or so, rooming-in has attracted much attention as a way to improve breastfeeding. This practice, however, dates back to the late 1940s.[45] Rooming-in positively correlates with demand feedings for breastfed infants[72] and has a greater impact on full breastfeeding in primiparas[72,73] and continuation of breastfeeding.[73]

During the antepartum period, show mothers how rooming-in is beneficial for mother and families, not just for infants. Rooming-in helps the mother to overcome many of the "common concerns" listed earlier because it gives her immediate access to her newborn (thereby increasing stimulation to her breasts and establishing a milk supply in a way that is most physiological) and because it helps her recognize her own infant's behaviors. There are multiple advantages to rooming-in and no apparent disadvantages. This may come as a surprise to some who presume that rooming-in will result in less sleep for the mother. The amount of sleep the mother gets should be viewed as a total rather than on a night-by-night basis. If she can have the benefit of rooming-in during the hospital stay, she is less likely to experience the many problems that emerge when infants do not have unrestricted access to their mothers' breasts.

After families express an eagerness to have rooming-in, become an advocate for this model as the standard of care. Furthermore, identify ways to help mothers achieve rest by decreasing the number of interruptions they experience during the hospital stay. Clustering care and facilitating daily nap times on postpartum units could arguably provide more benefits than removing newborns to central nurseries at night.

Evaluation

During the antepartum period, evaluate whether the woman and her partner are comfortable with the decision to breastfeed. Does she have the confidence to succeed? Does she harbor any lingering myths about disadvantages for breastfeeding mothers? Does she consistently voice her contentment with her decision to breastfeed, or is she consistently voicing misgivings, hesitations, or ambivalence? Ideally, these issues should be resolved in the antepartum period, but otherwise they should be communicated to the postpartum personnel involved in the mother's care.

Immediate Postpartum

Assessment

Determine whether the mother has decided to breastfeed and then identify her particular needs. Often the medical record indicates that she has chosen to breastfeed or bottle feed but contains no details about her knowledge of either. Worse still, the woman may have changed her mind since the information was recorded. For these reasons, ongoing assessment of her choice and knowledge level is essential.

If the woman's medical record indicates that she is planning to bottle feed, explore the issue with her further in a nonjudgmental way. Simply present the objective data and elicit from her the subjective feelings and responses. For example, say, "Mrs. X, I see from your chart that you are planning to bottle feed [baby's name]. But I know that sometimes pregnant women make a decision by default rather than from an informed choice; they know more about how to bottle feed than about how to breastfeed, or feel that others won't support breastfeeding. I'm here to give you support or information for either choice, but it would be helpful to me if you could tell me a little about your decision. What was the one main thing that made bottle feeding attractive to you?" Often, mothers will give reasons for why they did not choose breastfeeding rather than why they chose bottle feeding.

If the infant has just been born, check the medical record to determine if the mother has chosen to breastfeed. If she has, start off with a positive message that will reinforce her decision and provide information about her particular needs. Some lead-in statements might be: "Congratulations! You must be very excited that [baby's name] has finally arrived! I'll bet he is as hungry as you are. Are you feeling confident that you can get him latched on, or would you rather that I help you get started?" In a bottle-feeding culture, this approach shows support for her decision and presumes that breastfeeding is the next logical step. It enables the experienced mother to proceed unassisted, or offers help to the mother who might not otherwise ask for it.

Later on, ask more broad-based questions that indicate the mother's knowledge level and her feelings about the breastfeeding experience. Talking with the woman, however beneficial it may be, is never a substitute for direct observation of

TABLE 4-6

CARE MAP FOR BREASTFEEDING

	Before 24 hr	24-48 hr	48-72 hr
Alertness	Alert sometimes	Alert most times	Alert for all feedings
Alignment	Mother correctly aligns infant in 1 or 2 positions with assistance	Mother correctly aligns infant in 1 position independently; aligns infant in 2-3 positions with help	Mother correctly aligns infant for 3 positions independently
Areolar grasp	Mother verbalizes importance of *open wide*	Mother reassured by open wide	Baby consistently opens wide
Areolar compression	Mother identifies difference in sucking patterns (nonnutritive vs. nutritive sucking)	Infant exhibits long, slow, rhythmic sucks at most feedings	Infant exhibits long, slow, rhythmic sucks at all feedings
Audible swallowing	Mother verbalizes importance of audible swallowing; presence of audible swallowing	Infant audibly swallows	Infant audibly swallows
Frequency/milk supply	Feed/stimulate q 2-3 hours	Feed/stimulate q 2-3 hours; mother begins to recognize hunger cues	Feed/stimulate q 2-3 hours or mother responds to hunger cues

breastfeeding. To assess whether milk transfer is occurring, watch the feeding and use a care map to document observations. Building on the ideas of alignment, areolar grasp, areolar compression, and audible swallowing, and adding the ideas of alertness and frequency, a care map for breastfeeding is presented in Table 4-6. Note that the presence of infant *sucking* is not considered a reassuring sign; *swallowing* is the key (see Chapter 5).

During the immediate postpartum period, also determine whether the woman will begin lactating for a full-term, appropriate-for-gestational age, healthy newborn or if she will be lactating under more difficult circumstances. Sections III and IV address special needs, and these should be incorporated into the overall assessment of the families' teaching/learning needs.

Planning/Implementation

The goal in the immediate postpartum period (i.e., during the hospital stay) is to have appropriate latch-on and transfer of milk. Without this, all other efforts, explanations, and encourage-

ment are futile. Otherwise stated, breastfeeding will never continue unless it is begun, and latch-on and milk transfer provide the cornerstone of successful breastfeeding.

Other topics surface and can be addressed, but unless milk is transferred to the infant, and unless the woman has a way to find help when she needs it, breastfeeding efforts are sure to fail. Similarly, avoid a list of don'ts and an overemphasis on potential problems. Problems can and do arise, but concentrating on normal adaptations serves two purposes. First, it reduces the amount of content taught during the hospital stay; second, it gives the mother a positive message about breastfeeding.

Nurses sometimes ask if women should be given a breast pump if they are discharged from the hospital with a sleepy infant or one who has not successfully breastfed. This is a difficult question that could be argued from either perspective. One could rightfully say that the stimulation provided by expressing helps establish milk supply, relieves maternal discomfort, and makes the milk available for the infant to

RESEARCH HIGHLIGHT
Does early discharge interfere with breastfeeding?

Citation: O'Leary A, Koepsell D, Haller S. Breastfeeding incidence after early discharge and factors influencing breastfeeding cessation. *JOGNN* 1997;26:289-294.

Focus: This two-group descriptive survey was designed to investigate the correlation between early discharge and cessation of breastfeeding. One hundred one vaginally delivered primiparas and their healthy, full-term newborns were studied at 6 to 8 weeks postpartum through a structured telephone interview. They were divided into two groups: group 1 mothers had been hospitalized for less than 48 hours without any home visits; group 2 had been hospitalized for 24 hours with one home visit on day 3. The infants were categorized as exclusively breastfeeding (milk from the breast only), complete human milk (human milk either from the breast or the bottle), partial breastfeeding (human milk and artificial milk), or bottle feeding (artificial milk only.)

Results: Whether or not women were breastfeeding at 6 to 8 weeks postpartum was not associated with the length of their hospital stay. Women did, however, give reasons for discontinuing breastfeeding. In both groups, the most frequently identified reason for discontinuing breast-

feeding was the perception that the infant was not getting enough milk (23% of the 48-hour stay mothers and 42% of the 24-hour stay mothers). Furthermore, a greater percentage (27%) of infants from group 2 were completely breastfeeding at 6 to 8 weeks, whereas only 16% from group 1 were exclusively breastfeeding.

Strengths, limitations of the study: The investigators ensured that the subjects were not demographically different in terms of age, years of education, or marital status—factors known to be associated with greater incidence and duration of breastfeeding. The study had many limitations. The subjects were recruited from a birthing center, and it is difficult to generalize the results to other populations. Further, one group had a home visit on day 3, when all mothers may have been more receptive to learning.

Clinical application: Numerous studies have suggested that mothers' perceptions of "not enough milk" result in discontinuation of breastfeeding. The results of this study encourage clinicians to concentrate efforts not on lengthening hospital stay but on helping mothers to build both their milk supply and their confidence early in the postpartum period.

take from a bottle. This reasoning, however logical it may seem, overlooks some other compelling points. First, the challenge of presenting more information in less time becomes more overwhelming; teaching the woman to pump in addition to teaching her to breastfeed only adds to the list of skills she must master. Second, it perpetuates the idea that one needs equipment to breastfeed, which is tantamount to saying that the woman herself is inadequate for the task—hardly a message that would increase her confidence. Finally, and perhaps most important, an infant who is not alert or does not suckle vigorously needs further one-on-one follow up, either for breastfeeding management or to determine if there is a more worrisome underlying pathology. Unless a successful feeding has been observed and documented, nurses cannot presume that it will eventually occur after discharge.

During this period the focus of breastfeeding education should be on the psychomotor learning of "how-to" and finding help after discharge. More specifically, assist the woman to become independent in getting her infant latched on, and be sure that she can identify at least three people whom she can call after hospital discharge if problems arise. Give plenty of nurturing and only a few well-focused expectations about independence.

Evaluation

During the early postpartum period, resist the commonly held belief that early hospital discharge interferes with breastfeeding continuation; this belief has no scientific basis. (See Research Highlight.) Instead, evaluate whether milk transfer is occurring, whether the mother has adequate information and confidence to seek help for urgent problems, and whether she has an adequate support network to help her with less urgent but genuine concerns.

Long-Term Postpartum

The primary goal for the long-term postpartum period is to assist the mother to continue breastfeeding until she wishes to wean, and to get adequate help for problems that may arise. A good way to help mothers know when they need help is to design a card for them to receive at discharge. The card should list reassuring signs and symptoms on one side, and worrisome signs and symptoms on the other side. There should be a space for numbers to call when the mother or infant exhibits worrisome signs. Secondary goals relate to making choices that enhance breastfeeding and overall health during lactation. During the hospital stay, focus on recognizing the *questions*, not providing the *answers*; detailed answers to these questions during hospitalization sacrifice attention to the primary goal. Create a second card that gives her ideas for questions she might need to ask in the future. Topics might include the relationship between fertility and lactation, the impact of employment on lactation, and other matters related to general health and lifestyle that are not critical to breastfeeding success during the first 2 weeks or so.

Assessment

Assessment for the long-term postpartum period includes three aspects. The first relates to immediate *problems* that can be anticipated: are there any red flags that require aggressive follow-up? Second, what are the most common *concerns* that are expressed by breastfeeding mothers and that might be overcome or minimized by anticipatory guidance? Third, what are the woman's support systems that will enable her to overcome either the problems or the concerns?

Problems are those issues that have some immediate or serious consequence—signs of dehydration, increasing jaundice, and other urgent matters. These require prompt, professional follow-up. Concerns, on the other hand, are less urgent. These might include the am-I-doing-this-right type of question, anxieties about insufficient milk supply, and so forth. There certainly is some overlap, but the important thing is that the woman realizes that urgent problems with potentially serious consequences need prompt, medical attention, not simply social support.

Most healthy, full-term infants will do well if staff nurses are competent in simple breastfeeding management, if the mother is adequately advised of when to call for professional help, and if the AAP criteria[75] are met prior to discharge. Some maternal-infant situations, however, raise red flags requiring nurse-initiated follow-up.

- Any unresolved problem for mother or infant—impending or increased risk for hyperbilirubinemia, lack of alertness, sore or damaged nipples, or other problems
- Any complexity—the infant is preterm, has a cleft defect, or various other pathology
- Lack of social support
- Poor maternal self-esteem and confidence, or frequently expressed self-doubts about breastfeeding

Planning/Implementation

Rather than assume that the hospital nurse can answer every question or give every piece of advice that the breastfeeding mother will ever need, establish collaborative systems where others in the community can take over where the hospital nurse left off. These systems work only when the mother has a clear directive, however. Tell a new mother whom to call when. Whom she should call depends on whether she has a problem or a concern.

Communication and collaboration with colleagues are essential. Alert other health professionals to any "red flag" situations that relate to breastfeeding. Colleagues who may be helpful include the pediatrician, obstetrician, office nurse-practitioner, community health nurse, or local Women, Infants and Children (WIC) breastfeeding coordinator. For more complex problems, a neonatal dietitian or lactation specialist may be required. The idea here is to avoid having the woman rely on one professional, but to encourage multiple professionals to provide support for breastfeeding as an ongoing process.

Some system needs to be in place whereby the staff nurse or clinical nurse specialist calls all mothers who have a "red flag" upon discharge. Patients who have been identified as needing to receive a nurse-initiated call should have their name and pertinent data entered into a special notebook upon discharge.

The mothers, sisters, and women relatives who might be willing and able to offer breastfeeding support to new mothers frequently live far away. The mother, therefore, is left not only to learn new skills but also to overcome any lack of self-confidence she may have. These points cannot be minimized, as discontinuation of breastfeeding has been associated with lack of support[76] and intercorrelated with perceived self-confidence in breastfeeding.[10] Provide mothers with phone numbers of consumer support groups in their geographic area, and encourage them to form networks with other breastfeeding mothers.

Evaluation

During the later postpartum periods, identify untoward situations that are likely to occur or recur, and determine if they are the result of "breastfeeding problems" or are more related to the transition to parenthood or to some unknown pathology. Good breastfeeding management should promote infant health and well-being and contribute to the mother's sense of pleasure and accomplishment. Usually, breastfeeding problems are transient and solvable.

Completing the Reproductive Cycle

The time and reasons for weaning are driven more by cultural norms and practices than by nutritional needs. Most authorities agree that infants can exist on human milk without supplementation until at least 4 months of age; some solids may be added after that time.

Process of Weaning

Give careful thought before teaching the mother about weaning. First, the timing of instruction about weaning is critical. It is completely inappropriate to teach about weaning before the milk supply has been well established! Assure the mother that when she and her child are ready to wean, help is available. Support the idea of child-led weaning where the child, rather than the mother, initiates and controls weaning.

Gradual weaning is ideal. This involves eliminating one feeding at a time. The first feeding to be eliminated is a matter of personal preference. Usually, however, the last feeding to be eliminated is the night feeding because the focus at that time is more on comfort than on nutrition.

Deliberate weaning is sometimes initiated by the mother when she perceives that her life circumstances or the infant's developmental age require it. For example, when the infant is walking, teething, or becoming easily distracted by visual stimuli and suddenly detaches from the breast, some mothers initiate deliberate weaning. Similarly, if the woman is going back to work or sustaining a new pregnancy, she may initiate deliberate, rather than child-led, weaning.

Abrupt weaning happens because of severe necessity or after frustration that gradual weaning did not result in complete weaning as expected. So, for example, the mother who is suddenly rushed to the hospital and requires major surgery or is severely debilitated may be forced to experience abrupt weaning. In this case, suggest ice packs and decreased stimulation to the breast. Sometimes abrupt weaning may take place when the mother simply wishes to call a halt. Over the years, mothers have been known to put all sorts of substances on their breasts—such as pepper, vinegar, and onion—to discourage the infant from suckling. These practices should be discouraged.

Closet nursing is a phenomenon that occurs because society is not accepting of an older child at the mother's breast. Hence, the mother carries our her mission in secret, or in the "closet," because she fears disapproval from others. Mothers and children seem to enjoy this secret bond and often have a special word for breastfeeding. As one mother said, "We called it 'ma.' And when we were in the supermarket and he said 'I want ma' people just thought that he wanted his mother." After a prolonged breastfeeding experience, one little girl announced to her mother, "When I grow up, I'm going to give my baby tahtah just like you gave me!"

References

1. Wlodkowski R. *Enhancing Adult Motivation to Learn.* San Francisco: Jossey-Bass; 1985.
2. Ellis A. *Reason and Emotion in Psychotherapy.* New York: Lyle Stuart; 1962.
3. Losch M, Dungy CI, Russell D, Dusdieker LB. Impact of attitudes on maternal decisions regarding infant feeding. *J Pediatr* 1995;126:507-514.
4. Rousseau EH, Lescop JN, Fontaine S, Lambert J, Roy CC. Influence of cultural and environmental factors on breast-feeding. *Can Med Assoc J* 1982;127:701-704.
5. Mackey S, Fried PA. Infant breast and bottle feeding practices: some related factors and attitudes. *Can J Public Health* 1981;72:312-318.
6. Ekwo EE, Dusdieker LB, Booth BM. Factors influencing initiation of breast-feeding. *Am J Dis Child* 1983;137:375-377.
7. Holt GM, Wolkind SN. Early abandonment of breast feeding: causes and effects. *Child Care Health Dev* 1983;9:349-355.
8. Jones DA, West RR. Effect of a lactation nurse on the success of breast-feeding: a randomised controlled trial. *J Epidemiol Community Health* 1986;40:45-49.
9. Goodine LA, Fried PA. Infant feeding practices: pre- and postnatal factors affecting choice of method and the duration of breastfeeding. *Can J Public Health* 1984;75:439-444.
10. Coreil J, Murphy J. Maternal commitment, lactation practices, and breastfeeding duration. *J Obstet Gynecol Neonatal Nurs* 1988;17:273-278.
11. Institute of Medicine. *Nutrition During Lactation.* Washington, DC: National Academy Press; 1991.
12. Worthington-Roberts B, Williams SR. *Nutrition in Pregnancy and Lactation.* 6th ed. St. Louis: Mosby; 1996.
13. Mennella JA, Beauchamp GK. Maternal diet alters the sensory qualities of human milk and the nursling's behavior. *Pediatrics* 1991;88:737-744.
14. Lust KD, Brown JE, Thomas W. Maternal intake of cruciferous vegetables and other foods and colic symptoms in exclusively breast-fed infants. *J Am Diet Assoc* 1996;96:46-48.
15. Dusdieker LB, Booth BM, Stumbo PJ, Eichenberger JM. Effect of supplemental fluids on human milk production. *J Pediatr* 1985;106:207-211.
16. Dusdieker LB, Stumbo PJ, Booth BM, Wilmoth RN. Prolonged maternal fluid supplementation in breast-feeding. *Pediatrics* 1990;86:737-740.
17. Morse JM, Ewing G, Gamble D, Donahue P. The effect of maternal fluid intake on breast milk supply: a pilot study. *Can J Public Health* 1992;83:213-216.
18. Johnston EM. Weight changes during pregnancy and the postpartum period. *Prog Food Nutr Sci* 1991;15:117-157.
19. Potter S, Hannum S, McFarlin B, Essex-Sorlie D, Campbell E, Trupin S. Does infant feeding method influence maternal postpartum weight loss? *J Am Diet Assoc* 1991;91:441-446.

20. Schauberger CW, Rooney BL, Brimer LM. Factors that influence weight loss in the puerperium. *Obstet Gynecol* 1992;79:424-429.

21. Dewey KG, Heinig MJ, Nommsen LA. Maternal weight-loss patterns during prolonged lactation. *Am J Clin Nutr* 1993;58:162-166.

22. Prentice A. Should lactating women exercise? *Nutr Rev* 1994;52:358-360.

23. Lovelady CA, Nommsen-Rivers LA, McCrory MA, Dewey KG. Effects of exercise on plasma lipids and metabolism of lactating women. *Med Sci Sports Exerc* 1995;27:22-28.

24. Lovelady CA, Lonnerdal B, Dewey KG. Lactation performance of exercising women. *Am J Clin Nutr* 1990; 52:103-109.

25. Dewey KG, Lovelady CA, Nommsen-Rivers LA, McCrory MA, Lonnerdal B. A randomized study of the effects of aerobic exercise by lactating women on breast-milk volume and composition. *N Engl J Med* 1994;330:449-453.

26. Wallace JP, Inbar G, Ernsthausen K. Infant acceptance of postexercise breast milk. *Pediatrics* 1992;89(6, pt 2):1245-1247.

27. Dewey KG, Lovelady C. Exercise and breast-feeding: a different experience. *Pediatrics* 1993; 91:514-515.

28. Vio F, Salazar G, Infante C. Smoking during pregnancy and lactation and its effects on breast-milk volume. *Am J Clin Nutr* 1991;54:1011-1016.

29. Andersen AN, Lund-Andersen C, Larsen JF, et al. Suppressed prolactin but normal neurophysin levels in cigarette smoking breast-feeding women. *Clin Endocrinol (Oxf)* 1982;17:363-368.

30. Hill PD, Aldag JC. Smoking and breastfeeding status. *Res Nurs Health* 1996;19:125-132.

31. Matheson I, Rivrud GN. The effect of smoking on lactation and infantile colic. *JAMA* 1989;261:42-43.

32. Mennella JA, Beauchamp GK. The transfer of alcohol to human milk: effects on flavor and the infant's behavior. *N Engl J Med* 1991;325:981-985.

33. American Academy of Pediatrics Committee on Drugs. The transfer of drugs and other chemicals into human milk. *Pediatrics* 1994;93:137-150.

34. Graef P, McGhee K, Rozycki J, et al. Postpartum concerns of breastfeeding mothers. *J Nurse Midwifery* 1988;33:62-66.

35. Mogan J. A study of mothers' breastfeeding concerns. *Birth* 1986;13:104-108.

36. Bevan ML, Mosley D, Solimano GR. Factors influencing breast feeding in an urban WIC program. *J Am Diet Assoc* 1984;84:563-567.

37. Gunn TR. The incidence of breast feeding and reasons for weaning. *N Z Med J* 1984;97(757):360-363.

38. Hawkins LM, Nichols FH, Tanner JL. Predictors of the duration of breastfeeding in low-income women. *Birth* 1987;14:204-209.

39. Hill PD. Effects of education on breastfeeding success. *Matern Child Nurs J* 1987;16:145-156.

40. Hill PD, Humenick SS. Insufficient milk supply. *Image J Nurs Sch* 1989;21:145-148.

41. Quickfall J. Can the duration of breast feeding be extended? *Health Visit* 1979;52:223-225.

42. Chapman JJ, Macey MJ, Keegan M, Borum P, Bennett S. Concerns of breast-feeding mothers from birth to 4 months. *Nurs Res* 1985;34:374-377.

43. Quinn AO, Koepsell D, Haller S. Breastfeeding incidence after early discharge and factors influencing breastfeeding cessation. *J Obstet Gynecol Neonatal Nurs* 1997;26:289-294.

44. Beske EJ, Garvis MS. Important factors in breast-feeding success. *MCN Am J Matern Child Nurs* 1982;7:174-179.

45. Jackson EB, Olmsted RW, Foord A, Thoms H, Hyder K. A hospital rooming-in unit for four newborn infants and their mothers: descriptive account of background, development and procedures with a few preliminary observations. *Pediatrics* 1948;1:28-43.

46. Anderson GC. Risk in mother-infant separation postbirth. *Image J Nurs Sch* 1989;21:196-199.

47. Yamauchi Y, Yamanouchi I. The relationship between rooming-in/not rooming-in and breast-feeding variables. *Acta Paediatr Scand* 1990; 79:1017-1022.

48. Keefe M. The impact of infant rooming-in on maternal sleep at night. *J Obstet Gynecol Neonatal Nurs* 1988;17:122-126.

49. Keefe M. Comparison of neonatal sleep-wake patterns in the nursery versus rooming-in environments. *Nurs Res* 1987;36:140-144.

50. Wiles LS. The effect of prenatal breastfeeding education on breastfeeding success and maternal perception of the infant. *J Obstet Gynecol Neonatal Nurs* 1984;13:253-257.

51. Hall JM. Influencing breastfeeding success. *J Obstet Gynecol Neonatal Nurs* 1978;7:28-32.

52. Hellings P. A discriminant model to predict breastfeeding success. *West J Nurs Res* 1985;7:471-478.

53. Arafat I, Allen DE, Fox JE. Maternal practice and attitudes toward breastfeeding. *J Obstet Gynecol Neonatal Nurs* 1981;10(2):91-95.

54. Janke JR. Breastfeeding duration following cesarean and vaginal births. *J Nurse Midwifery* 1988;33:159-164.

55. Ryan AS, Martinez GA. Breast-feeding and the working mother: a profile. *Pediatrics* 1989;83:524-531.

56. Wright HJ, Walker PC. Prediction of duration of breast feeding in primiparas. *J Epidemiol Community Health* 1983;37:89-94.

57. Rentschler DD. Correlates of successful breastfeeding. *Image J Nurs Sch* 1991;23:151-154.

58. Locklin MP, Naber SJ. Does breastfeeding empower women? insights from a select group of educated, low-income, minority women. *Birth* 1993;20:30-35.

59. Jelliffe DB, Jelliffe EFP. *Human Milk in the Modern World.* Oxford: Oxford University Press; 1978.

60. Moore ML, Givens SR. *Window of Opportunity.* White Plains, NY: March of Dimes Foundation; 1994.

61. Bryant CA. The impact of kin, friend and neighbor networks on infant feeding practices: Cuban, Puerto Rican and Anglo families in Florida. *Soc Sci Med* 1982;16:1757-1765.

62. Lawrence RA. *Breastfeeding: A Guide for the Medical Profession.* 2nd ed. St. Louis: Mosby; 1985.

63. Biancuzzo M. Breastfeeding education for early discharge: a three-tiered approach. *J Perinat Neonat Nurs* 1997;11:10-22.

64. Littman H, Medendorp SV, Goldfarb J. The decision to breastfeed: the importance of father's approval. *Clin Pediatr (Phila)* 1994;33:214-219.

65. Freed GL, Fraley JK, Schanler RJ. Accuracy of expectant mothers' predictions of fathers' attitudes regarding breast-feeding. *J Fam Pract* 1993;37:148-152.

66. Freed GL, Fraley JK. Effect of expectant mothers' feeding plan on prediction of fathers' attitudes regarding breast-feeding. *Am J Perinatol* 1993; 10:300-303.

67. Sciacca JP, Dube DA, Phipps BL, Ratliff MI. A breast feeding education and promotion program: effects on knowledge, attitudes, and support for breast feeding. *J Community Health* 1995;20:473-490.

68. Giugliani ER, Bronner Y, Caiaffa WT, Vogelhut J, Witter FR, Perman JA. Are fathers prepared to encourage their partners to breast feed? a study about fathers' knowledge of breast feeding. *Acta Paediatr Scand* 1994;83:1127-1131.

69. Freed GL, Fraley JK, Schanler RJ. Attitudes of expectant fathers regarding breast-feeding. *Pediatrics* 1992;90(2, pt 1):224-227.

70. Barnes GR, Lethin AN, Jackson EB, Shea N. Management of breastfeeding. *JAMA* 1953;151:192-199.

71. Janke JR. Development of the Breast-Feeding Attrition Prediction Tool. *Nurs Res* 1994;43:100-104.

72. Perez-Escamilla R, Pollitt E, Lonnerdal B, Dewey KG. Infant feeding policies in maternity wards and their effect on breast-feeding success: an analytical overview. *Am J Public Health* 1994;84:89-97.

73. Perez-Escamilla R, Segura-Millan S, Pollitt E, Dewey KG. Effect of the maternity ward system on the lactation success of low-income urban Mexican women. *Early Hum Dev* 1992;31:25-40.

74. Lindenberg CS, Cabrera Artola R, Jimenez V. The effect of early post-partum mother-infant contact and breast-feeding promotion on the incidence and continuation of breast-feeding. *Int J Nurs Stud* 1990;27:179-186.

75. American Academy of Pediatrics. Committee on Fetus and Newborn. Hospital stay for healthy newborns. *Pediatrics* 1995;6:788-790.

76. Ekwo EE, Dusdieker L, Booth B, Seals B. Psychosocial factors influencing the duration of breastfeeding by primigravidas. *Acta Paediatr Scand* 1984;73:241-247.

5

Technique: The Mother-Baby Connection

The key to successful breastfeeding is instilling confidence in the mother and providing good counseling. As the saying goes, nothing succeeds like success. The mother gains confidence in herself when she sees her infant happily breastfeeding. Most newborns and their mothers, however, require some assistance in learning techniques that will result in a satisfying experience. This chapter is based on the premise that all nurses have a responsibility to teach mothering skills and promote good infant nutrition—breastfeeding is both.

BREASTFEEDING AS A RECIPROCAL PROCESS

Chapter 3 discussed human milk as a product with multiple components that is synthesized through complex neurophysiological mecha-

nisms. The key component of breastfeeding as a process, however, is the reciprocal interaction of the infant and the mother. Maternal milk production and milk ejection reflex have been discussed in Chapter 3; this chapter will address milk transfer to the newborn.

The Sucking Sequence

Several studies have shown the movements associated with feeding. Ardran, Kemp, and Lind performed two landmark studies, the first on artificially fed infants[1] and the second on breastfed infants.[2] Movements of the nipple, jaw, and tongue were clearly seen. Later, using ultrasound, Woolridge visualized the movements involved in suckling the breast and had an artist create drawings to replicate the ultrasound image of the suck cycle.[3] Figure 5-1 shows the sucking cycle and

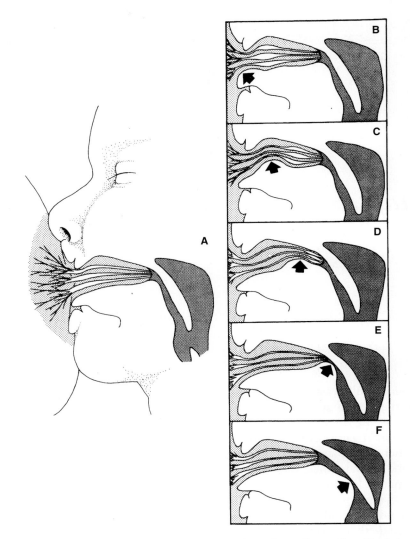

Fig. 5-1 Shows a complete "suck" cycle; the baby is shown in median section. The baby exhibits good feeding technique with the nipple drawn well into the mouth, extending back to the junction of the hard and soft palate (the lactiferous sinuses are depicted within the teat though these cannot be visualised on scans).

A, "Teat" is formed from the nipple and much of the areola, with the lacteal sinuses, which lie behind the nipple, being drawn into the mouth with the breast tissue. The soft palate is relaxed and the nasopharynx is open for breathing. The shape of the tongue at the back represents its position at rest, cupped around the tip of the nipple.

B, The suck cycle is initiated by a welling up of the anterior tip of the tongue. At the same time, the lower jaw, which had been momentarily relaxed (not shown) is raised to constrict the base of the nipple, thereby "pinching off" milk within the ducts of the teat (these movements are inferred as they lie outside the sector viewed in ultrasound scans).

Fig. 5-1, cont'd

C, The wave of compression by the tongue moves along the underside of the nipple in a posterior direction, pushing against the hard palate. This roller-like action squeezes milk from the nipple. The posterior portion of the tongue may be depressed as milk collects in the oropharynx.

D and **E,** The wave of compression passes back past the tip of the nipple and pushes against the soft palate. As the tongue impinges on the soft palate the levator muscles of the palate contract raising it to seal off the nasal cavity. Milk is pushed into the oropharynx and is swallowed if sufficient [enough] has collected.

F, The cycle of compression continues and ends at the posterior base of the tongue. Depression of the back portion of the tongue creates negative pressure drawing the nipple and its milk contents once more into the mouth. This is accompanied by a lowering of the jaw which allows milk to flow back into the nipple.

In ultrasound scans it appears that compression by the tongue, and negative pressure within the mouth, maintain the tongue in close conformation to the nipple and palate. Events are portrayed here rather more loosely to aid clarity. *(From Woolridge MW. The "anatomy" of infant sucking. Midwifery 1986;2:164-171.)*

---

gives a description. A few points are especially notable.

Nipple

The nipple and areola are drawn into the mouth, and a teat is formed that is approximately three times the length of the resting nipple. Despite technology's attempts to manufacture a teat to mimic the human nipple, no artificial nipple lengthens like the human nipple.[4]

Jaw

The jaw should move up and down in a rhythmic motion when milk transfer is occurring. The observer will also see the ears wiggling. The cheeks should be full and rounded, not sucked in.

Lips

Both upper and lower lip should be flanged, although not too far. Sometimes, particularly in preterm or hypotonic infants, the lower lip folds inward, resulting in a sucking blister for the infant and sore nipples for the mother.

Tongue

The tongue should look troughed—cup-shaped or scoop-shaped—and should begin at the bottom of the mouth, extending over the lower alveolar ridge. When the lateral aspects of the tongue are troughed in this way, the tongue can correctly draw in the nipple, press it against the hard palate, and form a teat. The tip of the tongue does not create friction along the teat (like fingers squeezing the length of a nearly empty tube of toothpaste). Rather, the tongue humps up from back to front in an undulating movement when milk is transferred.

Reflexes

Reflexes are important factors in milk transfer. Rooting, sucking, and swallowing help the newborn to initiate and sustain milk transfer.

Rooting

The rooting reflex, usually defined as a one-component operation, is more accurately described by Woolridge as a two-component reflex.[3] Woolridge says the rooting reflex has two components: "(1) tactile stimulation of the skin around the mouth causes the infant to turn his head towards that source of stimulation, and (2) his mouth gapes in preparation to accept the nipple." This second component is called the *oral searching reflex* by Righard and Alade.[5] The term used for this action is unimportant; what is important is that the newborn exhibit the gaping, open-wide behavior before attaching to the breast.

Sucking

The sucking reflex is elicited by tactile or chemical stimulation of the *palate*, not the tongue.[3] Although we are tempted to assume that the sweet taste of the milk stimulates sucking, Woolridge emphasizes that the lower jaw and tongue are the motive force for milk expulsion; therefore the palate—situated above the jaw and tongue—provides a target for stimulation by the nipple.

The sucking reflex is often misunderstood because it is poorly named. The word *suck* conjures up a notion of negative pressure. For example, sucking through a straw creates suction (i.e., negative pressure). The sucking reflex occurs at the breast; however, the suction or negative pressure associated with breastfeeding is only related in small part to milk transfer; transfer of milk is accomplished mostly by the positive pressure of the jaw and tongue in an undulating motion compressing the teat against the hard palate.

A landmark study of infants using artificial teats showed that they were not able to fully compress the rubber teat.[1] Admittedly, nowadays rubber nipples are more pliable than those used in the study, but it is still likely that the infant using an artificial teat obtains milk transfer primarily through negative pressure. An example may help to illustrate this concept of negative and mechanical pressure. Assume for a moment that the plastic-liner type of bottle is being used. If the infant could exert enough negative pressure, he could presumably use only this method to obtain milk from the container. If he could not, an adult could use her cupped hand to alternately compress and release the plastic bag—exerting mechanical pressure only—and the milk would shoot out; with either type of pressure, milk would be transferred from one place to another.

During breastfeeding, mechanical pressure is the primary method of obtaining milk; the infant's jaws and tongue are beneath the lactiferous sinuses, compressing them (much as the adult's hand would compress the bag in the preceding example). The negative pressure that the infant exerts is used primarily to hold the nipple and the areola in place, resulting in a good seal, but contributes only minimally to obtaining milk.

Lawrence[6] differentiates between *suckling* and *sucking*. Suckling means "to take nourishment at the breast and specifically refers to breastfeeding in all species. Sucking, on the other hand, means to draw into the mouth by means of a partial vacuum, which is the process employed when bottle feeding. Sucking also means to consume by licking."[6(p216)] Here and in most other texts the terms are used somewhat interchangeably. There must be a clear understanding, however, that milk transfer while breastfeeding is dependent on mechanical, not negative, pressure. The terminology helps to delineate the two feeding modes, nutritive and non-nutritive, used by the infant.

Wolff[7] first identified two different modes of sucking, nutritive and non-nutritive. Although his classic study was conducted with artificially fed infants, he defined non-nutritive sucking as that which occurs in the absence of fluid. At the beginning of a feeding session, the infant exhibits non-nutritive sucking characterized by a pattern of short bursts of fast sucking (rate of about two per second). Wolff concerned himself with two basic premises: presence or absence of palatable fluid, and the rate of sucking in relation to the presence or absence of fluid.

As soon as palatable fluid enters the mouth, nutritive sucking begins for the artificially fed infant. Wolff's study showed that nutritive sucking occurs at a slower, more continuous rate of about one per second with the presence of fluid, and later studies confirmed that this initial nutritive sucking and faster sucking rate occur in breastfed infants as well.

Similarly, breastfed infants begin with a faster, two-per-second type of suck, which helps the mother to have a milk-ejection reflex. At this time, the infant is exerting only negative pressure, and in the absence of fluid in the oral cavity, the negative pressure will be highest (and therefore pressure on the mother's nipple greatest). When the mother has a milk-ejection reflex, nutritive suckling begins. This is exhibited by a slow, rhythmic suck of about one per second, with no pauses in the early stages. After the milk-ejection reflex, there is a decreased need for negative pressure because of fluid in the oral cavity, and hence maternal discomfort disappears.

As the feeding progresses, however, there are some notable differences between the breastfed and artificially fed infant. Artificially fed infants show a distinct difference between non-nutritive and nutritive sucking, eventually returning to the faster suck exhibited at the beginning of the feed. Unlike artificially fed infants, breastfed infants have a less clear distinction between the nutritive and non-nutritive modes after the feeding has progressed for a while. The change in sucking rate varies inversely with milk flow; the higher the milk flow, the slower the rate.[8] As the milk flow decreases toward the end of the feed on each breast, the sucking rate within sucking bursts increases, but there are more and longer rests between bursts.[9] For this reason, the observer or mother can see when the milk starts to flow, as the infant's suckling rate slows down when the mother experiences a milk-ejection reflex. Similarly, suckling will return to a more rapid rate as milk becomes less abundant and flow diminishes. Suckling will terminate with sleep (in infants less

than 12 weeks old). Both the behavior (satiation ending with sleep) and age (less than 12 weeks old) are important factors to determine whether the feeding has been successful. Infants younger than 12 weeks who continue to suckle and do not terminate the feeding with sleep should be carefully evaluated; these infants are probably not latched on well and not achieving milk transfer.

Swallowing

Swallowing is really a continuation of the sucking reflex; that is, sucking can occur apart from swallowing, but swallowing cannot occur apart from sucking. The up-and-down movements of the larynx are associated with swallowing and have been used to identify swallowing in studies.

During the first 5 to 9 days, breastfed infants consume a relatively small volume even when supply is plentiful; infants consume a mean of 34.2 g on the first breast and 26.2 g on the second breast at each feeding. Each suck yields 0.14 ml at the beginning of the feed and 0.01 ml by the end.[10] Important clinical implications emerge from this data: (1) newborns consume more milk from the first breast than from the second, and (2) newborns obtain more milk per suck at the beginning of a feeding but continue to suck even when intake is negligible.

Coordination of Sucking, Swallowing, and Breathing

While the rooting, sucking, and swallowing reflexes are somewhat easier to describe, the coordination of the reflexes, together with breathing, is more difficult to explain. One study[11] gave particular attention to this coordination.

Coordination of Sucking and Swallowing

In the first 2 to 3 days after birth, breastfed infants may need to suck several times before they swallow. For this reason, it is sometimes difficult to hear swallowing because the nurse or mother may need to observe several sucks—perhaps as many as 20—before the infant obtains a volume of fluid great enough to stimulate the swallowing reflex. Furthermore, because of the low volume of fluid, the swallowing is generally very quiet. It is critical to note, however, that swallowing can be heard long before the mother's milk "comes in," although it is easier to hear after her milk becomes abundant. At 4 days and thereafter, the newborn will generally swallow with every suck in the beginning of the feeding, and will have about two sucks for every swallow toward the end of the feeding.

Coordination of Swallowing and Breathing

Newborns must pause to swallow. However, the pause is different for the newborns at 2 days of age than for those at 4 days of age. A study[11] showed that 2-day-olds paused, held their breath, and swallowed. Those who were 4 days old paused but swallowed at the end-expiratory pause (the pause between expiration and inspiration).

Coordination of Sucking and Breathing

Similarly, the 2- and 3-day-old newborns breathed in a somewhat more uncoordinated rhythm, while the 4- or 5-day-olds had a smoother pattern of breathing and sucking. The newborn's breathing was faster when it occurred in the presence of sucking only (no swallow component) and slower when the suck-swallow occurred. Recognizing these behaviors helps the observer to determine that milk transfer is taking place.

Influences on Supply and Demand

The concept of supply and demand starts with the first feeding. As described in Chapter 3, the body signals for milk production to begin as soon as the placenta is delivered. However, milk production will not continue unless suckling is initiated, and sooner is most definitely better than later.

Supply and Maternal Production

Supply may be used synonymously with *production*, and both words seem simple enough to comprehend. When reading the literature, however, it is important to distinguish between milk production, which refers to "*volume* of milk removed from the breast either by breastfeeding or expression" in contrast to milk *synthesis*, which refers to "the accumulation of milk within the breast."[12] A good analogy might be this: A spring in your backyard can produce X amount of water, but whether or not you consume it is quite another matter. Similarly, the breast may have synthesized plenty of milk, but whether or not the infant consumes it is another matter.

Demand (Infant Need)

The statement that milk supply is based on demand is somewhat oversimplified. It first raises the question of what constitutes demand. "Demand" is often erroneously thought of as when the infant cries; such a definition carries a negative connotation and does not reflect a clear understanding of infant behavior. Rather, the "demand" is really about a need.

Demand feedings, or feeding on cue, are most physiological. Infants who are given "demand" feedings do eat more frequently than their schedule-fed cohorts,[13] but infants appear to self-regulate their intake.[14,15] This self-regulation should be the basis for understanding the concept of demand and for defining it in a positive light.

Maternal supply and infant demand must also be understood in terms of the age of the infant. Breastfeeding is not considered to be "well established" until around 3 or 4 weeks after birth. Maternal supply of milk is clearly correlated to frequency of feedings until that time. In other words, milk production will increase as the frequency of stimulation increases *during that month.*[13] After milk supply is well established, however, milk production does *not* correlate with frequency of feeding.[16-18]

It appears that the critical factor in having supply meet demand is breast emptying.[12] The lactating breast is never completely "empty." If, indeed, frequency has a great influence on supply during the first few weeks but has little influence after lactation is well established, milk volume increases could be explained by the idea that infants self-regulate their intake; they may indeed empty the breast more completely during the first few weeks, and during "growth spurts." This concept forms the basis for recommendations about early contact, a dwindling milk supply, and so-called "growth spurts."

Full, Partial, and Token Breastfeeding

Maternal supply best meets infant demand when the parent offers no food or drink to the infant other than human milk. Breastfeeding can be defined as full, partial, or token.[19] Figure 5-2 describes the subdivisions of these patterns. Full breastfeeding—exclusive or almost exclusive—

has many benefits for both the mother and the infant, as described in Chapter 3. Partial breastfeeding, while not as beneficial as full breastfeeding, may be a necessary or desirable alternative under certain circumstances. Token breastfeeding provides little nutritional value and is more suited for older infants or toddlers who come to the breast primarily for comfort rather than nutrition. Particularly during the newborn period, exclusive breastfeeding is preferable to partial breastfeeding.

There are two styles of partial breastfeeding. *Supplemental feeding* means that the infant consumes human milk at one feeding and human milk substitutes or water at another feeding. *Complemental feeding* means that the infant is first fed human milk (either at the breast or pumped human milk from a bottle), followed by artificial milk or water. This is sometimes called "topping off" or "p.c." (after meals) feeding. Complementary feedings are deleterious to breastfeeding from both a physiological and a psychological standpoint. First, complementary feedings rob the infant of the full benefits of the mother's milk. Furthermore, mothers implicitly state that they feel

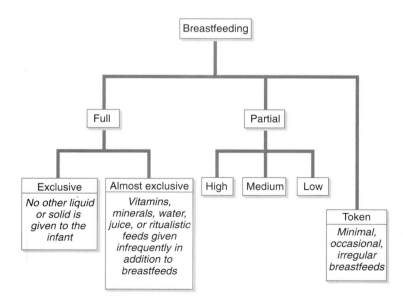

Fig. 5-2 Schema for breastfeeding definition. *(From Labbok M, Krasovec K. Toward consistency in breastfeeding definitions. Stud Fam Plann 1990;21:226-230.)*

Box 5-1
Acceptable Medical Reasons for Supplementation

A few medical indications in a maternity facility may require that individual infants be given fluids or food in addition to, or in place of, breastmilk.

It is assumed that severely ill babies, babies in need of surgery, and very low birth weight infants will be in a special care unit. Their feeding will be individually decided, given their particular nutritional requirements and functional capabilities, although breastmilk is recommended whenever possible. These infants in special care are likely to include:

- Infants with very low birth weight (less than 1500 g) or who are born before 32 weeks gestational age
- Infants with severe dysmaturity with potentially severe hypoglycemia, or who require therapy for hypoglycemia, and who do not improve through increased breastfeeding or by being given breastmilk

For infants who are well enough to be with their mothers on the maternity ward, there are very few indications for supplements. In order to assess whether a facility is inappropriately using fluids or breastmilk substitutes, any infants receiving additional supplements must have been diagnosed as:

- Infants whose mothers have severe maternal illness (e.g., psychosis, eclampsia, or shock)

- Infants with inborn errors of metabolism (e.g., galactosemia, phenylketonuria, maple syrup urine disease)
- Infants with acute water loss, for example, during phototherapy for jaundice, whenever increased breastfeeding or use of expressed breastmilk cannot provide adequate hydration
- Infants whose mothers require medication which is contraindicated when breastfeeding (e.g., cytotoxic drugs, radioactive drugs, and antithyroid drugs other than propylthiouracil)

When breastfeeding has to be temporarily delayed, interrupted, or supplemented, mothers should be helped to establish or maintain lactation, for example, through manual or hand-pump expression of milk, in preparation for the moment when full breastfeeding may be begun or resumed. If the interruption is due to problems with the infant, milk can be expressed, stored if necessary, and provided to the infant as soon as medically advisable. If it is due to a maternal medication or disease which negatively affects the quality of milk, the milk should be pumped and discarded.

From WHO/UNICEF. Baby-Friendly Hospital Initiative. Part 2: Hospital-Level Implementation, 1992.

---

less than adequate in their breastfeeding efforts when, after feeding at the breast, the infant is offered the bottle and, as one mother said, "takes it like a champ." Generally, when clinicians use the word "supplementation" they mean either supplementing or complementing. Ideally, newborns should be exclusively breastfed at least until lactation is well established (i.e., from birth until about 28 days thereafter).

The risk of artificial feeding clearly outweighs any possible advantage, as outlined in Chapter 3. There are few reasons for supplemental or complemental feedings; medically indicated reasons are listed in Box 5-1. Unless such a reason indicates otherwise, newborns should not be given any supplemental or complemental artificial milk or

water. Supplementing the newborn interferes with the natural symbiosis of supply and demand, and reduces suckling time, which in turn reduces intake at the breast. Total suckling time (min/day) and supplementary food intake (kcal/day) are significant predictors of breastfeeding intake after allowing for the age of the infant.[20]

CLINICAL MANAGEMENT: FEEDING PATTERNS

The breastfeeding process, as described in the previous section, is best accomplished when it is begun immediately and continued exclusively. Parents and health care providers can capitalize on the newborn's natural inclinations at this time.

Early Initiation of Breastfeeding

Early initiation of breastfeeding has many benefits as listed in Box 5-2. Women who initiate breastfeeding continue breastfeeding for a longer period than those with delayed contact.[21-24] Multiparas and mothers who deliver vaginally initiate breastfeeding earlier than primiparas or mothers who have had cesarean deliveries.[25] Breastfeeding is seldom contraindicated (see Chapter 8), so the woman who is committed to breastfeeding should offer her breast to the newborn immediately after delivery. Ideally, the newborn should go to breast within the first hour when he is in the alert state, as shown in Figure 5-3. Most newborns will happily suckle—or at least lick and explore—immediately after birth.

The newborn's capabilities during the first hour are remarkable. When labor is unmedicated and infants are placed on the mother's abdomen, they will make crawling motions to get to the breast, find the nipple, and attach themselves.[26] (Newborns may or may not exhibit this behavior if mothers have been medicated intrapartally.) A common misconception is that newborns are unable to "do much" at the breast immediately after delivery. This is not true, however. A rubber nipple transducer has been used to determine the pressure exerted by the newborn. Immediately after birth, newborns exert a pressure of 5 mm Hg in the non-nutritive mode; 90 minutes after birth this pressure peaks to about 103 mm Hg.[27]

After the first hour the newborn wants to sleep, as does his mother. The hour immediately following birth is a sensitive period, not a critical period, however, so if breastfeeding is delayed somewhat beyond one hour, a positive outcome can still be achieved, as described in the Clinical Scenario. If it is anticipated that the infant is too ill to tolerate oral feeding for a substantial time,

Box 5-2

Benefits of Exclusive Breastfeeding During First Few Days

Exclusive breastfeeding during the first few days provides many benefits for the mother, which include the following:

- Helps milk come in earlier
- Decreases severity of engorgement
- Enhances supply of milk (related to supply and demand)
- Helps uterus to involute
- Bolsters mother's confidence that she can be sole provider for her infant
- Gives mother plenty of practice in the hospital

Exclusive breastfeeding includes many benefits for the infant as well:

- Prevents/minimizes nipple confusion
- Baby can practice sucking at the breast
- Decreases likelihood of allergies and diarrhea
- Baby obtains colostrum first 2 days or so; the colostrum acts as a laxative on the gut, thereby minimizing the risk of jaundice
- Illness is reduced because colostrum is rich in immunoglobulins
- Colostrum is high in protein, concentrated in volume and easily digestible
- Breastfeeding is more likely to continue for several months

Modified from Biancuzzo M. *Breastfeeding the Healthy Newborn: A Nursing Perspective.* White Plains, NY: March of Dimes Foundation; 1994.

the mother should express milk as soon as possible, but should not delay beyond 6 hours after delivery. Whether the first breastfeeding experience is immediate or delayed, the nurse should provide information and enthusiastic support for the mother.

It is highly likely that feeding is the first "mothering" task a mother performs. She should therefore find it a pleasurable and successful experience. Before the mother actually puts the newborn to the breast, help her to see that the

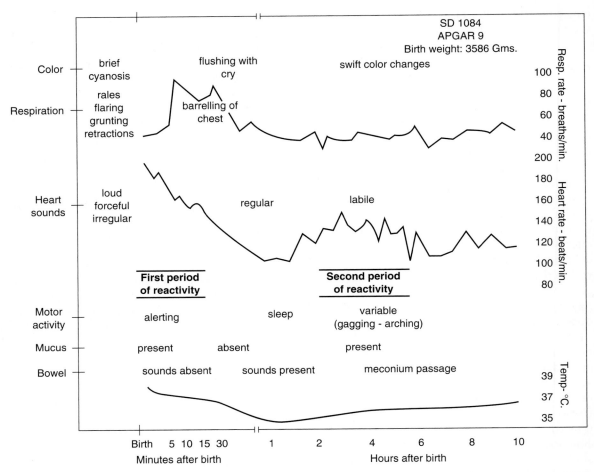

Fig. 5-3 Periods of reactivity during the first 10 hours of life. *(From Desmond M, Rudolph A, Phitakspharaiwan P. The transitional care nursery.* Pediatr Clin North Am *1966;13:656.)*

experience is successful if her newborn only licks and explores; suggest that suckling is a bonus, not a requirement. This approach will help her to view the initial experience as positive rather than disappointing if the newborn does not suckle. Praise her for her interaction with the newborn, and point out any especially positive aspects of the interaction. Give positive, reinforcing messages to the mother that highlight her capabilities as a new mother rather than her limitations.

Mothers are unable to absorb much information immediately after delivery, so carefully prioritize the information that is given. The greatest priority is to help the newborn to have a gaping, open-wide mouth and good positioning, and to offer praise and instill confidence in the woman. The importance of the second point should not be underestimated. Throughout the early days, keeping the focus on *doing* rather than *knowing* helps to build the mother's confidence.

Short-Term Tactic Supports Long-Term Goal

Mrs. P., G1 P1, had a full-term healthy male, Steven, by cesarean delivery at 9:31 PM. She had an uneventful recovery and was admitted to the postpartum floor around 11:00 PM. At 12:30 AM you are again assessing Mrs. P.'s vital signs, incision, and flow; her blood pressure is elevated somewhat, but otherwise her clinical status is within normal limits. She emphatically tells you that she does not want to feed the baby; she wants you to feed him in the nursery. You are struck by how adamant she is, and you feel conflicted because of the benefits of early breastfeeding.

How would you respond to her request? If and when you do take the newborn from the nursery to his mother, what would your priorities be for helping him and his mother to have a positive experience?

A Management Strategy

Mrs. P.'s elevated blood pressure is your first clue that she is in pain. Ask her open-ended questions about how she is feeling. She will then reveal that she is experiencing a high level of pain, and she is very discouraged and fatigued after her all-day induction. Medicate the mother and feed Steven in the nursery. When you do take him to his mother, however, suggest a position that is most comfortable for the mother; this is likely to be the side-lying position. Place the infant so that the mother can use the hand that does not have the IV line. Use plenty of pillows to get her body into good alignment, and use a rolled-up baby blanket to keep Steven facing his mother directly, not rolling partially onto his back. Keep the instructions simple; focus on nuzzling and opening wide. If the baby seems interested in the second breast, "tuck" the mother's breast under her and help him to suckle the top breast so that the mother can feed him without having to change her position.

Outcome

Flexibility seemed to be the key to managing this woman's breastfeeding experience. Nearly a year after her hospitalization, I learned that she was still happily breastfeeding Steven.

The effects of this early experience seem to have some imprinting effect. When newborns go to the breast immediately after delivery, they are more likely to consistently exhibit correct sucking techniques than are those who have been separated from their mothers.[26] Furthermore, early initiation has been positively correlated with better continuation of breastfeeding; it appears to be even more influential than frequent feeds.[28]

Frequency of Feedings

The general concept that influences clinical management is the understanding that during the first month or so, increased frequency of feeding correlates with increased supply. However, *increasing the frequency will not increase the supply unless transfer of milk is successfully occurring;* the best reassurance of transfer of milk is *audible swallowing.*

Scheduled Feedings

Imposing any schedule on a breastfed infant is most unnatural and counterproductive. When the natural symbiosis is replaced by the clock, the principle of supply and demand is violated, usually resulting in difficulties with milk supply for the mother, and frustration and hunger for the infant.

During the last half of this century, hospitals routinely fed all infants—breastfed and artificially fed—on a 4-hour schedule. Presumably, this practice began when knowledge about artificial feeding was used to determine hospital practices. It takes about 4 hours for newborns to digest artificial milk but less than 3 hours to digest human milk. Four-hour feeding schedules persisted long after there was a clear understanding of the differences in digestion time for artificially fed versus breastfed infants, probably because it was convenient for the staff.

Scheduled feedings contradict what is known about the anatomy and physiology of the newborn. Newborns have a stomach capacity of about 30 ml; one can envision the newborn's stomach as about the size of a golf ball. Because human milk is more easily digested than artificial milk, owing to a low ratio of casein to whey, the stomach is empty within about 3 hours. Therefore, the breastfed infant who has an interval of more than 3 hours between feeds may require further follow-up.

Demand Feedings

Many people think that the infant "demands" to be fed by crying. Actually, crying is the last sign of hunger (see Box 5-3 which lists hunger cues). Infants should generally be fed whenever they are hungry. It is not unusual for hunger cues to be exhibited 90 minutes after the last feeding. Demand feedings are best accomplished by having an awareness of the sleep-wakefulness continuum and a respect for night feedings.

Sleep-Wakefulness Continuum

Feeding can be accomplished any time that the infant is awake. However, infants are not simply asleep or awake; Figure 5-4 shows the sleep-wakefulness continuum. Ideally, infants should go to the breast when they are in the quiet alert state. A simple concept governs breastfeeding management here: it is difficult to get a hungry infant to sleep, and it is difficult to get a sleepy infant to eat. Keeping the infant unwrapped sometimes helps him to stay awake. It also allows him to maintain his temperature through skin-to-skin contact with his mother.

Night Feedings

Breastfeeding at night might be considered optional by hospital staff and a chore by mothers after they return home. This negative view is based more on cultural perceptions than on the known biological benefits.

Skipping night feedings in the hospital is a deterrent to establishing a good milk supply; in an effort to "let mothers sleep" in the hospital, problems are only delayed until they return home. The resulting difficulties, including initial engorgement (see Chapter 8) and later insufficient milk supply, are direct consequences of skipped or infrequent feedings. Efforts to "let mothers sleep" should be aimed at helping them to sleep undisturbed during the day; women who deliver in hospitals are more frequently awakened on the first postpartum day by nurses and visitors than by the newborn.[29] Reexamining protocols that awaken mothers for "routine" vital signs, clustering care, and limiting visitors would be infinitely more beneficial than limiting or discouraging night feedings.

Although breastfed newborns generally need to be fed more often than their artificially fed counterparts, the natural and learned processes help night feedings to be tolerable for tired parents. First, the fat content of milk is higher in the evening,[30,31] which may help the infant to consume more calories and therefore feel more satiated. Second, infants who consume more milk in the morning can be socialized to sleep for substantial periods during the night around 8 weeks, although not during the hospital stay.[32]

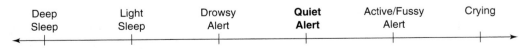

Deep Sleep	Light Sleep	Drowsy Alert	**Quiet Alert**	Active/Fussy Alert	Crying

Fig. 5-4 The consciousness continuum. The quiet alert state is optimal for breastfeeding.

Duration of Feedings

Beliefs and Recommendations

It is commonly believed that limiting time at the breast will minimize or prevent sore nipples. There is no research to document this common myth, however.[33] Sore nipples are almost always the result of poor latch-on (see Chapter 8 for a discussion of sore nipples). Quoting Chloe Fisher, one source says, "Unlimited sucking time + no nipple trauma = no pain, no damage. Any length of sucking + nipple trauma = nipple pain, nipple damage."[34]

Mothers frequently ask how long to allow the newborn to suckle. The best answer is, "Watch the baby, not the clock." As described previously, what the infant is doing at the breast is a good indicator of milk transfer, whereas the time spent at the breast gives little information about the milk actually obtained. Nonetheless, some mothers insist on a recommended time. If it is not possible to persuade the mother to watch the baby instead of the clock, suggest 10 minutes or so on the first side (after the mother experiences a milk-ejection reflex) and as long as the baby wishes on the second side. This is a rather arbitrary number, however, based on the idea that *some* infants are able to get most of the milk within the first 10 minutes.[35,36] However, newborns with different sucking styles take different amounts of time to "empty" the breast.

Sucking Styles

It is seldom helpful to make determinations about milk transfer by looking at the clock. Different infants exhibit different characteristics when they go to the breast; some take more time, while others take less. Early researchers identified five basic styles of sucking and used the terms *barracuda, excited ineffective, procrastinator, gourmet,* and *rester* to describe the associated characteristics.[37] Helping the mother recognize the style—*not* the term—the nurse can suggest actions that help rather than hinder breastfeeding efforts.

Barracudas

Barracudas promptly grasp the nipple and suckle with energy and vigor for 10 to 20 minutes. The barracuda is likely to exert unrelieved negative pressure on the nipple, making the mother's nipple sore for a few days.

Excited Ineffectives

The excited ineffective infant alternately grasps and loses the nipple, then starts screaming. This behavior usually makes the mother tense and can greatly interfere with her milk-ejection reflex. It is sometimes helpful to remove the infant from the breast, soothe him until he becomes quieter, and then try again.

Procrastinators

Procrastinators put off for tomorrow what they could have done today. With early discharge, nurses and mothers worry about these infants. Prodding them, however, does little to speed up the process. They will breastfeed when they are ready. In the meantime, watch for signs of hypoglycemia and hypothermia. The full-term newborn who has no risk factors may be fine; those with other health problems may require medical referral and supplementation.

Gourmets (or Mouthers)

Typically, the gourmet tastes the milk and may even smack his lips before starting to suckle. Hurrying or prodding the gourmet often results in his screaming. Allow the infant to try a taste, and in a few minutes he will usually settle down.

Resters or Snackers

Resters suckle a few minutes and then rest a few minutes. Mothers are often inclined to jiggle these infants, but that is not helpful. Advise the mother that breastfeeding may take a little longer, but these infants will usually do just fine when

they are unhurried. The rester is the extreme opposite of the barracuda; for this reason, the number of minutes spent at the breast provides little
information about how the infant breastfed; the
rester might suckle every bit as effectively as the
barracuda, but the time it takes to do so differs
significantly.

The behavior of the rester or snacker can be
better understood by realizing that the fetus is fed
continuously via the umbilical cord. In some cultures, the infant is continually at the mother's
breast, allowing him to "snack" in a way that
mimics the continuous feeding that occurred via
the umbilical cord before birth.

Others

There are a variety of other sucking styles, but
they are usually some combination of those described here.

CLINICAL MANAGEMENT TO PROMOTE EFFECTIVE SUCKLING

Positioning

Good positioning is paramount to achieving good
latch-on and effective suckling. Furthermore,
good positioning promotes comfort for both
mother and infant.

Basic Positions for Mother

Body Position for Mother

Good positioning starts with good maternal posture. It is best for the mother to be in a chair,
rather than in bed, because the chair facilitates
good posture. Some simple items help with good
alignment. If the woman's feet do not touch the
floor, use a footstool beneath her feet to help
maintain good posture. Pillows, especially during
the very early days, should be positioned beneath

the woman's arms so that mother's neck, arm,
shoulder, and back muscles do not need to support the weight of the infant. A pillow can also be
placed beneath the infant so that he is not
"reaching" for the breast. The idea is to bring the
baby to the breast, not the breast to the baby, and
pillows help raise the baby to the height of the
breast in some circumstances. Women with especially large breasts may need to use a rolled-up
diaper between their breast and torso so that the
weight of the breast does not rest on the infant's
chin.

Unfortunately, the first breastfeeding experience usually takes place in the bed, and achieving
good posture there is a challenge at best. When
the mother leans back—as in a semi-Fowler's position in bed—her nipples point upward; this may
be acceptable in a special circumstance, but it
usually makes it more difficult for the infant to
grasp as much of the nipple/areola complex as he
otherwise might. Leaning forward—bringing the
breast to the infant rather than the infant to the
breast—results in the nipples pointing downward.
When the woman's back is straight, the nipples
are in a position where the newborn can best
achieve good latch-on.

Some simple actions and observations help to
get breastfeeding off to a good start. Remind the
mother to relax her shoulders—otherwise she will
soon become uncomfortable. Note the mother
who hunches over when breastfeeding; instruct
her to bring the baby to the breast, not the breast
to the baby. An important part of positioning is
making sure that the infant's skin is touching the
mother's skin. Unswaddle the infant to get skin-
to-skin contact, which helps maintain or improves thermoregulation and highlights the
chest-to-chest idea.

If the woman has had a cesarean delivery,
comfort and good positioning are essential. Administer ordered analgesics to the mother who
needs them; if the woman is in agony, depriving
her of medication will not enhance the breast-

feeding experience. Before suggesting a position for breastfeeding, determine her level of comfort and mobility. The mother who has delivered by cesarean section may find that sitting is difficult and puts pressure on her suture line. To reduce pressure on the suture line using this position, the woman's knees should be flexed and feet flat. A bedpan, turned upside down in the bed, can serve as a "footstool" for this purpose. Or she may wish to use the side-lying position (see Figure 5-9). An older article written by a master clinician still offers many practical hints for positioning the mother and infant for breastfeeding after a cesarean delivery.[38]

Hand Positions for Mother

There are few rules about the mother's hand position or body posture. Some techniques work better for some mothers, and it may not be possible to immediately identify the best one. The guiding light about hand position is fit. The position used should not allow the fingers to occlude the lactiferous sinuses. The hand position used by a woman with a small hand and a large breast will usually not work well for a woman with a large hand and small breast. Encourage the woman to experiment to find which hold works best; eventually at least one of them will become second nature.

Either of two hand positions can be used to support the breast while breastfeeding. There are two basic ways to support the breast: (1) *palmar grasp,* also called the *C-hold,* (Figure 5-5, A) shows how the mother's thumb is on top and her fingers below, allowing the mother to support the breast; and (2) *scissors hold,* also called the *V-hold* or *cigarette hold* (Figure 5-5, B shows how the mother supports the breast using the index finger on top and third finger below the breast). Either position is acceptable, although several years ago the scissors hold fell out of favor. Some breastfeeding advocates have claimed that this position was wrong, but to date no research has shown that this position is less effective than the palmar

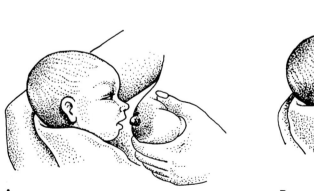 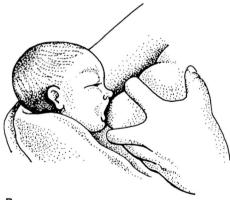

A   **B**

Fig. 5-5 Supporting the breast using palmar grasp **(A)**; scissors hold **(B)**. Thumb and fingers are outside the areola. *(From Spangler A. Amy Spangler's Breastfeeding: A Parent's Guide. 6th ed. Atlanta, GA: Amy Spangler; 1995.)*

grasp. The important thing to remember is that the mother's fingers should not obstruct the lactiferous sinuses. This obstruction can indeed happen with the scissors hold, but it can also happen with the palmar grasp. In general, the palmar grasp works better for women with larger breasts, probably because their fingers are not large enough to grasp the breast without obstructing the lactiferous sinuses. Contrary to popular advice, the mother should not use her finger to push the breast tissue out of the way of the infant's nose. Sometimes this technique is suggested as a way to "allow the baby to breathe." Rather than pushing the breast tissue with her finger, which can interfere with good latch-on, the mother should use her other hand to bring the infant's buttocks in closer. This should alleviate the problem, and the infant will be able to breathe freely.

For the first week or so, the mother will need to hold her breast in place during the feeding. After that time, she should be able to get the feeding started and then let go, unless her breasts are unusually large. Certainly, the large breast should not at any time rest on the infant's chin. The infant who requires continuous breast support throughout the feeding after week 1 may need further evaluation.

These basic techniques work for most infants. If the infant has any sort of hypotonia or craniofacial abnormality, however, some special techniques, described in Chapter 7, can be used.

Basic Positions for the Newborn

Three basic positions can be used when breastfeeding: (1) *cradle hold* (sometimes called *Madonna hold*), (2) *side-lying hold* (sometimes called *parallel hold*), and (3) *football hold* (sometimes called *clutch hold*). Regardless of which position is used, the infant's trunk should always be skin-to-skin with the mother; this is generally referred to as "tummy-to-tummy," or "chest-to-chest." This chest-to-chest technique permits the newborn's head and neck to be in good alignment; if the in-

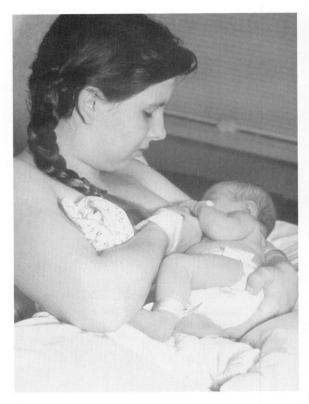

Fig. 5-6 Cradle hold, with correct chest-to-chest positioning and no space between the mother's body and newborn's body. This adolescent mother is supporting her newborn's buttocks close to her body, holding him skin-to-skin. (© *Debi Bocar, Lactation Consultant Services, Oklahoma City, Oklahoma. Used with permission.*)

fant is not chest-to-chest, he will need to turn his head in order to breastfeed, which interferes with swallowing. Teach the mother to recognize the difference between chest-to-chest as shown in Figure 5-6 and chest-to-ceiling, shown in Figure 5-7. When the infant is not chest-to-chest, point it out to the mother. Help her to visualize a camera that is hanging from the ceiling; if the camera would "see" the infant's skin between his nipples and umbilicus, he is not chest-to-chest.

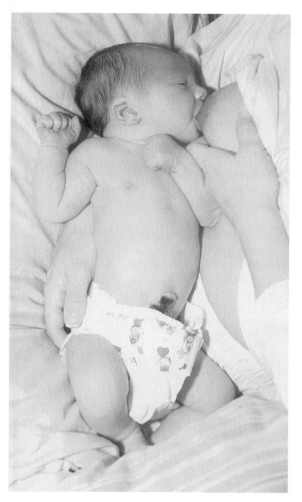

Fig. 5-7 Cradle hold, **incorrect.** Newborn is mostly on his back, making it necessary for him to turn his head to the breast. (© *Debi Bocar, Lactation Consultant Services, Oklahoma City, Oklahoma. Used with permission.*)

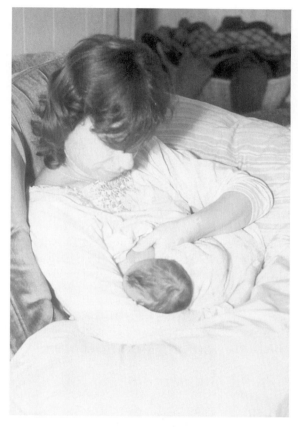

Fig. 5-8 Cradle hold. Newborn is curled around mother's abdomen in cradle hold with pillow support. Mother supports breast with palmar grasp. (© *Debi Bocar, Lactation Consultant Services, Oklahoma City, Oklahoma. Used with permission.*)

Cradle Position

The cradle position, shown in Figure 5-8, is used most frequently in America. This position works well for most mothers. It is important to remember, however, that this is only one option; mothers may need to use a different position, but they will generally identify this one first because it is similar to the position they have seen used by bottle-feeding mothers. A few important points that are frequently overlooked include the following:

- Make sure infant is chest-to-chest.
- Discourage the mother from holding the infant above the level of the nipple; the milk would need to overcome gravity to be transferred to the infant.

- Alert the mother to not hold the infant below the level of the nipple; this will cause a "drag" on the nipple and subsequent bruising.
- Point out that the infant's head should not be directly in the antecubital fossa, as bottle-fed infants are held. Rather, the infant should rest slightly lower on the mother's forearm, so that he will be better aligned.

Side-Lying Position

The side-lying position, shown in Figure 5-9, works well for nighttime feeding, when the mother does not want to get up and sit in a chair, or for the mother who has delivered vaginally and is trying to avoid sitting on her "sore bottom." It also works for mothers who have had cesarean deliveries. Furthermore, the mother who has had a cesarean delivery may be able to use both breasts without rolling over. Instruct the woman to feed first from the bottom breast (the one nearest the mattress); then, when the infant has finished on that side, she can "tuck" the first breast under her torso and offer the upper breast. This works reasonably well for mothers who have neither especially large nor especially small breasts. Use a rolled-up receiving blanket behind the baby to maintain his position and a pillow tucked behind the mother's back to maintain her position and comfort.

Football Position

The football hold, shown in Figure 5-10, is useful for mothers who have had a cesarean delivery because it eliminates the fear that the infant will

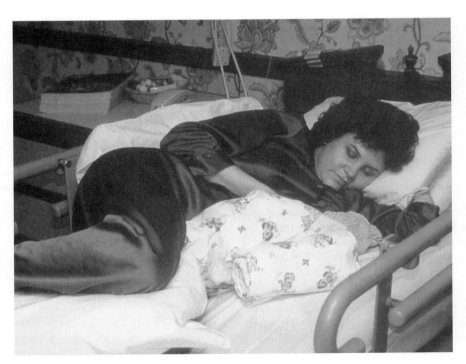

Fig. 5-9 Side-lying hold. *(© Debi Bocar, Lactation Consultant Services, Oklahoma City, Oklahoma. Used with permission.)*

kick the mother's incision. The football hold is also useful if the mother needs better visualization of the latch-on process. It can also be used when the mother wishes to offer a second breast without moving her own position; she can move the infant from a cradle position on the left breast to the football position on the right breast.

These common positions should work well under most circumstances. Special circumstances require other techniques, discussed in Chapter 7.

All of the basic positions can be used by mothers after vaginal or cesarean births, but the mother should be encouraged to find the one that is most comfortable for her, given her set of circumstances. A summary of advantages, disadvantages, and important tips is provided in Table 5-1.

The Nurse's Role in Achieving Effective Latch-On

The nurse plays a key role in helping the mother and infant achieve effective latch-on and milk transfer. It is the nurse's responsibility to watch for early feeding cues, assist with latch-on, determine if suckling is effective, and answer feeding-related questions.

Watch for Early Readiness Cues

Ideally, the infant should go to the breast in the quiet alert state. Box 5-3 summarizes early hunger cues that occur during this quiet alert state. Typically, licking movements will precede the rooting reflex; when this happens, the tongue is correctly placed in the bottom of the mouth cavity. However, if the infant is forced to the breast before licking and rooting occur, the rooting reflex may be abolished, resulting in the tongue being placed in the palate and consequently, improper attachment. Also see Chapter 6, which describes interventions to assist the sleepy newborn.

Assist With Latch-On

Good latch-on is prerequisite for milk transfer. When latched on properly, as shown in Figure 5-11, the infant will successfully obtain a quantity of milk adequate to meet his needs, and the mother will be free of sore nipples. Proper latch-on results in audible swallowing, a hallmark of successful milk transfer.

The nipple should be centered. The mother can easily visualize this as a nose-to-nipple idea. If the infant's nose is directly in line with the mother's nipple, he is centered. Instruct the mother to

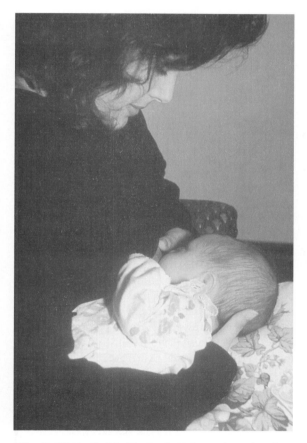

Fig. 5-10 Football hold. *(© Debi Bocar, Lactation Consultant Services, Oklahoma City, Oklahoma. Used with permission.)*

T A B L E 5-1
ADVANTAGES AND LIMITATIONS OF BASIC POSITIONS

Position	Advantages	Limitations	Pertinent Points
Cradle hold	• Women are most likely to have seen this position used • Works best for most situations	• Difficult to achieve good sitting position in hospital bed; use chair if possible • Requires sitting; cesarean incision or hemorrhoids may make sitting a less desirable position	• Be sure that infant is chest-to-chest rather than chest-to-ceiling • Infant should be at the level of the nipple
Side-lying	• Helpful after cesarean birth • Great for nighttime feedings	• Difficult to visualize latch	• Be sure that infant is chest-to-chest rather than chest-to-ceiling • Use folded receiving blanket behind infant to maintain chest-to-chest position • Mother's body should be at a slight angle to the mattress, leaning backward just a bit against a pillow
Football	• Helpful after cesarean birth • Helpful for women with especially large breasts • Provides better visualization of latch-on process	• Often difficult to do sitting up in hospital bed	• Be sure that infant is chest-to-chest rather than chest-to-ceiling

Box 5-3
Signs of Hunger and Satiety

Signs of Hunger
- Rooting
- Sucking motions
- Motor activity; hands-to-mouth, flexion of arms, legs moving as though riding a bicycle
- Posture/affect: tense; clenched fists
- Crying is the *last* sign of hunger

Signs of Satiety
- Audible swallowing during the feeding
- Cessation of audible swallowing; increased non-nutritive sucking and longer pauses between sucking bursts
- Infant takes himself off from the breast, rather than being taken off
- Disappearance of hunger cues
- Posture/affect: arms and legs relaxed, drowsy
- Sleeping

use her fingers to tilt the nipple; it should be aimed toward the roof of the infant's mouth. He should be ready to go to the breast chin first, and as soon as he has adequately grasped the nipple, the mother should stop aiming the nipple upward.

Show the mother how to stimulate the infant with her nipple; allow him to search and make progressively more active movements to grasp the nipple. Explain that she may need to alternately offer and withdraw the nipple before he opens wide. It is imperative, however, to wait until the infant has opened *wide*, as shown in Figure 5-12. This open-wide concept is central to achieving effective latch-on. The tongue should be troughed, or scoop-shaped. If the infant latches on before his mouth is gaping open, show the mother how to insert her finger between the mouth and her nipple to break the suction (to prevent sore nipples).

When the infant is ready—nipple centered,

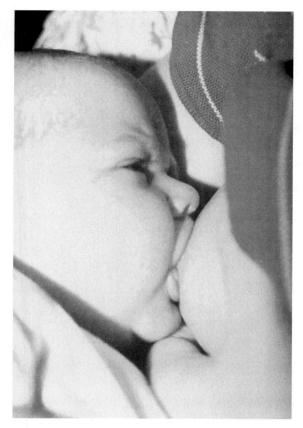

Fig. 5-11 Excellent latch-on. (© *Debi Bocar, Lactation Consultant Services, Oklahoma City, Oklahoma. Used with permission.*)

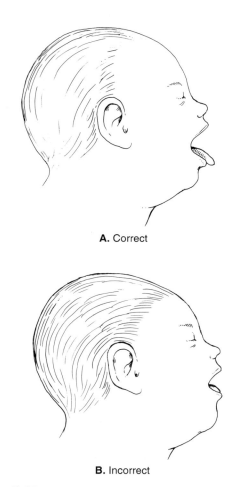

A. Correct

B. Incorrect

Fig. 5-12 Wait until the infant's mouth is opened wide before he grasps the breast. **A,** Shows how the mouth should be gaping with tongue troughed and extended over the lower alveolar ridge and lower lip. **B,** Shows mouth that is not completely gaping, with a flat tongue, resulting in poor latch-on.

mouth gaping open, tongue troughed—quickly move the mother's arm to bring the infant onto the nipple/areola complex. Note that the directive here is to move the mother's arm, not to push the baby's head onto the breast. Such an action stimulates the infant's reflex to hyperextend the neck, which is not desirable. Also, swiftly moving the mother's arm gives her the kinesthetic feeling of how to accomplish latch-on, and, in the absence of the nurse, she will not feel a need for an extra hand.

Show the mother how to bring the infant onto the breast chin first. While we frequently preach that the infant should "take as much of the areola as possible," this might not be the best advice; one experienced clinician points out that this advice causes women to bring the infant's mouth farther *up* onto the breast, rather than having the chin indent the breast *below* the

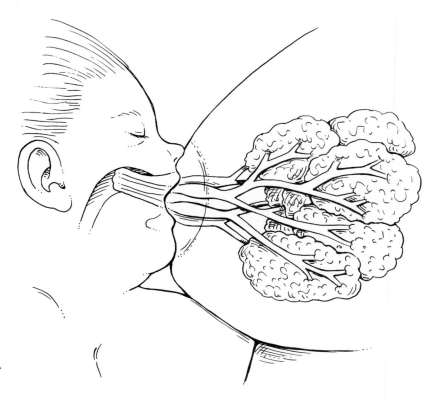

Fig. 5-13 Lateral view of breast (with anatomy) and position of infant's mouth.

nipple.[39] If properly positioned, the chin should slightly indent the breast as shown in early x-rays.[2] Remember that at first the mother relies on visualization; because she cannot see the underside of her breast, bringing the infant on chin first increases the likelihood that his gums will compress the lactiferous sinuses properly, as shown in Figure 5-13.

Explain Ramifications of Effective and Ineffective Latch-On

Effective latch-on is easy to achieve with only a small amount of practice. When infants are latched on incorrectly, multiple problems result. If the problems are left uncorrected, women whose infants have ineffective suckling techniques are more likely to wean early than those who receive help.[5] Effective latch-on prevents most of the problems associated with sore nipples (see Chapter 8). Furthermore, mothers who experience problems with breastfeeding and use compensatory strategies (including supplementation) to overcome them are more likely to discontinue breastfeeding.[40]

Determine If Suckling Is Effective

The infant's mouth on the mother's breast does not equal breastfeeding; audible swallowing is required for breastfeeding! Swallowing can occur at the very first breastfeeding episode moments after birth, but it may be difficult to hear. First, it doesn't happen very often because it takes many, many sucks to yield a sufficient volume of fluid required to trigger the swallowing reflex. Second, when it does happen, it is not very loud—to hear it, it helps to have an ear very close to the newborn. If the newborn is latched on correctly, most parents can hear swallowing during the first few hours if it is pointed out to them. During the first 24 hours or so, the infant may be sleepy and have few sustained periods of audible swallowing so it may be difficult to hear swallowing. After this time, however, absence of audible swallowing requires follow-up. *Audible swallowing is one of the most important evaluation criteria.* The presence of swallowing may not guarantee that all is well, but absence of swallowing is a sure sign that something is wrong. Audible swallowing is evidence that milk is being removed from the breast; without this removal, more milk will not be produced.

Nonpathological Causes of Ineffective Suckling

Most of the problems with ineffective suckling are likely to be caused by poor positioning and latch-on, and all are likely to result in sore nipples (discussed in Chapter 8). Most times, ineffective suckling at the breast is the result of poor latch-on related to inexperience of the infant, the mother, or both. Perhaps the most telling visual cue is the pistonlike motion (jaws move up and down in a choppy motion rather than a smooth, undulating motion), gumming the nipple or areola. In all of these cases, the tongue is positioned behind the gum line rather than over the lower alveolar ridge. Sometimes, clicking or smacking can be heard as well.[41] The most telling auditory cue is lack of swallowing; if audible swallowing is present, milk transfer is occurring.

In a healthy, full-term newborn, most of these problems can be swiftly resolved with some simple interventions. Signs of ineffective suckling are listed in Table 5-2. Most frequently, *the root of the problem is that the infant has not opened wide.* Instruct the mother to break the suction and elicit a wide-open mouth before latching the infant onto the breast. If the tongue is indeed over the lower alveolar ridge during latch-on, the po-

sition of the tongue is not the problem. Introduce a little glucose water or milk via a dental syringe at the corner of the mouth while the infant is at the breast. This bolus of fluid helps to initiate the suck/swallow reflex and encourages the infant to use his tongue in an undulating motion.

In the past decade or so, anecdotal reports have described suck training, a deliberate manipulation of the newborn's oral cavity, to alleviate the problems associated with suckling during the early days.[42] There have not, however, been any controlled studies that show that suck training is effective. With a few simple interventions, such as those just described, and a little time and experience, ineffective suckling frequently disappears.

Pathological Causes of Ineffective Suckling

Sometimes, ineffective suckling is the result of more generalized problems. The data the nurse gathers can assist in determining whether this observation is a breastfeeding problem or a symptom of pathology. For example, a newborn who has a neurological deficit will have poor rooting and other reflexes, and may not be able to exert enough negative pressure to hold the nipple/areola in place. Infants with these sorts of problems will be discussed in Chapter 7.

Answer Feeding-Related Questions

Mothers raise numerous questions to which nurses must respond. The most important guideline to answering questions is this: keep it simple! Creating too many "rules" for breastfeeding only dissuades women from continuing. The following are some common questions.

One Side or Two?

It is ideal for the infant to stimulate both breasts, particularly during the first month, but it is not imperative. Sometimes, removing the newborn from the first breast for the sole purpose of stimu-

T A B L E 5-2
EVALUATING THE EFFECTIVENESS OF LATCH-ON AND SUCK

Proper Alignment:

- Helps keep nipple and areola in infant's mouth
- Reduces traction on mother's nipples
- Facilitates swallowing

Proper Alignment	Improper Alignment	Nursing Interventions
Infant is flexed and relaxed	Muscular rigidity	Comfort and calm the infant Try a football hold to get flexion
Head and body are at breast level	Head and body sagging; baby "reaching" for the breast	Provide pillows to facilitate baby's head and body at breast level
Head squarely facing breast	Head turned: • Laterally • Hyperextended • Hyperflexed	Help mother to adjust her hold on infant Do not force baby's head against the nipple. Instead, help mother to move arm to align infant
Infant's body aligned from shoulder to iliac crest	• Trunk facing the ceiling instead of skin-to-skin with mother • This results in poor compression of the sinuses and obstructed swallowing	Hold "tummy-to-tummy"

Areolar Grasp:

Peristaltic motions of tongue result in effective areolar compression, i.e., compression of the lactiferous sinuses.

Proper Areolar Grasp	Improper Areolar Grasp	Nursing Interventions
Infant's mouth opens widely to cover lactiferous sinuses	Pursed lips indicate that mouth is not open wide enough	Tickle lips with nipple or finger Move mother's arm quickly toward breast when baby finally opens wide (see text)
Lips flanged outward	Lips pursed: lip(s) curled under	As above
Complete seal formed around areola; strong vacuum	Incomplete seal; baby can be easily pulled away from nipple	Hook your finger (or have mother hook her finger) under infant's chin
Approximately 1.5 inches of areolar tissue is centered in infant's mouth	Only nipple is in mouth, or nipple is not centered	Break suction and reposition
Tongue is troughed and extends over lower alveolar ridge	Tongue partially inside mouth Nurse has "biting" sensation if she inserts her finger in infant's mouth Results in sore nipples and diminished milk supply Likely to happen if infant does not open wide	Break suction and reposition

Note: Data in left column expanded from Shrago L, Bocar D. The infant's contribution to breastfeeding. *J Obstetr Gynecol Neonatal Nurs* 1990;19(3):209-215. Table from Biancuzzo M. *Breastfeeding the Healthy Newborn* 1994:31-32. Copyright 1994 by March of Dimes Birth Defects Foundation. Reprinted by permission.

T A B L E 5-2

EVALUATING THE EFFECTIVENESS OF LATCH-ON AND SUCK—cont'd

Areolar Compression:

Removes milk from breast

Proper Areolar Compression	Improper Areolar Compression	Nursing Interventions
Mandible moves in a rhythmic motion	Mandible moves in tiny motions up and down; appears more like "chewing" instead of gliding	Break suction and reposition
If indicated, a digital suck assessment reveals a wave-like motion of the tongue from the anterior mouth toward the oropharynx; tongue is cupped or "troughed"	Incorrect tongue motions include: • Side-to-side movement • Deviation of the tongue to one side • Peristaltic movement from the posterior region to the anterior region of the tongue • Frank tongue thrusting (actively pushing the finger out of the mouth with the tongue) • Diminished negative pressure • Absence of seal around lips • Tongue not troughed	Digital suck assessment is not routinely performed Break suction and reposition Suck training has been advocated[42] but has not been proven effective in well-controlled, scientific studies Sucking is a reflex, and deviations in reflexes should be followed up with a complete neurologic assessment
Checks full and rounded when sucking	Cheeks dimple when sucking	Break suction and reposition

Audible Swallowing:

(Most reliable indicator of milk intake)

Proper	Improper	Nursing Interventions
Audible swallowing present	Lack of audible swallowing	Reevaluate alignment, areolar grasp, areolar compression
Quiet sound of swallowing is heard	No swallowing is heard	Break suction; take baby off breast and try again. Be sure to get baby to open wide, which frequently solves the problem
May be preceded by several sucking motions, especially in first few days	Even after many rapid sucks, infant does not display rhythmic sucking motion and swallowing is not heard	Reevaluate latch-on Evaluate milk supply Evaluate milk ejection reflex
May increase in frequency and consistency after milk ejection reflex occurs	No change in observable pattern after milk ejection occurs; flutter-sucking more common	Reevaluate latch-on Evaluate milk supply Evaluate milk ejection reflex

lating the second breast may deprive him of the hindmilk that, left to his own efforts, he would have happily suckled. When interrupted before finishing, preterm newborns may "forget" what they were doing when offered the second breast. Infants exhibit no differences in restlessness, crying, frequency of feedings, wet diapers, or loose stools when fed from one rather than two breasts.[43]

Sometimes, stimulating both breasts is not possible if the infant falls asleep. Instruct the mother to start on the side where she left off last time because infants suck most vigorously on the first side. One way to remember this is for the mother to attach a pin to her bra on the side where she left off.

Starting on the side where she left off might not always be practical, however. If, for example, the mother has an awkward IV site, it would do no harm to start on the side where she is most comfortable until after the IV is removed. This strategy would increase her chances for feeling successful and would increase the likelihood of successful milk transfer to the infant. If the mother has a sore breast, correct the root of the problem, but meanwhile start on the least sore side first, since the infant suckles more vigorously on the first side.

Mothers frequently comment that the infant has a "favorite" side. In reality, the mother probably is more comfortable holding the infant on one side—usually the left side, regardless of which hand is dominant. Mothers may ask what will happen if the infant feeds more often or more vigorously at the same side over a period of time. Reassure the mother that nothing "bad" happens; the uneven stimulation may result in one breast being slightly larger than the other, but there are no negative effects for the infant.

Rotating Positions

Frequently, mothers are told that they must always alternate the position they use—cradle hold this time, side-lying next time, and football hold the next time. This advice is based on the idea that pressure from the infant's mouth will cause soreness to the mother's nipple. This advice is not necessarily bad, but it usually is superfluous. First, it requires the mother to learn several positions when she may be struggling to learn just one. Second, poor latch-on, in any position, is usually the cause for sore nipples; rotating the position will not prevent sore nipples if this is the root of the problem. Rotating positions may, however, be useful if the infant has a barracuda style of sucking.

Burping and Sleep Positions

Typically, mothers think that infants should be positioned over their shoulder and patted vigorously for burping. This is usually unnecessary. Infants can be burped simply by keeping their torso straight—explain that the baby's "food pipe" needs to be straight. If the infant is crying, however, put him over the shoulder. An infant can also be burped by sitting him on the caregiver's lap with a hand on his chest, leaning forward a bit. Recommend to mothers that they give the newborn the opportunity to burp after nursing at one breast, but if the infant does not burp, don't worry about it; some infants don't take in much air and won't need to burp. Signs that the infant needs to burp include arching the back, throwing out the legs, and pulling away from the breast.

Nipple Confusion

Much controversy has come about over so-called nipple confusion. Nipple confusion supposedly happens when the newborn is introduced to artificial nipples (and bottles) and then "forgets" how to suckle the breast correctly, or, rather, uses the pistonlike tongue motion and negative pressure to attempt transfer of milk. Some self-help books imply that as little as one bottle will result in this so-called confusion, while a well-controlled prospective study showed that mothers who are highly motivated to nurse can give one bottle per day with no significant impact on the duration of breastfeeding.[44] Perhaps both are right, and the difference lies in the skill of the infant or the motivation of the mother.

Well-respected experts have suggested that the term *nipple confusion* should be limited to describing only newborns who have not learned to nurse well (not older infants). Furthermore, they specify that the term be used only for those situations where an infant may or may not have breastfed successfully but was offered an artificial nipple and subsequently had difficulty achieving good latch-on at the breast, rather than using it

Box 5-4
Hypotheses to Explain Nipple Confusion

1. A neonate may have limited ability to adapt to various oral configurations. When a newborn infant who has been breastfed is given an artificial teat to suck, such as a pacifier, bottle nipple, or adult finger, this stimulus may intercept the physiological action of normal breastfeeding, and the infant may readjust to a sucking pattern that compresses and controls the teat. In addition, if a higher volume and faster flow of fluid is obtained by bottle feeding than by breastfeeding, the infant may adapt his or her oral configuration to control the increased fluid flow.

2. A form of "imprinting" may occur in the immediate postpartum period. If the first feeding after birth is given by bottle, the artificial nipple may be imprinted in the infant and make subsequent attempts at breastfeeding more difficult.

3. Newborn infants may be vulnerable to nipple confusion because of the relatively low volume of colostrum available with breastfeeding in the first few days of life. Before full lactogenesis, the amount of colostrum available is small, and even after the true milk comes in, infants must nurse correctly to obtain generous quantities during breastfeeding. Measurements of milk intake by breastfed newborn infants have documented intakes of about 1 oz (30 ml) in the first 24 hours after birth. Thus if a neonate is given the opportunity to feed from a 3- or 4-oz (90- to 120-ml) bottle on the first day of life, at a time when only a minimum quantity of milk would be available during a single breastfeeding session, the infant might act fretful during attempts at breastfeeding.

4. Infants who have difficulty with their initial attempts at breastfeeding may be more prone to manifest nipple confusion. Not only is the poorly feeding infant more likely to receive supplemental bottle feedings, but an infant who has not learned to grasp and suckle the maternal nipple correctly is likely to perceive bottle feeding as easier and more rewarding than the breast.

From Neifert M, Lawrence R, Seacat J. Nipple confusion: toward a formal definition. *J Pediatr* 1995;126:S126-S127.

for the infant who displays a primary inability to suckle the breast effectively without prior exposure to an artificial teat.[45] These researchers have formulated the only hypotheses to date; their hypotheses to explain the phenomenon of nipple confusion are summarized on Box 5-4. The reader is strongly encouraged to read the original source, since it is the only work to date that deals with this phenomenon from a scientific standpoint, completely unadulterated by personal experience and myth.

Pacifiers
During the last few decades, hospital personnel have regularly given pacifiers to newborns. The use of pacifiers, however, has been associated with early termination of breastfeeding.[46-50] Furthermore, mothers of infants who use a pacifier for more than 2 hours per day experience more breastfeeding problems.[5,46,50] These studies, however, do not substantiate a cause-and-effect relationship; there is only an association. One study,[50] described further in the Research Highlight, has addressed the characteristics of the mothers who use the pacifier more and other studies have been published as this book goes to press.

A few commonsense ideas guide clinical recommendations. First, pacifiers should never be used to replace or "hold off" a feeding. Second, the mother should be fully informed that there is a clear relationship between using a pacifier and early termination. Third, forbidding the use of the pacifier will not necessarily increase the length of time that an infant is breastfed. Rather, there must be a clear emphasis on letting the infant control the feeding frequency, pace, and termination rather than having the mother control these factors by using the pacifier or some other method.

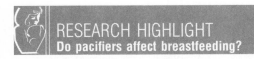

RESEARCH HIGHLIGHT
Do pacifiers affect breastfeeding?

Citation
Victora CG, Behague DP, Barros FC, Olinto MTA, Weiderpass E. Pacifier use and short breastfeeding duration: cause, consequence, or coincidence? *Pediatrics* 1997;99: 445-453.

Focus
This prospective study used a combination epidemiological and ethnographic approach. The epidemiological aim was to (1) describe pacifier use and breastfeeding patterns; (2) investigate the association between pacifier use and subsequent breastfeeding; (3) check reverse causality; (4) understand the mechanisms mediating the association; (5) rule out a large number of possible confounding variables; and (6) identify factors that may modify the relation of pacifiers to breastfeeding. The ethnographic study aimed to explore (1) how much and why mothers value pacifier use; (2) how mothers stimulated pacifier use; (3) how readily the infants actually take the pacifiers; and (4) the presence of self-selection.

Results
Almost half of the mothers took the pacifiers to the hospital, and about 85% of mothers were using pacifiers 1 month after birth. Some who did not use pacifiers while they were breastfeeding used them after weaning, suggesting reverse causality. Bottles were a possible confounding factor, as more than 84% of 1-month-old infants used bottles. There was a strong relationship between pacifier use at 1 month and breastfeeding discontinuation; greater use of the pacifier (more hours per day) varied directly with discontinuation of breastfeeding. Further, mothers saw the pacifier as a "luxury," and many strongly stimulated the infant to accept the pacifier, even after he refused it. Mothers who used the pacifier with greater intensity (more hours per day and more stimulation to get the infant to accept it) had breastfeeding behaviors that restricted infant-led feeding.

Strengths, Limitations of the Study
A large sample size (605 subjects) and the careful attention to confounding variables were clear strengths of this study. The study was conducted in Brazil, and few of the infants were exclusively breastfed, both of which limit the generalizability of the findings to other populations.

Clinical Application
Like earlier studies, this study shows an association between pacifier use and early discontinuation of breastfeeding. However, this is the first study to suggest that pacifiers may not be the culprit in early discontinuation of breastfeeding. Rather, the observation that the woman values the pacifier and uses it as one way to restrict infant-led breastfeeding interaction underscores the need to increase consumer education and change the cultural paradigm. Professionals need to help mothers develop realistic expectations about newborns' need for frequent feedings and comfort.

EVALUATION OF BREASTFEEDING

There is no substitute for direct observation of the breastfeeding process. Every mother—primipara or multipara—should have a nurse evaluate whether breastfeeding is going well.

Determining the effectiveness of breastfeeding is the nurse's responsibility, and shifting this responsibility to anyone else is negligence. As in the adult patient, where the nurse is responsible for observing, recording intake and output—and intervening if the intake or output is inadequate—so, too, the nurse has a responsibility to assess the intake (breastfeeding) of the newborn. Similarly, the nurse is responsible for assessing many other parameters of the newborn's physical well-being.

Documenting Appraisal of Breastfeeding Efforts

Traditionally, documentation of the breastfed infant's intake has been grossly inadequate. Most hospitals use a subjective good-fair-poor rating, or reporting of the number of minutes of

T A B L E 5-3

COMPARISON OF BREASTFEEDING ASSESSMENT TOOLS

Characteristic	IBFAT	MBA	LATCH	SAIB
Focus on	Infant	Infant and mother	Infant and mother	Infant and mother
Scored by	Mother or nurse	Nurse	Mother or nurse	Nurse
Time frame	Progressive: beginning to ending	Progressive: beginning to ending	Static	Any point in the feeding
Analysis of sequential scores	Use mean of scores	Use best of scores	Expect increase in scores	Does not apply; this is a yes-no tool
Measures	Signaling Rooting Suckling	Readiness Position Latch-on; milk transfer Outcome	Latch-on Audible swallowing Nipple comfort Assistance needed with positioning	Alignment Areolar grasp Areolar compression Audible swallowing

Modified from Riordan JM, Koehn M. Reliability and validity testing of three breastfeeding assessment tools. *J Obstet Gynecol Neonatal Nurs* 1997;26:183.

breastfeeding. Good-fair-poor works well if the observer is well trained in breastfeeding management and if the clinician rating the feeding is actually present when it takes place. Documenting the number of minutes is virtually meaningless. First, it delivers a mixed message—telling mothers that they should watch the newborn, not the clock, and then asking them how many minutes he fed on each side. And, because it is a self-report system, the mother's reporting is accurate only if she uses a watch, which defeats the "watch the baby, not the clock" directive. Finally, the number of minutes the newborn was at the breast may be completely irrelevant. Resters will take longer than barracudas, for example. More important, however, if there was no milk transfer, any amount of time spent at the breast does not help to determine adequacy of intake.

A more objective method of determining intake is therefore needed. If the newborn has a clinical condition that requires close monitoring, test-weighing, described in the next section, is one way to quantify intake. Under most circumstances, however, it is best to use a tool that sim-ply documents the observation of the feeding. Numerous tools for evaluating and documenting the infant's breastfeeding efforts have been developed to overcome the subjectivity of good-fair-poor and time. Each of the following documentation tools was designed to provide some objective data, and most require direct observation, rather than relying on self-report. Table 5-3 compares four tools.

In order to be clinically useful, however, these tools must be clinically reliable (consistently measuring the concept or behavior they intend to) and valid (the extent to which the tool measures what it says it measures). So far in their development, the Infant Breastfeeding Assessment Tool (IBFAT), Mother-Baby Assessment (MBA), and LATCH tools described below were shown to be neither valid nor reliable according to one study.[51] The SAIB was not studied for reliability and validity. Further studies are needed.

SAIB

Shrago and Bocar developed the Systematic Assessment of the Infant at Breast (SAIB).[52] They

T A B L E 5-4

INFANT BREASTFEEDING ASSESSMENT TOOL

Score	3	2	1	0
Readiness to feed	Baby starts to feed readily without effort (alert)	Needs mild stimulation to start feeding	Needs more stimulation to rouse and start feeding	Cannot be roused
Rooting	Roots effectively immediately	Needs some coaxing, prompting, or encouragement to root	Roots poorly, even with coaxing	Did not try to root
Fixing ("latch-on")	Starts to feed immediately	Takes 3-10 minutes to start	Takes over 10 minutes to start	Did not feed
Sucking pattern	Sucks well on one or both breasts	Sucks on and off, but needs encouragement	Weak suck, suck on and off for short periods	Did not suck
Maximum possible	12	8	4	0

Data derived from Matthews MK. Developing an instrument to assess infant breastfeeding behavior in the early neonatal period. *Midwifery* 1988;4(4):154-165. Table adaptation reprinted from Biancuzzo M. *Breastfeeding the Healthy Newborn: A Nursing Perspective*. White Plains, NY: March of Dimes Birth Defect Foundation; 1994.

have identified criteria for evaluating the effectiveness of infant's breastfeeding behavior: alignment, areolar grasp, areolar compression, and audible swallowing. This tool's underlying principle is that when alignment, areolar grasp, areolar compression, and audible swallowing are present, breastfeeding is usually going well. The strength of this tool is that it is simple and straightforward to use, and it captures the most important points that the nurse should be observing in the breastfeeding couplet. The original criteria are found on the first column of Table 5-2; the other columns describe signs and symptoms of incorrect technique. Recommendations for correcting the problems associated with incorrect technique have been added to help the reader implement corrective strategies. A limitation is that, unlike the others, this tool has not been studied for reliability or validity.

IBFAT

Matthews developed the Infant Breastfeeding Assessment Tool (IBFAT).[53] This system assigns a score of 0, 1, 2, or 3 to behaviors such as readiness, rooting, fixing (latching on), and sucking.

The tool as written in the original text may be cumbersome to use; Table 5-4 summarizes the text that describes the scoring system. The tool has a clear advantage over others in that one of the criteria is readiness to feed. The tool's greatest strength is that it recognizes behavior that happens before the infant gets to the breast—the display of alertness and rooting behavior. A strong limitation of the system, however, is that the criteria do not address swallowing. If used, this tool should be modified to include information about the infant's swallowing.

LATCH

Jensen and colleagues developed the LATCH system.[54] This system assigns a score of 0, 1, or 2 to key elements, including latch-on, audible swallowing, type of nipple, comfort of the mother, and help mother needs. Table 5-5 describes the scoring. This documentation tool has some merits, including identification of key criteria and simplicity. A limitation is that the tool may overemphasize how much assistance the mother needs and minimize the actual observations of whether the infant is properly latched on.

TABLE 5-5

THE LATCH SCORING SYSTEM

	0	1	2
Latch	• Too sleepy or reluctant • No latch achieved	• Repeated attempts • Hold nipple in mouth • Stimulate to suck	• Grasps breast • Tongue down • Lips flanged • Rhythmic sucking
Audible swallowing	• None	• A few with stimulation	• Spontaneous and intermittent, 24 hours old • Spontaneous and frequent >24 hours old
Type of nipple	• Inverted	• Flat	• Everted (after stimulation)
Comfort (breast/nipple)	• Engorged • Cracked, bleeding, large blisters, or bruises	• Filling • Reddened/small blisters or bruises • Mild/moderate discomfort	• Soft • Tender
Hold (positioning)	• Full assist (staff holds infant at breast)	• Minimal assist (i.e., elevate head of bed; place pillows for support) • Teach one side; mother does other • Staff holds and then mother takes over	• No assist from staff • Mother able to position/hold infant

From Jensen D, Wallace S, Kelsay P. LATCH: a breastfeeding charting system and documentation tool. *J Obstet Gynecol Neonatal Nurs* 1994;23:29.

Mother-Baby Assessment

Mulford has devised the Mother-Baby Assessment (MBA),[55] as described in Table 5-6, to evaluate and document the infant's breastfeeding efforts using a score fashioned after the Apgar score. A strength of this tool is that it evaluates maternal recognition of and response to feeding cues, as well as how the feeding ends. A limitation is that, like the others, it has not been shown to be reliable or valid.

Parameters Beyond the Breastfeeding Interaction

There is no substitute for direct observation of the breastfeeding interaction. To more completely evaluate milk transfer and correct unmet needs, however, other parameters such as weighing and growth spurts should be monitored.

Test Weighing

Routine test weighing—weighing before and after a feeding—should be reserved for cases where the infant is not healthy. Otherwise, the procedure may erode the mother's confidence by emphasizing the outcome rather than the process of breastfeeding. If test weighing is indicated, it is acceptable to use electronic scales, since they are more accurate than other methods.[56] Prior to the 1980s, objections to test-weighing prevailed, and these objections had a sound rationale. In those days, test-weighing was accomplished using the balance scales, which did not have the accuracy that modern-day electronic scales now provide.

Weight Gain/Loss

A parent or professional frequently asks, "How much weight did he gain?" This question is a good

TABLE 5-6

USING THE MBA SCORING SYSTEM

Steps	Points	What to Look For/Criteria
1. Signaling	1	Mother watches and listens for baby's cues. She may hold, stroke, rock, talk to baby. She stimulates baby if he is sleepy, calms baby if he is fussy.
	1	Baby gives readiness cues: stirring, alertness, rooting, sucking, hand-to-mouth, vocal cues, cry.
2. Positioning	1	Mother holds baby in good alignment within latch-on range of nipple. Baby's body is slightly flexed, entire ventral surface facing mother's body. Baby's head and shoulders are supported.
	1	Baby roots well at breast, opens mouth wide, tongue cupped and covering lower gum.
3. Fixing	1	Mother holds her breast to assist baby as needed, brings baby in close when his mouth is wide open. She may express drops of milk.
	1	Baby latches on, takes all of nipple and about 2 cm (1 in) of areola into mouth, then suckles, demonstrating a recurrent burst-pause sucking pattern.
4. Milk transfer	1	Mother reports feeling any of the following: thirst, uterine cramps, increased lochia, breast ache or tingling, relaxation, sleepiness. Milk leaks from opposite breast.
	1	Baby swallows audibly; milk is observed in baby's mouth, baby may spit up milk when burping. Rapid "call-up sucking" rate (two sucks/second) changes to "nutritive sucking" rate of about one suck/second.
5. Ending	1	Mother's breasts are comfortable; she lets baby suckle until he is finished. After nursing, her breasts feel softer; she has no lumps, engorgement, or nipple soreness.
	1	Baby releases breast spontaneously, appears satiated. Baby does not root when stimulated. Baby's face, arms, and hands are relaxed; baby may fall asleep.
	$\overline{10}$	

This is an assessment method for rating the progress of a mother and baby who are *learning* to breastfeed.

For every step, each person—both mother and baby—should receive a "+" before either one can be scored on the following step. If the observer does not observe any of the designated indicators, score "0" for that person on that step.

If help is needed at any step for either the mother or the baby, check "Help" for that step. This notation will not change the total score for mother and baby.

From Mulford C. The mother-baby assessment (MBA): an "Apgar score" for breastfeeding. *J Hum Lact* 1992;8:82.

one, but it sometimes implies that weight gain is the sole means of quantifying infant well-being or breastfeeding success; it is a factor, but not the sole indicator. Neither does it imply maternal failure or success; mothers frequently worry that they "don't have enough milk." These two issues are certainly related, but problems with weight gain are not necessarily caused by an insufficient milk supply. Determining the adequacy of infant weight gain involves more than simply putting the infant on the scales. Observing the infant at the breast is the best indicator for determining whether milk transfer occurs; other clinical parameters, such as weight, length, and head circumference, help to form a broader picture of the infant's overall well-being. The Historical Highlight identifies several subjective and objective data to observe and record when weight gains are inappropriate.

Weight from Birth to 1 Week

Most healthy, full-term newborns weigh between 2250 and 3900 g at birth (for a discussion of weight in relation to gestational age, see Chapter 7). Newborns weighing 1500 to 2499 g are considered low-birth weight, and those who weigh

Historical Highlight

Milk Ejection Reflex and the Mother-Baby Connection

A descriptive study was undertaken in 1949 at the Hospital of the University of Pennsylvania to determine whether the milk-ejection reflex influenced exclusive breastfeeding past 4 days postpartum. A total of 127 breastfeeding women were recruited for the study and were asked about their signs of milk ejection during the first 4 days. The investigator looked for both objective and subjective signs of the milk-ejection reflex. Objective signs included (1) uterine cramps, (2) contralateral dripping, (3) dripping when the infant was not suckling, and (4) cessation of nipple pain after the infant had sucked for a few seconds. The objective sign was the test-weighing of the infant to determine milk intake. Those with more signs and symptoms of milk-ejection reflex were more likely to be exclusively breastfeeding by the fourth day postpartum.

This study raises many questions for today's nurse, who may be seeing mothers immediately postpartum or following up later in a home visit, clinic visit, or telephone assessment. When we see infants with inappropriate weight gains, do we ask about signs of milk ejection? Do we routinely ask mothers about the presence of uterine cramping while breastfeeding, contralateral dripping, dripping at times other than breastfeeding, or cessation of nipple pain after the infant has suckled? Where on our flow sheet can we record these signs and symptoms of milk ejection? We often become focused on objective and subjective indicators associated with other bodily processes or diseases, but we are less aware of the signs and symptoms of milk ejection. It is important to keep in mind that "the [milk ejection reflex] is a psychosomatic mechanism which influences the expulsion of milk which has already been secreted," (p 726). Even if milk is secreted, without milk ejection, there can be no transfer. The nurse often has the opportunity to reduce environmental factors that interfere with the milk-ejection reflex, such as stress or distraction, or to enhance factors that promote the reflex, such as relaxation.

From Newton NR, Newton MN. Relation of the let-down reflex to the ability to breastfeed. *Pediatrics* 1950;5:726-733.

less than 1500 grams are considered very low birth weight. It is not at all uncommon for newborns to lose weight during the first few days, since they are born with extra fluids "on board" to compensate for the fact that the mother's rich colostrum does not provide much fluid. Assuming that the infant goes to breast frequently during the first couple of days, a volume of milk will be available before the third day.

It is unlikely that the newborn will gain weight during the first week or so of life. A 5% weight loss during this time is acceptable, if all is going well, but beware of any mother or newborn factors that signal trouble. A 10% weight loss is the outside limit of what is acceptable. By 7 to 10 days the newborn should start to "turn the corner," gradually gaining a little weight.

Weight from 7 to 28 Days

By 2 weeks, the newborn should have completely regained his birth weight. As a general rule, a weight gain of at least 1/2 ounce per day during the first month is appropriate.[6] Infants who gain less than this amount require medical follow-up.

Continued Weight Gains

It has often been assumed that unless breastfed infants gained weight according to the standard growth charts, they were underfed. Breastfed infants do not gain weight at the same rate as bottle-fed infants. For this reason, breastfed infants sometimes receive supplemental feedings because they are not gaining weight as rapidly as their bottle-fed cohorts. It is important to remember that the graphs used to determine adequacy of

Box 5-5
Helpful Points for the First Month of Life

Infant Weight Gain
- Baby will probably lose 5% to 10% of birth weight the first week. By 7 to 10 days, baby should "turn the corner" and start to gain.
- Baby will gain approximately ½ to 1 oz per day after that, during the first month.

How Much Is Enough?

Maintaining Weight
100 kcal/kg/day

Gaining Weight
120 kcal/kg/day

Mother's Milk

Calories
- Colostrum = 20 kcal/oz
- Mature Milk = 22 kcal/oz

Pumping Time
If pumping, mother should achieve a total pumping time of 90 to 100 minutes per day.

Total Volume
Mother will produce about 750 g of milk per day by 1 month. (This, of course, varies with the number of times per day that the breast is stimulated.)

Calculating Weight Loss From Birth
- Identify birth weight
- Subtract present weight from birth weight; this will give you the difference.
- Multiply the *difference* by 100, and divide by the birth weight. This will give you the *percentage* of weight lost.

Approximate Equivalents
28 g = 1 oz (approximately)
1 kg = 2.2 lb

Conversions
To convert baby's weight to metric:
- Multiply the number of pounds by 16, so that you have the total *ounces* that the baby weighs.
- Multiply that by 28. This will be the approximate number of grams that the baby weighs.

Example: Baby weighs 8 lb 4 oz
Calculation:
8 lb × 16 = 128 oz. Add 4 oz. Baby weighs a total of 132 oz.
(132 × 28) = 3584 g

---

weight gain were based on studies conducted during the 1950s, when most infants were bottle fed. More recent studies that focus on the difference between breastfeeding and bottle feeding show that breastfed infants gain weight more rapidly during the first 2 months and less rapidly from month 3 to 12 than bottle-fed infants.[57] Box 5-5 contains helpful information for determining intake and needs in relation to weight gain.

"Growth Spurts"
Unlike in the teenage boy who suddenly grows out of his trousers, "growth spurts" in newborns—usually around 2 weeks, 6 weeks, and 3 months—reflect the infant's need for increased calories. This situation is best handled by forewarning the mother that it will occur. Advise her to put the

infant to the breast as often as he is hungry; usually the mother's supply will meet the infant's need within about 72 hours.

Output

During the first few days, two or three wet diapers per day is probably sufficient, since the mother's milk has not become abundant and the infant is born with a supply of extra fluids. If the mother has had a particularly long labor, multiple episodes of vomiting during labor, or other factors that would cause her to be somewhat dehydrated, the infant is likely to have diminished urine output during those first few days. For the remainder of the first month, advise the mother to look for at least six wet diapers, with one really soaked—

eight wet diapers per day would be preferable— and to report any smaller output. Discourage mothers from using ultraabsorbent diapers during the first month because these make it difficult to accurately determine voiding patterns.

The newborn has a strong gastrocolic reflex and usually produces stools with each feeding. At minimum, however, he should have at least one stool per day during the first month of life; the stool should be fairly loose and nonmalodorous.[6] Tell the mother that if during the first month the newborn does not have at least three stools per day that look like cottage cheese and mustard, she should call the pediatrician. During the newborn period, lack of at least one stool per day is a marker for inadequate weight gain. Reassure the mother, however, that after the first month of life, it is not at all uncommon for breastfed infants to go several days without stooling.

SUMMARY/CONCLUSION

Breastfeeding is truly a reciprocal process. Mothers produce and eject milk, and the milk is transferred to the infant when he suckles effectively. Maternal milk supply best meets infant's demand when breastfeeding is initiated early and is not restricted in any way. Achieving good positioning and latch-on is critical, and the nurse has a responsibility to assist the mother with these efforts. Immediate evaluation of the breastfeeding interaction is best accomplished through direct observation, but ongoing evaluation is also needed.

References

1. Ardran GM, Kemp FH, Lind J. A cineradiographic study of bottle feeding. *Br J Radiol* 1956;31:11-22.
2. Ardran GM, Kemp FH, Lind J. A cineradiographic study of breast feeding. *Br J Radiol* 1958;31:156-162.
3. Woolridge MW. Aetiology of sore nipples. *Midwifery* 1986;2:172-176.
4. Nowak AJ, Smith WL, Erenberg A. Imaging evaluation of artificial nipples during bottle feeding. *Arch Pediatr Adolesc Med* 1994;148:40-42.
5. Righard L, Alade MO. Sucking technique and its effect on success of breastfeeding. *Birth* 1992;19:185-189.
6. Lawrence RA. *Breastfeeding: A Guide for the Medical Profession*. 4th ed. St. Louis: Mosby; 1994.
7. Wolff PH. The serial organization of sucking in the young infant. *Pediatrics* 1968;42:943-956.
8. Bowen-Jones A, Thompson C, Drewett RF. Milk flow and sucking rates during breast-feeding. *Dev Med Child Neurol* 1982;24:626-633.
9. Drewett RF, Woolridge M. Sucking patterns of human babies on the breast. *Early Hum Dev* 1979;3:315-321.
10. Woolridge MW, Baum JD, Drewett RF. Does a change in the composition of human milk affect sucking patterns and milk intake? *Lancet* 1980;2:1292-1293.
11. Weber F, Woolridge MW, Baum JD. An ultrasonographic study of the organisation of sucking and swallowing by newborn infants. *Dev Med Child Neurol* 1986;28:19-24.
12. Daly SE, Hartmann PE. Infant demand and milk supply. Part 2: The short-term control of milk synthesis in lactating women. *J Hum Lact* 1995;11:27-37.
13. DeCarvalho M, Robertson S, Friedman A, Klaus M. Effect of frequent breast-feeding on early milk production and infant weight gain. *Pediatrics* 1983;72:307-311.
14. Daly SE, Kent JC, Huynh DQ, et al. The determination of short-term breast volume changes and the rate of synthesis of human milk using computerized breast measurement. *Exp Physiol* 1992;77:79-87.
15. Dewey KG, Lonnerdal B. Infant self-regulation of breast milk intake. *Acta Paediatr Scand* 1986;75:893-898.
16. Dewey KG, Heinig MJ, Nommsen LA, Lonnerdal B. Maternal versus infant factors related to breast milk intake and residual milk volume: the DARLING study. *Pediatrics* 1991;87:829-837.

17. Butte NF, Garza C, Smith EO, Nichols BL. Human milk intake and growth in exclusively breast-fed infants. *J Pediatr* 1984;104:187-195.

18. Butte NF, Wills C, Jean CA, Smith EO, Garza C. Feeding patterns of exclusively breast-fed infants during the first four months of life. *Early Hum Dev* 1985;12:291-300.

19. Labbok M, Krasovec K. Toward consistency in breastfeeding definitions. *Stud Fam Plann* 1990; 21:226-230.

20. Drewett RF, Woolridge MW, Jackson DA, et al. Relationships between nursing patterns, supplementary food intake and breast-milk intake in a rural Thai population. *Early Hum Dev* 1989;20: 13-23.

21. Ferris AM, McCabe LT, Allen LH, Pelto GH. Biological and sociocultural determinants of successful lactation among women in eastern Connecticut. *J Am Diet Assoc* 1987;87:316-321.

22. Salariya EM, Easton PM, Cater JI. Duration of breast-feeding after early initiation and frequent feeding. *Lancet* 1978;2:1141-1143.

23. DeChateau P, Holmberg H, Jakobsson K, Winberg J. A study of factors promoting and inhibiting lactation. *Dev Med Child Neurol* 1977;19:575-584.

24. Taylor PM, Maloni JA, Brown DR. Early suckling and prolonged breast-feeding. *Am J Dis Child* 1986;140:151-154.

25. Humenick SS. The clinical significance of breast-milk maturation rates. *Birth* 1987;14:174-181.

26. Righard L, Alade MO. Effect of delivery room routines on success of first breast-feed. *Lancet* 1990;336:1105-1107.

27. Anderson GC, McBride MR, Dahm J, Ellis MK, Vidyasagar D. Development of sucking in term infants from birth to four hours postbirth. *Res Nurs Health Care* 1982;5:21-27.

28. Salariya E, Easton P, Cater J. Breast-feeding: the natural way. Early and often for best results. *Nurs Mirror* 1979;148:15-17.

29. Lentz MJ, Killien MC. Are you sleeping? sleep patterns during postpartum hospitalization. *J Perinatal Neonatal Nurs* 1991;4:30.

30. Jackson DA, Imong SM, Silprasert A, et al. Circadian variation in fat concentration of breast-milk in a rural northern Thai population. *Br J Nutr* 1988;59:349-363.

31. Stafford J, Villalpando S, Urquieta Aguila B. Circadian variation and changes after a meal in volume and lipid production of human milk from rural Mexican women. *Ann Nutr Metab* 1994;38: 232-237.

32. Pinilla T, Birch LL. Help me make it through the night: behavioral entrainment of breast-fed infants' sleep patterns. *Pediatrics* 1993;91:436-444.

33. L'Esperance C, Frantz K. Time limitation for early breastfeeding. *J Obstet Gynecol Neonatal Nurs* 1985;14:114-118.

34. Woolridge MW. The "anatomy" of infant sucking. *Midwifery* 1986;2:164-171.

35. Lucas A, Lucas PJ, Baum JD. Pattern of milk flow in breast-fed infants. *Lancet* 1979;2:57-58.

36. Lucas A, Lucas PJ, Baum JD. Differences in the pattern of milk intake between breast and bottle fed infants. *Early Hum Dev* 1981;5:195-199.

37. Barnes GR, Lethin AN, Jackson EB, Shea N. Management of breastfeeding. *JAMA* 1953;151: 192-199.

38. Frantz KB, Kalmen BA. Breastfeeding works for cesareans, too. *RN* 1979;42(12):39-47.

39. Minchin MK. Positioning for breastfeeding. *Birth* 1989;16:67-73.

40. Ramsay M, Gisel EG. Neonatal sucking and maternal feeding practices. *Dev Med Child Neurol* 1996;38:34-47.

41. Widstrom AM, Thingstrom-Paulsson J. The position of the tongue during rooting reflexes elicited in newborn infants before the first suckle. *Acta Paediatr* 1993;82:281-283.

42. Marmet C, Shell E. Training neonates to suck correctly. *MCN Am J Matern Child Nurs* 1984;9:401-407.

43. Righard L, Flodmark CE, Lothe L, Jakobsson I. Breastfeeding patterns: comparing the effects on infant behavior and maternal satisfaction of using one or two breasts. *Birth* 1993;20:182-185.

44. Cronewett L, Stukel T, Kearney M, et al. Single daily bottle use in the early weeks postpartum and breast-feeding outcomes. *Pediatrics* 1992;90:760-766.

45. Neifert M, Lawrence R, Seacat J. Nipple confusion: toward a formal definition. *J Pediatr* 1995;126:S125-S129.

46. Barros FC, Victora CG, Semer TC, Filho ST, Tomasi E, Weiderpass E. Use of pacifiers is associated with decreased breast-feeding duration. *Pediatrics* 1995;95:497-499.

47. Victora CG, Tomasi E, Olinto MT, Barros FC. Use of pacifiers and breastfeeding duration. *Lancet* 1993;341:404-406.

48. Ford RP, Mitchell EA, Scragg R, Stewart AW, Taylor BJ, Allen EM. Factors adversely associated with breast feeding in New Zealand. *J Paediatr Child Health* 1994;30:483-489.

49. Righard L, Alade MO. Breastfeeding and the use of pacifiers. *Birth* 1997;24:116-120.

50. Victora CG, Behague DP, Barros FC, Olinto MT, Weiderpass E. Pacifier use and short breastfeeding duration: cause, consequence, or coincidence? *Pediatrics* 1997;99:445-453.

51. Riordan JM, Koehn M. Reliability and validity testing of three breastfeeding assessment tools. *J Obstet Gynecol Neonatal Nurs* 1997;26:181-187.

52. Shrago L, Bocar D. The infant's contribution to breastfeeding. *J Obstet Gynecol Neonatal Nurs* 1990;19:209-215.

53. Matthews MK. Assessments and suggested interventions to assist newborn breastfeeding behavior. *J Hum Lact* 1993;9:243-248.

54. Jensen D, Wallace S, Kelsay P. LATCH: a breastfeeding charting system and documentation tool. *J Obstet Gynecol Neonatal Nurs* 1994;23:27-32.

55. Mulford C. The Mother-Baby Assessment (MBA): an "Apgar score" for breastfeeding. *J Hum Lact* 1992;8:79-82.

56. Butte NF, Garza C, Smith EO, Nichols BL. Evaluation of the deuterium dilution technique against the test-weighing procedure for the determination of breast milk intake. *Am J Clin Nutr* 1983;37:996-1003.

57. Dewey KG, Peerson JM, Brown KH, et al. Growth of breast-fed infants deviates from current reference data: a pooled analysis of US, Canadian, and European data sets. World Health Organization Working Group on Infant Growth. *Pediatrics* 1995;96(3, pt 1):495-503.

6

Managing Newborns With Common Breastfeeding Challenges

BASIC NEEDS FOR WELL INFANTS

Feeding is one of multiple tasks that must be established and integrated for the infant's successful adaptation to extrauterine life. The newborn must accomplish *biological tasks*—establishing and maintaining respiration, circulatory changes, thermoregulation—in addition to ingesting, retaining, and digesting nutrients. Furthermore, the newborn must accomplish *behavioral tasks*: establishing a regulated behavioral tempo, processing, storing and organizing multiple stimuli, and establishing a relationship with caregivers and the environment.[1]

Biological Tasks

Throughout life, organisms must maintain homeostasis. The fetus, however, uses different mechanisms to maintain homeostasis than the newborn. The transition to extrauterine life has some points that are pertinent to feeding in general and breastfeeding in particular.

Gastrointestinal and Metabolic Needs and Function

Prior to birth, the fetus obtained all of its nutrients through the placenta. After birth, however, the nutrients from human milk must first pass through the digestive tract and are then used for metabolism. The normal functioning of the digestive tract and the newborn's metabolic needs and function are briefly reviewed here to provide a basis for clinical management.

Metabolism and Hormonal Regulation

Metabolism is the *use* of the nutrients from food after it has been digested, absorbed, and circulated to the cells.[2] Metabolism—the use of nutrients—can be either catabolic (decomposition, or breakdown) or anabolic (synthesis, or building of molecules). The basal metabolic rate is the rate of nutrient use under basal conditions, that is, being awake but resting and being in a postabsorptive state (not digesting food) and a thermoneutral environment.

During metabolism, energy is expended. Energy is defined as "the capacity to do work or to produce a change in matter. Applied to nutrition, energy deals mostly with the chemical energy obtained from foods."[3] One kilocalorie of energy is the amount of energy required to raise the temperature of 1 kg of water from 14.5° to 15.5° C (i.e., 1° Celsius). The term *kilocalorie* is usually used to describe energy needs with respect to nutrition. The commonly used *calorie* (e.g., 1 oz of artificial milk has 20 calories) refers to the scientifically correct term, *kilocalorie* (abbreviated kcal).

Energy is required for the basic needs of metabolism, including respiration, circulation, maintenance of electrochemical gradient across cell membranes, and maintenance of body temperature.[3] Infants use nutrients to maintain this basic metabolic rate, but they also use nutrients for growth and activity. During the first 4 months after birth, about 50% to 60% of kilocalories are used to maintain the infant's basic metabolic rate, 25% to 40% are for growth, and 10% to 15% are for activity.

Metabolism—the use of digested nutrients—has two central concepts that are critical to breastfeeding management. First, there must be an understanding of how metabolism is regulated and, second, how metabolism is related to the newborn's energy requirements and the macronutrients that human milk provides.

REGULATION OF METABOLISM

Metabolism must be regulated in some way. The neurological and endocrine systems are regulatory in nature, but both are immature at birth. Reflexes, part of the neurological system, are primitive, but they are sufficiently developed to sustain extrauterine life. The endocrine system has hormones that regulate the two processes of metabolism—catabolic and anabolic.

Hormones, although present and functioning, sometimes may be produced in limited quantities or may be unable to fully meet the dynamic changes associated with the transition to extrauterine life. Hormones related to food and fluid regulation predispose the newborn to some risks. For example, antidiuretic hormone (ADH), which inhibits diuresis, is produced in limited quantities, resulting in many voidings per day, and hence a higher susceptibility to dehydration. Glucagon and insulin are the hormones most closely associated with glucose regulation.

ENERGY REQUIREMENTS

Well infants require 90 to 120 kcal/kg/24 hr.[3] About 40 to 60 of those kilocalories are needed to maintain basic metabolic functions. It is important to remember, however, that basal metabolism requirements are measured at room temperature when the subject has an empty stomach and is physically and emotionally quiet. Therefore, when food is ingested and assimilated, metabolic needs increase. The well infant also has activity and growth needs, so sufficient kilocalories should be ingested to support these needs.

MACRONUTRIENTS IN HUMAN MILK

Macronutrients vary in human milk as described in Chapter 3. The macronutrients—carbohydrates, proteins, and fats—can be either broken down or synthesized through metabolic processes, as shown in Table 6-1. Proteins are synthesized from other substances, while carbohydrates and fats are broken down.

TABLE 6-1

DEFINITIONS

Term	Definition	Key Point
Glucagon	A hormone, produced by alpha cells in the islets of Langerhans, that stimulates the conversion of glycogen to glucose in the liver	Hormone
Glucose	Monosaccharide; major source of energy occurring in human and animal body fluids	Simple sugar
Glycogen	A polysaccharide that is the major carbohydrate stored in animal cells; it is formed from glucose and stored chiefly in the liver and, to a lesser extent, in muscle cells	Complex sugar
Glycogenolysis	The breakdown of glycogen to glucose	Breakdown of complex sugar to simple sugar
Glycogenesis	The synthesis of glycogen from glucose	Formation of complex sugar from simple sugar
Glycolysis	A series of catalyzed reactions, occurring within cells, by which glucose and other sugars are broken down to yield lactic acid or pyruvic acid, releasing energy in the form of adenosine triphosphate; may be aerobic (accomplished with oxygen) or anaerobic (accomplished without oxygen)	Breakdown of simple and complex sugars
Glyconeogenesis	The formation of glycogen from fatty acids and proteins rather than carbohydrates	Formation of complex sugar from noncarbohydrates

Source: *Mosby's Medical Nursing and Allied Health Dictionary.* 4th ed. St. Louis: Mosby; 1994.

Carbohydrates. Carbohydrates (sugars) supply energy; they spare the metabolism of protein and fat. Glucose, a monosaccharide (simple sugar), is the form of carbohydrate used by cells for energy. This simple sugar is derived from the digestion and metabolism of disaccharides and more complex carbohydrates such as starch and glycogen. There are 4 kcal in each gram of carbohydrate. About 38% of the calories in human milk are supplied by the disaccharide lactose.

Carbohydrate metabolism is both catabolic and anabolic. Through catabolism, more complex carbohydrates are broken down into simple sugars; through anabolism, simple sugars are synthesized into glycogen. The catabolic process breaks down human milk lactose into glucose and galactose, so that it can be used in cells. The anabolic process synthesizes glycogen, stored in the liver beginning at around 9 weeks gestation. Glycogen stores are used for such events as hypoxia during labor, or the work of breathing, or for cold stress. Newborns use stores from gestation because they have a limited ability to produce glucose from glycogen. Hence their blood sugar levels can drop rapidly.

Blood glucose levels are regulated by hormonal and neural influences. The sugar-regulating hormones include insulin (secreted by beta cells of the pancreas), glucagon (secreted by alpha cells of the pancreas), epinephrine, adrenocorticotropic hormone (ACTH), growth hormone, thyroid-stimulating hormone, and thyroid hormone. Ideally, the newborn should have blood sugar levels above 60 mg/dl, but a blood sugar level above 40 mg/dl is acceptable.

Proteins. In contrast to carbohydrates and fats, whose primary function is to provide energy, proteins are primarily concerned with building tissue (anabolism). There are 4 kcal in each gram of protein. Although the amount varies with the stage of lactation, about 7% of the calories in human milk are supplied by protein (whereas 9% to

11% are supplied by protein in artificial milk).[3] Metabolizing protein increases the basal metabolic requirement for kilocalories by as much as 30%, while the metabolism of carbohydrate and fat increases it by only 4% and 6%, respectively.[4] Simply stated, it takes more energy to metabolize protein than to metabolize carbohydrate or fat. This is yet another reason that breastfeeding is advantageous. Human milk is significantly lower in protein than cow's milk, home-prepared evaporated milk formulas, or commercially prepared artificial milks, and therefore minimizes the increase in the basal metabolic requirement.

Fats. Like carbohydrates, fats are used for energy. Although the consumption of fats adds to a feeling of satiety in adults and early studies suggested this effect occurred in newborns also, this was refuted in later research. Fats are essential for infants; cholesterol in particular is important during early infancy because it contributes to brain development. There are about 9 kcal per gram of fat in human milk. In the breastfed infant, about 55% of the calories consumed are from fat, whereas only about 48% of the calories in artificial milk are from fat.

Lipid metabolism can be either catabolic or anabolic (lipogenesis). Most lipids can be synthesized through lipogenesis, including triglycerides, cholesterol, phospholipids, and prostaglandins. Some, however, are essential fatty acids, which are used for growth and tissue maintenance (rather than energy only). Fat in human milk is easier for infants to digest than the fat in cow's milk because of the position of the fatty acids on the glycerol molecule and because of natural lipase activity.

Gastrointestinal Function

The gastrointestinal tract makes essential nutrients available to all cells throughout the body. This is accomplished by ingestion (taking in), digestion (breaking down), motility (movement—peristalsis and segmentation of *undigested* nutrients), secretion of digestive juices, ab-

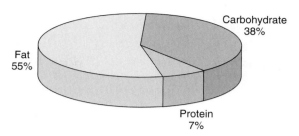

Fig. 6-1 High fat is needed for brain development. Lactose, the carbohydrate in human milk, is easily broken down into simple sugars for energy. Low protein requires little energy to metabolize.

sorption (movement of *digested* nutrients), and elimination.

INGESTION

Ingestion—the transfer of milk—is discussed in Chapter 5. Through ingestion of human milk the infant takes in six main substances: carbohydrates, proteins, fat, vitamins, minerals, and water. Human milk provides energy: a total of about 67 kcal/100 ml (20 kcal/oz).[5] Very little energy (calories) comes from protein, while the greatest amount is provided by fat, as shown in Figure 6-1.

DIGESTION

Digestion, or the breakdown of food, is accomplished by either mechanical or chemical means. It occurs in the mouth, stomach, pancreas, and intestines. Mechanical digestion involves mastication (chewing—for solid foods only), deglutition (swallowing), peristalsis (the undulating movement), and segmentation (mixing movement). As described in Chapter 5, the newborn digests human milk primarily by swallowing and an undulating movement that begins in the tongue and continues throughout the gastrointestinal tract. Chemical digestion promotes the breakdown of carbohydrate, fat, and protein to absorbable units through hydrolysis. Chemical digestion relies on digestive enzymes (see the Clinical Scenario).

CLINICAL SCENARIO

Kilocalorie Requirements

A mother says that her newborn weighs 7½ pounds and feeds 10 times in a 24-hour period. She would like to know how many ounces he would need to consume at each feeding in order to get the minimum amount of calories for his current weight.

1. What is the answer to her question?
2. She doubts that she has that much milk. How could you help her to visualize what a small amount this is?

Answer

As specified earlier, the well newborn needs 90 to 120 kcal, (or, as the mother would say, "calories") per kilogram per 24 hours. First, there are about 2.2 lb/kg, so the newborn weighs 3.41 kg. Human milk varies, but for the sake of simplicity, figure that there are 20 kcal per ounce of milk (and there are exactly 20 kcal per ounce of standard artificial milk). Using the formula of 90 to 120 kcal per kg of body weight per 24 hours, this newborn would require about 307 to 409 calories per 24 hours. This would be supplied in 15.4 to 20.5 ounces of milk per day. If the newborn feeds 10 times per day, he would need to consume 1.5 to 2.1 ounces each time.

Mothers frequently fear that they do not have enough milk. It would be helpful to fill a medicine cup with 23 ml and tell the newborn's mother that is all she would need to have in each breast for each feeding. Another way to visualize this is by the teaspoon. One and a half ounces is approximately equivalent to 9 teaspoons, or 4½ teaspoons per breast.

Secretion

The presence of secreted enzymes promotes the chemical digestion of food. Digestive enzymes are secreted into the lumen of the gastrointestinal tract. Important enzymes for digestion include salivary amylase, lingual lipase, gastric lipase, peptidases, and pancreatic amylase. But pancreatic amylase, lipase, and saliva are scarce at birth. In human milk, the presence of mammary amylase (highest in colostrum) compensates for the decreased pancreatic amylase. Bile salts in human milk are critical for the emulsification and absorption of fats.

Motility

The undulating movements of the gastrointestinal tract start with the tongue (see Chapter 5) and continue throughout. Colostrum is important because it acts as a laxative on the gut, therefore facilitating the excretion of unneeded substances, most notably bilirubin, as described later in the chapter.

Absorption

As the digested nutrients move through the gastrointestinal tract, they cross the intestinal wall into the internal environment through the process of absorption. The newborn is unable to absorb some nutrients that are ingested. For example, infants can take in great quantities of iron in iron-fortified artificial milk, but they absorb them rather inefficiently, as described in Chapter 3. Substances that are indigestible and not needed are not absorbed into the internal environment but instead move into the external environment for elimination.

Elimination

Newborns have three distinct types of stools as described in Table 6-2. The first stool is called *meconium*. The next stool is a *transitional stool*, and the last is a *milk stool*. Infants who are exclusively breastfed will have softer stools because of the whey-to-casein ratio in human milk. The stools of artificially fed infants are more rubbery, owing to the more rubbery curd produced by the comparatively greater amounts of casein in artificial milk.

Cardiopulmonary Function

For the fetus, the placenta provides both nutrients and oxygen. In contrast, the newborn has two separate systems: one for nutrients, and one

T A B L E 6-2
STOOL PATTERNS OF NEWBORNS

Stool Pattern	Appears	Composed of	Clinical Description	Teaching Implications
Meconium	Within first 24 hours	• Amniotic fluid and related constituents • Sluffed-off mucosal cells • Possibly blood; from maternal vaginal vault or from minor bleeding of alimentary tract	Black or dark green, very sticky	Stools should *not* continue to be dark brown/black for more than 3-5 days
Transitional stools	By 2-3 days after initiation of feeding	• Meconium • Milk curds	Greenish brown to yellowish brown, pasty, less sticky than meconium	Should not continue more than 4-7 days
Milk stools	By 4-7 days after initiation of feeding	Milk curds; higher in whey than in curd content, hence human-milk stools are less rubbery than those excreted by artificially fed infants	Stools from breastfed infants are yellow (look like cottage cheese and mustard mixed together) with a nonoffensive odor Stools from artificially fed infants are pale yellow to light brown, with more rubbery consistency, and a more offensive odor	During the newborn period, it is common for stooling to occur with nearly every feeding; thin milk stools do not mean the baby has diarrhea; later in infancy, thin stools may indicate there has been more consumption of hindmilk than foremilk

for oxygen. After birth, the transition from fetal to postnatal circulation involves the immediate functional closure of the foramen ovale, followed by the ductus arteriosus around the fourth day after birth, and later the ductus venosus. If the ducts fail to close, various types of congenital heart defects result. Cardiac defects do not preclude breastfeeding (see Chapter 7), but they do increase the metabolic rate and therefore the amount of energy needed to maintain basal metabolic rate, activity, and growth.

The newborn obtains oxygen through the lungs; this requires inhalation—breathing. This process becomes important in breastfeeding because the infant must be able to coordinate suckling, swallowing, and breathing. Usually, infants with a respiratory rate exceeding 60 breaths per minute have difficulty coordinating breathing and suckling and are considered tachypneic; most hospital protocols do not allow these infants to take oral feedings. Usually, however, newborns can and do coordinate sucking, swallowing, and breathing. The suckling results in the ingestion of nutrients and fluid, as well as the digestion and elimination of food.

Thermoregulation

To prepare for the transition to extrauterine life, "brown fat" is deposited in the fetus around the 28th week of gestation. This specialized fat is highly vascular and is specifically designed for heat production. Deposits of this brown fat are located in the axilla, the area of the scapula, the neck muscles, and around the kidneys and adrenals. Prior to birth, the fetus's temperature is dependent on the mother's temperature. Usually, the fetus's temperature is approximately 0.5° C (0.9° F) higher than that of the mother—around 37.6° to 37.8° C (99.7° to 100.0° F).[6] Immediately upon birth, the newborn is thrust into a significantly colder environment. Typically, delivery rooms are cool, and the newborn arrives covered with amniotic fluid, which makes him colder because of evaporative heat loss than if he were dry. The newborn's thermoregulatory system is not as well developed as that of adults. Therefore, hypothermia, as discussed later in the chapter, frequently develops.

Fluid Balance

For newborns, small fluctuations have a great impact on fluid balance. To avoid or minimize problems, clinicians involved in breastfeeding management need to understand water requirements and observe water losses.

Normal infants require about 80 to 100 ml of water per kilogram of body weight per 24 hours.[4] Generally, newborns who are ingesting human milk do not need additional fluids. Human milk consists of about 87% water. Exclusively breastfed healthy infants less than 4 months old do not require extra water even if they are in a hot, dry climate.[7-11]

Water loss is the total of insensible water loss and renal water loss. It is more difficult to determine insensible losses—for example, losses that occur through the normal functions of breathing—but fairly simple to observe urine output. If the newborn is less than 48 hours old, total urinary output should be 250 to 400 ml/day; after 48 hours of age, output of less than 15 to 60 ml/kg/day is considered oliguria.[6]

Newborns have some special characteristics related to fluid balance. Under normal circum-

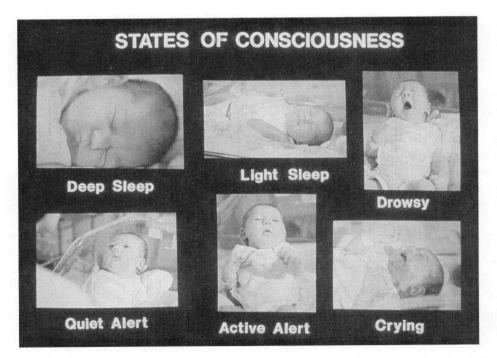

Fig. 6-2 Summary of sleep-wake states of newborn. States of consciousness: deep sleep, light sleep, drowsy, quiet-alert, active-alert, crying. *(From Early Parent-Infant Relationships [video]. White Plains, NY: March of Dimes Birth Defects Foundation; 1991. Used with permission.)*

stances, infants are born with extra fluids "on board," and therefore they have some fluid loss (and therefore weight loss) the first few days after birth. Sometimes, however, these extra fluids are diminished or depleted because the mother has been dehydrated during the childbearing experience—a long labor, multiple episodes of vomiting, or large blood losses all contribute to maternal dehydration. Therefore, before making judgments about the infant's fluid needs or losses, it is important to consider the labor history.

Behavioral Tasks

Sleep-Wakefulness Continuum

Infants are not simply asleep or awake. Rather, the sleep-wakefulness continuum, shown in Figure 5-4, ranges from deep sleep or lethargy to extreme irritability or crying.[12] How or whether an infant controls or modifies his response varies according to which particular sleep or awake state he is experiencing. Note the facial "brightness" of the newborn, since this is usually the most distinguishing factor that alerts the caregiver to the infant's state, as shown in Figure 6-2. Clues as to which state the infant is in include body activity, eye movements, facial movements, breathing pattern, and level of response as summarized in Table 6-3.[13]

Sensory Needs, Stimuli, and Relationship With Caregivers

The five senses are developed to varying degrees in the newborn. At birth, *visual* acuity is limited. The newborn can best see objects that are about 8 inches away—about the distance of the mother's face from the infant while at the breast. *Hearing* acuity for a newborn is similar to that for an adult. Newborns are readily consoled by familiar sounds, such as the mother's heartbeat, that have

been audible during breastfeeding. *Smell* is well developed and more functional than in adults; newborns can smell their mother's milk, and—if left to their own instincts—will find the breast to get the milk. The sense of *taste* is fully functioning at birth, with newborns able to distinguish between sweet, sour, bitter, and tasteless solutions. The sweetness of the mother's milk will usually elicit an eager suck because of the pleasant taste the newborn experiences. *Touch* is especially important for the newborn. He perceives tactile sensation in any part of the body, but the perioral area is the most sensitive.

Happily, one notes that breastfeeding provides not only nutrition but also positive stimuli. The newborn's sensory capabilities are designed to capitalize on the pleasant sensory experiences associated with breastfeeding.

Assessing Risks for Well Infants

Most newborns accomplish the biological or behavioral tasks easily and quickly. Some, however, have slight deviations or delays that have an impact on breastfeeding.

Lethargy or Sleepiness

Often the newborn who is lethargic or sleepy does not feed well. This sleepiness or reluctance to feed is seldom a breastfeeding "problem" but rather is the result of the normal physiological state that the infant experiences. Breastfeeding can be best accomplished when the infant is in the optimal state of alertness.

Impact on Breastfeeding
Breastfeeding should commence when the infant is in the quiet-alert state. Infants who are in deep sleep or light sleep will not breastfeed. Infants who are drowsy may begin to breastfeed but may return to sleep states. These infants may benefit

T A B L E 6-3

INFANT STATE CHART (SLEEP AND AWAKE STATES)

STATE is a group of characteristics that regularly occur together: body activity, eye movements, facial movements, breathing pattern, and level of response to external stimuli (e.g., handling) and internal stimuli (e.g., hunger)

	Characteristics of State					
	Body Activity	Eye Movements	Facial Movements	Breathing Pattern	Level of Response	*Implications for Caregiving*
Sleep States						
Deep sleep	Nearly still, except for occasional startle or twitch	None	Without facial movements, except for occasional sucking at regular intervals	Smooth and regular	Threshold to stimuli is very high, so that only very intense or disturbing stimuli will arouse infants	Caregivers trying to feed infants in deep sleep will probably find the experience frustrating. Infants will be unresponsive, even if caregivers use disturbing stimuli (flicking feet) to arouse infants. Infants may only arouse briefly and then become unresponsive as they return to deep sleep. If caregivers wait until infants move to a higher, more responsive state, feeding or caregiving will be much more pleasant.
Light sleep	Some body movements	Rapid eye movements (REM); fluttering of eyes beneath closed eyelids	May smile and make brief fussy or crying sounds	Irregular	More responsive to internal and external stimuli; when these stimuli occur, infants may remain in light sleep, return to deep sleep, or arouse to drowsy	Light sleep makes up the highest proportion of newborn sleep and usually precedes wakening. Due to brief fussy or crying sounds made during this state, caregivers who are not aware that these sounds occur normally may think it is time for feeding and may try to feed infants before they are ready to eat.

Adapted from Brazelton TB, Nugent JK. *Neonatal Behavioral Assessment Scale*. 3rd ed. London: MacKeith Press; 1995.

T A B L E 6-3

INFANT STATE CHART (SLEEP AND AWAKE STATES)—cont'd

STATE is a group of characteristics that regularly occur together: body activity, eye movements, facial movements, breathing pattern, and level of response to external stimuli (e.g., handling) and internal stimuli (e.g., hunger)

	Characteristics of State					
	Body Activity	Eye Movements	Facial Movements	Breathing Pattern	Level of Response	*Implications for Caregiving*
Awake States						
Drowsy	Activity level variable, with mild startles interspersed from time to time; movements usually smooth	Eyes open and close occasionally, are heavy-lidded with dull, glazed appearance	May have some facial movements, often there are none, and the face appears still	Irregular	Infants react to sensory stimuli although responses are delayed; state change after stimulation frequently noted	From the drowsy state, infants may return to sleep or awaken further. In order to awaken, caregivers can provide something for infants to see, hear, or suck, as this may arouse them to a quiet alert state, a more responsive state. Infants left alone without stimuli may return to a sleep state.
Quiet alert	Minimal	Brightening and widening of eyes	Faces have bright, shining, sparkling looks	Regular	Infants attend most to environment, focusing attention on any stimuli that are present	Infants in quiet alert state provide much pleasure and positive feedback for caregivers. Providing something for infants to see, hear, or suck will often maintain this state. In the first few hours after birth, most newborns commonly experience a period of intense alertness before going into a long sleeping period.
Active alert	Much body activity; may have periods of fussiness	Eyes open with less brightening	Much facial movement; faces not as bright as quiet alert state	Irregular	Increasingly sensitive to disturbing stimuli (hunger, fatigue, noise, excessive handling)	Caregivers may intervene at this stage to console and to bring infants to a lower state.
Crying	Increased motor activity, with color changes	Eyes may be tightly closed or open	Grimaces	More irregular	Extremely responsive to unpleasant external or internal stimuli	Crying is the infant's communication signal. It is a response to unpleasant stimuli from the environment or from within infants (fatigue, hunger, discomfort). Crying tells us the infant's limits have been reached. Sometimes infants can console themselves and return to lower states. At other times they need help from caregivers.

from alerting techniques, as shown in Box 6-1. The infant who is in the active-alert state is distracted by his own hunger; these infants may need to be consoled before they can successfully breastfeed, as shown in Box 6-2. It is extremely difficult to coax the crying newborn to breastfeed. He is often so frustrated that he is disinterested in any further stimuli. Furthermore, lengthy periods of crying will cause him to take in air, and hence he may have the feeling of a full stomach. Therefore, he needs time to burp before feeding. Breastfeed-

ing can be thought of as the infant's "job" in life. Just as an adult is not very good at performing his daily job when he is tired or frustrated, so too a newborn is considerably less effective at breastfeeding when he has been asked to do his "job" under less than optimal circumstances. These suboptimal circumstances can be avoided with good clinical management.

Clinical Management Strategies

One simple guideline should govern clinical management: a sleepy baby will not eat, and a hungry baby will not sleep! Be aware of the *early* hunger cues described in Chapter 5 (see Box 5-3). Ideally, the infant should go to the breast when he is in the quiet-alert state; this is most likely when the infant has easy access to the breast, as shown in Box 6-3. When the care provider, parents, and environment foster easy access to the breast, breastfeeding will go well. Frequently, both mothers and nursing staff question whether a newborn should be awakened for a feeding if he appears to have a prolonged sleep period. Newborns sleep the majority of the time during the first 24 hours. Waking them will not necessarily result in a good feeding during this first day. The WHO states, "Interval between feeds varies considerably particularly in the first few days of life. There is no evidence that long interfeed intervals adversely affects health of newborns who are kept warm and who are breastfed when they show signs of hunger."[37] Infants who have risk factors for hypoglycemia should be awakened every 3 hours using the alerting techniques shown in Box 6-1.

Food-Fluid-Warmth Relationship

Thermoregulation is critical for newborns. Similarly, nutrients and fluids are essential to maintain survival. However, the thermoregulatory mechanism and the ingestion, digestion, and utilization of nutrients and fluids are interrelated. Not only are these processes interrelated, but their relationship is influenced by breastfeeding, which supplies calories, fluids, and skin-to-skin warmth.

Box 6-1
Alerting Infants

General Principles of Alerting Infants
- Infants tend to be alert immediately after birth and then move into a deep sleep. This is followed by highly individualized sleep-wake patterns.
- Infants tend to sleep much of the first 2 weeks (especially the first 2 to 3 days).
- An infant in deep sleep does not breastfeed well. Maternal analgesia, anesthesia, sedatives, and magnesium sulfate, as well as infant jaundice, may augment sleepiness.
- Noxious stimuli should not be used to alert infants. Noxious stimuli include pinching, thumping feet, and so on. Infants should associate feedings with pleasure, not discomfort. Frantically crying infants do not breastfeed effectively.

Techniques for Alerting Infants
- Unswaddle, undress to diaper
- Change diaper
- Talk to infant
- Gently stimulate extremities by stroking, massaging
- Apply cool cloth to face
- Hold infant upright
- Use motion; simulate motion within the uterus by gently bouncing infant (never shake infant)
- Turn infant from side to side
- Elicit "doll's eye reflex" but avoid jackknifing

Modified from Bocar D. *Breastfeeding Educator Program Resource Notebook.* Oklahoma City: Lactation Consultant Services; 1997. Used with permission.

Box 6-2
Consoling Infants

General Principles of Consoling

- *Frantically crying* infants need consoling before they go to the breast.
- *Fussy* infants can be consoled at the breast.
- If an infant has his tongue elevated against the hard palate, consoling techniques should be used before offering the breast.
- Respond quickly to signs of discontent; infant calms more rapidly and learns trust.
- Infants may need interactions and/or stimulation (stimulation may distract from discomfort).
- Always rule out hunger; if infant responds to rooting reflex, offer breast; use consoling techniques to calm infant prior to breastfeeding, but not as a substitution for a feeding.
- No technique works every time; try different techniques at different times, or combine techniques.

Techniques for Consoling Infants

Provide Kinesthetic Stimulation
- Keep infant in warm, humid environment
- Physical security: swaddling, flexion with head support, "nesting" with soft, supportive linens creates physical security
- Holding
- Gentle motion in all three planes: side to side, up and down, front to back (amount of motion similar to intrauterine motion)
- Carry, rock, swing, gently bounce (never shake infants!)
- Skin-to-skin contact
- Tactile stimulation
- Massaging/stroking: massaging or stroking in the direction of hair growth is consoling; massaging or stroking against hair growth is stimulating

Provide Auditory Stimulation
- Parent's voice (infants are more responsive to familiar parental voices)
- Talking (infants are more responsive to high-pitched voice tones)
- Soft, rhythmic sounds at about 60 to 100 beats per minute; singing, humming, nursery rhymes, metronome
- White noise (monotone constant sound that reduces stimulation from other sounds (e.g., sound of clothes dryer, vacuum cleaner, TV "off" channel)

Provide Visual Stimulation
- Human face with eye contact
- Mirrors, lights, ceiling fans, mobiles
- Pictures with black-and-white geometric figures
- Primary colors (especially red and yellow)

Provide Gustatory and Olfactory Stimulation
- Expressing colostrum
- Placing colostrum or mother's milk on lips
- Offering clean parental finger to suck (health care providers should use glove)
- If parent is unavailable, caregiver may wear parent's unwashed clothing

Combine Consoling Techniques
- Place in infant seat on top of an operating clothes dryer within parental view; moist, warm area with rhythmic motion and sounds
- Car ride with infant seat (physical security, gentle motion, white sound)

Modified from Bocar DL. *Breastfeeding Educator Program Resource Notebook.* Oklahoma City: Lactation Consultant Services, 1997. Used with permission.

Box 6-3
Priorities for Care: Access to the Breast

- Encourage mothers and newborns to share a room.
- Watch for signs of alertness as shown in Figure 6-2.
- Teach parents to watch for *early* hunger cues (see Box 5-3).
- Encourage mothers to breastfeed at night.
- Be an advocate for decreasing other interactions and treatments occurring in hospitals that interfere with the breastfeeding experience (visitors, discharge photos, routine hearing tests).
- Discourage time-limited feedings.
- Emphasize importance of adequate help at home so that mother can focus on newborn's needs.

Therefore, any alteration in breastfeeding can positively or negatively affect the infant's serum glucose level or temperature. Conversely, any alteration in the infant's serum glucose level or temperature can affect breastfeeding behavior. The following sections aim to explain the physiological basis for the food-fluid-warmth relationship.

Hypoglycemia

Glucose needs and regulation start long before birth. During pregnancy, glucose is delivered to the fetus via the placenta. Typically, fetal glucose levels are about 70% to 80% of the maternal serum levels. (Hence, the importance of regulation for diabetic mothers.) For example, if the gravida's serum glucose is 70 to 80 mg/dl as it should be, the fetal level will be around 49 to 64 mg/dl. The glucose supports not only fetal metabolism but also growth and development. After about 24 weeks gestation, glycogen is stored in the liver and the muscles, and it increases in quantity as term gestation approaches.

Glucose supply from the placenta is abruptly terminated once the umbilical cord is severed. After birth, glucose supplies depend on a multitude of factors, including heat loss. Fortunately, newborns also have glycogen stores, but these stores are used up within about 2 to 3 hours after birth. Although the stores of glycogen do exist, glycogenolysis appears to be depressed in newborns, resulting in a decreased serum blood glucose. Also, after the glycogen stores are used, the newborn uses fat for metabolism. Hence, the adaptation to extrauterine life results in fluctuations in newborn glucose supply and utilization while regulatory mechanisms are still immature. Clinical signs and symptoms of hypoglycemia are listed in Box 6-4.

RISK FACTORS

Some newborns are at especially high risk for hypoglycemia, as shown in Box 6-5. Unless there are risk factors for hypoglycemia, it is not

Box 6-4
Signs and Symptoms of Hypoglycemia

- Jittery and tremors
- Hypothermia
- Difficulty in feeding
- Apathy, limpness, lethargy
- Intermittent apneic spells or tachypnea
- Weak or high-pitched cry
- Sudden pallor
- Eye rolling
- Episodes of cyanosis
- Convulsions
- Cardiac arrest and failure

Source: Behrman RE, Kleighman RM, Arvin AM, eds. *Nelson Textbook of Pediatrics*. 15th ed. Philadelphia: Saunders; 1996.

necessary to routinely test for it.[37] Furthermore, results of tests may be more or less accurate, depending on what is used for the test. Many brands of reagent strips do not give an adequate reading of the *newborn's* glucose level. The reagent strips are affected by the subject's hematocrit level, and because they were designed to be used with adults, the strips yield inaccurate results when used with newborns, who have higher hematocrits. The reagent strips can be considered only a screening device. They are, however, a useful screening device, if used properly. In general, no further action is needed if the newborn's glucose level is at least 47 mg/dl, but a normal range for blood glucose values for breastfed infants has not been well-defined.[37]

IMPACT ON BREASTFEEDING AND CLINICAL MANAGEMENT STRATEGIES

An infant who is mildly hypoglycemic is usually willing to suckle. Instruct the mother to keep him skin-to-skin; cover his back with a receiving blanket to keep away any drafts. Moderate hypoglycemia can also cause lethargy, so some nursery protocols call for giving the infant some artificial milk (assuming expressed human milk is unavail-

Box 6-5
Risk Factors for Hypoglycemia

- Maternal history of diabetes
- Maternal history of eclampsia
- Maternal history of compromised health status (e.g., smoking)
- Birth events suggestive of hypoxia
- Use of forceps, vacuum, presence of nuchal cord, shoulder dystocia
- Twins, especially the smaller of discordant twins
- Large for gestational age
- Small for gestational age
- Preterm infant (less than 37 completed weeks of gestation)
- Cold-stressed infants
- Infant with respiratory distress
- Intrauterine growth retardation
- Postterm infants
- Erythroblastosis fetalis
- Polycythemia (hematocrit greater than 60)
- Low Apgar scores
- Sepsis

Infants with these risk factors should be watched for *early* signs of hypoglycemia!

able) until he perks up enough to suckle. If the infant is extremely hypoglycemic, however, he will require more aggressive interventions as ordered by the physician or primary health care provider. Furthermore, the infant who is hypoglycemic is at risk for hypothermia. The WHO summarizes recommendations for newborns with hypoglycemia;[37] especially pertinent points include the following:

- Hypoglycemia is most likely to occur in the first 24 hours of life
- Newborns who have risk factors for hypoglycemia, including those who are preterm or neurologically impaired, should be awakened every 3 hours

- Newborns at risk for hypoglycemia should have their blood glucose levels measured around 4 to 6 hours after birth. Thereafter, blood glucose levels should be measured at 1 hour before and 3 hours after feedings, until stable

Hypothermia

Hypothermia commonly occurs in newborns. An understanding of the newborn's thermoregulatory mechanisms helps the nurse avoid the potential consequences of heat loss, and recognize its impact on breastfeeding.

THERMOREGULATORY MECHANISMS

The newborn tries to maintain homeostasis with a temperature of about 36.5° to 37.5° C (97.7° to 99.5° F), but he may easily lose heat and need to produce heat. One concept is central to the understanding of heat production: heat is produced through the metabolism of foods. It follows, then, that if one does not have enough food for metabolism, a decreased body temperature results. The thermoregulatory mechanism strives to maintain homeostasis in the presence of heat production and heat loss.

Infants can produce a little heat simply by increasing activity. The main way of producing heat in the neonate, however, is through nonshivering thermogenesis through the metabolism of brown adipose tissue. Contrary to the adult, in whom nonshivering thermogenesis is controlled by epinephrine, nonshivering thermogenesis in the neonate is controlled through norepinephrine. When norepinephrine is released, it increases the body's metabolic rate and stimulates brown fat to release glycerol and fatty acids that act as fuel. In essence, the newborn burns fat to keep warm. This mechanism indeed keeps the infant warm, but once supplies of brown fat are exhausted, they are not replenished. Hypothermia becomes a real threat.

Newborns are especially at risk for heat loss because of their larger body surface area in

T A B L E   6-4

COMPARISON OF HYPOTHERMIA AND HYPERTHERMIA

	Hypothermia	Hyperthermia
Definition	**Temperature** <**36.5° C (97.7° F)**	**Temperature** >**37.5° C (99.5° F)**
Possible causes	*Physiological problems*	*Physiological problems*
	• *Hypoglycemia*	• *Tachypnea*
	• *Prematurity*	• *Septicemia*
	• *Sepsis*	• *Dehydration*
	• *Hypoxia*	
	• *SGA or IUGR*	
	Conduction: infant has been on a cold surface	*Conduction:* infant has been on a warm surface or wrapped in warm blankets
	Radiation: isolette or room too cold	*Radiation:* warmer or isolette temperature is too high
	Convection: drafts in room, portholes of isolette open	
	Evaporation: giving a bath or not drying thoroughly after bath, wet diapers, clothes, blankets; not drying the newborn immediately after birth	
Physical signs	• Mottling	• Tachypnea
	• Cold extremities	• Red skin (plethoric)
	• Lethargy	• Low serum blood glucose
	• Poor feeding	• Occasionally, infant will have sweat on forehead
	• Low serum blood glucose levels	
Corrective strategies	Dependent on cause, but some general suggestions include:	Hyperthermia happens infrequently in newborns; corrective strategies depend on cause, but some general suggestions include:
	Hypoglycemia: feed infant and listen for swallowing; check blood glucose 1 hour later, then after feeding every 3 hours until stable	Check setting if infant is in warmer or isolette; it is especially easy for isolettes to overheat
	Hypoxia: work with physician to identify and ameliorate cause	Check pulse and respirations; this infant may be ill
	Conduction losses: pad cold surfaces with blankets	Undress infant; wipe with cool cloth if indicated
	Radiation losses: keep room warmer, use a second blanket	Refer to primary health care provider if above actions do not correct the hyperthermia
	Convection losses: decrease drafts, or move infant away from drafts	
	Evaporation losses: dry immediately after birth; keep under warmer for bath; cover dry head with cap; keep in dry clothes and diapers; use upside-down T-shirt as "pajama" bottoms.	
	Refer to primary health care provider if hypothermia persists	

relation to their body mass, the close proximity of their blood vessels to the skin, and their immature thermoregulatory mechanisms. Because heat is produced through only one means—the metabolism of nutrients—the infant who is *hypothermic* will soon become *hypoglycemic*. Hypothermia triggers increased metabolism—the infant will be burning calories just to keep warm—resulting in hypoglycemia. Never be complacent about hypothermia or hypoglycemia; both can be life-threatening to a newborn.

Heat loss occurs because of stresses on metabolism—the infant has an increased basal metabolic rate for whatever reason—or through the environment. Common examples of metabolic stressors include prematurity, cardiac defects, acidosis, and infection. After birth, the infant is exposed to various environmental stressors. Infants lose heat through four processes in the environment: evaporation, radiation, conduction, and convection. Heat loss can result in hypothermia, as described previously. The skin is the primary site of sensory receptors that alert the body to environmental temperature changes. These receptors relay the information to the hypothalamus in the brain. The hypothalamus is the control center for thermoregulation; it coordinates both heat production and heat loss, but its function is immature in the newborn. Usually, this "thermostat" works reasonably well to keep the infant within the normal range (i.e., from 36.5° to 37.5° C). It can, however, be impaired by oxygen deprivation, alterations in central nervous system functioning (e.g., birth trauma), or maternal drug consumption.

Consequences of Heat Loss

Newborns who are exposed to heat loss can quickly become hypothermic. Infants lose heat by one of four mechanisms: conduction, radiation, convection, or evaporation. Aside from losing heat, however, infants can become hypothermic

if they are hypoglycemic. For this reason, it is imperative to recognize that these conditions are likely to coexist, and an effective breastfeeding session is likely to prevent or minimize either condition. Table 6-4 summarizes physiological problems associated with hypothermia and hyperthermia.

Impact on Breastfeeding and Clinical Management Strategies

Infants who are on the low side of normal temperature should be put to the breast in order to obtain additional energy (calories) and skin-to-skin warmth. Hypothermia in the presence of a warm environment and adequate breastfeeding requires medical follow-up; such a situation may indicate that the infant has a higher metabolic need, as is seen with cardiac defects, sepsis, and other problems.

Hyperthermia

Hyperthermia is somewhat uncommon in newborns and frequently is the result of overdressing the infant. If it is accompanied by the signs and symptoms listed on Table 6-4, it may be a sign of inadequate fluid intake, or it at least requires further follow-up. This does not mean that the infant should be supplemented with water; human milk contains an adequate amount of water to provide good hydration for the infant, as described earlier in this chapter. Rather, it should be a signal to re-dress an overdressed infant or to explore other possible explanations for the hyperthermia.

Hyperbilirubinemia and Jaundice

A direct relationship between breastfeeding and jaundice was established in early studies; breastfed infants have elevated bilirubin levels ($\geq$ 12 mg/dl) three to four times more often than their artificially fed cohorts.[14-18] It is important to realize, however, that these studies were con-

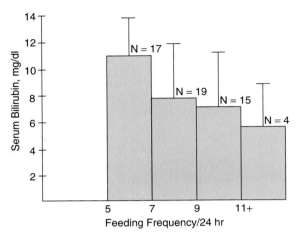

Fig. 6-3 Relationship of mean frequency of feedings during first 3 days of life and serum bilirubin concentrations ($r = .361$, $p < .01$). Vertical bars represent standard deviations. *(From DeCarvalho M, Klaus MH, Merkatz RB. Frequency of breast-feeding and serum bilirubin concentration.* Am J Dis Child *1982;136:737-738.)*

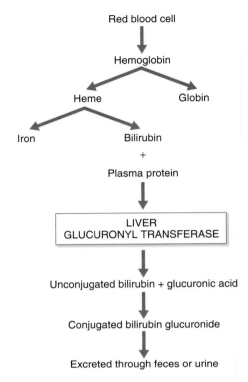

Fig. 6-4 Formation of bilirubin from red blood cells. Bilirubin is excreted primarily through the feces; it can be reabsorbed if feces remain in the colon too long. *(From Wong D.* Whaley and Wong's Nursing Care of Infants and Children. *5th ed. St. Louis: Mosby; 1995.)*

ducted when breastfed infants were typically restricted in terms of frequency. Studies have also shown an inverse relationship between frequency of feeding during the first few days and incidence of jaundice,[19,20] so it would appear that frequency of feeding was the key to minimizing the incidence of jaundice for breastfed infants (Figure 6-3).

Definitions and Descriptions

Many misconceptions exist about jaundice and the breastfed infant. To clarify these misconceptions, it is important to understand the relevant terms. *Bilirubin* is the orange-yellow pigment of bile, and it is created through the breakdown of red blood cells. Bilirubin, an end product of digestion, is not used for anything; the body is trying to excrete it. *Jaundice* is a symptom of increased levels of bilirubin, which are caused by problems with production, transport, metabolism, and excretion.

Bilirubin

Bilirubin is present in the developing fetus from the first trimester, with most of it formed by the breakdown of hemoglobin. Hemoglobin catabolizes into the heme and the globin (protein) components; the heme component is then converted into *biliverdin*, which is later reduced to *bilirubin* by enzymes.

PRODUCTION

The major sites of bilirubin production are the spleen and the liver, but all body tissues can form bilirubin from hemoglobin. Figure 6-4 summarizes the processes. The amount of bilirubin produced

T A B L E 6-5

COMPARISON OF DIRECT AND INDIRECT BILIRUBIN

	Direct Bilirubin	Indirect Bilirubin
Terms	"Bilirubin diglucoromide"	"Bilirubin"
Status	Conjugated	Unconjugated
Soluble	Soluble in aqueous solution	Insoluble in aqueous solution
Deviations	May be increased in the following conditions: • Biliary atresia • Biliary hypoplasia • Hepatitis • Cystic fibrosis • Trisomy 18 • Dubin-Johnson syndrome • Choledochal cysts • Galactosemia • Alpha$_1$-antitrypsin deficiency	**Increased Production of Bilirubin** Extravascular hemolysis • Bruising • Petechiae • Enclosed hemorrhage (intracranial bleed) Intravascular hemolysis • Polycythemia • Rh incompatibility • ABO incompatibility • Intrinsic red cell abnormalities • Hemolysis from drug toxicity **Transport Deficiencies** • Acidosis • Prematurity • Hypoglycemia • Hypothermia **Increased Conjugation in the Liver** • Prematurity • Hypoxia **Decreased Intestinal Excretion** • Antibiotic therapy • Intestinal obstruction **Metabolic Problems** • Infants of diabetic mothers • Hypothyroidism • Amino acid deficiency diseases

varies inversely with gestational age; the lower the gestational age, the more bilirubin that is produced. Furthermore, the amount of bilirubin that is considered "normal" varies according to how many days old the infant is. Although there are two forms of bilirubin, direct and indirect, serum levels are frequently calculated as "total" when one is speaking of the normal range for serum levels in the newborn.

TRANSPORT

Table 6-5 describes pertinent differences between direct and indirect bilirubin. Bilirubin produced outside the liver is transported to the liver via the plasma; there it undergoes conjugation. Then bilirubin is converted into water-soluble, direct bilirubin. Indirect bilirubin is transported via the plasma and is bound to albumin.

METABOLISM

In the small intestine, conjugated (i.e., water-soluble) bilirubin undergoes further catabolism in the intestinal tract to form urobilinogen and sterocobilinogen. This accounts for the yellow-orange color that contributes to the color of feces.

EXCRETION

Indirect bilirubin is not readily excreted in the urine because it is fat-soluble. Direct bilirubin is a major component of bile and feces; it is excreted through the intestines. Understanding that bilirubin is excreted primarily in the feces helps to explain why giving breastfed infants water does not prevent or minimize jaundice; one cannot "flush" the bilirubin out through the urinary tract. In breastfed infants, greater stool output has been associated with greater excretion of bilirubin in the feces and lower serum bilirubin concentrations.[21]

Hyperbilirubinemia

Elevated levels of bilirubin will result in an observable symptom called *jaundice*. Jaundice is a symptom; it is the yellowish color that results when the infant's skin is blanched. Usually, jaundice is visible when bilirubin levels are above 5 mg/dl. Newborns, with their higher-than-adult hematocrit levels (normal is about 57% to 58% for newborns) and immature livers, have increased levels of bilirubin. Determining the severity of the bilirubin level is day-dependent. Generally, medical treatment is recommended for a total bilirubin level $\geq$12 mg/dl during the first 25 to 48 hours, $\geq$15 mg/dl if the infant is 49 to 72 hours old, or $\geq$17 mg/dl if the infant is over 72 hours old.[22] A slightly elevated bilirubin level results in jaundice in the upper part of the body; higher levels affect the upper and lower body. In other words, the lower on the body that the jaundice can be observed, the higher the bilirubin level. Elevated levels are treated medically with blood transfusions (for pathological jaundice) and/or phototherapy.

Four types of jaundice exist: idiopathic jaundice, pathological jaundice, breastfeeding jaundice, and breast-milk jaundice. It is important to distinguish between these types because clinical management, including breastfeeding management, differs. Table 6-6 compares three types of jaundice.

Idiopathic Jaundice

Idiopathic jaundice is frequently referred to as "physiological jaundice," although describing any increase beyond the normal limits as "physiological" is probably a misnomer. Idiopathic jaundice, which appears after the infant is 24 hours old, indicates a sluggish bilirubin excretion. Asian and American Indian infants are at increased risk for developing idiopathic jaundice.

Pathological Jaundice

Pathological jaundice appears before the newborn is 24 hours old and usually indicates increased serum bilirubin *synthesis* or decreased clearance. Pathological jaundice in the newborn frequently is due to a blood disorder, such as Rh or ABO incompatibility, or to a pathological condition of the hepatic system. These ill newborns require intervention directed by their primary health care provider.

Breastfeeding Jaundice

Breastfeeding jaundice should be distinguished from breast-milk jaundice. Breastfeeding jaundice is indeed related to the *feeding*, not the milk. It has an onset earlier than 5 days. Gartner[23] describes it as the equivalent of adult "starvation jaundice." Although the mechanism of this type of jaundice is poorly understood, the resulting increase in bilirubin is due simply to an inadequate intake of milk. This type of jaundice is not compared with other types of jaundice on the accom-

T A B L E 6-6
COMPARISON OF TYPES OF JAUNDICE*

	Idiopathic Jaundice (Physiological Jaundice)	Pathological Jaundice	Breast-Milk Jaundice
Onset	About 48 hr after birth	<24 hr after birth	About 7 days
Peak	72 hr in term infant	24 hr in term infant	2 weeks
Duration	Variable; recedes after 72 hr	Variable; rapid rise in bilirubin that recedes with treatment	Variable; 2-16 weeks
Cause	Alteration primarily in bilirubin excretion	As a result of pathological condition, alteration in bilirubin 1. Production 2. Transport 3. Conjugation 4. Excretion	Substance in some mothers' milk that exhibits certain enzyme activity in baby's liver, resulting in a slower breakdown and secretion of bilirubin
	These alterations are due to physiological conditions, and require monitoring and possible intervention	These alterations are due to pathological conditions and require additional medical evaluation and treatment	
Risk factors	Prematurity, delayed passage of stool	Hemolytic disease of newborn, some maternal diseases or drug ingestion, other	Mothers who have had previous baby with breast-milk jaundice
Treatment	Day-dependent	Phototherapy Blood transfusion	Phototherapy if bilirubin >15 mg/dl

*Breast*feeding* jaundice is described and discussed in the accompanying text. Breastfeeding jaundice is caused by poor intake and is best managed by the techniques described in Chapter 5.
Modified from Biancuzzo M. *Breastfeeding the Healthy Newborn: A Nursing Perspective.* White Plains, NY: March of Dimes Foundation; 1994.

panying tables because its causes and cures are usually fairly simple. Using the strategies described in Chapter 5, identify infants who may not have an adequate milk intake and offer early, frequent feedings; listen for audible swallowing to be sure the infant is taking in a sufficient volume of milk. A delayed passage of meconium also is likely to increase the rise of serum bilirubin levels because feces that remain in the colon will be reabsorbed.

Breast-Milk Jaundice
Breast-milk jaundice is a condition related to the milk, not the feeding (or lack thereof). Its onset is after 5 to 7 days, and it is due to the enhanced absorption of unconjugated bilirubin. Some theories suggest that an enzyme in some mothers' milk causes this condition to exist.

Impact on Breastfeeding and Clinical Management Strategies

There are frequent misconceptions about how to manage the breastfed infant who has been diagnosed with jaundice. Priorities for breastfed infants are listed in Box 6-6. Some mothers may recall that their last jaundiced infant was forbidden to breastfeed, or they were encouraged to give the infant water between feedings. Both of these strategies are outdated and are not based on research results or physiological principles. It has long been established that there is no difference in peak serum bilirubin levels between those who have been supplemented with water and those who have not,[24] as shown in the Research Highlight.

Mothers with jaundiced infants may have

Box 6-6
Priorities for Care: The Jaundiced Newborn

- Discourage the use of water supplementation. The practice of giving supplementary water continues, despite the landmark study nearly two decades ago showing that water supplements did not lower the serum bilirubin level.[24] Furthermore, the American Academy of Pediatrics states that "supplementing with water or dextrose water does not lower the bilirubin level in jaundiced, healthy, breast-feeding infants."[22]

- Advocate for continuation of breastfeeding. The American Academy of Pediatrics clearly states, "The AAP discourages the interruption of breastfeeding in healthy term newborns and encourages continued and frequent breastfeeding (at least eight to ten times every 24 hours)."[22]

- Explain the importance of frequent feedings. Infants who breastfeed more than eight times per 24 hours have significantly lower bilirubin levels than those whose feedings are limited.

- Promote early feedings at the breast. Colostrum has a laxative effect on the gut, which helps bilirubin to be excreted.

- Monitor intake and output. Note the time of the first stool. Continue to note the quantity and quality of voidings and stools, and weight loss. Call the pediatrician or primary care provider about data that appear worrisome.

- Lead efforts to minimize maternal-infant separation when the hyperbilirubinemia is treated with phototherapy. Ideally, the newer fiberoptic treatment is more conducive to keeping the mother and infant together. Separation in and of itself can breed problems with breastfeeding, so keeping the dyad together is optimal.

- Teach the parents how to blanch for jaundice. In addition, provide a card describing worrisome signs, and a clear idea of when to call the primary health care provider.

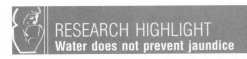

RESEARCH HIGHLIGHT
Water does not prevent jaundice

Citation
DeCarvalho M, Hall M, Harvey D. Effects of water supplementation on physiological jaundice in breast-fed babies. *Arch Dis Child* 1981;56:568-569.

Focus
This prospective study of 175 healthy full-term newborns was designed to determine the effects of water supplementation on bilirubin levels. Fifty-five newborns were given no water; 120 were given water ad libitum at the end of each breastfeeding.

Results
There was no significant difference between the two groups when peak serum bilirubin levels and incidence of phototherapy were compared. Bilirubin peaked at 4 days in both the control and the study groups.

Strengths, Limitations of the Study
Only infants who had no risk factors for jaundice were included in this study conducted in London. All newborns began breastfeeding within the first 3 hours of life and continued to breastfeed on demand, although the number of feedings per day was not specified.

Clinical Application
The practice of giving water to newborns was begun without any scientific evidence to support the claim that it prevents or minimizes jaundice, yet it still exists in some hospitals. The results of this study should be considered when updating jaundice protocols in hospitals. Giving water probably interferes with the mechanisms that *do* minimize or prevent jaundice. For example, when the infant consumes water, he is likely to breastfeed fewer times in a day, and a later study by the same author[19] shows that frequent feedings are beneficial in minimizing bilirubin levels. Furthermore, the same author[21] shows that lower serum bilirubin levels are associated with greater stool output—which is enhanced by colostrum, not water—and lowered bilirubin levels.

T A B L E 6-7

COMPARISON OF BREASTFEEDING MANAGEMENT STRATEGIES FOR DIFFERENT TYPES OF JAUNDICE

	Idiopathic Jaundice	Pathological Jaundice	Breast-Milk Jaundice
Onset (clue)	About 48 hr after birth	Anytime after birth	About 7 days
Initiation of breastfeeding	Early initiation decreases threat	Early initiation desirable	Unrelated to condition
Weaning	Not necessary	Not necessary	Not necessary
Interruption of breastfeeding	Not necessary	Not necessary	Rarely, if ever, necessary to interrupt breastfeeding for diagnosis[23]
Supplementation			
• Indication	If baby is too lethargic to suckle	If baby is too lethargic to suckle	Likely to be ordered if bilirubin levels are greater than 25 mg/dl
	Dependent on hydration status and/or phototherapy	Dependent on hydration status and/or phototherapy	May need formula to dilute effect on bilirubin
• With water?	No	No	No
• With artificial milk?	Acceptable if supplementation is indicated and human milk is unavailable	Acceptable if supplementation is indicated and human milk is unavailable	Yes, every other feeding
• With expressed mother's own milk	If supplementation is indicated, this is best option	If supplementation is indicated, this is best option	Not appropriate
• With banked donor milk	Yes, if mother has insufficient volume	Yes, if mother has insufficient volume	Yes, if available
Expressing breast milk			
Frequency	Express milk after any skipped or partial feedings	Express milk after any skipped or partial feedings	Express milk after any skipped or partial feedings
Save and feed	Yes	Yes	No—may be unusable after 1 month of age
Discard	No	No	Yes
Helpful devices			
Wallaby phototherapy unit	Safe and effective; improves mother's access to baby	Safe and effective; improves mother's access to baby	No data to determine effectiveness with this group; good for home care
Nursing supplementers (see Chapter 12)	Probably not indicated if infant can suckle	May be helpful for baby who is lethargic or who has weak suck	May be helpful for supplementation

Modified from Biancuzzo M. *Breastfeeding the Healthy Newborn: A Nursing Perspective.* White Plains, NY: March of Dimes Foundation; 1994.

questions about "pumping and dumping" their milk; Table 6-7 answers some of these and other related questions with respect to which type of jaundice the infant is experiencing. Appendix B lists patient education materials on the topic of jaundice.

Inadequate Fluids

Generally speaking, infants who are taking in adequate amounts of milk are consuming adequate amounts of fluids. Infants can and do get dehydrated, however. There are three types of dehydration: *isotonic* (also called *isonatremic*), *hypotonic (hyponatremic),* and *hypertonic (hypernatremic).* Most descriptions of a dehydrated infant refer to isotonic dehydration, which is usually associated with the use of artificial milk. The important thing is not the label but the early recognition that there is a problem.

Reports of hypernatremic dehydration[25,26] have been associated with breastfeeding, but the reader is cautioned to read these reports with the insight that breastfeeding was not the cause of dehydration. Rather, a series of clinical management errors, including poor breastfeeding management, a delay in seeking help for worrisome factors, and not being seen by a physician were all apparent in those cases that resulted in serious morbidity. Similarly, scare stories in the popular press describe desperate scenarios in which newborns have been severely dehydrated,[27] and, as a result, mothers have been frightened that breastfeeding will have deleterious effects. It is therefore important to emphasize that if breastfeeding is going well, as described in Chapter 5, dehydration is unlikely to occur.

Clinical Signs of Dehydration

Typically, professional education emphasizes a sunken fontanel as a sign of dehydration in the newborn. However, this is a very late sign. Like other problems that can be detected, dehydration is easier to manage in the early phases. Several earlier signs of dehydration are clues that, if left uncorrected, indicate a dangerous situation. Table 6-8 shows that most clinical signs of isonatremic dehydration appear "normal" during the early phases of dehydration; signs and symptoms of hypernatremic dehydra-

T A B L E 6-8
SIGNS AND SYMPTOMS RELATED TO DEGREE OF DEHYDRATION

Parameter	Mild	Moderate	Severe
Weight loss	3-5%	10%	15%
Skin color	Pale	Gray	Mottled
Skin turgor	May be elastic	Decreased elasticity	Tenting
Mucous membranes	Slightly dry	Dry	Dry, parched, collapse of sublingual veins
Eyes	Probably normal	Decreased tears	Sunken; absence of tears, soft globes
Central nervous system	Alert but calm	Irritable	Lethargic
Pulse: Quality	Probably normal	Somewhat increased	Markedly tachycardic
Rate	Norm (<2 sec)	2-4 sec	>4 sec
Blood pressure	No change	Orthostatic decrease	Decreased while supine
Urine	Probably normal or slightly decreased volume	Elevated specific gravity, decreased volume	Less than 0.5 ml/kg/hr over past 12-24 hr; may be anuric
Clinical implications	Assess closely; implement preventative measures Notify primary health care provider and record observations	Initiate interventions as ordered; goal is to avoid severe problem Continue to assess; record observations Help mother and family understand impact on feeding	Continue to implement medical interventions as ordered Help mother to continue breastfeeding efforts, even if separated from infant (see Chapter 11)

The table is best used to judge severity in infants with isonatremic dehydration; those with hypernatremic dehyration have the same signs, but they are more subtle and therefore are more likely to be underestimated.
Modified from Hoekelman RA, Friedman SB, Nelson NM, Seidel HM, Weitzman ML. *Primary Pediatric Care.* 3rd ed. St. Louis: Mosby; 1997.

tion are less obvious, which means the clinical assessment usually *underestimates* the magnitude of hydration.[28] Note that one of the earliest signs of dehydration is *pallor,* which warrants follow-up.

Impact on Breastfeeding and Clinical Management Strategies

Dehydration is a medical diagnosis that should be managed by the pediatrician or primary care provider. Indeed, it is possible that good breastfeeding management may alleviate the problem. However, supplementation may be indicated.

Supplementation can be a therapeutic intervention, or it can be a risk for breastfeeding. As discussed previously, supplementation may indeed upset the supply-and-demand phenomenon, so the benefit of supplementation must always outweigh the cost. Infants do not routinely need extra fluids.

WELL INFANTS WHO NEED EXTRA HELP

Normal, full-term, healthy newborns and their mothers can usually breastfeed with little assistance. Some situations, however, may require a little extra help. Mothers who breastfeed multiple-birth infants and those who tandem breastfeed are common examples.

Multiple Gestation

Breastfeeding two offspring poses multiple challenges. The greatest problem, however, is usually not breastfeeding per se. Multiple gestation may result in preterm birth; hence, the mother may arrive home with one but not all infants. In these cases, base breastfeeding management on information in Chapters 7 and 11. Whether the infants are ill or well, discourage the mother from

breastfeeding one and artificially feeding another; she may experience differences in bonding/attachment, and all infants benefit from and deserve human milk. Similarly, discourage her from always putting the same infant to the breast before his sibling; if one sibling suckles more vigorously, he may consistently obtain more milk.

The percentage of multiple births is the highest reported in at least 50 years.[29] Of those infants born in 1996, 2.7% were multiple births, the most frequent type of which is twins. Frequently, mothers of multiple infants assume that breastfeeding is not a realistic possibility. Multiple gestation does not preclude breastfeeding, however. The mother should be counseled about breastfeeding as soon as she realizes that she has multiple fetuses.

Impact on Breastfeeding and Clinical Management Strategies

The principles that promote a balance of supply and demand for a singleton become even more important with multiple birth. With adequate stimulation, a mother of twins will produce more than 800 ml of milk per day.[30] Advise the mother to avoid artificial milk if possible—since supplementing or complementing will decrease her milk supply—and increase the number of times the infants are at the breast. There is a direct relationship between frequency of breastfeeding sessions and milk production for singletons,[31-33] as well as for twins and triplets.[30] Quadruplets have successfully breastfed and have made mean weight gains of 30 to 54 g per day.[34] While the inverse seems implicit—that discouraging or curtailing breastfeeding will result in lower milk supply for multiple infants—it bears emphasis. If artificial milk is introduced, suckling is decreased and milk synthesis is decreased as well. This is usually accompanied by the cascade of deleterious effects that occur with milk stasis.

Some women are reluctant to breastfeed twins because they have heard that doing so will make their nipples twice as sore as breastfeeding a singleton. This may be true, but only if the soreness is the result of poor latch-on or incorrect use of a pump, but it should not be the result of multiple infants suckling at the breast. Some breast and nipple problems, however, do seem to be more prevalent in mothers of multiples. Mastitis, for example, is frequently seen in these situations. It is likely that mastitis occurs because of increased milk synthesis and incomplete removal of milk at each feeding (see Chapter 8). Thrush that occurs in one infant requires immediate treatment not only of that infant but of the others as well. There is, however, no reason to "assign" a breast to a particular infant when there is an outbreak of thrush (see Chapter 8).

The newborns may suckle simultaneously or separately. There are advantages and disadvantages to both strategies, and there are no rules for how to accomplish breastfeeding multiples. Simultaneous feedings save time, however, so encourage mothers to at least learn this option. Several positions for simultaneous feedings offer specific advantages, as shown in Table 6-9, and include[35]: (1) the double football (or double clutch hold); (2) the cradle-football (or parallel hold) and (3) the double cradle (crisscross or V-hold), as shown in Figures 6-5 to 6-7.

Feeding one twin and then the other is referred to as *alternate feeding*. In alternate feeding, the hungrier infant demands to be fed and therefore sets the pace as the mother then wakens the second infant. Some mothers have successfully breastfed for several months using alternate feedings and enjoy the one-on-one contact. This

TABLE 6-9

BREASTFEEDING MULTIPLES: COMPARING STRATEGIES

Positioning for More Than One Infant	Advantages	Limitations
Alternate The mother feeds first one infant and then the other	• May be easier for mother to manage in the beginning • Gives "private time" with each infant	• More time-consuming • Difficulty letting down when other baby is waiting to eat and crying • More difficult to meet needs of both babies at once; may require another person to feed the other baby who is hungry but not at the breast
Simultaneous Feeding Two infants are fed at the same time; these include:	• More time-efficient • Easier to meet the needs of both babies at once	• Requires more coordination to latch-on and reposition infants
• Double football (double clutch)	• Allows mother better head control of smaller, fussier infants, since her hands are more free • Hands more free to position both infants, since pillows function as a sort of extra "hand" • Usually able to support each breast for latch-on and/or throughout the feeding	• Requires a couch or large chair for support on both sides
• Cradle/football (parallel hold)	• Can alternate positioning; thus each infant exercises both eyes for eye contact	• Hands not free to reposition infants • Difficult for mother to support her breasts prior to latch-on
• Double cradle (crisscross or V-hold) both infants in cradle position	• Allows for eye contact between mother and both infants	• Difficult to use until after infants have gained more head control

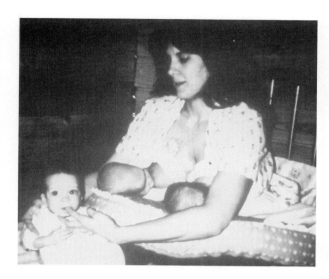

Fig. 6-5 Double football hold. *(Courtesy Jane Bradshaw.)*

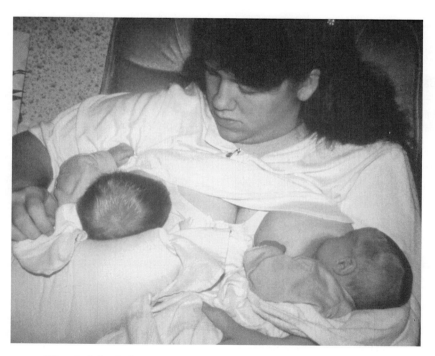

Fig. 6-6 Cradle/football (or parallel) hold. *(Courtesy Jane Bradshaw.)*

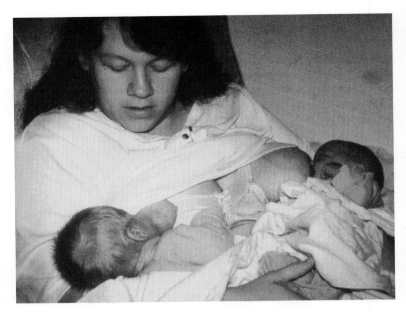

Fig. 6-7 Double cradle (crisscross or V-hold) an infant and his older sibling are suckling at the same time. *(Courtesy Jane Bradshaw.)*

Box 6-7
Priorities for Care: Breastfeeding Education for Mothers of Multiples

- Applaud mother's breastfeeding efforts and help her to find lifestyle adjustments that facilitate breastfeeding.
- Teach the mother about adequate rest and nutrition and about positions for simultaneous breastfeeding.
- Verify proper latch-on to avoid sore nipples and other problems that become magnified with multiple infants.

- Access material and human resources: find support services in the community and provide helpful literature before hospital discharge. Help mother to ask for practical help from family and friends.
- Emphasize that adequate stimulation is critical to adequate milk supply and that adequate consumption of hindmilk by all infants is critical; pump if indicated. Provide list of reassuring signs.
- Refer to support services; TWINLINE offers national telephone counseling for parents of multiples (see Appendix C).

approach is quite acceptable, and breastfeeding may continue nicely despite the extra time required.

Sometimes the mother assigns one breast to one infant and one to the other, but this is not recommended. A more abundant supply may be created on one side if one infant sucks more vigorously and removes more milk there.

Priorities for teaching mothers of multiples are listed in Box 6-7. Professional literature about breastfeeding multiples is somewhat limited. However, Gromada[36] describes in detail the importance of prenatal preparation (including the decision to breastfeed, social support assessment, and developing goals and plans specific to multiples); circumstances surrounding the initiation of lactation for multiples; interventions to promote maintenance of lactation; and alternative plans for carrying out the feedings. This article, although somewhat dated, is still well worth reading. Suggestions for educational materials for parents of multiples are listed in Appendix B.

Tandem Breastfeeding

Tandem breastfeeding means that the mother is breastfeeding two siblings of different ages at the same time (Figure 6-8). Usually the mother becomes pregnant while breastfeeding a toddler or preschooler and then wishes to breastfeed the newborn upon his arrival. The mother may feel uneasy about lactating while she is pregnant and may require reassurance and approval. Some women experience contractions when they are breastfeeding, and for mothers at high risk for preterm labor, breastfeeding may be contraindicated. Many mothers may experience increased nipple soreness due to the hormonal changes of pregnancy and positioning the older child at the breast with the enlarging abdomen may be awkward.

Impact on Breastfeeding and Clinical Management Strategies

Colostrum is produced as the pregnancy advances to term, but the colostrum tastes saltier than the milk the older child was accustomed to. The older child may have loose stools because of the colostrum's laxative effect. Sometimes the older child weans himself at this point. If he does not, however, tandem breastfeeding can continue as long as the mother wishes. After delivery, these mothers will experience some degree of postpartum engorgement, although less than mothers who are not tandem breastfeeding. The most important priority is the mother's nutritional status; sufficient stores of nutrients—most notably calcium—are needed, and the mother's own body becomes deficient in response to the extra demands to make milk. (See Clinical Scenario in Chapter 1.)

There are no rules about the pattern of breast-

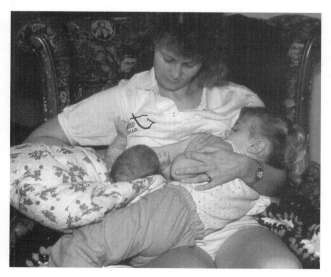

Fig. 6-8 Tandem nursing. *(Courtesy © Debi Bocar.)*

feeding—frequency, duration, whether the siblings suckle simultaneously or separately; encourage the mother to find what works best for her and her family. Some recommendations to aid in successful tandem breastfeeding are described in Box 6-8. Some consumer education materials are listed in Appendix B.

Tandem breastfeeding is for some people but not for others. Some men and women may consider this practice natural and acceptable; others are repulsed by it. Support whatever decision the mother makes, and avoid any cultural biases. If the mother approaches the idea of tandem breast-feeding enthusiastically but later decides that it isn't for her, help her to gently wean the older child.

SUMMARY

The transition to extrauterine life requires several adaptations for the newborn. The newborn's metabolism is immature, and he may need changes in the environment or food to meet his biological needs and achieve homeostasis. Human milk provides nutrients, including energy, to help the newborn establish and maintain circulatory, respiratory, thermoregulatory, and gastrointestinal function. Behavioral tasks such as sleep-wake cycles and sensory needs are an integral factor in the breastfeeding experience. Newborns are especially at risk for hypoglycemia, hypothermia, and hyperbilirubinemia. These conditions, however, can be minimized or overcome by good breastfeeding management. Newborns who are generally healthy but have some special situation—for example, those whose mother is breastfeeding a twin or an older sibling—can breastfeed successfully if their mothers adapt good breastfeeding principles to the special situation.

Box 6-8
Priorities for Care: Tandem Breastfeeding

- The newborn has priority at the breast. The older sibling can increase intake of solid foods during the first 3 to 5 days after birth so that the newborn receives adequate colostrum. The mother may fear that the older child will consume the younger child's portion, but this is unlikely, given that human milk is synthesized according to supply and demand.

- Reassure the mother that any change in behavior from the older child—being repulsed by the engorgement or being thrilled with the bountiful supply—is okay. Things will return to "normal" in a few days.

- Suggest many different ways to position two siblings at the breast if the mother wishes to breastfeed simultaneously, as described in Figures 6-5 to 6-7.

- Reassure the mother that it is not necessary to discontinue breastfeeding or limit feedings to one breast if one child becomes ill. After the onset of symptoms, the siblings have already been sharing the breast for several days.

- Help the mother to identify ways to get some time to herself, since she may be feeling that her body is no longer her own. Even a short walk alone can be helpful.

- Identify calcium-rich food and encourage the mother to consume these foods in substantial quantities.

References

1. Bobak IM, Jensen MD. *Maternity and Gynecologic Care.* 5th ed. St. Louis: Mosby; 1993.

2. Thibodeau GA, Patton KT. *Anatomy and Physiology.* 3rd ed. St. Louis: Mosby; 1996.

3. Committee on Nutrition, American Academy of Pediatrics. *Pediatric Nutrition Handbook.* Elk Grove Village, IL: American Academy of Pediatrics; 1993.

4. Behrman RE, Kliegman RM, Arvin AM, eds. *Nelson Textbook of Pediatrics.* 15th ed. Philadelphia: Saunders; 1996.

5. Vorherr H. Human lactation and breast feeding. In: Larson BL, ed. *Lactation*. New York: Academic Press; 1978:216-217.

6. Blackburn S, Loper DL. *Maternal, Fetal, and Neonatal Physiology: A Clinical Perspective*. Philadelphia: Saunders; 1992.

7. Almroth SG. Water requirements of breast-fed infants in a hot climate. *Am J Clin Nutr* 1978;31:1154-1157.

8. Almroth S, Bidinger PD. No need for water supplementation for exclusively breast-fed infants under hot and arid conditions. *Trans R Soc Trop Med Hyg* 1990 84:602-604.

9. Ashraf RN, Jalil F, Aperia A, Lindblad BS. Additional water is not needed for healthy breast-fed babies in a hot climate. *Acta Paediatr* 1993;82:1007-1011.

10. Goldberg NM, Adams E. Supplementary water for breast-fed babies in a hot and dry climate—not really a necessity. *Arch Dis Child* 1983;58:73-74.

11. Sachdev HP, Krishna J, Puri RK, Satyanarayana L, Kumar S. Water supplementation in exclusively breastfed infants during summer in the tropics. *Lancet* 1991;337(8747):929-933.

12. Brazelton TB. *Neonatal Behavioral Assessment Scale*. Philadelphia: Lippincott; 1984.

13. Barnard K. *Early Parent-Infant Relationships*. White Plains, NY: March of Dimes Foundation; 1978.

14. Butler DA, MacMillan JP. Relationship of breast feeding and weight loss to jaundice in the newborn period: review of the literature and results of a study. *Cleve Clin Q* 1983; 50:263-268.

15. Johnson CA, Lieberman B, Hassanein RE. The relationship of breast feeding to third-day bilirubin levels. *J Fam Pract* 1985; 20:147-152.

16. Kivlahan C, James EJ. The natural history of neonatal jaundice. *Pediatrics* 1984;74(3):364-370.

17. Maisels MJ, Gifford K. Normal serum bilirubin levels in the newborn and the effect of breastfeeding. *Pediatrics* 1986;78(5):837-843.

18. Schneider AP 2d. Breast milk jaundice in the newborn. A real entity. *JAMA* 1986;255(23):3270-3274.

19. DeCarvalho M, Klaus MH, Merkatz RB. Frequency of breast-feeding and serum bilirubin concentration. *Am J Dis Child* 1982;136:737-738.

20. Yamauchi Y, Yamanouchi I. Breast-feeding frequency during the first 24 hours after birth in full-term neonates. *Pediatrics* 1990;86:171-175.

21. DeCarvalho M, Robertson S, Klaus M. Fecal bilirubin excretion and serum bilirubin concentrations in breast-fed and bottle-fed infants. *J Pediatr* 1985;107:786-790.

22. American Academy of Pediatrics: Provisional Committee for Quality Improvement and Subcommittee on Hyperbilirubinemia. Practice parameter: management of hyperbilirubinemia in the healthy term newborn. *Pediatrics* 1994;94(4, pt 1):558-565.

23. Gartner LM. Neonatal jaundice. *Pediatr Rev* 1994;15:422-432.

24. DeCarvalho M, Hall M, Harvey D. Effects of water supplementation on physiological jaundice in breast-fed babies. *Arch Dis Child* 1981;56:568-569.

25. Thullen JD. Management of hypernatremic dehydration due to insufficient lactation. *Clin Pediatr (Phila)* 1988;27:370-372.

26. Cooper WO, Atherton HD, Kahana M, Kotagal UR. Increased incidence of severe breastfeeding malnutrition and hypernatremia in a metropolitan area. *Pediatrics* 1995;96(5, pt 2):957-960.

27. Helliker K. Some mothers, trying in vain to breast-feed, starve their infants. *Wall Street Journal*. July 22, 1994:1, 4.

28. Hoekelman RA, Friedman SB, Nelson NM, Seidel HM, Weitzman ML. *Primary Pediatric Care*. 3rd ed. St. Louis: Mosby; 1997.

29. United States Bureau of Statistics. *Monthly Vital Statistics Report*. 1998;46(11):21.

30. Saint L, Maggiore P, Hartmann PE. Yield and nutrient content of milk in eight women breastfeeding twins and one woman breast-feeding triplets. *Br J Nutr* 1986;56:49-58.

31. DeCarvalho M, Robertson S, Merkatz R, Klaus M. Milk intake and frequency of feeding in breast fed infants. *Early Hum Dev* 1982;7:155-163.

32. Egli GE, Egli NS, Newton M. The influence of the number of breastfeedings on milk production. *Pediatrics* 1961;27:314-317.

33. Illingworth RS, Leeds MD, Stone DGH. Self-demand feeding in a maternity unit. *Lancet* 1952;1:683-687.

34. Mead LJ, Chuffo R, Lawlor Klean P, Meier PP. Breastfeeding success with preterm quadruplets. *J Obstet Gynecol Neonatal Nurs* 1992;21:221-227.

35. Sollid DT, Evans BT, McClowry SG, Garrett A. Breastfeeding multiples. *J Perinat Neonatal Nurs* 1989;3:46-65.

36. Gromada KK. Breastfeeding more than one: multiples and tandem breastfeeding. *NAACOGS Clin Issu Perinat Womens Health Nurs* 1992;3:656-666.

37. WHO. *Hypoglycaemia of the Newborn: Review of the Literature*. Geneva: World Health Organization.

3

Breastfeeding Under Difficult Circumstances

7

The Compromised Infant: Impact on Breastfeeding

*B*reastfeeding occurs within the context of the many biological and behavioral tasks the infant must accomplish. Similarly, when an infant is compromised in some way, breastfeeding—both a biological and a behavioral task—is impacted. Unlike the healthy infant who can breastfeed with little assistance, the compromised infant should have special assistance based on an understanding of how his associated pathophysiology affects his ability to breastfeed.

The purpose of this chapter is to frame breastfeeding within the broader context of the health-illness continuum. It would not be practical to list every disease entity here, but pathophysiology is discussed in relation to breastfeeding (the activity) and human milk (the source of nutrition). Breastfeeding management is described within the broader context of the infant's capabilities and limitations.

The first part looks at infants who have alterations in nutrient requirements, in neurological function, and in structural anatomy in general. One specific prototype is given to demonstrate specific needs and management strategies. The second part looks at the preterm infant, who frequently has multiple problems that require special management of breastfeeding.

ALTERATIONS IN NUTRIENT REQUIREMENTS

Nutrients—source of energy, vitamins, and minerals—are essential for survival. Sometimes the infant's *need* for nutrients is about normal, but his net intake is insufficient to meet a normal need. Otherwise stated, his processes of ingestion, digestion, and absorption are inadequate to meet his needs. For example, if the infant cannot ingest adequate food (perhaps he has a structural defect of the oral cavity, or inadequate neuromuscular capabilities to suckle effectively) or if he has a disorder that impedes digestion, absorption, or retention of food (e.g., diarrhea or vomiting) good nutrition becomes central to good clinical outcomes. The clinical implication in all three situations is clear: feeding must be carried out in a way that meets the infant's nutrient requirements.

The normal, full-term, healthy infant requires about 108 kcal/kg/day (see Chapter 6 for details) for basal needs, growth, and activity. Energy requirements are greater, however, when infants have an increased metabolic rate. The term *metabolic rate* means "the amount of energy released in the body in a given time by catabolism. It represents energy expended for accomplishing various kinds of work. In short, metabolic rate actually means catabolic rate, or rate of energy release."[1] In the presence of certain conditions (infection, cardiac dysfunction, prematurity, surgery), the metabolic rate is accelerated; more energy is released in order to meet the increased need for nutrients to the cells. To meet these demands, these infants also need an increase in intake. Furthermore, energy—kilocalories—alone will not suffice. Compromised infants usually need an increase in other nutrients, such as vitamins and minerals.

Infections

Infants who have infections require a greater amount of energy because their metabolic rate is increased. Preterm infants are 10 times more likely to experience infection, and boys are more vulnerable than girls. The clinical signs and symptoms of sepsis are listed in Box 7-1; these are subtle and often overlooked. "Poor feeding" and "disinterested" behavior should not be mistaken

Box 7-1
Signs of Neonatal Sepsis

Signs may be subtle and nonspecific. They include:

- Respiratory distress
- High-pitched cry
- Lethargy
- Temperature instability (hypothermia or hyperthermia)
- Hypotonia
- Vomiting
- Jaundice
- Diarrhea
- Abdominal distention
- Poor feeding
- Apnea
- Cyanotic spells
- Seizures
- Poor perfusion
- Petechiae
- Purpura

Source: Seidel HM, Rosenstein BJ, Pathak A. *Primary Care of the Newborn.* St. Louis: Mosby; 1993.

for breastfeeding problems. These manifestations, especially when they occur in the presence of other signs of sepsis or in a newborn at risk for infection, should be reported to the primary caregiver.

Often, infants have been exposed to infections in utero, as is the case with amnionitis, endometritis, or a urinary tract infection. If so, these infants can experience respiratory distress and apnea, and hence feeding is hampered. Whether the infection was transmitted from the mother in utero or was acquired by the infant postnatally, good lines of communication between the physician, the mother, and the nursing staff will enhance breastfeeding efforts. In most cases, transmission of the infection is not exacerbated by breastfeeding. See Chapter 8 for further discussion of common maternal infections.

Alterations in Gastrointestinal Function

Alterations in gastrointestinal function cause obstruction and result in differing symptoms. Lawrence[2] discusses various disorders along with their clinical manifestations and treatment, so details of each disorder will not be described here. Alterations in gastrointestinal function often result in separation from the mother, at least temporarily. Chapter 10 suggests strategies to deal with separation issues.

When a gastrointestinal problem exists, the nurse's role becomes that of expert observer, parent educator, and breastfeeding advocate. Some common gastrointestinal disorders affect the breastfeeding mother-infant couple, either because the diagnosis has not yet been made or because the clinical interpretations of the problem differ according to whether the infant is breastfed or bottle fed. Problems that may not be immediately diagnosed include tracheoesophageal fistula and tracheoesophageal atresia. Data about problems such as diarrhea and regurgitation are interpreted differently, depending on the method of feeding.

Diarrhea

It is unusual for a breastfed newborn to have diarrhea. Stools are typically very soft, as described in Chapter 6. Excessively thin stools may indicate that there is not an adequate consumption of the hindmilk. If diarrhea is observed in the infant, prompt referral for medical diagnosis and treatment is needed.

Colic

The etiology of colic is poorly understood, but it is apparently related to a combination of biological and psychosocial factors that lead to a fussy period each day. Typically the fussy period—with loud crying and drawing the legs up to the abdomen—occurs in the evening and lasts for a few hours.

Unfortunately, when infants exhibit signs of colic, parents often become fretful about breastfeeding and switch to artificial feeding. Infants do not improve with the artificial feeding.[3] If anything, their symptoms become exacerbated. It may be helpful for the mother to avoid ingesting milk products because the infant may have gastrointestinal distress from dairy products the mother has ingested. Usually, however, colic runs its course, and breastfeeding should be continued.

Regurgitation, Spitting Up, Esophageal Reflux, Vomiting

Both breastfed and artificially fed newborns may spit up a little milk. Artificially fed newborns are likely to spit up a significant amount, whereas those who are breastfed spit up a relatively small amount. Regurgitation and esophageal reflux, while common in the artificially fed newborn, are possible but unlikely for the breastfed newborn. The breastfed newborn who exhibits esophageal reflux requires further evaluation. Gastrointestinal reflux is sometimes helped by an upright position. Vomiting—especially projectile vomiting—is not normal in the breastfed infant; this infant needs immediate medical follow-up.

Tracheoesophageal Fistula and Tracheal Atresia

Tracheoesophageal fistulas (TEFs) and esophageal atresias (EAs) are rare congenital defects of the gastrointestinal tract that occur around the 4th week of gestation. During fetal development the foregut usually lengthens and separates longitudinally, and each longitudinal portion separates to form two channels, the esophagus and the trachea. In normal development (1) both proximal and distal segments of the esophagus *connect* to the stomach, and (2) the esophagus completely *separates* from the trachea or bronchus.

When these two channels do not separate properly, a *fistula* and/or *atresia* results. A TEF is an abnormal opening between the trachea and

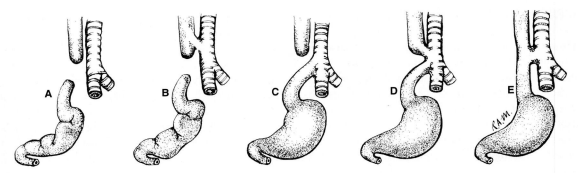

Fig. 7-1 Five most common types of esophageal atresia and tracheoesophageal fistula. *(From Wong D.* Whaley and Wong's nursing care of infants and children. *5th ed. St. Louis: Mosby; 1995.)*

the esophagus—the trachea fails to separate from the esophagus. An atresia is an abnormal occlusion, or discontinuous character of a channel. There are five types of EA and TEF, as shown in Figure 7-1. The most common situation is where the proximal segment of the esophagus dead-ends (an atresia), and a fistula (abnormal opening) exists between the distal segment of the esophagus and the trachea (or primary bronchus). Clinical symptoms include the following:

- Frothy saliva in the mouth and nose
- Drooling, frequently accompanied by choking and coughing
- Swallowing milk normally, followed by sudden coughing and gagging, with fluid returning through the nose and mouth
- Becoming cyanotic and apneic as the overflow of milk or saliva is aspirated into the trachea or bronchus, when there is a proximal esophageal pouch (most cases)[4]

Any infant who has a known or suspected TE fistula should not be put to the breast. TE fistulas are known if they are seen on ultrasound and are suspected if the mother has polyhydramnios. If the mother has polyhydramnios, wait for a feeding tube to be passed to confirm esophageal pa-

tency before suggesting that the newborn go to the breast. The objective is to have the infant undergo surgery as soon as possible, so feeding is contraindicated in order to avoid aspiration of milk, which is likely.

Necrotizing Enterocolitis

Infants who are born preterm are particularly at risk for developing necrotizing enterocolitis, an inflammation of the bowel. This condition can be life-threatening. In one study, infants who were exclusively artificially fed were 6 to 10 times more likely to develop necrotizing enterocolitis than those who were exclusively fed human milk, while those who were fed human milk and artificial milk were 3 times more likely to be affected than those who were exclusively fed human milk.[5] Infants who are unable to feed at the breast should be given their own mother's milk or donor milk to decrease the threat of necrotizing enterocolitis.

Weight Gain Problems

Weight gain is only one consideration of well-being and should be considered along with other measurements, including length, head circumference, and skinfold thickness. While Chapter 5 discusses normal weight gains in more detail, it is important to keep in mind a few principles with respect to the compromised infant: (1) the preterm infant should be gaining in length, weight, and circumference at approximately the same rate as he would be experiencing if he was still in utero; (2) the compromised infant should be ingesting, digesting, and retaining enough calories to support not only basal requirements but also activity and growth; and (3) patterns of weight gain in breastfed infants are not identical to those in artificially fed infants. Full-term healthy newborns, as well as compromised infants, may not achieve their expected weight gains. These infants can be classified as either failing to thrive or slow to gain.

Failure to Thrive

Failure to thrive (FTT) is defined generically, as is seen in this classic reference: (1) "The rate of gain in weight is less than the −2SD value during an interval of 2 months or longer for infants less than 6 months of age or during an interval of 3 months or longer for infants over 6 months of age," and (2) "the weight for length is less than the 5th percentile."[6]

This definition, however, is not entirely applicable to the breastfed infant. Lawrence[2] defines failure to thrive in the breastfed infant as:

- Continuing to lose weight after 10 days of life
- Not regaining birth weight by 3 weeks
- Gaining at a rate below the 10th percentile for weight gain beyond 2 months of age

Four types of FTT are delineated in the pediatric literature:[6] (1) organic—due to pathological causes; (2) psychosocial—formerly called inorganic and due to psychosocial causes; (3) combined organic and psychosocial; and (4) undetermined. The distinctions of "organic" and "psychosocial," however, are probably meaningless for the breastfed infant; breastfeeding is a bio-psycho-social process. Although delineating these categories for the breastfed infant is not clinically relevant, the astute consumer of research needs to understand that studies describing FTT may have limited relevance to the breastfed infant.

Lawrence[2] identifies causes of FTT in the breastfed infant, shown in Figure 7-2. Failure to thrive in the breastfed infant may be due to maternal causes (poor milk production caused by diet, illness, or fatigue) or poor let-down (related to psychological factors, drugs, or smoking.) Frequently, however, it is due to infant causes, including poor intake (the result of poor suck, infrequent feeds, or structural abnormality), low net intake (vomiting and diarrhea, malabsorption, or infection), or high energy requirements (due to central nervous system pathology, congenital heart disease, or small for gestational age). Most frequently, FTT in the breastfed infant is caused by poor infant intake.

It is important to recognize that FTT may be a symptom of pathology rather than a breastfeeding problem! Not all worrisome signs and symptoms can be corrected by better breastfeeding management; rather, they should be reported and medical follow-up should be initiated.

Slow to Gain

Some infants are "slow to gain." Unlike FTT infants who show worrisome signs, infants who are slow to gain generally show signs of wellness along with slow but steady progress as shown in Table 7-1. They do gain weight, but their rate of weight gain is considerably slower than expected. Regardless of the label—FTT or slow to gain—it is the nurse's role to recognize the problems and initiate corrective strategies.

Nurse's Role in Weight-Gain Problems

The nurse may be the giver or the receiver of information about a diagnosis of FTT or slow to gain infants. Generalized "feeding problems" may

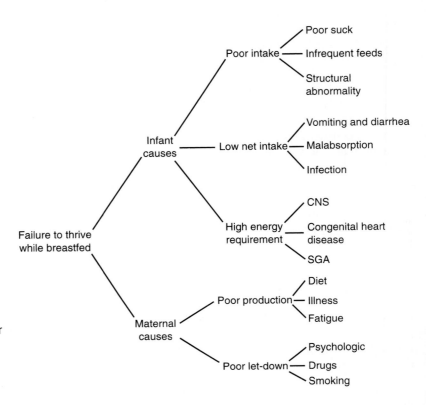

Fig. 7-2 Diagnostic flowchart for failure to thrive. *(From Lawrence, RA. Breastfeeding: A Guide for the Medical Profession. 4th ed. St. Louis: Mosby; 1994.)*

signal the need for further follow-up; these infants require referral to the primary health care provider. In other situations, infants may have already been diagnosed as failing to thrive or being slow to gain, and the physician refers the infant to the breastfeeding specialist for a comprehensive teaching session. In either event, good assessments, a plan of action with thorough implementation, and an evaluation mechanism will be invaluable in the management of these infants.

ASSESSMENT

Whether a diagnosis has already been made or is pending, ongoing data gathering leads to better clinical management. The following sections describe the nurse's responsibility in gathering data.

Perform an infant physical assessment. Perform a head-to-toe physical assessment of the infant. Typically, this begins with measuring the infant's weight, length, and head circumference. Weight loss is not the only factor to consider, but it is often the trigger for action. Unfortunately, the action is sometimes based on data that are obtained incorrectly or recorded inaccurately. Therefore, a few commonsense rules bear repeating when weight discrepancies are noted:

• Weigh the infant on the same scale, and with approximately the same amount of clothing each time a weight is assessed. (Nude weights are generally done during at least the first month of life.)

T A B L E 7-1
PARAMETERS FOR EVALUATION OF BREASTFED INFANTS

Infant Who Is Slow to Gain Weight	Infant With Failure to Thrive
Alert, healthy appearance	Apathetic or crying
Good muscle tone	Poor tone
Good skin turgor	Poor turgor
At least 6 wet diapers/day	Few wet diapers
Pale, dilute urine	"Strong" urine
Stools frequent, seedy (or if infrequent, large and soft)	Stools infrequent, scanty
8 or more nursings/day, lasting 15-20 minutes	Fewer than 8 feedings, often brief
Well-established let-down reflex	No signs of functioning let-down reflex
Weight gain consistent but slow	Weight erratic—may lose

From Lawrence RA. *Breastfeeding: A Guide for the Medical Profession.* St. Louis: Mosby; 1994.

- Be sure that the electronic scale is in proper working order.
- Verify that the last weight was recorded correctly. A simple but frequent error occurs when converting metric to U.S. measurements, and vice versa.

If a significant and otherwise unexplained discrepancy occurs, reweigh the infant. There is no shame in having made a simple mistake, but time, resources, and anxiety will have been wasted if the only problem is human error. If the discrepancy still exists after double-checking, follow up with appropriate data gathering and physical assessment.

Perform a *complete* physical assessment. Assume nothing. There are, for example, infants who have been discharged from the hospital with undiscovered small clefts. Neuromuscular problems—lack of vigorous reflexes, poor muscle tone, and so forth—and any deviations in normal maxillofacial anatomy deserve special attention. A complete assessment will help to determine if the observed problems are the result of breastfeeding management or if they are symptoms of pathology. Priorities for physical assessment include the following:

- *Vital signs:* Remember that vital signs are indeed *vital;* if the infant's vital signs are outside of normal parameters, further follow-up is imperative. For example, hypothermia may indicate an inadequate caloric intake; tachycardia may indicate a high metabolic rate; tachypnea may be a clear sign that the infant cannot successfully eat and breathe at the same time.
- *Signs of dehydration* (described in Chapter 6) result from insufficient fluid. Remember that sunken fontanels are one of the last signs of dehydration, so look for more subtle signs early on.
- *Worrisome signs:* As discussed earlier in this chapter, several pathological conditions put the infant at risk for weight gain problems. Signs such as sustained apathy or crying, poor tone, poor skin turgor, and poor output need prompt medical follow-up. Also, a digital exam of the oral cavity is indicated if any of the following are observed: poor infant weight gain; absence of or limited audible swallowing; persistently sore maternal nipples.

Obtain history and perform maternal physical assessment. All too frequently, there is no recognition that the infant's history is the mother's history. Furthermore, good history taking cannot be overemphasized and starts when the client walks in the door (or, perhaps, when you walk in her door). Usually, several cues about the overall situation become evident long before the history taking, physical assessment, or observation of a feeding has begun. When making a home visit, walking into a room that is blue with smoke probably contradicts the woman who reports that she smokes two or three cigarettes per day. Or, the infant who comes into the office with a pacifier in his mouth may require more vigorous inquiries about the number of feedings per day and the intervals between feedings.

Conduct a thorough interview with the mother about her medical and obstetric history, social habits, and environments, and how she perceives the breastfeeding experience. Similarly, obtain information about the infant's feeding and elimination patterns, perinatal problems, or exposure to prescribed or illicit drugs, and any problems the mother has noted. Frantz, Fleiss, and Lawrence[7] have developed an excellent history form that captures pertinent points of the mother's social and health habits, infant's behaviors, birth history, and family history. This comprehensive but easy-to-use form is shown in Figure 7-3.

Make no assumptions as the mother relates pertinent history. This is especially true now that hospital discharge is occurring so early and typically the infant comes for a follow-up visit 2 to 3 days after birth. For example, a woman may readily volunteer that she has been diagnosed as hypothyroid; this condition does not preclude breastfeeding, but it must be treated. Inquire if the mother has resumed thyroid-replacement therapy after giving birth. It is not uncommon for women to go to the hospital without their routine medications, and then assume that the drug is contraindicated while they are lactating. Keep in mind that some women may have their hypothyroidism diagnosed after they present with clinical signs; producing insufficient milk is one possible sign. Inquire about "clots" because a woman who has retained parts of the placenta will have difficulty lactating. Again, make no assumptions; I once cared for a woman who passed pieces of placenta several days after her cesarean delivery.

Determine the adequacy of mammary tissue to support lactation. Ask about breast tissue development during pregnancy. If a woman did not experience an increase of at least one bra-cup size in both breasts during pregnancy, this is a cause for concern. Colostrum usually appears during the third trimester, and women who have not noted this require further investigation. Similarly, a woman who did not experience physiological engorgement during the first few days after birth warrants further follow-up. The mother's breasts should also be examined to determine if reassuring signs of lactation are present (see Chapter 8). However, lactation is not regulated by the mammary gland alone, and a complete physical examination may be required.

Elicit information about the frequency and duration of feedings, including the occurrence of night feedings. Restricting infant feeding, as described in Chapter 5, is likely to affect infant weight gains. Some data about frequency and duration can be obtained through the interview. Because mothers may want to respond with the "right answer," however, it is better to observe a feeding. There is no substitution for direct observation of a feeding.

Observe the feeding. Observe the breastfeeding interaction in order to obtain important clues about whether the weight-gain problem is related to breastfeeding management, or if instead a more serious pathological problem is present. Determine if good latch-on is achieved (as described in Chapter 5). Next, look for subtle signs that may indicate trouble. The infant who is always slightly hypothermic, for example, requires further investigation, as does the infant who seems overly fa-

No. _____
Date _____

Slow Gaining Special History

Mother

Name _____

A. Diet
1. Do you eat regular meals? _____ How do you rate the kind of food you eat?
   excellent ❑   good ❑   poor ❑
2. Do you take vitamins? _____ If so, what? _____
   _____
3. Do you take brewer's yeast? _____
4. Are you worried about your weight? _____

B. Health
1. Are you in good health? _____ If not, describe problems _____
   _____
2. Are you taking any medications? _____ Birth control pills? _____
   Prescriptions? _____ Nonprescription medicines? _____
3. Have you had any thyroid problems at any time in your life? _____
   Are thyroid medications being taken now? _____ What kind? _____
   _____
   Dosage _____ Last time you had your blood tested for thyroid _____
4. Do you have any blood pressure problems? _____

C. Habits
1. Do you smoke? _____ Which brand? _____
   How many per day? _____
2. Do you drink coffee? _____ How many cups per day? _____
   Do you drink caffeinated sodas? _____ How many caffeinated sodas per day? _____
3. Do you drink alcohol? _____ How much per day? _____
   week? _____ month? _____

D. Nursing
1. When the infant nurses, do you feel tingling ❑   burning ❑   filling feeling ❑
   leaking on other side ❑   nothing ❑
   other _____
2. Do you have a quiet environment for nursing? _____ If not, why? (describe)
   (Example, loud music, freeway noise, dogs barking) _____
   _____
3. Do you own a rocking chair? _____

E. Social environment
1. Do you have a busy life-style? _____ If so, why? (name activities) _____
   _____
   _____
2. Marriage relationship is good ❑   average ❑   poor ❑
3. Do you have other children? _____ Ages _____
   Breastfed? _____ How long? _____
4. Do you have any source of anxiety or tension? _____ If so, describe _____

Fig. 7-3 Slow-gaining special history. *(From Lawrence RA. Breastfeeding: A Guide for the Medical Profession. 4th ed. St. Louis: Mosby; 1994.)*

Continued

Infant

Name _____ Date of birth _____

1. How often is infant fed? _____
2. Breast milk only? _____ Other? _____
   Does he feed at each breast at each feeding? _____ How long on each breast? _____
3. How long does infant take to finish a feeding? _____ Does infant pause often during feeding? _____
4. Who initiates end of feeding? you ❑   infant ❑
5. How do you rate his sucking? poor ❑   weak ❑   average ❑   strong ❑
6. Is he burping easily? _____ What technique is used? _____
   When is he burped? _____
7. Is a pacifier used? _____ What kind? _____
   How much usage? _____
8. Number of wet diapers per day _____ Are ultra-absorbent diapers used? _____
9. Number of stools per day _____ consistency _____ color _____
10. Infant is active ❑   average ❑   placid ❑
11. Night sleep pattern: time put to bed _____ Is this on a regular basis? _____
    List awake times _____
12. Is infant healthy? _____ Any problems since birth? _____ If so, what? _____
    _____

    Jaundice? _____ How high was the bilirubin level? _____
    Had any medications? _____ If so, what? _____
13. Ever had a urinalysis? _____ When? _____
    Any other test (especially those for slow weight gain)? _____ If so, what? _____
    _____

    Where? _____

Birth history

1. Type of delivery: vaginal ❑   CS ❑   If CS, scheduled ❑   or emergency ❑?
2. Labor: yes ❑   no ❑   Length of time _____
3. Were medications given during labor or delivery? _____ If so, what? _____
   _____
4. Was it a difficult birth? _____ If so, describe problem _____
   _____
5. First time infant put to breast was _____ hr after birth. Did infant take it easily? _____
6. Where was the birth? Home birth ❑   Hospital with rooming-in ❑
   Hospital with infant only in the nursery ❑   Were you separated from infant for any length of time?
   _____ If so, why? _____
   _____
7. Any medications taken during pregnancy? _____ If so, what? _____
   _____
8. Any medications taken after birth? _____ If so, what? _____

Family history

1. Have previous infants or relatives with failure to thrive? yes ❑   no ❑
2. Have history of metabolic or malabsorption disease? yes ❑   no ❑
3. Infant has cystic fibrosis? yes ❑   no ❑
4. Infant has milk allergy? yes ❑   no ❑
5. Other _____

Fig. 7-3, cont'd For legend see p. 171.

T A B L E 7-2

SIMPLE MISMANAGEMENT OF BREASTFEEDING A NEWBORN

Assessment	Intervention	Rationale
Mother removes infant before he is finished or adheres to a preset time guideline	Encourage mother to let infant self-limit feedings by monitoring swallows; teach swallow sounds	Breastfed newborns take 10- to 60-minute feedings, mean of 31 min; length of feeding is equal to quantity of nutritive suckle
	Explain about overdressing; may need to unwrap and wake infant to finish feeding	Overheated infants decrease suckling; swaddled newborns assume sleep state
	Switch to second breast when swallows slow or stop, and back to first breast again *if* infant is interested	Offering both breasts stimulates better milk volume; pauses may not mean newborn is finished; feeding refusal when switched may mean newborn is finished
Consistently long intervals between feedings (4 hr or more for newborn)	Feed more *often;* do not adhere to formula-fed 4-hr schedule	Breastfed newborns usually feed every 2-3 hr; some infants "cluster feed" after a long sleep period
	Discourage pacifier during first weeks	Desire to suckle is a survival mechanism but may indicate real need to feed; more suckling equals more milk volume
	Wake sleepy infants, feed *at least* 8 times every 24 hr	Drugs during labor, maternal postpartum drugs, or hyperbilirubinemia may cause infant to sleep *too* much
Trying to get infant to "sleep through the night" before 8-12 weeks	Dispel myths that parents should promote long infant sleep periods by letting infant cry or using pacifier	Newborns need to feed throughout a 24-hour period; most do not sleep for a 6-hr stretch until 8-12 weeks of age
	Tell mother "power" feedings are at night the first 3 weeks; she should rest during the day	Prolactin levels are high when mother sleeps; newborns feed best at night during the first 3 weeks
Mother offering more water than breast milk, thinking she is supposed to or because of fear of jaundice	Discontinue water for more frequent breast milk feedings	No extra water is needed, because of the lower solute load of breast milk, if the infant is feeding frequently
		Water not proven to lower bilirubin levels faster than milk feedings; bilirubin also excreted in stool with milk feedings
Mother using nipple shield	Discontinue shield Use feeding tube device if infant will not breastfeed well	Shield reduces available milk by 22-66%

Frantz KB. The slow-gaining breastfeeding infant. *NAACOGS Clin Issu Perinat Womens Health Nurs* 1992;3:647-655. © Kittie Frantz.

tigued. Look for signs that are reassuring as well as those that are worrisome. Audible swallowing is a very reassuring sign that milk transfer is occurring; lack of audible swallowing is *always a worrisome sign.* Never underestimate the seriousness of FTT, but recognize that some problems are simple and can be easily corrected.

Frantz[8] outlines how simple mismanagement

contributes to weight-gain problems for the newborn. Restricted feedings, long intervals, sleeping through the night, offering water, and using nipple shields can all be corrected by some simple interventions, as listed in Table 7-2. Very often, it is likely that the primary cause for FTT is simple mismanagement of breastfeeding. Restricted feedings—either offering too few feedings or limiting the length of the time the infant suckles—set up circumstances in which failure to thrive is a likely consequence.

PLANNING/IMPLEMENTATION

If the primary care provider determines that no pathology is present, establish goals and priorities for the breastfed infant with weight-gain problems as shown in Box 7-2. Identify the two or three most pressing problems that interfere with transfer of adequate amounts of milk; correct these problems. Continue to gather data and monitor progress, and report any changes—those that are reassuring and those that are worrisome—to the primary health care provider.

Plan to work collaboratively with the primary health care provider, whose philosophy about supplementation may differ from your own. Avoid a turf battle; otherwise, the mother may get mixed messages about who is "right" or "wrong" in the management of the infant. This is no time to insist on exclusive breastfeeding. Rather, acknowledge that supplementation may be essential for sustaining life. Donor milk is the better alternative, but if it is unavailable, the benefits of artificial milk may outweigh any potential risks. Misgivings about the use of bottles and "nipple confusion" are understandable; this is a point for negotiation. Most primary health care providers prescribe only the supplementation, not the method by which it should be delivered. Help the parents to weigh the advantages of several alternative feeding methods and to identify one that will work (see Chapter 12). The point here is to expedite feeding—to provide adequate calories, nutrients, and fluids—not to have a philosophical discussion about the use of bottles.

Provide sensitive teaching and counseling for parents of infants with poor or slow weight gain. Discuss many assessment findings with the mother—not just weight gain or loss, or she may interpret weight-gain problems as her fault (i.e.,

---

Box 7-2
Goals and Priorities for Care: Weight-Gain Problems

Correct simple mismanagement: See discussion in the text. Poor latch-on or restricted feedings are a frequent cause of weight loss in the newborn.

Ensure complete evaluation: In some cases, failure to thrive may be a symptom of pathology rather than a breastfeeding problem.

Increase milk production: The simplest intervention here is to express milk after every feeding in which the infant was unsuccessful in "emptying" the breast.

Supplement as prescribed: Exclusive breastfeeding may not be the treatment of choice for an infant who has been diagnosed with failure to thrive. This may indeed be a time when supplementation is the safest approach. Supplementation however, does not need to occur via bottle. Several alternative feeding methods may be used, so consider the effect of feeding options (see Chapter 12).

Promote maternal food, fluid, and rest: While milk production is not dependent on the quantity or quality of food and fluids consumed, hormonal changes that occur when the mother is having a nourishing snack before or during breastfeeding do seem to improve milk production. A woman who is well rested can more readily have a milk-ejection reflex than one who is chronically fatigued.

Facilitate interdisciplinary collaboration: Frequently, this is a multifactorial clinical situation that requires everyone's expertise. It is imperative, however, that everyone give the mother the same message and that the members of the health care team do not have turf battles. Clear communication, negotiation, and respect for everyone's input—especially the mother's—are essential. Scaring the mother by suggesting that she is "starving" her infant is counterproductive, but a high degree of complacency is undesirable, too.

Offer appropriate guidelines: Create a simple 3 × 5 card that lists reassuring signs on one side and worrisome signs on the other. This card should be fairly brief and should use simple words. The card should also contain the names and phone numbers of three support people (list these on the reassuring side) and the names and phone numbers of three places to call in case of an emergency.

she blames herself for the infant's problems). It is extremely difficult for women to hear that their infants are not gaining weight satisfactorily; they often interpret this situation as a sign of their own inadequacy in providing nutrition for the infant. Mothers may be tempted to discontinue breast-feeding and to give a bottle, instead. Handle this issue carefully. On the one hand, certain circumstances may dictate that the infant receive at least some artificial milk, so if artificial milk is medically indicated, avoid giving the impression that it is "bad." On the other hand, if the mother's anxieties and frustrations have driven the decision to discontinue breastfeeding, help her to overcome these negative feelings. In all cases, give practical advice for achieving milk transfer, reassure her that she is doing the right thing, and give truthful information about her infant's status. Reinforce the importance of having the infant, not the mother, control the frequency and duration of feeding.

EVALUATION

Never assume that strategies for improving the infant's weight gain are successful. Evaluate and reevaluate whether milk transfer is actually occurring. If it is not, the short-term goal is to "empty" the mother's breast, and the longer-term goal is to achieve effective latch-on. In the meantime, supplementation may be appropriate. Weight checks should continue on a regular basis until the problems are satisfactorily resolved. This may be every 2 days or every 7 days, depending on the severity of the problem. The important thing is to make certain that the test-weighs are accurate.

Cardiac Defects

When observing a breastfeeding experience, the aim is usually to determine whether the newborn is well attached to his mother's breast and to offer assistance if he is not. However, the observer should realize that the newborn who is at the breast is really at his "job." Feeding, whether by breast or bottle, requires effort from the newborn, and those who struggle with the task may have a cardiovascular system that is not functioning adequately.

The cardiovascular system has a twofold purpose: (1) to deliver oxygen and nutrients to meet the metabolic needs of every cell in the body, and (2) to remove waste products such as carbon dioxide. Infants with cardiac defects have increased metabolic needs and therefore require more calories.

Infants with increased metabolism or those who tire easily are not overstressed by breastfeeding. Breastfeeding actually uses less oxygen than bottle feeding. Infants with cardiac defects can and should breastfeed; those with cyanotic defects will have more difficulties than those with

CLINICAL SCENARIO

The Breastfed Infant Who Fails to Thrive

The pediatrician, Dr. R., calls and asks you to do a home visit for a newborn whom she has diagnosed as having failure to thrive. The newborn has no known defects, anomalies, or unusual circumstances. You arrive at an upper-middle-class home and meet a married couple in their early 40s and their 3-week-old baby, Joshua. Mrs. A., a short woman, appears to be recovering from her cesarean delivery, but you notice that she has flat nipples and large breasts. She holds Joshua in a cradle position, and he arches his back, screams, and will not take the breast.

What are your first assessments for the mother-baby dyad?

What is your first intervention?

Assuming that you have corrected the basic technique, what else may help?

Readers are encouraged to discuss this scenario among their colleagues, since often there is no one right answer.

acyanotic defects, but bottle feeding those infants will be problematic also.

Infants with cardiac defects are likely to experience problems that will influence feeding practices, including low tolerance for activity and energy expenditure. Problems and goals vary slightly from one cardiac defect to another, but general goals and priorities for care are those listed in Table 7-3. Ventricular septal defects are discussed in the following section as a prototype to demonstrate care for the cardiac infant.

Ventricular Septal Defects

Incidence and Implications

Ventricular septal defect (VSD) is the most common congenital cardiac defect, occurring in about 25% of all cardiac defect cases. VSDs are congenital problems that result when the septum (wall) between the left and right ventricle of the heart fails to close completely at 4 to 8 weeks' gestation, creating an opening—or *communication*—between the ventricles through which blood can flow. This, of course, results in altered circulation. With a VSD, whether or not shunting occurs depends on several factors, but the size of the defect is the most important.

A small communication (<0.5 cm^2) is called restrictive; that is, the blood is largely restricted to one ventricle or the other and does not offer resistance to flow, and the pressures in the two ventricles may differ. Right ventricular pressure is normal, and left pressure is increased. Therefore, the higher left-sided pressure may shunt blood from left to right (left-to-right shunting), but the volume of shunted blood may be minimal because the communication is so small. Small defects usually do not have clinical signs and symptoms that are immediately evident, and they are likely to be identified when the examiner auscultates the newborn's heart on routine examination. These defects often close spontaneously, and surgery is not recommended under most circumstances.

Some communications may be so large (>1.0 cm^2) that the septum is completely absent and the infant has only one common ventricle. These larger defects are called nonrestrictive; that is, there is no resistance to blood flow. Here the severity and the direction of the shunting vary. These large defects result in feeding difficulties and dyspnea. The infant is usually not cyanotic—this is an acyanotic defect—but duskiness is likely to be seen, particularly when the infant feeds. A septal defect most commonly involves the membrane part of the septum, but it can involve the muscle part of the septum. In either case, the size of the defect can be relatively small or large, and the size of the defect is most influential in determining whether there is a left-to-right shunt.

Benefits of Breastfeeding

Feeding at the breast is more physiological for the newborn than feeding from the bottle. Oxygen saturation (SaO$_2$) during breastfeeding is higher, on the average, and less variable, than the SaO$_2$ of bottle-fed infants. Furthermore, in one study, cardiac-impaired infants had no episodes of desaturation (SaO$_2$ less than 90%) while breastfeeding, but some of those who were bottle feeding did.[9] Similarly, studies of preterm infants have examined the effects of breastfeeding and bottle feeding on oxygenation in newborns.[10,11] The transcutaneous oxygen pressure (tcPO$_2$) levels decreased while bottle feeding, but tcPO$_2$ levels returned to baseline or nearly to baseline while breastfeeding. These data form a basis for the recommendation that breastfeeding appears to offer relatively few difficulties in maintaining oxygenation, as opposed to bottle feeding, and obliterates the myth that breastfeeding is more "work" than bottle feeding.

Human milk, while ideal for all infants, is especially important for the infant with cardiac defects. These infants are especially vulnerable to infections, and the immunoglobulins found in human milk help protect them.

T A B L E 7-3

POSSIBLE PROBLEMS AND BREASTFEEDING MANAGEMENT FOR NEWBORNS WITH ALTERATIONS IN CARDIAC FUNCTION

Problem	Clinical Strategy	Rationale
Activity intolerance	Short, frequent feeds	To minimize fatigue and decrease cardiac demands
	Stop feeding if signs of fatigue develop:	
	• Cyanosis	
	• Tachypnea	
	• Dyspnea	
	• Oxygen saturation below 87%	
	• Infant takes himself off the breast but looks exhausted rather than peaceful (a well newborn who is satiated would take himself off the breast, but he looks peaceful, not exhausted)	
	If infant exhibits the above signs for three consecutive feedings, stop feeding and call physician or primary care provider	
	Consider using a nursing supplementer which may conserve energy	Infant has better chance of getting greater intake with less energy exerted
	Keep drafts off the infant; place blanket over infant's back, and use skin-to-skin contact with mother	Cold stress increases oxygen consumption
Tachypnea and/or dyspnea	Infant may be NPO if respiratory rate is greater than 70 (or per hospital policy); initiate gavage feeding	To minimize risk of aspiration, as coordination of suck/swallow/breathe is more difficult
Fluid volume excess (if congestive heart failure develops)	Encourage use of human milk	Greater volume of artificial milk is needed to gain the same amount of nutrients, as nutrients are better absorbed from human milk
	Monitor intake and output; consider test-weighing	
	Explain rationale for use of powder fortifier, if ordered	Powdered milk fortifier minimizes fluid volume given
Possible hypothermia	Keep infant warm	Conserves oxygen and nutrients
	Encourage breastfeeding	Milk is at body temperature, and lactating breast is warm
Risk for slow growth or failure to thrive	Be sure infant gets the hindmilk! "Emptying" one breast completely to get the hindmilk is better than going to both breasts, but not getting hindmilk	Rich in fat and calories
	Listen for audible swallowing	To verify milk transfer
	Monitor weight: infant should have at least 143 ml/kg/day to maintain weight and at least 171 ml/kg/day to gain weight during the first month of life	To ensure that infant is getting enough calories
	Explain rationale for artificial supplementation to mother if it is ordered	Infant may not be able to get all needed nutrition from the breast
Risk for hypoxia	Encourage feeding at the breast if mother is available	PO_2 of oxygen is less labile when feeding at the breast, rather than using a rubber nipple
	Respond and offer other breast promptly when infant is hungry	Crying increases oxygen consumption
	Encourage intake of human milk	Iron is better absorbed from human milk than from artificial milk; Fe is necessary for O_2
Risk for respiratory infection	Encourage intake of human milk	Presence of immunoglobulins mobilizes infant's natural defenses and minimizes threat of infection
Risk for separation from mother	Suggest creating a supply of frozen mother's milk if infant is scheduled for surgery	To facilitate use of human milk and preserve breastfeeding relationship

Prenatal Assessment and Counseling

Thanks to advances in fetal imaging and ultrasound, including echocardiography, fairly accurate prenatal diagnosis of cardiac defects is now possible.[12] Parents who are anticipating an infant with VSD should be told that breastfeeding is possible for their child, and that the benefits of breastfeeding and human milk are particularly suitable for the infant with a cardiac defect. Prenatal information should include information about anticipated feeding difficulties that the infant may experience.

Immediate Postpartum Period

ASSESSMENTS

Sometimes the VSD is not so obvious and may not be detected until the routine physical. Or difficulties in feeding may hasten the physical examination, as the infants generally do become dyspneic. The newborn who has not been diagnosed with a cardiac defect may exhibit mild symptoms or difficulties; he may breastfeed immediately after birth, and these symptoms are unlikely to interfere with continued efforts to breastfeed. Newborns with more dramatic symptoms need a complete medical evaluation before further feeding—by breast or bottle—occurs. Symptoms can be subtle or severe, and the severe symptoms may indicate a life-threatening problem.

VSDs can occur as isolated defects or associated with other congenital cardiac defects. A VSD might go undetected for the first 3 or 4 days after birth, and then the infant starts to exhibit symptoms when he is home. Because feeding is the time when the infant increases his activity and hence his oxygen consumption, parents may wonder about the behavior the infant is manifesting.

POSSIBLE CONCURRENT PROBLEMS

Infants who have VSD occasionally experience endocarditis. Infants who have large defects may experience multiple episodes of respiratory infection and congestive heart failure. They may also experience pulmonary hypertension, which is a result of high pulmonary blood flow. Their risk for pulmonary vascular disease is prevented when surgery is performed within the first year.[13] These infants are especially at risk for failure to thrive.

The degree of difficulty with feeding and whether or not surgery is performed vary with the type and severity of the defect. Small defects do not require surgery, and generally feeding progresses without problems. The infant may, however, show signs of difficulty. Large defects require medical management and/or surgery. The aim of medical management is to control episodes of congestive heart failure, and the goal of surgery—ideally performed within the first year—is to prevent pulmonary vascular disease. The goal of therapeutic management is maintenance of normal growth.

CLINICAL MANAGEMENT

Feeding should be carried out with the recognition that it requires expenditure of energy for the infant. He should not be hurried or prodded; in fact, jiggling or prodding any infant who eats slowly is often counterproductive. However, watch for signs that the infant is too tired to continue breastfeeding. These signs might include the following: dyspnea; marked tachypnea; cyanosis; and the infant stops, but looks exhausted (in contrast to the well infant, who spontaneously comes off the breast but looks peaceful).

Conclusions about Breastfeeding Management

Infants with cardiac impairment can breastfeed. The stress these infants experience relates to the expenditure of energy during the feeding. Breastfeeding, however, should be thought of as an intervention for these infants as it conserves oxygen, and provides needed amounts of nutrients and anti-infective properties. With good observation skills and some very simple interventions to enhance the experience, breastfeeding can often continue with few if any problems.

ALTERATIONS IN NEUROLOGICAL FUNCTION

The transition from intrauterine to extrauterine life puts full-term newborns at risk for fluctuation in neurophysiological responses. After an uneventful birth, relatively common alterations—for example, hypothermia and hypoglycemia—are merely a result of the normal newborn's adaptation to extrauterine life and have little impact on breastfeeding.

Newborns may also have transient alterations in neurological status that are related to unfavorable perinatal events. Hypoxic-ischemic brain injury, resulting in birth asphyxia and later some residual hypoxia, is the most common cause of neurological impairment in newborns. Infants who have experienced decreased oxygenation during labor, poor Apgar scores, respiratory difficulties due to respiratory distress syndrome or recurrent apnea, or any type of cardiac insufficiency (defects, persistent pulmonary hypertension, respiratory failure secondary to sepsis) are at risk for neurological impairment. (Preterm infants may experience several of these problems.) These factors may preclude or hamper initial breastfeeding sessions, and the severity and duration of the clinical manifestation will be directly related to the severity and duration of the oxygenation deprivation.

Some newborns have diseases or defects that result in long-term alterations in neurological function. These problems require some special management in terms of the nutrition required and the feeding technique. Some commonly encountered examples include infants with Down syndrome, hydrocephalus, and myelomeningocele. Breastfeeding is usually quite possible for infants with these and similar difficulties and is best managed with a sound understanding of how anatomy and physiology are affected.

Structure and Function

Breastfeeding is accomplished by intact structure and function of the oral cavity—the lips, cheeks, tongue, and hard and soft palates, as well as the jaw. When a *stimulus* occurs to the nerve in any one of these structures, it forms the beginning of a reflex arc. When a *nerve* impulse passes over the reflex arc, a predictable response to the stimulus, called a *reflex*, results. A reflex consists of either a muscle contraction (e.g., suckling) or glandular secretion (milk ejection is an example of a glandular reflex). Therefore, when a stimulus occurs (e.g., touching the infant's cheek), the message is carried to the spinal cord and a reflex—in this case, rooting—results. The reflex is accomplished by using *muscles*.

In the well infant, muscles involved in breastfeeding are innervated by several nerves. The *trigeminal* nerve (cranial nerve V) innervates muscles of the mandible (jaw). The *facial* nerve (cranial nerve VII) innervates muscles of the face, including the buccinator, lower lip, and chin muscles. The *glossopharyngeal* nerve (cranial nerve IX) innervates sensations of the tongue, while the *hypoglossal* nerve (cranial nerve XII) innervates tongue movements. The glossopharyngeal and the *vagus* (cranial nerve X) nerves innervate muscles of the posterior pharynx, palate, and epiglottis.

Oral, buccal, lingual, and pharyngeal muscles are directly involved in breastfeeding, as shown in Figure 7-4. The *masseter* and *temporalis* muscles elevate the jaw when the infant is latching on, then retract the jaw while compressing the tongue, a solid mass of skeletal muscles, against the alveolar ridge and hard palate. The *genioglossus* protrudes the tongue, and the *hypoglossus* depresses it. The glossopharyngeal muscle groups are

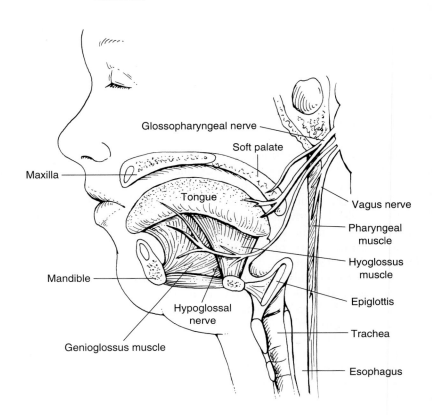

Glossopharyngeal nerve

Soft palate

Maxilla

Tongue

Vagus nerve

Pharyngeal muscle

Hyoglossus muscle

Mandible

Epiglottis

Hypoglossal nerve

Trachea

Genioglossus muscle

Esophagus

Fig. 7-4 Muscles and nerves used in suckling and swallowing. **A,** Sagittal section.

involved in swallowing and when the infant gags. If the infant has neurological impairments, these muscles may not be intact, or they may be too weak to initiate and/or sustain successful suckling. Similarly, the muscle response may be delayed, or the infant may be hypersensitive to stimuli, and the muscle response may therefore occur too early.

Muscles of the head and neck are less directly involved in breastfeeding, but they do influence feeding success. In the well infant, muscles that extend the neck are usually better developed than those that bring the head forward, requiring the caregiver to support the head in order to keep it aligned with the rest of the newborn's body. This head lag is even more pronounced in infants with weak head and neck muscles, as is typically found

in neurologically impaired infants. These weak muscles make positioning at the breast somewhat more difficult. Muscular deficits may or may not be associated with impaired reflexes.

Sucking, swallowing, gagging, and rooting are all somatic *reflexes* associated with breastfeeding. The breastfeeding infant needs not only the ability to suck and swallow—reflexes normally present very early in gestation—but also the ability to *coordinate* suck and swallow with breathing, which appears around 32 weeks' gestation. This coordination of suck and swallow is essential for milk transfer. Intact reflexes are an indication of normal neurological functioning. Conversely, impaired reflexes are generally a result of dysfunction of the central or peripheral nervous system for a variety of reasons.

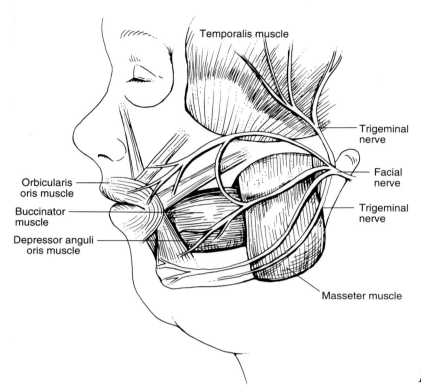

Temporalis muscle

Trigeminal nerve

Facial nerve

Trigeminal nerve

Orbicularis oris muscle

Buccinator muscle

Depressor anguli oris muscle

Masseter muscle

Fig. 7-4, cont'd **B,** Lateral view.

Preterm infants do not have "abnormal" reflexes, but because their nervous systems are immature, they will not exhibit reflexes equivalent to those of a term infant. Other situations that may interfere with neurological functioning include the events of labor (e.g., a particularly stressful labor that depletes the fetus's oxygen reserves) or neurological disease. In this case, the muscles of the oral, buccal, lingual, and pharyngeal musculature might not be intact or might be too weak to accomplish and sustain suckling.

Assessments

A few key assessments about neurological status should be part of routine care for the infant. General assessments may affect the decision to initiate feedings or to discontinue a feeding that is in progress. More specific observations related to breastfeeding will provide the basis for breastfeeding management of the infant who has alterations in neurological functioning.

General Assessments

Sometimes infants are diagnosed at or before birth as having a neurological deficit. Other times, however, neurological limitations are not immediately evident. Before and during a feeding—when the infant is interacting and using muscles and reflexes associated with feeding—is an opportune time to identify signs of neurological impairment. The following observations[14] are critical for the infant's general well-being and to breastfeeding management in particular: altered states of consciousness, eye responses, abnormal posture and tone, abnormal reflexes, and abnormal movements, described in Table 7-4, are all clues to possible neurological deficits. In assessing an infant it is important to first determine if he is a candidate for oral feedings; sometimes those with neurological damage are not. Those who are candidates for oral feedings should be offered the breast, and the feeding should be monitored to see how the infant tolerates the activity.

State of consciousness is particularly important to observe; those who have an altered state of consciousness are at risk for aspiration. Eye responses are also important; for example, the preterm infant whose eyes appear glassy may be overstimulated and unable to continue the feeding. The infant's posture may also influence the feeding decision. For example, hypotonia may be dif-

T A B L E 7-4
NEUROLOGICAL STATUS AND FEEDING DECISIONS

Assessment/Observation	Normal	Abnormal	Feeding Implications for Abnormal Reflexes
State of consciousness	Infant should respond to noxious stimuli and should become quiet after soothing or a successful feeding (see Chapter 6 for full discussion of states of consciousness)	Infant does not respond to noxious stimuli and does not become quiet after successful feeding or after attempts to soothe the infant; infants who are comatose or have alterations in their level of consciousness are very worrisome	Question whether these infants should be NPO; evaluate for other signs of neurological impairment before initiating feeding for infants who are unresponsive or exhibit signs of alterations in consciousness
Eye responses	Around 32 weeks' gestation, infants should blink, and should have extraocular movements	A fixed stare may indicate that the infant is having a seizure; "glassy" eyes while feeding may indicate that the infant is overstimulated	Term infants who stare are worrisome and require further evaluation before initiating feeding; glassy eyes, particularly in the preterm infant, suggest that the infant is tired and needs to rest
Posture and tone	Flexion of the arms, knees, and hips should be present in term infants; varying degrees of flexion will be present in the preterm infant	Hypotonia or hypertonia; hypotonia is particularly relevant to the feeding experience; the infant has a "floppy" posture, making it difficult to achieve and maintain a good position at the breast	Positioning, described in the text and in boxes in this chapter, enhances feeding
Reflexes	Reflexes associated with breastfeeding (e.g., rooting, sucking, swallowing, and gagging) are indeed part of a larger assessment; observe other reflexes, including Moro, grasp, blink, tonic neck; reflexes are not fully developed in the preterm infant	Reflexes may be absent or weak, as described in the text; the infant may also have difficulty coordinating the suck and swallow reflex with breathing	Report abnormal reflex activity to the physician because the problems encountered may be beyond the scope of a "breastfeeding problem"; trying to correct a "breastfeeding problem" is futile if other reflexes are not functioning optimally
Movements	Infants should have organized movement in response to stimuli; movement should also reflect symmetry	Clonic, tonic, myoclonic, and subtle seizures	Infants who are seizing should not be fed

ficult to distinguish from lethargy, particularly in the preterm infant. Usually, however, the lethargic infant appears disinterested in the feeding; the hypotonic infant is more likely to appear interested and willing, but unable to successfully accomplish feeding.

Infants who have any abnormal movement, including jitters or seizures, require medical follow-up. There are four types of neonatal seizures: clonic, tonic, myoclonic, and subtle. Subtle seizures may develop in either the term or preterm infant; they can be easily overlooked or mistaken for jitteriness. It is critical to distinguish jitters from seizures; infants who are jittery are likely to be hypoglycemic and should be immediately put to the breast. Infants who are having seizures may be hypoglycemic, although multiple other causes are also possible. Unlike infants with jitters, infants with suspected seizures should not receive oral feedings, pending medical confirmation, because they are at risk for aspiration. They at least require further investigation; they may also have difficulties sucking. Box 7-3 differentiates ocular movements, dominant movement, sensitivity to stimulation, and duration of jitters and seizures.[4]

Assessments Related to Breastfeeding

Infants who are neurologically impaired may have structural problems, functional problems, or both. Successful breastfeeding management will depend on accurate assessment of the infant's capabilities and limitations, especially with respect to suckling.

Infants who have sucking difficulties may have alterations of structure, function, or both. Structural problems may involve the face, jaw, posterior pharynx, palate, epiglottis, and tongue. Muscles of the oral, buccal, lingual, and pharyngeal *musculature* might not be intact, or they might be too weak to accomplish and sustain sucking. Infants may have dysfunction of the central or peripheral nervous system and musculature; therefore, the sucking *reflex* will not be optimal. Sometimes the muscular and reflex problems are interrelated.

Infants with neurological impairments may have a variety of sucking disorders. These might include (1) an absent or decreased sucking reflex, (2) weakness of suckling, (3) nonrhythmic suckling, or (4) uncoordinated suck/swallow/breathe.[15] An absent sucking reflex simply means that when the infant is stimulated to suck, he does not. (He may not even have a rooting reflex.) A decreased sucking reflex occurs when he is presented with stimulation but cannot establish an adequate suck. He responds with little sucking, or only a flutter-suck, although he may continue that sucking pattern for an extended time. In contrast, a weak suck means that the infant can establish sucking but cannot sustain it. Nonrhythmic suckling means that the infant does not

Box 7-3
Distinguishing Between Jitters and Seizures

	Jitters	*Seizures*
Ocular movement	Absent	Present
Dominant movement	Tremors—repetitive movement of both hands at frequency of 2 to 5 per second lasting more than 10 minutes	Clonic jerking that cannot be stopped by flexion of the affected limb
Sensitivity to stimulation	High	Low
Persist beyond 4th day	No	Yes

Source: Wong DL. *Whaley and Wong's Nursing Care of Infants and Children*. 5th ed. St. Louis: Mosby; 1995.

CLINICAL SCENARIO

The Infant with Neurological and Structural Alterations

Baby Thomas was born at 40 weeks' gestation. His mother is a gravida 4, para 4, and has successfully breastfed three other infants for a substantial period of time. You are called to the pediatric floor to see Thomas when he is about 5 days old. He has been diagnosed with Pierre Robin syndrome, as shown in Figure 7-5. He has been readmitted to the hospital for apneic episodes.

What are the three *greatest* difficulties you could anticipate for Thomas, and what recommendations could you make?

Problem	Recommendation

What are the three *greatest* difficulties you could anticipate for his mother, and what are your discharge priorities?

Problem	Recommendation

Readers are encouraged to discuss this scenario among their colleagues, since often there is no one right answer.

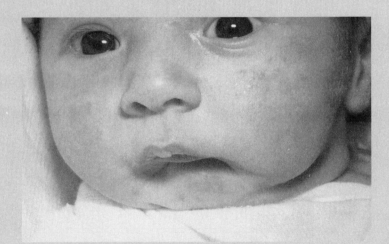

Fig. 7-5 Infant with Pierre Robin syndrome. *(Photo taken with assistance of Ruth A. Lawrence, M.D.)*

suck in a rhythm; he sucks in a disorganized way. Uncoordinated suck/swallow/breathe means that the infant may suck—and may even suck well—but cannot coordinate his efforts to take in food with his efforts to take in air. These infants frequently sputter and may even become cyanotic.

Clinical Management

Infants with neurological deficits may be unable to achieve an adequate suckling mechanism because their tongue muscles are too weak to form a trough to perform the undulating motion necessary for obtaining milk. The negative pressure, necessary for holding the nipple/areola complex in place, is inadequate, so the infant cannot achieve a good seal. Interventions that aim to overcome weak muscles and inadequate negative pressure and to organize suck patterns are most helpful for the infant who is neurologically impaired.

If sucking is *absent*, initiate pumping, but if the sucking reflex is *present but decreased*, ensure that the infant and the mother receive adequate stimulation. To stimulate the infant, use stroking and/or a cold washcloth in and around the mouth, as well as other interventions. Then, try the Dancer hand or try pressing the chin inward slightly (see later discussion of special techniques). Use pillows for the hypotonic infant, and position him so that the mouth is fairly high up on the breast. In this way, an active milk ejection reflex will not "choke" the infant who suckles poorly. Likewise, the mother needs adequate stimulation. Suggest a nursing supplementer (see Chapter 12) so that she receives stimulation when the infant suckles, but keep the pump handy if the breast needs further stimulation.

Interventions should be timed so that they correspond with the infant's quiet-alert state.[16] Table 7-5 describes some specific interventions that enhance suckling mechanisms for infants who have alterations in neurological function; the categories are delineated rather arbitrarily,

and each difficulty described is likely to coexist with another difficulty. For example, the Clinical Scenario describes an infant with Pierre Robin syndrome; this infant exhibited neurological difficulties as well as structural difficulties.

Several congenital and acquired problems are associated with neurological impairment. Down syndrome, myelomeningocele, and hydrocephalus are but a few of the more common problems.

Down Syndrome

According to the National Down Syndrome Society, the risk of having a child with Down syndrome is about 1 in 1000 births for mothers in their 20s. The risk increases dramatically, however, if the mother is over 35, to about 1 in every 350 births, and to about 1 in every 100 births for women who are over 40. It is important to remember, however, that about 75% of infants born with Down syndrome are born to mothers who are under age 35, so this is not a deviation reserved only for the elderly gravida. This statistic reflects the greater number of infants delivered by younger women.

Down syndrome is a congenital defect. Usually, the somatic cell nucleus contains 46 chromosomes arranged in 23 pairs; the members of each pair are virtually identical. Sometimes, however, the cell contains three, rather than two, copies of one chromosome; this is called a *trisomy*. In trisomy 21, or Down syndrome, as it is frequently called, the infant has extra chromosomal material on the 21st chromosome. This extra genetic material alters the course of growth and development (Figure 7-6).

Benefits of Breastfeeding an Infant With Down Syndrome

Breastfeeding is advantageous for all infants but especially for infants with Down syndrome. From an emotional perspective, the breastfeeding expe-

T A B L E 7-5

POSSIBLE PROBLEMS AND BREASTFEEDING MANAGEMENT FOR NEWBORNS WITH ALTERATIONS IN NEUROLOGICAL FUNCTION

Problem	Clinical Strategies	Rationale
Impaired sucking reflexes Decreased sucking reflex	If sucking or rooting is *absent,* express milk Offer the breast so that it is positioned in center of mouth Press chin down as infant latches on Encourage nonnutritive sucking • Offer textured teething toy, even for newborn • Offer breast or pacifier to suck Consider equipment (e.g., nursing supplementer; see Chapter 12)	Helps infant to *establish* and optimize (or prepare) response to reflex stimulus
Weakness of sucking	Try different positions: across lap with pillow, specially designed pillows, football hold Try Dancer hand (see Figure 7-19) Consider infant sling Burp frequently Encourage short, frequent feeds	Helps newborns to *sustain* sucking reflex after they have established it
Nonrhythmic sucking	Hold infant across lap; use two pillows Try infant sling Burp frequently	Helps infant to maintain *rhythmic* suck
Uncoordinated suck/swallow	Position nipple so that back of neck and throat are higher than mother's nipple Have mother recline at about 30° angle if milk flows too fast Sit baby on extra pillows	Improves ability to exhibit long, slow, rhythmic sucks *interspersed* appropriately with breathing; milk flow is unaided by gravity when mother reclines
Low muscle tone (generalized), weak head and neck muscles	Use pillows to get infant nearer to breast instead of having infant use muscles to "reach for breast" Tap, stroke lips, cheeks, and tongue (use circular mouth exercise) Offer clean, textured teething toys dipped in breast milk Consider help of special therapist	Helps overcome or promote *muscle* tone that in turn promotes milk transfer
Hyperreflexia	Use infant sling or football hold; keep baby flexed! Tonic bite: try Dancer hand	Helps infant to flex, rather than extend, muscles
Risk for failure to thrive	Listen for audible swallowing! Emphasize importance of having infant obtain the hindmilk	Emphasizes milk transfer and promotes adequate nutrients for growth

rience enhances bonding. This may be particularly helpful if the mother is having difficulty accepting her newborn's condition. From a biological perspective, breastfeeding and human milk help the infant with Down syndrome to reduce the risk of morbidity associated with concomitant problems.

Human milk is especially beneficial for these infants because of problems that may accompany Down syndrome. About 30% to 40% of children with Down syndrome also have cardiac defects, predisposing them to respiratory difficulties and infection. The act of breastfeeding is beneficial to these infants because it conserves their cardiopulmonary resources and contributes to better speech development.

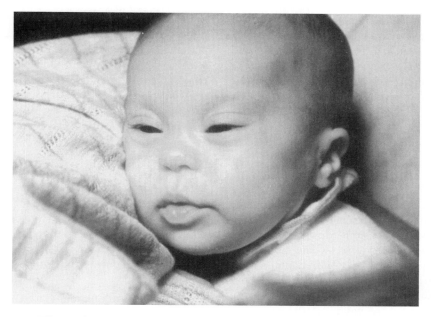

Fig. 7-6 Infant with Down syndrome. *(Courtesy Sarah Coulter Danner.)*

Prenatal Assessment and Counseling

Down syndrome can be suspected from results of prenatal blood testing (alpha-fetoprotein), but conclusive prenatal diagnosis is determined from the results of an amniocentesis. Women who have been told that their infants have Down syndrome may not be immediately interested in discussing feeding methods, but the topic should be addressed as soon as possible because these infants may have special feeding difficulties. Goals during the antepartum period include those listed in Box 7-4.

Prenatal education and counseling can be extremely helpful for the parents of a child with Down syndrome. First, because it is so common for Down syndrome to be detected prenatally—and because abortion is legalized in the United States—in most cases the parents have made a conscious decision to birth and care for the infant. Therefore, early discussion about effective ways to help the infant overcome his potential limitations gives a strong message of support for the parents' decision and expresses confidence in their caregiving skills. Infants with Down syndrome are more like other infants than they are different, and parents can maximize their child's potential by not placing limits on their own expectations. Second, early planning gives the entire health care team an opportunity to mobilize personnel and equipment that will optimize the breastfeeding experience.

Postpartum Period Assessment and Management

These days, infants with Down syndrome are frequently born to parents who are aware of the condition prenatally. However, many infants with

Down syndrome are also born to parents who do not have prior knowledge of the infants' condition, especially to younger mothers who have little or no prenatal care or did not opt for an amniocentesis. With or without the advanced warning, mothers may need to simultaneously grieve for the loss of a perfect child and bond with their infant. Goals and priorities during the antepartum period include those listed in Box 7-4.

Assessments

Assess strength and organization of suck, but be careful not to overstimulate because infants with Down syndrome may "shut down." Typically, infants born with Down syndrome are hypotonic; hypotonicity not only will hamper their ability to position themselves at the breast, but it also will affect their ability to compress the tongue against the hard palate. If the tongue is hypotonic, the infant will therefore be unable to form the trough necessary to good areolar compression. Furthermore, the tongue often falls to the back of the mouth; this impairs sucking motions, and may result in apneic periods as well. Use assessment findings to form a basis for clinical management.

Clinical Management

The infant with Down syndrome may have some generalized difficulties, as well as some feeding-related difficulties that will make the feeding experience frustrating whether the infant is breastfed or bottle fed. Typically the infant has generalized hypotonia, making it difficult to position him at the breast. His tongue is also hypotonic and is likely to fall to the back of his mouth when he feeds. To minimize this problem, advise the mother to hold the infant more upright so that gravity does not add to the problem. Frequently, the tongue protrudes, having the appearance of not quite fitting into the mouth.

SUCKLING AT THE BREAST

Follow all of the directives listed in Chapter 5 to achieve good positioning and latch-on. Infants with Down syndrome are likely to have problems that make it more difficult to achieve an adequate seal, adequate negative pressure, and adequate suckling mechanisms. These include hypotonia and frequent drooling.

POSSIBLE CONCURRENT PROBLEMS

In about 30% to 50% of the cases, infants with Down syndrome have an accompanying congenital heart defect, which can range in severity from mild to severe (see section on cardiac defects). This makes them more vulnerable to respiratory infections and fatigue. Other concurrent problems may include the following:

- Hyperbilirubinemia related to liver dysfunction
- Congenital cataracts
- Intestinal anomalies—duodenal atresia/stenosis, Hirschsprung's disease
- Thyroid dysfunction
- Hearing loss
- Prematurity
- Childhood leukemia

EDUCATION, COUNSELING, AND SUPPORT

Mothers who choose to breastfeed their infants with Down syndrome may have some difficulties that may not immediately be apparent. They may experience chronic sorrow, a continued wish for the perfect child, or guilt feelings related to the infant's condition. Increased social isolation is a continuing problem; hence, the mother may never go out of the house or seek companionship with other breastfeeding mothers. A sense of decreased family self-esteem may further affect her stress level, and marital difficulties frequently come to a head when families have a child with a

The Infant With Down Syndrome

Baby Jeffrey was born at 37 weeks' gestation. His mother (23 years old and a gravida 1, para 1) has delivered about 2 hours ago. She is quietly resting in bed, but is asking about Jeffrey. She says, "What will we do to feed him?" What are the three *greatest* difficulties you could anticipate for Jeffrey, and what recommendations could you make?

Problem	Recommendation

What are the three *greatest* difficulties you could anticipate for his mother, and what are your discharge priorities?

Problem	Recommendation

Readers are encouraged to discuss this scenario among their colleagues, since often there is no one right answer.

serious deviation. Although there are no easy remedies to help these mothers, sensitivity, compassion, and acceptance of the infant's capabilities and limitations will go a long way to support not only the breastfeeding efforts but also the family dynamics surrounding this birth. It is often helpful for parents to link with a local parent support group. The National Down Syndrome Society, listed in Appendix A, can refer parents to local groups.

Help the mother to deal with issues of separation and modesty. Frequently, infants with Down syndrome go to "school" within the first few months. To maintain breastfeeding, help the mother identify ways to be present for the breastfeedings—in which case she will need to know how to breastfeed discretely—or to express and save milk in order to maintain supply.

GOALS OF BREASTFEEDING MANAGEMENT
All of the goals and priorities for the compromised infant (Box 7-4) are appropriate for the infant with Down syndrome. In addition, establish the goals and priorities found in Box 7-5.

Conclusions About Breastfeeding Management

Infants with Down syndrome can breastfeed. Various interventions, largely aimed at overcoming the difficulties associated with hypotonia, will improve the breastfeeding experience. Active support, instruction, and collaboration among members of the health care team are essential for breastfeeding success.

ALTERATION IN STRUCTURAL ANATOMY

Structural defects influence breastfeeding. Perhaps the most important question for infants with structural defects is: Does the infant have an adequate seal, adequate suckling mechanism, and adequate negative pressure? Whether or not the infant can breastfeed depends on the extent of the problem, but in many cases he can. Infants with significant structural alterations frequently have as much or more difficulty bottle feeding as

Box 7-4
Goals and Priorities for Compromised Infants

Antepartum Period
- Assist mother to recognize that breastfeeding is not only possible but optimal.
- Facilitate contact with local support groups, especially mothers who have successfully breastfed similarly affected infants (see Appendix A).
- Collaborate with other members of the health care team to identify strategies and options for supplemental feeding.
- Mobilize equipment: be sure that a suitable pump will be available both in the hospital and after discharge.
- Ensure that educational media will be available and accessible at the hospital when the infant is delivered (see Appendix B).

Immediate Postpartum Period
- Initiate or reinforce actions listed for the antepartum period.
- Assist newborn to achieve good latch-on.
- Teach mother to pump or supplement, if indicated.
- Provide mother with a list of worrisome signs and a list of phone numbers to call for help.
- Give suggestions to overcome problems of engorgement in early period and diminished supply later on.
- Provide a list of pump rental depots and become the mother's advocate for getting a prescription for a pump. This prescription may enable the mother to obtain reimbursement from her health insurance company.

Discharge Planning
- Assist the couplet to achieve excellent latch-on and audible swallowing prior to hospital discharge; this may not be entirely achieved because infants are being discharged early nowadays.
- Provide anticipatory guidance to help parents with the most common concerns.
- Plan for some mechanism for weighing infant to determine appropriate weight gains. How frequently the infant will need to be weighed will depend largely on the infant's weight at discharge and his nutritional and general health status. Electronic scales can be rented for accurate test-weighing at home.
- Recommend appropriate resources in the community, and list phone numbers where parents can find information and support.
- If appropriate, coordinate efforts so that an electric pump can be available at home, and parents can successfully demonstrate how to use it prior to discharge.
- Create a list of danger signs and reassuring signs.
- Schedule follow-up visits or telephone consultation within the first week after discharge and plan for ongoing support and follow-up.

Time Preceding and Following Surgery, If Needed
- Support mother's decision to continue breastfeeding or to wean.
- Anticipate the need for milk after surgery and initiate an appropriate pumping regimen about 10 days prior to the schedule.
- Assist the family to ask questions pertinent to feeding after the surgery.
- Facilitate rooming-in, if feasible.

Box 7-5
Goals and Priorities: Down Syndrome

- Ensure adequate intake. Make sure the infant gets the hindmilk.
- Remember that growth patterns are different for infants with Down syndrome than for other infants,[17] and current charts describing growth in infants with Down syndrome do not differentiate between breastfed and bottle-fed infants.
- Champion breastfeeding as ideal for this infant, who is at greater risk for cardiac defects and infection.
- Promote family self-esteem and self-confidence.
- Foster family education and support through use of pamphlets, such as those listed in Appendix B and consumer organizations.

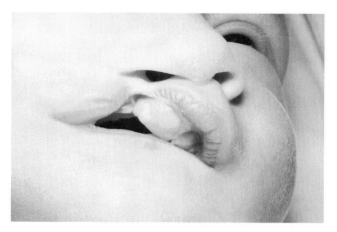

Fig. 7-7 Cleft of lip only. *(Photo taken with assistance of Ruth A. Lawrence, M.D.)*

they do breastfeeding. A broad overview of a common craniofacial defect is used here to show how to apply this idea of achieving adequate suck, seal, and negative pressure.

Cleft Lip and Palate

Incidence and Implications

Clefts occur about once in every live 700 births.[18] Sometimes a cleft lip is immediately obvious, but a small cleft palate may go undetected for a while. Breastfeeding specialists may be called for an obvious case; at other times they may be called for "breastfeeding problems" and discover the need for a thorough examination of the oral cavity.

Clefting is a congenital problem. It can occur in isolation, but it is also seen in over 150 syndromes, including Pierre Robin syndrome, Turner's syndrome, and Van der Woude's syndrome. Cleft lip, a congenital failure of fusion of the upper lip, occurs during the fifth week of gestation. The cleft may be unilateral or bilateral and may involve the alveolar ridge (gum), as shown in Figure 7-7. When the left and the right palatal

shelves fail to fuse during the seventh or eighth week of embryonic development, a cleft palate results. Cleft palates may involve the hard palate, the soft palate, or both, as shown in Figure 7-8. Clefts of the soft palate may involve either the back of the soft palate, as shown in Figure 7-9, or the complete soft palate, as shown in Figure 7-10. Pregnant mothers frequently fear this congenital problem and its impact on breastfeeding. The dearth of research related to feeding infants with clefts—either by breast or by bottle—makes this problem especially difficult to manage. A basic understanding of the defect's impact on structures and functions associated with breastfeeding can help allay those fears and overcome the associated feeding difficulties.

The degree of difficulty in feeding varies with the severity of the lesion. If the infant has only a small notch on the lip or a split uvula, feeding may not be a problem. A complete clefting of the lip, which may occur in conjunction with a cleft palate, as shown in Figure 7-11, complicates clinical management. Clefting poses both structural and functional difficulties; the alteration in oral-facial structure impacts dental, speech, and hearing function as well as feeding. Perhaps the great-

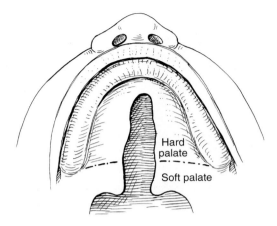

Fig. 7-8 Cleft of soft and hard palates.

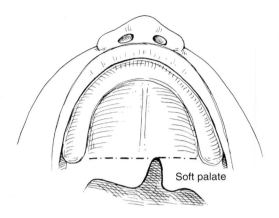

Fig. 7-10 Cleft of the soft palate.

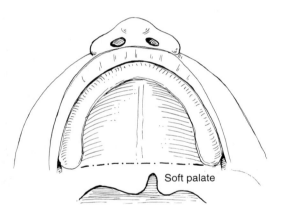

Fig. 7-9 Cleft of the posterior soft palate.

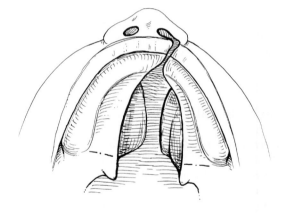

Fig. 7-11 Complete cleft of lip and palate.

est difficulty is convincing the mother that breastfeeding is not only possible but optimal.

Benefits of Breastfeeding Infants With Cleft Lip or Palate

Breastfeeding is advantageous for all infants, but especially for infants with clefts. From an emotional perspective, breastfeeding is an ideal way to promote bonding for these infants whose faces are not intact. From a biological perspective, problems associated with clefts can be overcome or minimized through breast milk and the act of feeding at the breast.

Human milk has immunologic, biospecific, and infection-protection advantages, and infants who consume it have fewer digestive problems and fewer allergies. These advantages are magnified for the infant with a cleft. The anti-infective property of lysozyme, a property of human milk but not artificial milk, is beneficial; the lysozyme acts as a healing balm on the incision postoperatively. Infants with cleft palates have more ear infections because the eustachian tubes easily fill with liquid when the infant swallows; breastfeeding creates less pressure in the middle ear than bottle feeding, thereby lessening the risk of otitis media and, ultimately, hearing loss. Otitis media occurs significantly more often when the infant is fed artificial milk than when he is fed breast milk, and duration of breastfeeding is positively correlated with an occurrence of effusion.[19]

Breastfeeding provides benefits to the infant with a cleft. The act of compressing the human nipple and areola promotes better muscle development of the face, mouth, and tongue. Certainly, the breast molds to minimize the effect of the cleft, whereas an artificial nipple is less malleable. All of these fairly objective reasons for breastfeeding should be considered in light of the more subjective benefits of closer mother-infant interactions.

Prenatal Assessment and Counseling

Prenatal assessment and counseling are pivotal for successful breastfeeding. Unless a mother has successfully breastfed before, she may lack confidence in her ability to breastfeed even under the best of circumstances. This problem escalates if clefting occurs.

For most parents, the risk of having a child with a cleft is about 0.14%; this increases to 2% to 5% if they have already had a child with a cleft, and to 10% to 12% if they have had more than one child with a cleft. Similarly, increased risk occurs if the gravida or her partner has a cleft, or if their siblings or other family members are affected.[20] Fetuses with cleft lips can now be detected on ultrasound. If a routine ultrasound is performed, encourage the gravida to specifically ask the technician to visualize the facial features. The ultrasound may not give a good indication of the width of the cleft, but this forewarning of the defect will mobilize the cleft team and help the

family recognize some of the infant's capabilities and limitations.

As soon as the presence of a cleft is established, initiate ways to overcome the difficulties that will accompany breastfeeding. Collaborate with other members of the cleft team to deliver a clear, consistent message about long-range feeding strategies. Goals and priorities during the antepartum period can be found in Box 7-6.

Box 7-6
Goals and Priorities for the Infant With Cleft Lip

Antepartum Period

- Assist mother to recognize that breastfeeding is not only possible but optimal.
- Facilitate contact with local support groups, especially mothers who have successfully breastfed cleft infants. La Leche League or About Face can help.
- Collaborate with other members of the cleft team to identify strategies and options for supplemental feeding.
- Mobilize equipment: be sure that a suitable pump will be available both in the hospital and after discharge.
- Ensure that educational media will be available and accessible at the hospital when the infant is delivered (see Appendix B).

Immediate Postpartum Period

- Initiate or reinforce actions listed for the antepartum period.
- Assist the newborn to achieve good latch-on.
- Teach mother to express milk or use donor or artificial milk, if indicated.
- Provide parents with a list of worrisome signs and a list of phone numbers to call for help.
- Give suggestions to overcome problems of engorgement in the early postpartum period and diminished supply later on.
- Provide a list of pump rental depots and ask the plastic surgeon, neonatologist, or other physician to write a prescription. This prescription may enable the mother to obtain reimbursement from her health insurance company.

Immediate Postpartum Period Management

Without the benefit of prenatal encouragement and planning, breastfeeding might not be initiated. When a mother discovers that her infant has been born with a cleft she frequently says, "I had planned to breastfeed until this happened . . ." immediately assuming that breastfeeding is no longer an option. In some cases, exclusive breastfeeding may not be realistic, but even partial or short-term breastfeeding is laudable. Some mothers may not wish to start breastfeeding infants with cleft lips, since they feel that the interruption of breastfeeding caused by anticipated reconstructive surgery is too difficult. Help the mother to reevaluate or modify her choice of feeding method in the context of the infant's capabilities and risk factors. Goals and priorities for the immediate postpartum period are found in Box 7-6.

Assessments

Sometimes, cleft palates are not obvious. Look for clues; for example, note if the infant makes a clucking noise. Although a clucking sound can be heard when a well infant is latched on incorrectly, it may also signal the possibility of a cleft. One multipara complained of extremely sore nipples and had not experienced such intense pain when breastfeeding a normal infant. More generalized signs—chronic hypothermia, poor weight gain, lack of swallowing—require further investigation to determine the cause; sometimes clefting can be the root of these problems. Some infants who have experienced "feeding problems" have had undetected clefts for years.[21]

Cleft lips are quite obvious at the time of delivery. Mothers who have been forewarned about the cleft may be inclined to put the infant to the breast immediately. Encourage this, because it gives the infant an opportunity to experiment with latching on and suckling when the breast is soft. The goal of the first feeding, however, is for

warmth, bonding, and stimulation of milk supply; whether or not colostrum is obtained is less important. In subsequent feedings, however, the mother and the infant will need to learn how to successfully suckle. A good assessment improves chances for success.

First, assess the extent of the defect and its impact on feeding success. Determine whether the newborn can accomplish the three factors necessary for successful breastfeeding. First, the *seal* must be not only present but adequate. The seal creates negative pressure and holds the nipple and areola in place, but it does not extract milk from the breast; an adequate seal can be difficult to achieve with a cleft defect. Second, the *negative pressure* must be adequate as described in Chapter 5; this is accomplished in part by the motion of the tongue upon the gum and lips and areola compressing the hard palate. When both cleft lip and cleft palate are present, an adequate negative pressure will not be generated.[22] Finally, the *suckling mechanisms* must be adequate; milk flows from the nipple and swallowing occurs as a result of reflex; normal infants with a cleft can swallow normally.[22] Problems with intraoral muscular movements are associated with bilateral cleft lips because the tongue does not stabilize the nipple. Similarly, wide cleft palates are problematic because the tongue cannot compress the nipple effectively (see Table 7-6).

Clinical Management

The visual impact of a cleft results in dismay and grief that require extensive support.[23] Infants with clefts of the lips and/or the alveolar ridge, however, look quite normal while breastfeeding because the breast tissue fills the cleft and camouflages it. During the first few days postpartum, help parents to develop realistic expectations of the breastfeeding experience. They may assume that the infant's less-than-enthusiastic approach to breastfeeding is a result of the cleft defect. Explain that some feeding behaviors are typical of any infant at the breast; many infants do not im-

T A B L E 7-6		
POSSIBLE PROBLEMS AND BREASTFEEDING MANAGEMENT FOR NEWBORNS WITH ALTERATIONS IN CRANIOFACIAL STRUCTURE OR FUNCTION		
Problem	Clinical Strategy	Rationale
Risk for aspiration	Determine if infant's respiratory status indicates or contraindicates oral feeding; withhold oral feedings if respirations are greater than 60-70, or if dyspnea is present, or per hospital protocol	Increased respiratory rate makes coordination of sucking and swallowing more difficult
	Have bulb syringe handy in case infant is unable to clear his own airway; aspirate contents of mouth first, then suction nose; show parents how to use the bulb syringe	Aspirating mouth first prevents inhalation of aspirate—infant will gasp if nares are stimulated first; avoid center of mouth because this stimulates gag reflex
	Cleft palate: use upright feeding position	Milk less likely to go into cleft
Inadequate seal	Help infant to open wide (tickle bottom lip; gently press chin inward)	Essential for all infants; improves likelihood of adequate areolar grasp, and ultimately, milk transfer
	Point nipple away from cleft	Minimizes the problem
	Try using Dancer hand as shown in Figure 7-19	Provides extra support for latch-on
	Try straddle position as shown in Figure 7-18	Facing breast head-on makes more tissue available
	Cleft lip: place index finger on top edge of areola and middle finger on bottom; nipple will protrude as if it were full of milk	Helps areolar tissue to mold to fill the cleft
	Cleft lip: fill the cleft with mother's thumb as shown in Figure 7-12	Minimizes amount of space that interferes with good seal
Inadequate negative pressure	Grasp both cheeks, pushing lips together	Helps to create negative pressure
	Burp more frequently	Infant may swallow more air; inadequate negative pressure leads to faulty seal
Inadequate suckling mechanisms	Consider pillow to help position infant	Decreases distance between infant and breast
	Make sure neck is flexed rather than extended	Difficult to swallow with extended neck
Milk let-down too slow; baby working too hard	Hand massage first	Enhances rapid milk-ejection reflex and hastens flow of milk
Milk let-down too fast; baby gagging	Consider Australian hold, as shown in Figure 7-16	Slows flow of milk; force of gravity pulls milk toward mother rather than toward infant

mediately latch on and suckle vigorously. Conversely, do not give the message that breastfeeding will be "difficult." Switching from breast to bottle does not eliminate the difficulty; infants with clefts continue to choke, gag, and sputter with the bottle, and bottle feeding may even exaggerate this problem.

Breastfeeding management depends on being sure that the basic techniques are not overlooked, and that specialized techniques are used to pro-

mote milk transfer. A SOAP note from an actual patient record is found in Box 7-7.

SPECIAL FEEDING CHALLENGES (BREAST OR BOTTLE) Whether they are breastfed or bottle fed, infants with clefts have some special difficulties. For example, they tire easily.[24] To overcome this, offer frequent feedings. Forewarn the parents that the infant may gag and have milk come back up through the nose. Reassure them that you will

Box 7-7
Sample Nurse's SOAP* Note for Cleft Lip Newborn

S: "It feels much better when we do that" (when baby opens wide and is positioned tummy-to-tummy).

O: A small reddened area (a few mm in diameter) on right nipple. Baby does not always open wide, and is not always tummy-to-tummy. Mom encouraged to elicit good open-wide before allowing latch-on and to position tummy-to-tummy. Multipara has breastfed two noncleft infants × 4-5 months each. Upon palpation, breasts do appear to be filling, congruent with mom's report of feeling full. Mom reports feeling let-down about the time that newborn has slower, rhythmic sucks. Audible swallowing. Unilateral cleft lip and cleft of alveolar ridge on right side—not a wide cleft. Shown how to tip nipple upward just until baby latches on chin first; then readjust. Also shown how to use straddle position. Dancer hand suggested as a possible option; reinforced idea of pointing nipple away from the cleft. Baby has lost 6% of birth weight and is jaundiced this morning. Sometimes takes baby off from breast and does switch-nursing; discouraged this and explained need for hindmilk. Mom and nursery staff instructed to use Asepto-type syringe or eyedropper if supplementation is ordered.

A: Infant has significant weight loss, but suckled and swallowed well at this feeding; asleep at end of feeding. Mom's milk is coming in; nipple breakdown due to baby not opening widely.

P: Reinforcement and anticipatory guidance/planning:
- Reinforce OPEN WIDE and good positioning; make sure baby gets hindmilk
- Give expressed pumped breast milk via Asepto syringe if supplement is ordered
- Reassure mom that 6% weight loss is okay at this point but will need to be reevaluated in context of entire clinical picture
- Reevaluate feeding success if mom becomes engorged
- Begin exploring possibility of Wallaby phototherapy unit for home use if this should become necessary.
- Call me if you have questions. Thanks.

M. Biancuzzo, R.N.

*The SOAP format—subjective and objective data, assessment and plan—is frequently used for nurses' notes.

stay with them; it can be very frightening to see the infant struggle. Suggest holding the infant upright as much as possible to reduce this problem. These infants may take in more air than others; burp them frequently.

SUCKLING AT THE BREAST

It is imperative to follow all of the principles of good positioning and latch-on when clefting is present. A few specialized techniques may be helpful, but none of the following are imperative; it is frequently a matter of trial and error (see Box 7-8).

An infant with a unilateral cleft may be most successful if the breast enters the mouth from the side on which the defect is located; this points the nipple away from the cleft. For example, instruct the mother whose infant has a right-sided cleft of the lip or palate to hold the infant so that his right cheek touches the breast. If this works, use the cradle hold on one side and the football hold on the other.[25]

An infant with a bilateral defect of the palate or alveolar ridge does best when he squarely faces the breast. This can be accomplished by using either a sitting or straddle position. Large defects may require that the breast be tipped downward or angled slightly to one side or the other.[25] Again, it is important to try multiple techniques and see which one works best. What works well for one infant may not work for another infant with a technically similar but clinically unique lesion.

It is all too easy to suggest intervention after intervention, only to learn much later that the infant is not gaining weight. The key is to evalu-

Box 7-8
Techniques for Special Feeding Challenge

- Encourage suckling when the breast is full and the nipple protrudes a bit.
- Consider using one breast at a feeding if the infant tires easily, since it improves the likelihood of obtaining the hindmilk before he gets too tired.
- Try the football position or the straddle position so that the infant squarely faces the breast. Because of the size of the infant's legs, the straddle position might be less successful during the neonatal period. Using a pillow underneath the infant's buttocks may help when using the straddle position.
- Point the nipple away from the cleft.
- Place the index finger at the top edge of the areola and the middle finger on bottom to make nipple protrude.
- Hold the infant semi-upright to prevent milk from coming out the nose.

- Massage or use warm compresses to improve the milk ejection reflex. Sometimes infants find it more gratifying to get the milk with less effort.
- Tickle the lips so that the infant opens wide! When the mouth is gaping and the tongue is troughed and over the lower alveolar ridge, quickly guide the mother's arm so that she brings the infant to the breast.
- Fill the cleft lip with the mother's thumb, as shown in Figure 7-12.
- Gently press chin inward, hook angle of the jaw as shown in Figure 7-20, or use the Dancer hand to maneuver when bringing infant onto the breast to augment intraoral suction.
- Make sure neck is flexed but not hyperflexed, rather than extended.

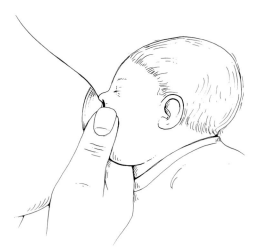

Fig. 7-12 Mother's thumb fills the cleft space.

ate each intervention. For example, the infant often appears to be latched on well, but further observation reveals that air can be heard going through the cleft. This produces a sort of soft hissing noise. Continue efforts to fill the cleft, either with a finger or with the breast tissue. This may be a trial-and-error process for a while. Audible swallowing is the one most reassuring sign that optimal latch-on has been achieved. If swallowing is not audible, or if air can be heard going through the cleft, the infant is not suckling effectively, even though he may appear to be making sucking motions.

POSSIBLE CONCURRENT PROBLEMS

If the seal, negative pressure, or suckling mechanisms are inadequate, the result will be an inadequate intake. The key, therefore, is to optimize milk intake through good intervention and evaluation. Inadequate intake can and does occur to some degree, however, so be alert to common problems that may accompany cleft defects.

Jaundice is a common problem. Because the infant may have particular difficulty suckling well in the first few days, he may be unable to gain the laxative effects of colostrum. Feed the colostrum to the newborn if possible. Sometimes an otherwise healthy infant needs to remain in the hospital for jaundice treatment after his mother has been discharged. This interruption in the normal breastfeeding relationship can be the difference between success and failure with cleft infants. Discharge planning should include a contingency plan to treat the jaundice at home if necessary so that potential separation of the mother and infant is avoided.

Breast engorgement is a likely problem in the early days because the infant may not be obtaining all the milk from the breast. In addition to helping the infant attain latch-on, suggest pumping after feedings. Any of the usual strategies for managing engorgement are appropriate.

A dwindling supply threatens breastfeeding if the infant is unable to suckle or becomes separated from the mother for several weeks or even months. For example, an infant with a cleft palate may be unable to suckle adequately for 8 to 10 months. Allowing the infant to nuzzle the breast, warm packs applied to the breast, and multiparity usually enhance success. The best strategy, however, is bilateral expression using an electric pump (see Chapter 10).

Failure to thrive is a threat to any infant who cannot suckle adequately. Cleft infants are particularly at risk not only because of feeding difficulties but also because of apparently increased metabolic rates. Those with isolated clefts, however, are less likely to be at risk for FTT than those who have clefts associated with a syndrome.[26] It is important to give the infant adequate time at the breast, since obtaining the hindmilk is critical for weight gain. If the infant is always hungry or hypothermic, he is not obtaining enough milk. Consider supplementation as one means to achieve the goal of adequate intake, but supplementing should not replace good clinical management.

SUPPLEMENTAL FEEDING

Many infants with cleft defects can suckle at the breast; some do as well as normal infants, while others need assistive devices. As early as possible, the cleft team should determine one or possibly two alternative feeding methods that can be used before and after surgery, rather than teach the parent one method and then another. A lactation supplementer can provide extra calories and promote stimulation to the breast (see Chapter 12). Each situation will require evaluation to determine what supplementation method will work best, but clear communication among the members of the cleft team and with the parents is critical to breastfeeding success. Rather than using bottles, consider alternative methods for giving supplemental feedings.

Various devices have been used in different facilities and in different countries. A few decades ago, the lamb's nipple and Brecht feeder, Mead-Johnson Cleft Palate Nurser, and Ross Cleft Palate Nurser were popular in the United States. In England and Australia the Rosti bottle (similar to the spoon-shaped devices distributed with liquid over-the-counter medications in the United States) has been used. Squeezable plastic bottles with narrow, long crosscut nipples have been used with cleft infants for decades, but infants appear to suckle and gain weight as well with a standard nipple that has been crosscut.[27] The Haberman feeder™ by Medela has recently gained popularity. Its elongated nipple can be compressed more easily than a traditional nipple, which may be helpful if the infant has difficulty getting adequate negative pressure, but no clinical studies are available to substantiate this. At the University of Rochester Medical Center, we used an Asepto-type syringe attached to a pediatric catheter-like tube. This device works well both before and after surgery. Variations on this idea might be a regular syringe, a dental syringe, or an eyedropper. Cup feeding, described in more detail in Chapter 12, has been used successfully in supplementing infants with clefts.[28]

EDUCATION, COUNSELING, AND SUPPORT

Patient education materials (Appendix B) offer little help unless they are available immediately after the infant is born. The pamphlet by Danner is outstanding; the photos are excellent and the approach is positive.

Intense support is required not only for initiating breastfeeding but also for continuing. Weaning is a continuous, recurring question. The mother may want to wean before cleft lip surgery because of a "quit-while-we're ahead" attitude, out of fear that it will be impossible to reestablish breastfeeding after the surgery. A mother who wants to wean before cleft palate surgery probably has many ambivalent feelings; her infant may have never suckled at the breast and/or may do markedly better after the palate is repaired. Breastfeeding can continue after surgery in any

case, but the challenge may seem insurmountable. Help the mother to identify her own goal, and together generate strategies to best accomplish it.

Mothers can become very discouraged. Despite good clinical management and the mother's valiant efforts, we saw an infant with a cleft lip and two cleft palates who was unable to suckle effectively and required supplementation. The mother saw this as not "really" breastfeeding, and she needed support to overcome her feelings of failure. Mothers in this situation need someone to acknowledge their disappointments and redefine their contribution and motivation. Reinforce the original idea that the mother is providing the best food for the infant, and emphasize that the goal is obtaining the *milk*, and that breast*feeding* is only one way to achieve that goal.

Assisting parents of cleft infants is truly a collaborative effort; tap the expertise of everyone on the cleft team. The Cleft Foundation (see Appendix A) can recommend a cleft team and a support group in every area of the United States.

Surgery for Cleft Lip or Palate Infant

Most surgical repairs are done after the infant is a month old. Goals and priorities for the time preceding and following surgery are listed in Box 7-4. When infants require surgery, parents will require teaching and support both preoperatively and postoperatively.

Preoperative Teaching and Support

Anticipate corrective surgery and provide teaching and support as soon as possible. Parents may ask how soon the cleft will be repaired. This varies dramatically from surgeon to surgeon, but the 10-10-10/10 guideline often applies. Some surgeons wait until the infant weighs 10 pounds and has a hemoglobin count of 10 dl; cleft lips are repaired before 10 weeks, and cleft palates are generally repaired before 10 months. This is by no means a rule, but it serves as a general guideline.

CLINICAL SCENARIO

The Infant With a Cleft Defect

You are the nurse-practitioner in the nursery. Baby George has a unilateral cleft lip, and appears to be breastfeeding well. However, he is losing weight. Here are his weights from the last few days:

Birth	3970
Day 1	3905
Day 2	3735
Day 3	3705
Day 4	3730

Would you order a supplement for this baby?

You are the lactation consultant, and the nursery staff nurses call you to see a baby with a fairly wide, unilateral cleft. You suggest that the mother try putting her thumb in the cleft, but this is not completely successful, as the cleft is so wide. What else might you try?

You are the staff nurse caring for baby Kurt who has a unilateral cleft lip. His mother successfully breastfed two other children. Kurt is a vigorous nurser, and has had about a 7% weight loss over the past 4 days. He is being discharged today with a bilirubin level of 12. What two priorities would you identify for Kurt's discharge planning?

You are the nurse practitioner in a busy pediatric office. Mrs. M. has been pumping for 6 months, as her son was born at 32 weeks' gestation with a significant cleft of the soft and hard palate. She is tearful; her supply is dwindling and she knows that the baby will have the cleft repaired at 8 months, but isn't sure she can continue pumping until then. She asks if she should quit. How would you respond, or what would you recommend?

Readers are encouraged to discuss this scenario among their colleagues, since often there is no one right answer.

Help parents to ask the right questions so they can adjust feeding accordingly. Parental concerns have been described,[29] and from these pertinent questions have been generated in Box 7-9.

Postoperative Management

Preferences vary widely, but many surgeons will not allow the infant to suck anything—a breast, a rubber teat, or a pacifier—for approximately 10 days after a cleft repair. (Again, note the "10" rule.) There is still a myth that delayed sucking reduces tension on the suture line of cleft lips, but a research study conducted in the United States shows that there were no detrimental effects when breastfeeding was initiated immediately after the surgery.[30] In the Third World, where breastfeeding is common, similar results have been noted and reported anecdotally to the author and in controlled studies.[31,32]

Mechanical trauma to the roof of the mouth—such as trauma caused by artificial nipples—may damage cleft palate repairs. If the surgeon insists on this delay, ask him to allow a Tommy-Tippy type of cup for supplemental feedings before the end of the 10 days. If surgeons prefer to delay sucking, the infant can be fed with a tube at the side of the mouth, allowing the infant to swallow the fluid. Pumped breast milk is superior to formula, so if a significant interruption in breastfeeding is anticipated, suggest expressing and freezing milk prior to the surgery. The mother's supply may be reduced during this hiatus, but assure her that her regular supply can be reestablished.

The Turner's bow, designed to reduce tension on the suture line, is no longer popular among plastic surgeons, probably because of its disadvantages. The bow is held in place with tape, which may cause trauma to the circumoral tissue, and the infant's drooling necessitates frequent retaping. Arm restraints, which hamper feeding efforts, are being ordered less frequently. It is doubtful that they serve a useful purpose.[33]

Box 7-9
General Concerns of Parents of Infants With Cleft

General Hospital Routines

- Is mother allowed to room-in with the baby?
- Are siblings allowed to visit?
- What routine procedures are performed prior to and after surgery?
- How long will my baby have nothing by mouth prior to surgery?
- How will my baby be anesthetized?
- Will I be able to visit my baby in the recovery area?

Postsurgical Restraints

- Will my baby be prevented from bending his elbow?
- Will any special positioning be necessary?

Lip Care

- Will I need to use normal saline and/or antimicrobial ointment on the suture line?
- Will a Turner's bow be used?

Feeding

- How soon will I be able to breastfeed my baby?
- Will you write an order for my baby to be fed my milk until he can go to breast?
- Will my baby be fed with an Asepto syringe or dropper? For how long?
- Will any obturator be used?
- How can I obtain a breast pump?

Postoperative Management

- Establish or resume breastfeeding as soon as the surgeon allows.
- Assist with latch-on and basic information if the infant has not previously suckled.
- Reestablish a full milk supply.

The palatal obturator is a prosthesis that is retained in the crevices of the mouth, providing a seal between the mouth and the nasal cavity. Few surgeons use palatal obturators these days. It is difficult to fit the device into the extremely small mouth of a newborn without the use of wires, which many surgeons object to. Dentists who make this prosthesis find that a proper fit is a difficult challenge even in older infants. Anecdotally, some nurses or mothers have suggested that breastfeeding is more effective with the use of the palatal obturator, but there have

been no studies to confirm this possibility. Mothers also report that the obturator causes sore nipples, but again, there is no conclusive research on this issue.

The infant's first postoperative feeding at the breast should proceed as normally as possible. Support the mother's efforts, and help her to realize that a little adjustment will be necessary for her and her infant. Focus on the real problem, which has become the *interruption* in breastfeeding, rather than breastfeeding per se. Help her to keep in mind that the repair should solve, not worsen, the feeding problems created by the cleft.

Conclusions About Breastfeeding Management

Infants with cleft defects can and should breast-feed. It is best to mobilize personnel, equipment, and educational materials and active support prior to delivery, if possible. Special techniques and community support help overcome problems immediately after delivery as well as in subsequent months prior to and after surgery. The breastfeeding specialist has a critical role in implementing interdisciplinary care and evaluating the effectiveness of interventions.

Short or Tight Frenulum

Infants are sometimes born with a short or tight frenulum. As with other structural defects, the extent of the problem determines the amount of difficulty that will be encountered in breastfeeding. The goal is for the infant to be able to extend his tongue enough so that he can adequately compress the mother's nipple, causing it to elongate into a teat (see Chapter 5). If this is happening, further intervention is probably not necessary. Having the mother lean back and use an Australian hold is sometimes helpful (see discussion later in chapter), since the infant's tongue is then "down" on the nipple rather than reaching upward. If the frenulum is particularly short, the pediatrician may recommend surgical repair. Various actions related to breastfeeding these infants have been reported anecdotally, but so far no valid and reliable assessment tools have been developed to assess the capabilities of these infants, and no controlled studies have demonstrated the impact on breastfeeding.

PRETERM AND LOW-BIRTH-WEIGHT INFANTS

Preterm birth affects feeding in general and breastfeeding specifically. Infants who are born before term are likely to have alterations in neurological function and in nutrient needs. These alterations, although not pathological, are transient, and require an understanding of the infant's increased needs and special breastfeeding management.

Incidence and Definition

Preterm birth is defined as less than 37 weeks' gestation.[34,35] Approximately 11% of births occur preterm; the percentage of preterm births has risen steadily since 1981.[35] A preterm birth is often preceded by months of maternal illness and/or hospitalization. These disruptions to the family can overshadow the joy of the birth event. When birth does occur, feeding the infant may be just one more challenge for the mother to meet.

No one method of feeding is easy for preterm infants, and the degree of difficulty they experience varies tremendously, depending on the exact gestational age and other factors. The closer to term birth occurs, the fewer the difficulties. Infants who are born at 35 to 37 weeks, for example, may need only a double blanket to keep warm, some encouragement to wake up for frequent feedings, and periodic assessment of serum glucose levels. Infants born before 35 weeks' gestation, however, require more vigorous interventions to compensate for immature functioning. In the more extreme cases, infants born between 24 and 30 weeks' gestation may spend weeks with no oral feedings, and their mothers will need to cope with the difficulties of establishing milk production without an infant to suckle.

Additionally, infants who are born prematurely are likely to have other factors that influence breastfeeding. For example, multiple gesta-

T A B L E 7-7

COMPARISON OF WEIGHT AND GESTATION STATUS

Gestation	Weight	Classification(s)			
		Full-Term	Preterm	Low Birth Weight	Very Low Birth Weight
≥37 wk	≥2500 g	●			
≥37 wk	<2500 g	●		●	
<37 wk	≥2500 g		●		
<37 wk	1500-2499 g		●	●	
<37 wk	<1500 g		●		●

Infants can be classified according to gestation (preterm, full-term, postterm), weight only (low birth weight or very low birth weight), and gestation in relation to age (appropriate for gestational age, small for gestational age, or large for gestational age).

- *Gestation* is merely the amount of time the infant has been in utero. Regardless of their weight, infants born before 37 weeks' (259 days') gestation are considered *preterm* according to the American Academy of Pediatrics and the American College of Obstetricians and Gynecologists.
- *Weight.* Regardless of their gestation, infants who weigh less than 2500 g at birth are *low birth weight* (LBW). Infants who weigh less than 1500 g at birth are considered *very low birth weight* (VLBW).
- Infants' weight and age are combined to form yet another category. *Appropriate for gestational age* (AGA) means that the infant's weight falls between the 10th and the 90th percentiles in comparison with other infants of the same gestational age. (The specific gestational age doesn't matter.) Infants who are *small for gestational age* (SGA) are those whose weight falls below the 10th percentile in relation to other infants of the same gestational age. (N.B: Infants who are SGA are not necessarily preterm!) *Large for gestational age* (LGA) means that the infant's weight falls above the 90th percentile in relation to other infants of the same gestational age at the same number of weeks' gestation, i.e., their weight is considered in relation to infants born at the same number of weeks' gestation.

Source: American Academy of Pediatrics and the American College of Obstetricians and Gynecologists. *Guidelines for Perinatal Care*. 4th ed. Elk Grove Village, IL: American Academy of Pediatrics; 1997 and Battaglia FC, Lubchenko LO. A practical classification of newborn infants by weight and gestational age. *J Peds* 1967;71:159-163.

tion is frequently associated with preterm birth. Infants born from multiple gestation, if born fairly close to term, can usually initiate and continue breastfeeding with relatively little assistance, as described in Chapter 6. However, infants with defects are often born before term, and these infants will experience many difficulties with breastfeeding as a result of their immaturity and their underlying pathology.

Because clinical decision making for breastfeeding is frequently based on data about the infant's age and/or weight, it is critical not to confuse issues of age with issues of weight. Infants can be classified according to gestation (preterm, term, postterm), weight only (low birth weight or very low birth weight), and gestation in relation to age (appropriate for gestational age, small for gestational age, or large for gestational age). A

summary of characteristics distinguishing gestation and weight classifications is presented in Table 7-7. Figure 7-13 shows infants of the same gestational age with different weights.

This section deals mainly with preterm infants, although an infant who weighs less than 2500 grams (low birth weight or LBW) is frequently born before term (i.e., preterm).

Benefits of Breastfeeding Preterm Infants

Unfortunately, families sometimes become focused on the limitations of the preterm infant rather than on his needs or his capabilities. While preterm infants may have difficulties with any type of feeding—breastfeeding or artificial feeding—the benefits of human milk as well as

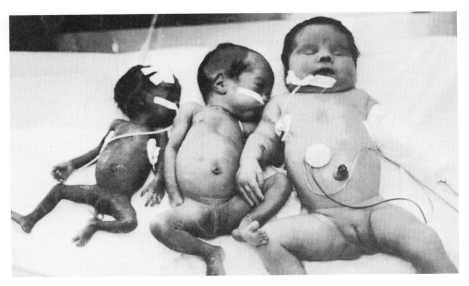

Fig. 7-13 Three infants, same gestational age, with weights of 600, 1400, and 2750 g, respectively, from left to right. *(From Korones SB.* High-Risk Newborn Infants. *4th ed. St. Louis: Mosby; 1986.)*

feeding at the breast (direct breastfeeding) are designed to meet his needs. Table 7-8 summarizes the benefits of human milk and direct breastfeeding.

Human Milk for Preterm Newborns

The American Academy of Pediatrics has determined that human milk is best for all infants, including those who are born preterm.[3] Expert clinicians strongly encourage the use of human milk for preterm or low-birth-weight infants.[36] More specifically, milk produced by mothers of preterm infants—called *preterm milk*—differs in composition from term milk, as shown in Box 7-10, and it has special benefits for the preterm infant.

In general, it is better to feed preterm infants preterm milk rather than term milk or artificial milk. In this chapter, only mother's own milk will be described; donor milk (discussed in Chapter 11) is another matter. Fortunately, the components of preterm milk differ from term milk and are better suited to meet the unique needs of the preterm infant during the first month or so. This is nature's way of precisely meeting the infant's unique and changing needs.

Preterm infants have nutritional needs that differ from those of the term infant. Like term infants, preterm newborns need nutrients that will provide energy sources, build tissue, and regulate body processes. However, the need is much greater for preterm than for term infants, as shown in Table 7-9.

Nutrients Provide Energy From Carbohydrates, Protein, and Fat

Preterm infants require more energy (from carbohydrates, proteins, and fats) because of their high metabolic rates. Preterm infants need at least 110 to 120 kcal/kg/day to support metabolic function and normal growth and development. To achieve this, the infant must take in 170 to 180 ml/kg/day of human milk. Infants with problems such as

TABLE 7-8

HEALTH OUTCOMES OF BREAST MILK AND BREASTFEEDING FOR PRETERM INFANTS

General Benefit	Specific Benefits	Source
Immunological	Decreased incidence and severity of infection	Narayanan et al. *Acta Paediatr Scand* 1982;71(3):441-445.
	Fewer hospital readmissions	Hagan et al. *Pediatr Res* 1991;29:1284.
Allergy	Decreased incidence of later allergy for infants at risk	Lucas et al. *BMJ* 1990;300:837-40.
Protection from necrotizing enterocolitis	In formula-fed infants, protection is 6-10 times higher than in infants fed only human milk	Lucas & Cole, *Lancet* 1990;336;1519-1523
	Rate 3.5 times higher when fed formula and human milk, compared to human milk alone	
Neurocognitive	Highly significant advantage in IQ score at 7½ to 8 years of age over children who did not receive mothers' own milk	Lucas et al. *Arch Dis Child* 1994;70:F141-6. Lucas et al. *Lancet* 1992;339:261-264. Lucas et al. *Arch Dis Child* 1989;64:1570-1578.
Retinal function	Decreased incidence of retrolental fibroplasia related to presence of Omega-3 fatty acids	Uauy RD et al. *Pediatr Res* 1990;28:485-92.
Direct breastfeeding	Longer, more rhythmic sucking bursts during breastfeeding when compared to bottle feeding	Dowling. University of Illinois at Chicago; 1996. Unpublished doctoral dissertation. Meier. Suck-breathe patterning during breast and bottle feeding for preterm infants. In T. David, ed. *Major controversies in infant nutrition.* London: Royal Society of Medicine Press Limited; 1996.
	Higher respiratory rate during sucking bursts in breastfeeding sessions	Dowling. University of Illinois at Chicago; 1996. Unpublished doctoral dissertation. Meier. *Nurs Res* 1988;37(1):36-41.
	More stable oxygen saturation during sucking bursts in breastfeeding sessions as compared to bottle feeding sessions	Bier et al, *J Pediatr* 1993;123:773-8. Meier. *Nurs Res* 1988;37(1):36-41. Bier et al. *Pediatrics* 1997;100: web page e3.

Dowling D, Danner SC, Coffey P. *Breastfeeding the Infant With Special Needs.* White Plains, NY: March of Dimes Foundation; 1997.

bronchopulmonary dysplasia or other serious problems will need a minimum of 120 to 150 kcal/kg/day.

Preterm milk is best for preterm infants who weigh more than 1500 grams. Preterm newborns may have difficulty consuming this amount of calories when suckling, however, because they often suckle only the foremilk and then become too tired to obtain the hindmilk. This is an important clinical consideration. Infants who do not get the energy-rich hindmilk—which derives most of its calories from fat—will make poor weight gains.

Preterm milk does not supply significantly more calories than term milk.[37]

Newborns who weigh less than 1500 grams will need supplementation. Extra nutrients (and therefore extra kilocalories) can be provided by using fortifiers added to human milk (see Chapter 11). Other ways to meet this requirement are through supplementation with standard (20-kcal/oz) artificial milk, or 150 ml/kg/day of specially designed (24-kcal/oz) artificial milk[38] or hindmilk only from expressed milk. (See Chapter 11 for full description.)

Box 7-10
Milk of Mothers Who Deliver Preterm

Level Increased in Preterm	Level Unchanged in Preterm
Total nitrogen	Volume
Protein nitrogen	Calories
Long-chain fatty acids	Lactose (? less)
Medium-chain fatty acids	Fat (?) by creamatocrit
Short-chain fatty acids	Linolenic acid
Sodium	Potassium
Chloride	Calcium
Magnesium (?)	Phosphorus
Iron	Copper
	Zinc
	Osmolality
	Vitamin B$_{(1-12)}$

From Lawrence RA: *Breastfeeding: A Guide for the Medical Profession.* 4th ed. St. Louis: Mosby; 1994.

T A B L E 7-9
GUIDELINES FOR DAILY ENTERAL FEEDING

Expressed in amounts per kilogram of body weight, unless otherwise stated

Newborn	Energy Requirements (kcal)	Protein (g)	Sodium (mEq)	Potassium (mEq)	Calcium (mg)	Phosphorus (mg)	Iron (mg)
Term (for 0-6 months)	108†	2.2	1-3	1-3	400*	300*	6*‡
Preterm (0-6 months)	110-120†	2.5-3.5	3-8	1-3	200-250	100-112	2*‡
SGA or critically ill	120-150	2.5-3.5	1-3	1-3	Up to 200	Approx. 100	2‡

†May need more due to underlying pathological condition.

‡Until the infant doubles his weight (approximately 1-2 months) unless being transfused repeatedly.

*Amounts of calcium, phosphorus, and iron needed for full-term infants are expressed as absolutes; all full-term infants need the specified amount per day, *not* per kilogram of body weight.

Note: Most amounts listed reflect the *minimum*. It is not always possible to achieve these minimum requirements through human milk only.

Preterm infants need to *build more tissue*, because the greatest amount of tissue accretion (growth or increase) occurs during the third trimester of gestation. In order to build tissue, the preterm infant needs greater amounts of protein. Preterm milk is dramatically higher in protein than term milk. Nitrogen, a building block of pro-

tein, is high in preterm milk and is especially suitable for the high rate of growth.

As for term infants, vitamins and minerals help preterm infants to *regulate body processes*. However, preterm infants need more calcium and phosphorus than term infants. Calcium is needed for bone mineralization because the greatest

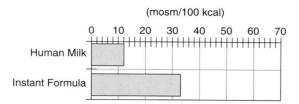

Fig. 7-14 Potential renal solute load for human milk and formula. *(Data from Committee on Nutrition, American Academy of Pediatrics. Pediatric Nutrition Handbook. Elk Grove Village, IL: American Academy of Pediatrics; 1993.)*

amount of bone mineralization happens during the last trimester of gestation—a time that is shortened for the infant who is born before term—and during early infancy. Phosphorus is needed, among other reasons, because it enhances the absorption of calcium and decreases urinary calcium and magnesium excretion.[39] When there is a deficit of phosphorus, calcium absorption is impaired; therefore, preterm infants especially need increased amounts of phosphorus. Unfortunately, the amounts of calcium and phosphorus are about the same in preterm and term milk, so the amount is inadequate to completely meet the needs of very preterm infants.

Easier Digestibility

Because they have immature digestive tracts, preterm infants have more difficulty digesting—breaking down—nutrients they have ingested. Human milk, with its lower curd ratio, is therefore ideal for these infants because it is more easily digested and absorbed than artificial milk. Accumulating evidence suggests that preterm infants are at lower risk for necrotizing enterocolitis when they are fed human milk rather than artificial milk.[5] The bifidus factor, available in human milk, results in gram-positive beneficial (normal) intestinal flora, rather than the gram-negative pathogenic bacteria found in the gut. Furthermore, constipation or "hard stools" are a common problem for preterm infants. Those who are fed artificial milk are more likely to have stools with a higher solid content than infants who are fed human milk.[40]

Lower Potential Renal Solute Load

Preterm infants have immature kidney functioning and are therefore less able to tolerate high renal solute loads. Human milk has a potentially lower renal solute load than artificial milk, as shown in Figure 7-14. This lower renal solute load occurs because there are lower levels of protein, sodium, phosphorous, and potassium in breast milk than in artificial milk. The relatively low levels of these ions require less water for excretion; hence, lower levels of water are lost when the infant consumes human milk. This water conservation results in a more stable body temperature because water is a factor in thermoregulation.

Protects Against Infection

The preterm infant's life is threatened by actual or potential infections; he is vulnerable not only because of preterm status but also because of invasive technology and exposure to staff who have cared for other potentially infected infants. His greatest protection is human milk—a living fluid that sustains life! Preterm infants, who are especially vulnerable to respiratory and gastrointestinal infection, particularly benefit from the infection protection properties—most notably secretory IgA, but also lysozyme, lactoferrin, and other protective components (see Chapter 3). Of course, because of the higher protein content of preterm milk (in comparison to term milk), antiinfective properties such as immunoglobulins (which are protein components) are greater. For example, sIgA, the antiinfective that provides so much protection against respiratory and gastrointestinal infection, is nearly doubled in preterm colostrum (about 310 mg/g of protein) compared with term colostrum (about 168, and therefore preterm). Furthermore, phagocytic cells—cells that engulf pathogenic organisms—are enhanced by colostrum. Preterm colostrum contains higher numbers of phagocytic cells than term colostrum.[41]

Better for Neurodevelopment

Preterm infants especially need cholesterol, which is a necessary component for brain development. Human milk appears to be the ideal food for neurodevelopmental needs.[42] Cholesterol is present in human milk but absent in artificial milk because it relies on vegetable oil. Lucas and colleagues' 1992 study caused quite a stir in the professional as well as the consumer literature; it showed that 7½ to 8-year-olds born preterm and fed mother's milk had higher intelligence quotients than their artificially fed cohorts.[43] This study was particularly significant because it showed the value of human milk only—not the process of breastfeeding (i.e., the infants were fed by tube). Retinal function also is improved when preterm infants are fed human milk, with its long-chain fatty acids, as opposed to artificial milk with corn oil–based fatty acids.[44]

Breastfeeding for Preterm Newborns

Not only is preterm milk advantageous for the preterm newborn, but the act of feeding at the breast has advantages for respiratory function and parent-infant attachment.

Facilitates Respiratory Function

Suckling at the breast is more physiological than sucking an artificial nipple. The common myth that breastfeeding is more "work" than bottle feeding is not supported by the research. To the contrary, preterm newborns can better maintain their transcutaneous oxygen pressure and body temperature while breastfeeding than while bottle feeding[11,45] as described in the Research Highlight. Because the preterm infant is likely to have weak or absent cough or gag reflexes, aspiration is possible, but it is less likely with breastfeeding than with bottle feeding. Furthermore, if the infant does aspirate, human milk is less irritating to the bronchial tree than artificial milk. Generally, however, infants with respiratory rates of over 60 to 70 are allowed nothing by mouth, and enteral or parenteral feeding must be implemented.

Provides Unique Maternal Benefits

Breastfeeding provides the mother with a special closeness to her newborn, as discussed in previous chapters. This is especially important when the infant is preterm because there are fewer opportunities to "mother" the infant who is attached to monitors, tubes, and other devices. When talking about breastfeeding, mothers frequently say, "Providing my milk is the only thing I can do for the baby." When newborns are finally free from monitoring and other devices, they need tactile, kinesthetic, and auditory stimulation.[46] Breastfeeding meets all of these needs, usually simultaneously.

Prenatal Assessment and Counseling

Often, a preterm birth can be anticipated. Mothers who have had a previous preterm birth are at risk for another. The many risk factors for preterm

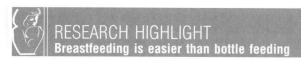

RESEARCH HIGHLIGHT
Breastfeeding is easier than bottle feeding

Citation

Meier P. Bottle- and breast-feeding: effects on transcutaneous oxygen pressure and temperature in preterm infants. *Nurs Res* 1988;37:36-41.

Focus

Five preterm infants who weighed less than 1500 g at the initial oral feeding were continuously monitored during 71 feeding episodes (32 bottle-feeding and 39 breastfeeding episodes). Each infant served as his own control; that is, the same infants were studied while breastfeeding and bottle feeding at different times. The investigator measured body temperature and qualitative and quantitative differences in transcutaneous oxygen pressure (tcPO$_2$).

Results

The tissue oxygenation of the infant's skin (tcPO$_2$) differed markedly from breastfeedings to bottle feedings during the episode, immediately postfeed, and 10 minutes postfeed. Typically, bottle-fed infants had a decline in tissue oxygenation during the period of intake, a return to near-baseline levels as sucking ceased, a plateau at or near baseline when the infant rested and burped, and a gradual decline in tissue oxygenation from the end of the feeding until about 10 minutes after the feeding was completed. The lowest oxygenation was always recorded while the infant was sucking the bottle nipple. In breastfed infants fluctuations in tissue oxygenation from baseline were minimal, as opposed to the large declines from baseline that occurred during bottle feeding. Breastfeedings generally lasted longer than bottle feedings; the author suggests that infants may be unable to tolerate longer bottle feedings because fatigue results from ventilatory disruption. Temperature increases were significant during breastfeeding but not during bottle feeding (Figure 7-15).

Clinical Application

This well-controlled study, although performed on only a few infants, looked at many feeding episodes. The dramatic difference in oxygenation while breastfeeding as opposed to bottle feeding gives strong direction for hospital protocols. Infants should not be required to tolerate bottle feeding before attempting breastfeeding. Caregivers and parents should recognize that breastfeeding is less disruptive to respiratory efforts and temperature is enhanced when the preterm infant is put to breast. The results from this study were similar to results in a 1997 study by Bier et al.

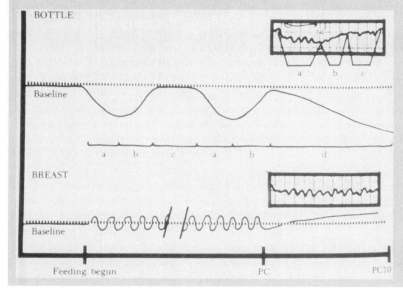

Fig. 7-15 Schematic of typical tcPO$_2$ patterns during bottle feeding and breastfeeding. Note in bottle feeding (BoF) (a) decline, (b) recovery, (c) plateau, and (d) decline between end of feeding (PC) and 10 minutes postfeeding (PC10). Both schematics have been magnified somewhat for clarity. Also note interruption in the breastfeeding (BrF) line to show that BrFs were generally longer than BoFs. Inserts are from actual tcPO$_2$ recordings. *(From Meier P. Bottle- and breast-feeding: effects on transcutaneous oxygen pressure and temperature in preterm infants. Nurs Res 1988;37:36-41.)*

birth are beyond the scope of this text, but when any of these risk factors is present, counseling, including the topic of infant feeding, should be addressed.

If a preterm delivery is anticipated, focus on ways to overcome the difficulties of initiating breastfeeding and lactation. These difficulties usually include the decision to breastfeed, the need to establish and maintain a milk supply by expressing milk, and concerns about an inadequate milk supply.[47] These difficulties can be minimized by implementing a plan of care based on priorities for counseling during the antepartum period (Box 7-11).

Immediate Postpartum Period

If the preterm birth was not anticipated, some mothers may feel bewildered and even defeated by the birth of an infant who is too weak to suckle or perhaps even too ill to hold. Other mothers may react differently; one study showed that 20% of mothers made the decision to breastfeed because the infant was born preterm. This may be explained by the frequent comment that mothers make, "This is the only thing I can do for my baby."

If the mother has made the decision to breastfeed, she may need some forewarning that breastfeeding might not progress ideally. In cases of extreme prematurity, direct breastfeeding will not be initiated for several weeks. In other cases, direct breastfeeding may be started, but full breastfeeding may not be realistic; supplements may be indicated. Help the mother to reevaluate or modify her choice of feeding method in the context of the infant's capabilities and risk factors. Goals and priorities for the immediate postpartum period are found in Box 7-11.

The preterm newborn should be assessed for his limitations but also, and more importantly, for his capabilities. If the infant is born *after* 35

weeks' gestation, he is technically classified as preterm and may also be low birth weight, but he is likely to have more capabilities than limitations. These infants may require only a little extra assistance or a few special interventions in order to obtain all or nearly all of their nutrition through direct breastfeeding. Many infants who are born *before* 35 weeks' gestation, however, have more limitations that may delay direct breastfeeding, or that may require special techniques and/or technology to meet all of their nutritional needs for survival.

All preterm infants, however, have varying degrees of problems with feeding at the breast. Often problems are minimal, and direct breastfeeding can begin immediately. Sometimes, however, breastfeeding must be delayed; if so, this should be dealt with in a positive way and indirect breastfeeding initiated. Chapter 10 describes many of the difficulties of providing human milk when the infant and mother are separated—which frequently happens with the preterm infant who is critically ill—and presents a plan for making the transition from indirect to direct breastfeeding.

Kangaroo care is a good strategy for preterm infants, especially if they are not breastfeeding directly, because it simulates some of the benefits of direct breastfeeding. Those mothers who feel they are "missing out" on the benefits of breastfeeding may feel comforted to know that the skin-to-skin contact that kangaroo care provides is one of the things that breastfeeding accomplishes. Skin-to-skin contact improves heart rate patterns, sleep-alert periods, and weight gains for preterm infants.[48] Fear that the infant will get cold when not under the warmer can be overcome by breastfeeding or by kangaroo care. Skin-to-skin contact was originally used to compensate for a lack of incubators.[49] Even very-low-birth-weight infants can maintain or even raise their temperatures during skin-to-skin contact with no increase in heat production.[50] Holding the infant skin-to-skin is an effective means to trigger the milk-

Box 7-11
Goals and Priorities for the Preterm Infant

Antepartum Period

- Assist the mother to recognize that breastfeeding is not only possible but optimal for a preterm infant.
- Acknowledge that direct breastfeeding—feeding the newborn directly at the breast—may not be possible at first. If it is not, indirect breastfeeding—expressing milk and giving it through a supplemental device—is an interim strategy.
- Facilitate contact with a local support group, especially one that includes mothers who have successfully breastfed preterm infants. La Leche League can help. Tertiary care centers that handle many preterm births may have established their own support group.
- Collaborate with other members of the health care team, including the registered dietitian, breastfeeding specialist, neonatologist, pediatrician and others to identify strategies and options for supplemental feeding. These should be thought of as options, not necessarily as closed cases.
- Mobilize equipment; be sure that a suitable pump—preferably with a double accessory kit as described in Chapter 10—will be available in the hospital and after discharge.
- Ensure that educational media will be available and accessible at the hospital when the infant is delivered.

Immediate Postpartum Period

- Initiate or reinforce actions listed for the antepartum period.
- Assist the infant who can coordinate suck/swallow/breathe to achieve good positioning and latch-on.
- Provide mother with a list of worrisome signs and a list of phone numbers to call for help.
- Give suggestions to improve milk supply (see Chapter 5).
- Provide a list of pump rental depots and ask the neonatologist to prescribe a pump. Having a prescription may enable the mother to obtain reimbursement from her health insurance company.

Continuation of Breastfeeding

- Bolster the mother's confidence in her ability to provide for her infant.
- Reinforce to the mother her infant's capabilities; suggest strategies that will help him overcome his limitations with suckling.
- Reassure mother that infant is "getting enough."
- Help the mother to understand why the neonatologist has ordered a quota of milliliters of milk that her infant must consume at each feeding; help her to understand that supplementation with fortifier or artificial milk may be necessary to meet this quota.
- Discuss devices, other than bottles, that can be used to supplement the preterm infant (see Chapter 11).
- Determine whether the infant has adequate weight gain by using test-weighing; collaborate with the entire health care team if he does not.
- Be sure that the infant can successfully ingest and retain enough human milk to make adequate weight and length gains. During the first 3 weeks of life, if the infant can successfully ingest and retain about 170 to 200 ml/kg/day, he will be able to achieve the expected intrauterine weight and length gains.[59,60] For a newborn who weighs 2000 g (2 kg), this would be a minimum of 340 ml of milk per day. How many milliliters he ingests can be determined by test-weighing.
- Ensure that the infant gets the hindmilk, since the high fat content of hindmilk is essential for energy needs and brain growth
- Determine whether the mother is developing an adequate supply of milk; initiate interventions if she is not (see Chapter 8). Kangaroo care can be especially helpful in developing an adequate milk supply for preterm infants.[52]
- Advocate for the use of banked donor milk if the mother's milk supply is insufficient to meet the infant's need.
- Anticipate discharge if the infant makes *consistent* weight gains, and if his weight approaches at least 2 kg and if other clinical factors are stable.

POSSIBLE PROBLEMS AND BREASTFEEDING MANAGEMENT FOR PRETERM NEWBORNS

Immaturity of Several Systems	Clinical Problem	Goals and Clinical Strategies	Rationale
Cardiopulmonary	Increased need for oxygen	Conserve oxygen: • Keep baby warm—skin-to-skin contact is effective • Breastfeed; this requires less oxygen than bottle feeding • Respirations >60-70; do not feed infant (per nursery protocol)	Hypothermia burns calories; when calories are spent, oxygen is burned for energy
	Unalert (sleepy) infant attempting to feed	Minimize factors that contribute to sleepy infant at breast: • Plan to breastfeed at baby's peak alert times • Use alerting techniques described in Chapter 6 • Unwrap baby if temperature is stable • Evaluate amount of supplementation infant has had	Stimulation may help infant to suckle successfully
	Baby tires easily when fed	Optimize chances for milk transfer at breast: • Use warm cloth or other techniques to elicit milk-ejection reflex • Offer frequent feedings (i.e., every 2-3 hours) • Limit infant to about 30-40 minutes of actively attempting to breastfeed	Best efforts are usually at beginning of feeding
Neuromuscular/ neuroendocrine (suck/swallow problems)	Poor coordination of suck-swallow reflex	If infant can coordinate suck/swallow, offer the breast rather than bottle	It is no more difficult to suck/swallow at breast than it is at bottle
	Absent or weak suck	Preterm infant may "practice" sucking between feedings Dancer hand is an option but not imperative Consider using a nursing supplementer (see Chapter 12)	
	Difficulty latching on	Make sure baby opens wide; tickle lower lip Decrease overfull nipple if mother is engorged	
	Nipple confusion	Ideally, offer only the breast; this is not always possible Alternatives include gavage, medicine cup, syringe	
Gastrointestinal/nutritional	Increased incidence, longer duration of jaundice	Increase feedings of colostrum	Bilirubin is excreted primarily through the gut, and colostrum acts as a laxative on the gut
	Need for calories, fluids, nutrients to support growth	Increase calories, fluids, and nutrients (see Chapter 11)	Milk fortifier provides nutrients and calories (see Chapter 11).
		Use combination plan: offer direct feeding and express milk for indirect feeding	Direct breastfeeding alone may be inadequate for newborn needs and/or maternal stimulation

ejection reflex, if pumping is the only alternative. Kangaroo care can help ease the transition from indirect to direct breastfeeding. Therefore, skin-to-skin contact should be encouraged if the infant is unable to suckle at the breast; as soon as he is able to feed orally, direct breastfeeding should commence.

Problems and Clinical Management for Direct Breastfeeding

Feeding problems can abound for the preterm infant. A discussion of the altered physiological functions associated with prematurity is beyond the scope of this text, but the reader is encouraged to gain this broader perspective. Preterm infants can and have breastfed successfully, however, and generations of preterm infants will continue to do so. Artificial feeding does not overcome the problems that preterm infants experience. Some feeding challenges exist whether the infant is breastfed or artificially fed.

Special Feeding Challenges (Breast or Bottle)

The preterm infant may begin his life with all his body systems underdeveloped to meet even basic survival needs. (The severity of the problem is directly proportional to the degree of prematurity.) The immaturity of some systems especially affects feeding, regardless of the method, and these, along with challenges to breastfeeding in particular, will be discussed here. Problems listed here are all interrelated, but to avoid repetition, the main problems are arbitrarily identified as alterations in (1) neuromuscular function, (2) neuroendocrine function, (3) cardiopulmonary function, and (4) gastrointestinal function. A summary of problems that affect preterm infants and breastfeeding management strategies is presented in Table 7-10.

Neuromuscular

Table 7-11 describes the normal sequence of motor development in the fetus. When the infant is born before term, therefore, some of the reflexes are not developed. The preterm infant's neuromuscular immaturity results in significant problems related to suckling. Reflexes, including gag, suck, swallow, and coordination of suck and swallow, are often inadequate and interfere with successful breastfeeding. Generalized hypotonia may make it difficult for the infant to maintain good positioning while feeding.

Neuroendocrine

Poor thermoregulation and increased metabolic needs usually result in an increased need for

T A B L E 7-11	
NORMAL SEQUENCE OF FETAL ORAL MOTOR DEVELOPMENT	
Gestational Age	Oral-Facial Reflex
9 weeks	Purposeful oral-buccal movement starts
10-14 weeks	Swallow develops; by the 12th week fluid can be swallowed by most fetuses
18-24 weeks	Suckling begins to appear
24-27 weeks	Gag reflex appears and becomes stronger until 40 weeks; strength diminishes to that of an adult by about 6 months of age
by 25 weeks	Phasic bite reflex and transverse tongue reflex appear
32 weeks	Rooting reflex appears and becomes stronger until 40 weeks; this reflex disappears by 3 months of age

From Dowling D, Danner SC, Coffey P. *Breastfeeding the Infant With Special Needs*. White Plains, NY: March of Dimes Foundation; 1997.

calories and specific components of milk. Hypothermia triggers increased metabolism, resulting in hypoglycemia (i.e., preterm infants are especially vulnerable to hypothermia and/or hypoglycemia). The general intervention is to keep the infant warm; specific strategies are discussed in Chapter 6.

Cardiopulmonary

Immaturity of the lungs makes it difficult or even impossible for the very preterm infant to breathe and suckle at the same time. He tires easily when fed (eating is an infant's only occupation!), but he needs increased calories, fluids, and oxygen. The preterm infant does best in situations where milk is available very early in the feeding. Milk immediately flows from a bottle or mothers can enhance their milk-ejection reflex and hence rapid availability of the milk, by using a few simple interventions. Sometimes it is helpful for the mother to apply warm compresses or to massage by hand just a bit before the infant goes to the breast; this will help her milk-ejection reflex so that the infant can get a more immediate reward for his efforts. The idea is to enhance milk *availability* early in the feeding, but this does not imply that milk *transfer* is more "work."

Gastrointestinal

Smaller stomach capacity, increased levels of bilirubin in the gut, and a lack of enzymes for metabolism all contribute to problems for the preterm newborn. Inadequate oxygenation in the intestinal tract complicates matters further.

Strategies to Promote Suckling

Before considering high-tech interventions, first provide good clinical management. Make sure that the infant has achieved good latch-on. Then make sure he gets the hindmilk. Weight gain improves when the infant consumes the energy-rich hindmilk; therefore, advise parents of its importance and ways to ensure its consumption. Some-

times the preterm infant stays at one breast long enough to get the hindmilk, but then falls asleep before feeding at the other breast. It is preferable, however, that he suckle long enough at one breast and obtain the hindmilk than suckle both breasts and not obtain hindmilk. If the infant does not suckle the breast but receives previously expressed milk, shake the container to mix the hindmilk with the foremilk. Human milk, consumed at the breast, is indeed the ideal source of infant nutrition, but the needs of preterm infants are so great that they are sometimes unable to consume sufficient quantities to support growth and development. In these cases, several helpful interventions can be used (see Chapters 10 and 11).

Infants who can coordinate suck and swallow should be assisted to breastfeed. Most of the strategies that help term infants are also helpful for preterm infants. Additionally, some specific strategies are helpful.

Note Readiness to Breastfeed

Traditionally, preterm infants have been denied access to their mothers' breasts until after they have successfully demonstrated their ability to bottle feed, or until they have attained an arbitrary weight deemed appropriate. However, it is better to base management on physiology rather than on tradition. If the infant can coordinate sucking, swallowing, and breathing, he can go to the breast. Usually, this occurs around 32 weeks' gestation; sometimes it happens a bit earlier.

Note when the infant starts to make sucking motions, because this is an indication of readiness. Suggest to the mother of the preterm infant that she offer her breasts as early and as frequently as possible. Because supply is driven by demand, lactation will be better established with early and frequent suckling. Also, colostrum has a greater percentage of immunoglobulins—which the preterm infant so desperately needs—than mature milk. For this reason, do not discard small

CLINICAL   SCENARIO

Breastfeeding Infants Born Preterm

Baby Megan and Baby Gretchen were born at 35 weeks' gestation. Baby Megan weighed 2245 g at birth, and baby Gretchen weighed 2740 g at birth. These fraternal twins went to the NICU for sepsis workups and were then admitted to the regular nursery at age 2 days. The infants are now about 72 hours old, floppy, and vigorously sucking 60 ml of artificial milk from a bottle at one feeding.

In checking the graph, you see that 10% of infants born at 35 weeks' gestation weigh less than 1750 g. Also, 10% of infants born at 35 weeks weigh more than 3000 g.

How would you classify Baby Megan?

❏ full-term   ❏ average for gestational age
❏ preterm   ❏ small for gestational age
❏ low birth weight   ❏ large for gestational age
❏ very low birth weight

The mother is about 72 hours postpartum and has seen the twins only briefly for one time. She was admitted to the high-risk postpartum floor and is making a steady recovery. She has a history of infertility × 19 years, and desperately wants to breastfeed these infants. What *immediate* priorities do you see?

1.
2.
3.

What problems could you anticipate for these twin girls, and what strategies would you use to overcome the difficulties?

Possible Problems	Strategies

Review your list of immediate priorities. Now, what do you see as critical priorities for discharge?

1.
2.
3.

What other issues might you want to address?
Readers are encouraged to discuss this scenario among their colleagues, since often there is no one right answer.

amounts of colostrum that the mother has expressed.[51]

Move Toward a Demand Feeding Schedule

As the infant moves closer to home discharge, it is best to work toward feeding him on demand. Feeding patterns are influenced by sleep-alert patterns, and those who would rather sleep than eat are managed with feedings every 3-hours rather than on demand. The trick, however, is to establish better sleep-alert patterns. This can often be accomplished through "kangaroo care" (i.e., skin-to-skin contact). Think of kangaroo care as "infant to chest" if "infant to breast" (i.e., suckling) is not feasible. When better sleep-alert patterns emerge, "on-demand" feeding patterns will be more easily established. Another benefit of kangaroo care is that it enhances the mother's milk ejection reflex if she wishes to express milk,[52] and it may help decrease her anxiety about putting her newborn to the breast.

Position Mother and Infant for Best Results

Encourage the mother to use whatever hand position she is comfortable with. Caution her, however, that her finger must not occlude the lactiferous sinuses (see Chapter 5). Sometimes the Dancer hand is helpful (see Figure 7-19), but it is by no means a "recipe" for success. Rather, use whatever means work best under the circumstances to achieve and maintain good latch-on.

Although positioning is important for all newborns in order to achieve milk transfer, good positioning is critical for the preterm infant to achieve transfer.[53] Rather than mandate a certain position for breastfeeding the preterm infant, try positions that provide extra support for the head and torso. The transitional hold and other special holds may be helpful; they are described later in the chapter.

Facilitate Effective Latch-on

All of the principles that are effective in helping the term infant to latch on are important with the preterm infant (see Chapter 5). Some techniques seem to be helpful for the preterm infant. Because of neurological immaturity, the tongue may be hypotonic. Be sure that the preterm infant has his tongue beneath the nipple/areolar complex when he latches on; sometimes his tongue will be on top of the breast, causing him to suck his tongue. If this happens, take the infant off the breast and try again. Help the mother entice him with the nipple until he opens wide with his tongue extended over the lower alveolar ridge, then quickly bring him to the breast, as discussed in Chapter 5.

Evaluate Clinical Management Strategies

It is tempting to assume that interventions are effective without truly evaluating each one. It is critical to evaluate all evidence of whether preterm infants are consuming enough milk. Clinical observation—observing the feeding—is helpful for identifying feeding difficulties and making recommendations about how to make feeding go better. However, clinical observations alone are inadequate for estimating milk intake.[53] Even if the tools described in Chapter 5 are perfected for evaluating term infant feeding behavior, their usefulness cannot be generalized to preterm infants. Weighing infants is essential for determining adequate milk intake in the preterm infant.

Newborns should be weighed every day, at the same time and either nude or with the same amount of clothing. (Typically newborns are weighed nude, while older infants are weighed with clothes; the aim is to be consistent.) Nursery protocols differ, but in general the LBW or VLBW infant should weigh about 1% more than he weighed a day earlier. For example, those who weigh 2000 g should gain 20 g/day. The infant should also make *consistent* weight gains.

Infants can also be test-weighed before and after breastfeeding to determine how much milk they have consumed. One milliliter of milk is approximately equivalent to 1 g of body weight. Most electronic scales are now sophisticated enough to provide valid and reliable data about milk intake during the feeding.[54] Although some clinicians fear that mothers will become anxious about test-weighing the infant, this fear has not been substantiated.[55]

Critical evaluation criteria related to breastfeeding the preterm infant include the following:

- *Weight gain:* during the first month, the LBW preterm infant should consistently gain about 1% of his weight daily.
- *Respiratory status:* No signs of respiratory distress should be noted while feeding.

• *Temperature regulation:* The infant's temperature should be within normal parameters. Adequate intake of milk will provide the calories necessary for thermoregulation. Remember the basic principle that hypothermia and hypoglycemia can and do occur as a cause or effect of one another.

Supplemental Feeding

Ideally, every infant would obtain all his nourishment directly at his mother's breast. Few would dispute the previously described benefits of human milk and breastfeeding for preterm infants, and most would agree that breastfeeding benefits for the infant who is relatively healthy, able to coordinate suck and swallow, and weighs more than 1500 g far outweigh any possible risks.

A more difficult issue, however, is the relative risk and benefit for infants who do not meet these criteria. Considerable controversy exists about whether human milk only is best for the preterm infant. In general, those who are classified as very-low-birth-weight infants require supplementation; those who weigh more than 1500 g (or 1800 g, depending on nursery protocol) may do fine but should be evaluated on a case-by-case basis.

Sometimes direct breastfeeding is impossible or impractical, but indirect breastfeeding is a good alternative. Chapter 10 discusses strategies to provide mother's milk when the mother and her infant are separated. If human milk alone does not completely meet the preterm infant's needs, supplementation will be required. Chapter 11 describes modified mother's milk (human milk fortifiers and hindmilk only), donor milk, and specially designed preterm artificial milk. Chapter 12 discusses devices to administer human milk or artificial milk when needed; readers are referred to these chapters for issues surrounding indirect breastfeeding.

Education, Counseling, and Support

The mother of a preterm infant will feel challenged whether she chooses breastfeeding or artificial feeding. The multiple concerns that are listed in Chapter 4 are magnified many times for the mother of a preterm infant. Like mothers of term infants, however, mothers of preterm infants have concerns about initiating and continuing breastfeeding.

Initiating Breastfeeding: Mother's Concerns

Sometimes mothers are less likely to initiate breastfeeding if their infants are preterm.[56] The woman who made the antepartum decision to breastfeed may feel overwhelmed, defeated, and unconvinced of the efficacy of breastfeeding after a preterm delivery. The hospital staff may have relatively little influence on the mother's choice of feeding method,[57] but the entire health care team must reinforce her decision to breastfeed once it has been made and must address her multiple concerns early on and continuously.

Review the advantages of breastfeeding which the mother identified for the well infant, and help her to see that these advantages are even more important for the vulnerable infant. Highlight the goodness and convenience of breastfeeding, and minimize any references to it being "more work" for infants in special circumstances. Forewarn her that the infant may consume very little at the breast during the first few feedings, and that he needs to practice breastfeeding and will gradually improve. After she reiterates her commitment to initiating breastfeeding, she will need support to continue.

Establishing and Maintaining Milk Supply and Feeding Patterns

Supply and demand are frequently a problem if the preterm infant is too sick, too weak, or separated from the mother. Supply is driven by demand; the preterm infant may be unable or unavailable to provide stimulation to the breasts. Getting the preterm newborn to the breast as soon and as frequently as possible will minimize the problem.

The "demand" cues may be subtle or absent in the sick or preterm infant. Frequently, he needs to be awakened every 3 hours for feedings but suckles after being awakened. As discharge approaches, it is best to work toward a demand pattern, but achievement of this goal may not be realistic in all circumstances. The mother, together with the health care team, needs to be alert to feeding cues but should also establish and follow a plan for feeding frequency when those cues are absent. Frequent feedings, of course, will benefit not only the infant but also the mother's milk supply.

Supply may be a problem when lactation occurs in the absence of the infant. In the early days the mother may be pathologically engorged due to milk stasis; later, she may have a dwindling supply if stimulation has been inadequate. Advise the woman to stimulate her breasts within the first 6 hours after birth with either the infant or the pump, and to continue stimulation as often as the infant would feed (i.e., about every 3 hours). Frequency and duration are less important than the total number of minutes pumping per 24 hours. Advise the woman to pump during the night once if she awakens, but otherwise enjoy a good night's sleep. Ideally, the mother should strive to achieve a minimum of 100 minutes per day pumping during at least five sessions.[58] (See also Chapter 10 for discussion of milk expression and strategies to improve milk supply in the absence of the infant.)

Continuing Breastfeeding

The mother who has begun breastfeeding her preterm infant may have misgivings and lose confidence. Not infrequently, she will be discharged from the hospital before her infant has had an opportunity to breastfeed directly. She needs reassurance that although indirect breastfeeding could provide for the infant's needs indefinitely, it is only a temporary situation. She will need support for her decision to breastfeed, as well as practical advice. Goals and priorities listed in Box 7-4 that address the needs of compromised infants apply to preterm infants as well. Additional goals and priorities for all breastfeeding preterm newborns are found in Box 7-11.

Discharge Planning

While we readily acknowledge that discharge planning starts upon admission, breastfeeding may get lost in the shuffle as survival and respiratory stability become the focus of care for the preterm infant. Teaching and learning objectives have been established for parents of breastfed preterm infants. These are helpful, but they are probably too lengthy to be practical.[61] For effective breastfeeding at home, the discharge planning process for preterm infants should include multidisciplinary involvement and strong links with the community.[62]

After hospital discharge, mothers of *term* infants frequently wonder if they "have enough milk,"[63-65] but mothers of *preterm* infants are more likely to express concerns about whether the infant consumes an adequate volume of milk.[66] This is an important distinction: the former questions what the *mother* has available; the latter questions what the *infant* has consumed. The same mothers also identified composition of the milk and mechanics of breastfeeding as their other most frequent concerns. To deal with their perceived problems, mothers complemented, supplemented, and looked for cues that the infants were "getting enough." Mothers identify the "turning point" as that time when the infant no longer exhibits signs that the mother had considered worrisome; for example, if the infant was previously falling asleep at the breast and is now staying awake, the mother feels reassured that he is "getting enough." Alert the mother to look for these reassuring cues around 36 weeks corrected age. Using this research as a basis for practice, initiate discharge planning as soon and as thoroughly as possible. Priorities for care in discharge planning can be found in Box 7-4.

Conclusions about Breastfeeding Management

Preterm infants can and should be fed human milk. Indirect breastfeeding may be a temporary strategy if the infant has been born very preterm, but a plan should be in place to promote direct breastfeeding that capitalizes on the infant's capabilities and overcomes his limitations. Various strategies can be used to enhance the initial breastfeeding session and to continue direct breastfeeding.

TECHNIQUES FOR DIRECT BREASTFEEDING OF NEWBORNS WITH SPECIAL NEEDS

Some techniques seem to work better than others when breastfeeding the compromised newborn. Frequently, however, the mother must experiment to see what works best for her infant. The most common positions—cradle hold, side-lying hold, or football hold—may work fine and should be encouraged. (See Chapter 5 for complete description.) For compromised infants, other alternatives sometimes need to be explored.

Australian Hold

In the Australian hold the mother lies fairly flat, and the infant squarely faces the breast; a modified Australian hold is shown in Figure 7-16. This

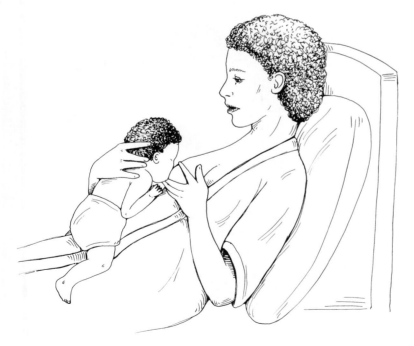

Fig. 7-16 Modified Australian hold.

position is useful for infants with anatomic anomalies—for example, a receding chin, a short tongue, or a tight frenulum. It is also useful if the mother has a milk-ejection reflex that is too fast for the infant to accommodate; for example, the preterm infant may not have reflexes that are quick enough to respond to this sudden rush of milk. The position is also helpful if the mother has a plugged duct; the infant simply needs to be positioned so that the tongue directly "milks" the plugged duct.

Transitional Hold

The transitional hold is known by a variety of other names: modified clutch position, cross-

clutch hold, cross-cradle hold, and across-the-lap hold. It has sometimes been used with preterm infants, as shown in Figure 7-17. This position is not mandatory for the preterm infant, but it should be considered if a horizontal cradle position is not working. The transitional hold allows the mother to have more control of the newborn's head, which is helpful with the preterm infant.

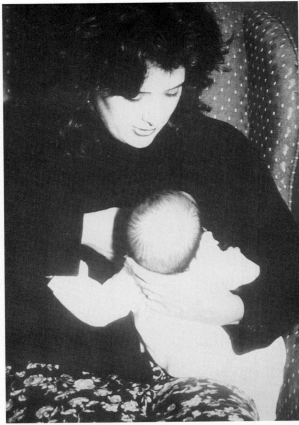

Fig. 7-18 Modified straddle hold. (© *Debi Bocar, Lactation Consultant Services, Oklahoma City, Oklahoma. Used with permission.*)

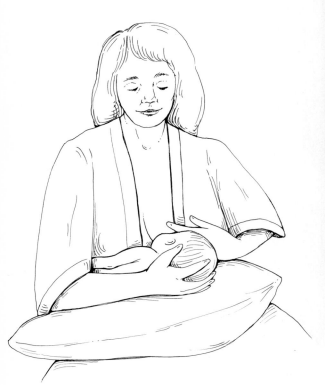

Fig. 7-17 Transitional hold.

Straddle Hold

The straddle hold, with the infant circling the mother's waist, is sometimes helpful for an infant with a bilateral cleft lip. This position, as shown in Figure 7-18, enables him to face the nipple head-on, and he is therefore more likely to get a good seal. A true straddle hold is difficult to accomplish with a newborn, and even more difficult to accomplish if the mother is obese. For newborns, a modified straddle, where the infant more or less "kneels" at the mother's side, is often effective.

Dancer Hand

The Dancer hand, so-named for nurse-midwife Sarah Danner and Dr. Edward Cerutti, is accomplished by having the mother form a "cup" with her hand; she then holds the breast with the lower fingers and the infant's face with her thumb and forefinger, as shown in Figure 7-19. This hold is helpful for the newborn who needs a little extra help getting an adequate seal around the breast. This may include preterm infants or infants with craniofacial defects. Sometimes the infant needs chin support only, as shown in Figure 7-20. This

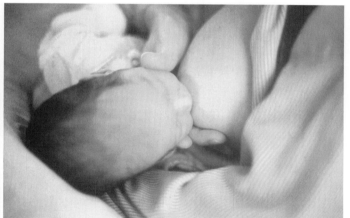

A

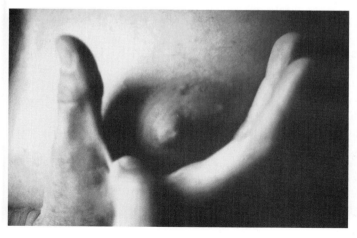

B

Figure 7-19 Dancer hand. **A,** Infant's chin rests in the V web between thumb and forefinger. **B,** The mother's finger is pointing to the place where the infant's chin should rest while breastfeeding. *(Courtesy Sarah Coulter Danner.)*

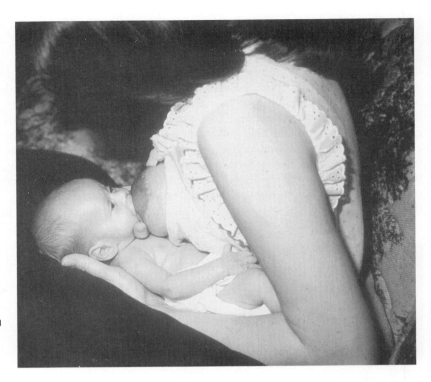

Figure 7-20 The infant's chin is supported by only the index finger. *(Courtesy Sarah Coulter Danner.)*

really is a variation of the Dancer hand. It supports only the chin, rather than the chin and cheeks.

SUMMARY

The newborn must quickly adapt to the extrauterine environment, and the processes used under most circumstances become more necessary but frequently less efficient when the infant has alterations in gastrointestinal, neurological, or cardiorespiratory function. Infants who are born preterm may have multiple alterations, and they will require many special interventions to reach or maintain homeostasis. In many of these cases, however, special techniques can be used to help the infant suckle at the breast, which promotes optimal functioning of all systems. If the infant is unable to suckle, or if breastfeeding must be interrupted for a time, the nurse needs to coordinate communication and clinical strategies to provide human milk and facilitate direct breastfeeding.

References

1. Thibodeau GA, Patton KT. *Anatomy and Physiology.* 3rd ed. St. Louis: Mosby; 1996.

2. Lawrence RA. *Breastfeeding: A Guide for the Medical Profession.* 4th ed. St. Louis: Mosby; 1994.

3. American Academy of Pediatrics Work Group on Breastfeeding. Breastfeeding and the use of human milk. *Pediatrics* 1997;100:1035-1039.

4. Wong DL. *Whaley and Wong's Nursing Care of Infants and Children.* 5th ed. St. Louis: Mosby; 1995.

5. Lucas A, Cole TJ. Breast milk and neonatal necrotising enterocolitis. *Lancet* 1990;336:1519-1523.

6. Foman SJ, Nelson SE. Size and growth. In: Foman SJ, ed. *Nutrition of Normal Infants*. St. Louis: Mosby; 1993:36-84.

7. Frantz KB, Fleiss PM, Lawrence RA. Management of the slow-gaining breastfed baby. *Keeping Abreast* 1978;3:287.

8. Frantz KB. The slow-gaining breastfeeding infant. *NAACOGS Clin Issu Perinat Womens Health Nurs* 1992;3:647-655.

9. Marino BL, O'Brien P, LoRe H. Oxygen saturations during breast and bottle feedings in infants with congenital heart disease. *J Pediatr Nurs* 1995;10:360-364.

10. Bier JB, Ferguson A, Anderson L, et al. Breastfeeding of very low birth weight infants. *J Pediatr* 1993;123:773-778.

11. Meier P. Bottle- and breast-feeding: effects on transcutaneous oxygen pressure and temperature in preterm infants. *Nurs Res* 1988;37:36-41.

12. Rossiter JP, Callan NA. Prenatal diagnosis of congenital heart disease. *Obstet Gynecol Clin North Am* 1993;20:485-496.

13. Behrman RE, Kliegman RM, Arvin AM, eds. *Nelson Textbook of Pediatrics*. 15th ed. Philadelphia: Saunders; 1996.

14. Oehler JM. *Family-Centered Neonatal Nursing Care*. Philadelphia: Lippincott; 1981.

15. McBride MC, Danner SC. Sucking disorders in neurologically impaired infants: assessment and facilitation of breastfeeding. *Clin Perinatol* 1987;14:109-130.

16. Danner SC. Breastfeeding the neurologically impaired infant. *NAACOGS Clin Issu Perinat Womens Health Nurs* 1992;3:640-646.

17. Cronk C, Crocker AC, Pueschel SM. Growth charts for children with Down syndrome: 1 month to 18 years of age. *Pediatrics* 1988;81:102-110.

18. Cleft Palate Foundation. Personal communication with Cleft Palate Foundation, 1998.

19. Paradise JL, Elster BA, Tan L. Evidence in infants with cleft palate that breast milk protects against otitis media. *Pediatrics* 1994;94(6, pt 1):853-860.

20. Cleft Palate Foundation. *The Genetics of Cleft Lip and Palate*. Pittsburgh: Cleft Palate Foundation; 1987.

21. Moss AL, Jones K, Pigott RW. Submucous cleft palate in the differential diagnosis of feeding difficulties. *Arch Dis Child* 1990;65:182-184.

22. Clarren SK, Anderson B, Wolf LS. Feeding infants with cleft lip, cleft palate, or cleft lip and palate. *Cleft Palate J* 1987;24:244-249.

23. Lynch MC. Congenital defects: parental issues and nursing supports. *J Perinat Neonatal Gynecol Nursing* 1989;2:53-59.

24. Styer GW, Freeh K. Feeding infants with cleft lip and/or palate. *J Obstet Gynecol Neonatal Nurs* 1981;10:329-332.

25. Danner SC. Breastfeeding the infant with a cleft defect. *NAACOGS Clin Issu Perinat Womens Health Nurs* 1992;3:634-639.

26. Avedian LV, Ruberg RI. Impaired weight gain in cleft palate infants. *Cleft Palate J* 1980;17:24-26.

27. Brine EA, Rickard KA, Liechty EA, Manatunga A, Sadove M, Bull MJ. Effectiveness of two feeding methods in improving energy intake and growth of infants with cleft palate: a randomized study. *J Am Diet Assoc* 1994;94:732-738.

28. Lang S, Lawrence CJ, Orme RL. Cup feeding: an alternative method of infant feeding. *Arch Dis Child* 1994;71:365-369.

29. Curtin G. The infant with a cleft lip or palate: more than a surgical problem. *J Perinat Neonat Nurs* 1990;3:80-89.

30. Weatherley-White RCA, Kuehn DP, Mirrett P, Gilman JI, Weatherley-White CC. Early repair and breast-feeding for infants with cleft lip. *Plast Reconstr Surg* 1987;79:879-887.

31. Fisher JC. Early repair and breastfeeding for infants with cleft lip. *Plas Reconstr Surg* 1987;79:886.

32. Fisher JC. Feeding children who have cleft lip or palate. *West J Med* 1991;154:207.

33. Jigjinni V, Kangesu T. Do babies require arm splints after cleft palate repair? *Br J Plast Surg* 1993;46:681-685.

34. American Academy of Pediatrics and the American College of Obstetricians and Gynecologists. *Guidelines for Perinatal Care*. 4th ed. Elk Grove Village, IL: American Academy of Pediatrics; 1997.

35. United States Bureau of Statistics. *Monthly Vital Statistics Report*. 1998;46(11):2.

36. Schanler RJ. Suitability of human milk for the low-birthweight infant. *Clin Perinatol* 1995; 22:207-222.

37. Anderson DM, Williams FH, Merkatz RB, Schulman PK, Kerr DS, Pittard WB III. Length of gestation and nutritional composition of human milk. *Am J Clin Nutr* 1983;37:810-814.

38. Schanler RJ, Tsang RC. Special methods in feeding the preterm infant. In: Tsang RC, Nichols BL, eds. *Nutrition During Infancy*. Philadelphia: Hanley and Belfus; 1988.

39. Tsang RC, Nichols BL. *Nutrition During Infancy*. Philadelphia: Hanley and Belfus; 1988.

40. Quinlan PT, Lockton S, Irwin J, Lucas AL. The relationship between stool hardness and stool composition in breast- and formula-fed infants. *J Pediatr Gastroenterol Nutr* 1995;20:81-90.

41. Straussberg R, Sirota L, Hart J, Amir Y, Djaldetti M, Bessler H. Phagocytosis-promoting factor in human colostrum. *Biol Neonate* 1995;68:15-18.

42. Uauy R, De Andraca I. Human milk and breast feeding for optimal mental development. *J Nutr* 1995;125(suppl 8):2278S-2280S.

43. Lucas A, Morley R, Cole TJ, Lister G, Leeson Payne C. Breast milk and subsequent intelligence quotient in children born preterm. *Lancet* 1992;339:261-264.

44. Hoffman J. Congenital heart disease: incidence and inheritance. *Pediatr Clin North Am* 1990; 37:25-43.

45. Meier P, Anderson GC. Responses of small preterm infants to bottle- and breast-feeding. *Am J Matern Child Nurs* 1987;12:97-105.

46. Klaus MH, Kennell JH. *Parent-Infant Bonding*. 2nd ed. St. Louis: Mosby; 1982.

47. Dowling D, Danner SC, Coffey P. *Breastfeeding the Infant with Special Needs*. White Plains, NY: March of Dimes Foundation; 1997.

48. Anderson GC. Current knowledge about skin-to-skin (kangaroo) care for preterm infants. *J Perinatol* 1991;11:216-226.

49. Whitelaw A, Sleath K. Myth of the marsupial mother: home care of very low birth weight babies in Bogota, Colombia. *Lancet* 1985;1:1206-1208.

50. Bauer K, Uhrig C, Sperling P, Pasel K, Weiland C, Versmold HT. Body temperatures and oxygen consumption during skin-to-skin (kangaroo) care in stable preterm infants weighing less than 1500 grams. *J Pediatr* 1997;130:240-244.

51. Mathur NB, Dwarkadas AM, Sharma VK, Saha K, Jain N. Anti-infective factors in preterm human colostrum. *Acta Paediatr Scand* 1990;79:1039-1044.

52. Hurst NM, Valentine CJ, Renfro L, Burns P, Ferlic L. Skin-to-skin holding in the neonatal intensive care unit influences maternal milk volume. *J Perinatol* 1997;17:213-217.

53. Meier PP, Brown LP. State of the science; breastfeeding for mothers and low birth weight infants. *Nurs Clin North Am* 1996;31:351-365.

54. Meier PP, Lysakowski TY, Engstrom JL, Kavanaugh KL, Mangurten HH. The accuracy of test weighing for preterm infants. *J Pediatr Gastroenterol Nutr* 1990;10:62-65.

55. Meier PP, Engstrom JL, Crichton CL, Clark DR, Williams MM, Mangurten HH. A new scale for in-home test-weighing for mothers of preterm and high risk infants. *J Hum Lact* 1994;10:163-168.

56. Ellerbee SM, Atterbury J, West J. Infant feeding patterns at a tertiary-care hospital. *J Perinat Neonatal Nurs* 1993;6:45-55.

57. Lucas A, Cole TJ, Morley R, et al. Factors associated with maternal choice to provide breast milk for low birthweight infants. *Arch Dis Child* 1988;63:48-52.

58. Hopkinson JM, Schanler RJ, Garza C. Milk production by mothers of premature infants. *Pediatrics* 1988;81:815-820.

59. Whyte RK, Haslam R, Vlainic C, et al. Energy balance and nitrogen balance in growing low birthweight infants fed human milk or formula. *Pediatr Res* 1983;17:891-898.

60. Chessex P, Reichman B, Verellen G, et al. Quality of growth in premature infants fed their own mothers' milk. *J Pediatr* 1983;102(1):107-112.

61. New York State Department of Health Breastfeeding Advisory Council. *Infant Feeding Education in the Hospital: A Resource Kit for Health Care Professionals.* Albany: New York State Department of Health Bureau of Child and Adolescent Health; 1994.

62. Biancuzzo M. *Breastfeeding the Healthy Newborn: A Nursing Perspective.* White Plains, NY: March of Dimes Birth Defects Foundation; 1994.

63. Chapman JJ, Macey MJ, Keegan M, Borum P, Bennett S. Concerns of breast-feeding mothers from birth to 4 months. *Nurs Res* 1985;34:374-377.

64. Kearney MH, Cronenwett LR, Barrett JA. Breastfeeding problems in the first week postpartum. *Nurs Res* 1990;39:90-95.

65. Mogan J. A study of mothers' breastfeeding concerns. *Birth* 1986;13:104-108.

66. Kavanaugh K, Mead L, Meier P, Mangurten HH. Getting enough: mothers' concerns about breastfeeding a preterm infant after discharge. *J Obstet Gynecol Neonatal Nurs* 1995;24:23-32.

8

Maternal Physical Assessment and Counseling

NORMAL PARAMETERS

Brief Review of Breast Structure

The breast consists of glandular, muscular, connective, and adipose tissue. The glandular tissue has 15 to 20 lobes, 20 to 24 lobules, and a complete ductal system. The breasts lie over the pectoral muscles (pectoralis major, pectoralis minor) and other muscles (serratus anterior, latissimus dorsi, subscapularis, external oblique, rectus abdominus). The mammary artery and the lateral thoracic artery provide most of the breast's vascular supply. Nerve supply is cutaneous (from the supraclavicular branches of the cervical plexus and the lateral perforating branches of the second, third, fourth, and fifth intercostal nerves) and deep (from branches of the fourth, fifth, and sixth intercostal nerves). The breasts are generally discussed according to quadrants (upper outer, upper inner, lower outer, lower inner); the tail of Spence is an extension of the upper outer quadrant, as shown in Figure 8-1.

Brief Review of Breast: Four Stages of Mammary Function

The breast undergoes four stages of mammary function: mammogenesis, lactogenesis, lactation, and involution. A more complete discussion is in Chapter 3. This brief review aims to provide background for the physical assessment of the

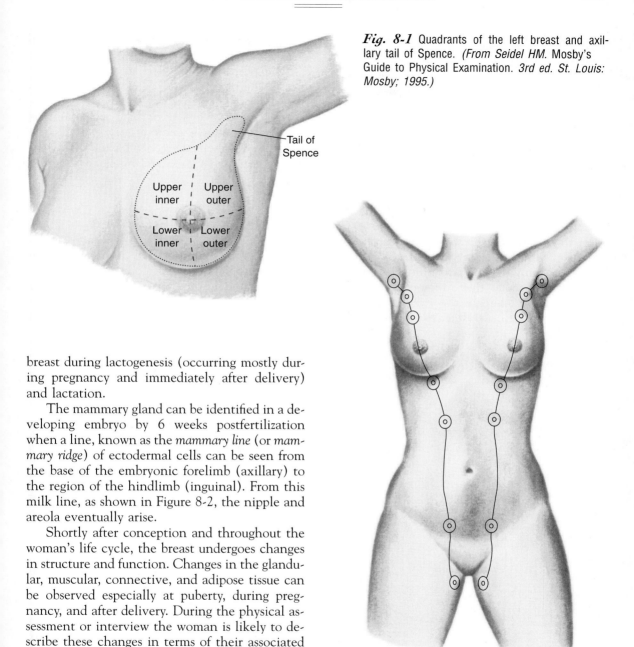

Fig. 8-1 Quadrants of the left breast and axillary tail of Spence. *(From Seidel HM.* Mosby's Guide to Physical Examination. *3rd ed. St. Louis: Mosby; 1995.)*

breast during lactogenesis (occurring mostly during pregnancy and immediately after delivery) and lactation.

The mammary gland can be identified in a developing embryo by 6 weeks postfertilization when a line, known as the *mammary line* (or *mammary ridge*) of ectodermal cells can be seen from the base of the embryonic forelimb (axillary) to the region of the hindlimb (inguinal). From this milk line, as shown in Figure 8-2, the nipple and areola eventually arise.

Shortly after conception and throughout the woman's life cycle, the breast undergoes changes in structure and function. Changes in the glandular, muscular, connective, and adipose tissue can be observed especially at puberty, during pregnancy, and after delivery. During the physical assessment or interview the woman is likely to describe these changes in terms of their associated discomforts. Talking with her provides an opportunity to reassure her of how these normal changes enable her to provide nourishment for her infant.

Fig. 8-2 Milk lines. *(From Thompson JM, McFarland GK, Hirsch JE, Tucker SM.* Mosby's Clinical Nursing. *4th ed. St. Louis: Mosby; 1997.)*

ASSESSMENT OF THE BREASTS AND NIPPLES

The discussion in this chapter is limited to those points that are most pertinent to the pregnant or lactating breast. It should be understood, however, that anything that can happen to a nongravid or nonlactating woman can also happen during pregnancy and lactation. Therefore, do not dismiss potentially pathological findings as a harmless change associated with lactation. Help the woman to become aware of how her breasts feel prior to lactation—and preferably prior to pregnancy—so that she can better identify pathological clues later. Teach or reinforce the technique for performing breast self-examination, since the hormones associated with pregnancy increase the risk for proliferation of malignant cells. Refer the woman to her physician or primary care provider for any suspicious findings.

The purpose of physical assessment of the breasts during pregnancy and lactation is to obtain information that will enhance the breast-feeding process. Inspection and palpation, as well as obtaining a good history, provide the basis for data about the general skin, areola and areolar skin, and nipple and nipple skin of the breast.

Assessment of Corpus Mammae

Early in the first trimester, hormones cause the ductular and lobular structures to begin proliferating, and the gravida may report swelling and tenderness in her breasts. As mammogenesis progresses internally, the external changes

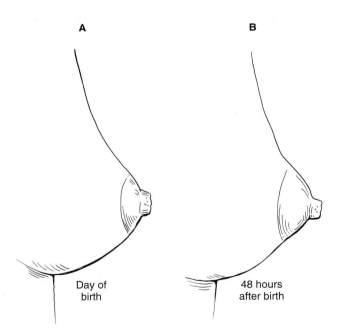

A   **B**

Day of birth   48 hours after birth

Fig. 8-3 Breast and nipple changes as lactation is established. **A,** Day of birth. **B,** 48 hours after birth.

Shape

Breasts can be described as having one of four different contours: conical, convex, pendulous, or large pendulous. These shapes remain largely unchanged during pregnancy and lactation, and the shape of the breast usually has no impact on the ability to breastfeed. These shapes are shown in Figure 8-4. The conical breasts are approximately equivalent to what some refer to as "tubular" breasts, although the latter is more extreme. Women with tubular breasts may be unable to fully lactate.[1]

Symmetry

The breasts should be more or less symmetrical, although the left breast is often slightly larger than the right. During pregnancy, however, note any marked asymmetry, since this may indicate that the glandular tissue is not proliferating properly. Refer the woman to her physician, but reassure her that even if one breast is not capable of fully lactating, unilateral breastfeeding is a possible option. Breasts that are symmetrical during pregnancy but asymmetrical during lactation suggest that the infant suckles more frequently or more efficiently on one side than the other. This is usually harmless, assuming that the infant is getting enough milk. Reassure the mother that this is common because infants frequently have a favorite side.

Assessment of General Skin

Appearance, Color, and Pigmentation

The skin should appear smooth, soft, and intact. During pregnancy, striae gravidarum (stretch marks) appear in various places throughout the body and may be especially noticeable at the outer aspects of the breasts. These are the result of stretching of the tissue and may be unsightly,

but they have no effect on breastfeeding. Note any lack of smoothness in the skin or any extraneous structures, such as supernumerary nipples, as shown in Figure 8-5. These appear as raised bumps anywhere along the milk line. They may secrete milk during lactation but will not interfere with breastfeeding. Upon palpation, the skin of the lactating breast should feel warm but not hot, and somewhat firm but not hard.

The skin should appear about the same color as the rest of the torso, and the color of the two breasts should be the same. During the postpartum period, any red streaking is a worrisome sign and requires follow up. Discoloration—usually ecchymotic areas—is the result of bruising, most probably from improper use of a breast pump or other equipment.

Antepartally, note any scarring around the areolae and determine the extent and origin of the scar. It is fairly common for women of childbearing age to have had previous breast surgery, but prior surgery does not necessarily preclude breastfeeding. Question the gravida about her history and retrieve previous medical records if further information is needed.

Scars caused by burns of the breast are a concern, as much from a psychological standpoint as from a milk synthesis standpoint. Even if the woman has come to terms with her body image, her self-confidence related to breastfeeding may be diminished. Reassure her that, in most cases, breastfeeding is possible after third-degree burns because the damage most often affects only the skin, not the glandular tissue beneath it. See the Clinical Scenario, which describes a case study.

Texture and Tautness

During the antepartum period, note the skin for texture and tautness. Inelastic skin, more likely to be noted in the primigravida, is tight and not easily picked up by the examiner's fingers. Elastic

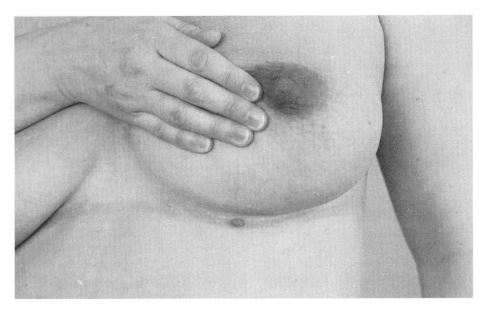

Fig. 8-5 Supernumerary nipple. *(From Seidel HM et al. Mosby's Guide to Physical Examination. 3rd ed. St. Louis: Mosby; 1995.)*

breast tissue, more common in the multigravida due to stretching from the previous pregnancy, is looser. If the breast tissue is inelastic antepartally, the woman is at greater risk for postpartum engorgement.[2] Instruct her to gently massage her breasts prenatally, which may help the skin to become less taut. Document the findings; these data will alert the postpartum clinician to be aware of the increased risk for engorgement. During the postpartum period, palpate for tautness also. Very taut and shiny skin suggests engorgement or infection. Other signs and symptoms of these conditions are discussed in the following.

Vascularity

Vascular changes are significant. During a single-ton pregnancy, total body blood volume increases by about 45%, and the richer supply available to the breasts dilates the vessels beneath the skin. Venous congestion may be more obvious in primigravidas. As pregnancy progresses, the general skin will appear very thin, and veins will be quite visible just beneath the skin.

Lesions

Various primary and secondary lesions may be present on the breast. Naming these lesions is somewhat unimportant unless the examiner is confident of well-honed physical assessment skills. It is more important to completely and accurately describe pertinent objective data about the lesion and to communicate that information to the physician or other primary health care provider. Note the location and distribution, color, pattern, edges, contour (flat, raised, or sunken), size, whether or not

CLINICAL SCENARIO

Mother with Third-Degree Burns

Mrs. X. age 28, gravida 1, para 1, had a spontaneous delivery of a full-term, appropriate-for-gestational age male. She was about 36 hours postpartum when I first encountered her. It was nighttime, but she was wide awake and appeared uneasy. I established rapport with her and asked what was keeping her awake.

She said that she longed to breastfeed but felt this was not a realistic option for her. When she was 7 years old, she had suffered third-degree burns from her neck to her knees. She had had multiple skin grafts over the years. Despite the extensive trauma, she seemed to have a positive self-image, and she displayed self-confidence.

She had put the infant to the breast several times, but nothing seemed to happen. She felt discouraged and was more or less resigned to the fact that this was just one more loss she would have to experience. We talked for a while about her feelings about breastfeeding, her feelings about her breasts, her relationship with her husband, and her infant's natural urge to suckle. I promised her nothing but asked to see her breasts.

The skin had the coarse, irregular appearance that typically follows severe burns. The nipples were small, but present and slightly everted. Upon palpation, it appeared that her breasts were beginning to fill with milk. We waited until the infant was hungry, and put him to the breast. Happily, the greatest impediment to breastfeeding was that she had not been taught how to latch the infant onto the breast. We were able to quickly overcome this problem, and the infant suckled until he was content. We could hear the infant swallowing. She was thrilled with the progress.

I had the great pleasure of caring for this woman a few years later when she delivered her second child. She reported that she had fed the first infant for more than 6 months and felt confident that she could nurse the new one as well.

the skin over the lesion is intact, and other characteristics (such as whether the lesion is hard, soft, or fluid-filled).[3] Thompson and Wilson identify and describe the various types of lesions on Table 8-1; some examples that are relevant for the lactating mother have been added. Some of these lesions may affect breastfeeding and will be discussed throughout the text.

Assessment of Areola and Areolar Skin

Appearance, Color, and Pigmentation

The areola should be centered on the breast. Hair on the areola is normal and harmless; absence of hair suggests that the mother may have been pulling it out, and this is a potential infection hazard.

The color of the areola varies according to the color of the woman's skin. Normally, however, the areola is somewhat lighter in color than the nipple, and it becomes more pigmented during pregnancy and lactation. During the postpartum period, the color of the areola should be only slightly lighter than the color of the nipple; a more marked difference commonly occurs when a fungal infection is present.

Size, Shape, and Symmetry

The areolae surround the nipples, and each should be the same in size and symmetry. During pregnancy, the areola increases in diameter from about 34 to 50 mm. The Montgomery's glands also become more prominent during pregnancy.

PRIMARY AND SECONDARY SKIN LESIONS

	Skin Lesion	Description	Example in Breast or Nipple Skin
Primary	Macule	A flat, circumscribed area that is a change in the color of the skin; less than 1 cm in diameter	Freckles, flat moles, petechiae, measles
	Papule	An elevated, firm, circumscribed area less than 1 cm in diameter	Wart
	Patch	A flat, nonpalpable, irregular-shaped macule more than 1 cm in diameter	Port-wine stains
	Plaque	Elevated, firm, and rough lesion with flat top surface greater than 1 cm in diameter	Usually candidiasis during lactation; other examples include psoriasis or seborrheic keratoses
	Wheal	Elevated, irregular-shaped area of cutaneous edema; solid transient; variable diameter	Allergic reaction; during lactation, most frequent cause is allergies to creams and ointment applied to the nipple/areola, especially lanolin
	Nodule	Elevated, firm, circumscribed lesion; deeper in dermis than a papule; 1-2 cm in diameter	
	Tumor	Elevated and solid lesion; may or may not be clearly demarcated; deeper in dermis; greater than 2 cm in diameter	Neoplasms, benign tumor, lipoma, hemangioma
	Vesicle	Elevated, circumscribed, superficial; not into dermis; filled with serous fluid; less than 1 cm in diameter	Varicella (chicken pox), herpes zoster
	Bulla	Vesicle greater than 1 cm in diameter	Sucking blister, sometimes found on nipple due poor latch-on
	Pustule	Elevated, superficial lesion; similar to a vesicle but filled with purulent fluid	Impetigo
	Cyst	Elevated, circumscribed, encapsulated lesion; in dermis or subcutaneous layer; filled with liquid or semisolid material	Galactocele
	Telangiectasia	Fine, irregular red lines produced by capillary dilation	Telangiectasia in rosacea (unlikely to be on breast, but possible)
Secondary	Scale	Heaped-up keratinized cells; flaky skin; irregular; thick or thin; dry or oily; variation in size	Flaking of skin following a drug reaction, or simply dry skin; eczema
	Lichenification	Rough, thickened epidermis secondary to persistent rubbing, itching, or skin irritation; often involves flexor surface of the extremity	Inflammatory response when allergic to products, such as lanolin cream; may also be due to rubbing breasts vigorously with wash cloth in an attempt to "prepare" the breasts
	Keloid	Irregular-shaped, elevated, progressively enlarging scar; grows beyond the boundaries of the wound; caused by excessive collagen formation during healing	Keloid formation following surgery; this is sometimes seen after reduction surgery on the breast and is more common in African-American and Asian women than in Caucasian women
	Scar	Thin to thick fibrous tissue that replaces normal skin following injury or laceration to the dermis	Healed wound or surgical incision; may be noted after breast surgery
	Excoriation	Loss of the epidermis; linear, hollowed-out crusted area	Abrasion or scratch; may also be result of improper use of a breast pump and is frequently accompanied by bruising
	Fissure	Linear crack or break from the epidermis to the dermis; may be moist or dry	Linear cracks in the nipple skin, usually due to poor positioning; white compression stripe on nipple is the first sign of a fissure
	Erosion	Loss of part of the epidermis; depressed, moist, glistening; follows rupture of a vesicle or bulla	Varicella, variola after rupture
	Abrasion	Friction that results in a rubbing away of the skin's surface	Rubbing nipple skin vigorously in an attempt to "prepare" the nipples
	Ulcer	Loss of epidermis and dermis; concave, varies in size	Tissue that is damaged; usually this is on the nipple as a result of poor latch-on; similar to fissures (ulcers are round); breast abscess is a type of ulcer

Adapted from Thompson J, Wilson S. *Health Assessment for Nursing Practice*. St. Louis: Mosby; 1996.

Assessment of Nipple and Nipple Skin

Appearance, Color, and Pigmentation

During pregnancy and lactation, nipples become more erectile due to the influence of hormones. Sebaceous glands keep the nipple lubricated, and the protective oils should therefore be preserved. Dissuade the woman from using soap, alcohol, or other products that have a drying effect on the areolar and nipple tissue.[4] Rinsing the nipples in the shower will suffice.

Color

The nipple should be only slightly darker than the areola, and it should be even in color. In the breastfeeding woman, make note if there is a white stripe, either vertical or horizontal; this compression stripe signals a poor latch-on. (See Chapter 5 for discussion of proper latch-on and later section of this chapter for discussion of "sore nipples.")

Lesions

All sorts of lesions may be present on the nipples or skin of the breast, as summarized in Table 8-1. During lactation, however, it is especially important to look for discoloration—the first warning sign of impending nipple skin breakdown—and cracks in the nipple. See discussion of sore nipples later in this chapter.

Size and Shape

Several nipple variations do exist, but they usually have little or no effect on breastfeeding. These include especially small nipples, large or elongated nipples, flat nipples, or other variations. Note and document these observations in the record, but remain optimistic that these variations will require little or no special management techniques postpartally. It is possible for women to breastfeed with nipples of various sizes and shapes.

Small or Flat Nipples

Flat nipples are neither well everted nor inverted. Generally, flat nipples have no impact at all on breastfeeding. The infant himself is likely to exert enough negative pressure so that the nipple is everted in his mouth and so that the nipple can be elongated and a teat formed when suckling. Similarly, flat nipples are usually best managed by putting the infant to the breast. Sometimes, it may be helpful to suggest the scissors hold, since this does help the nipple to protrude somewhat. Manual expression of a few drops may help the nipple to become more prominent. If these corrective actions are not enough, consider pumps or other devices to better evert the nipples (see next section). Small nipples are generally not a problem and can be managed using the same techniques described for flat nipples.

Large or Elongated Nipples

Like small or flat nipples, large or elongated nipples pose little or no problem for breastfeeding. Occasionally, a mother with very large or long nipples tries to suckle an infant with a very small mouth, and the infant may be somewhat overwhelmed by the amount of tissue. Encourage the infant to open wide because he may be tempted to latch on only to the nipple.

Symmetry

The nipple should be located in the center of the areola. Occasionally, it is not, but this is unlikely to hamper breastfeeding efforts. It does require a little more care in helping the infant latch on because the visual illusion may tempt the mother to center the areola, not the nipple. The nipple should always be centered in the infant's mouth when breastfeeding.

Discharge and Secretions

There is a clear difference between "nipple discharge" and "nipple secretions." Lawrence states,

"A discharge from the nipple is defined as fluid that escapes spontaneously. A secretion, on the other hand, is fluid present in the ducts that must be collected by nipple aspiration or by other means such as conventional breast pump or gentle massage and expression from the ducts."[2]

Discharges can be milky (e.g., galactorrhea), multicolored and sticky, purulent, watery, serous, or serosanguineous.[2] Galactorrhea is a condition where milk escapes from the nipples in a nonlactating woman. Some discharges may be worrisome and require follow-up. The focus of this text, however, is on the lactating breast, which secretes milk.

During pregnancy and lactation, there may be a bloody discharge from the nipple, which usually is harmless. In some cases, however, immediate medical follow-up is indicated. Table 8-2 shows pertinent assessment points to distinguish when the patient can be watched and reassured, and when immediate medical attention is indicated.

During pregnancy, *precolostrum*, a thin, clear, viscous fluid, is present and may be expressed from the nipples between 6 and 16 weeks' gestation. As the pregnancy progresses, the fluid thickens and becomes yellowish white. *Colostrum* can be expressed during the second and third trimester or may spontaneously leak in the multigravida. Production of colostrum continues until it is gradually replaced by transitional milk during the first week postpartum.

Occasionally, mothers secrete milk with various tints. Sometimes milk will have a red-orange tint, called a "rusty-pipe" appearance. The reason for this is unclear, but it appears to be the result of the increased vascularity and is harmless. Milk can have a green tint after the mother has consumed a large amount of green vegetables. In one reported case, milk was black, presumably due to the patient's minocycline therapy.[5] The various tints that have been identified in milk are harmless. Infants probably consume this colored milk more often than we realize, but it is most evident when the mother is expressing and saving her milk.

T A B L E 8-2
BLOODY DISCHARGE DURING PREGNANCY AND LACTATION

Physical Assessment Finding	Possible Explanation/Alteration During Pregnancy and/or Lactation	Clinical Implications
Bloody nipple discharge	During pregnancy, may be due to increased vascularity and epithelial proliferation; typically bilateral and not confined to a single duct	Ominous when woman is not pregnant or lactating; may be physiological during pregnancy and lactation
		Reassure mother that bloody discharge is not harmful to the infant
	During lactation, may be due to poor latch-on; typically accompanied by visible signs of trauma to the nipples; this typically resolves within the week	Persistent bloody nipple discharge, especially if from a single duct, requires further evaluation
Bloody nipple discharge and a breast mass	When both are present, this is an ominous sign	Prepare woman for mammography
		Galactography, used to localize the abnormality to assist with excision, has not been used during pregnancy and lactation

Source: Berens P, Newton ER. Breast masses during lactation and the role of the obstetrician in breastfeeding. *ABM News and Views* 1997;3(2):4-6.

Protractility

Visual inspection of the nipple is not enough to determine adequacy for breastfeeding; palpation is essential. To properly palpate, compress the nipple/areola between the thumb and forefinger, as shown in Figure 8-6. Normally, nipples should be well everted, which means that when the base of the nipple is compressed between the thumb

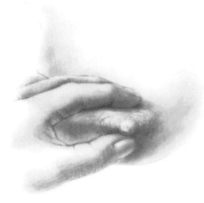

Fig. 8-6 Normal nipple everts with gentle pressure. *(From Lawrence RA.* Breastfeeding: A Guide for the Medical Profession. *4th ed. St. Louis, Mosby; 1994.)*

and forefinger, it will protrude. With inspection only, some nipples may appear everted, but compression may reveal that the nipples will retract; these are inverted nipples.

Inverted Nipples
DEFINITION, DESCRIPTION, AND ETIOLOGY

Inverted nipples are those that do not evert with gentle compression. During fetal development, the woman's nipple is formed. Usually the lactiferous ducts open into a shallow depression called the *mammary pit.* From this pit, cells proliferate to form the nipple and the areola, and the pit elevates. When the cells proliferate but do not elevate, the nipple fibers become "tied" and the nipple is inverted; this is also called an *invaginated nipple,* as shown in Figure 8-7. Plastic surgeons report that patients with invaginated nipples have been known to breastfeed, although the duration or success of the experience has not been described. Apparently, however, the degree of nipple inversion and the strength of the infant's suck determine whether breastfeeding is possible. These researchers have stated that "there is no way to predict whether a woman with invaginated nipples will be able to breastfeed or not."[6]

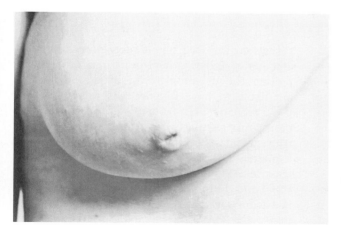

Fig. 8-7 Simple nipple inversion with lifetime history. *(From Seidel HM et al.* Mosby's Guide to Physical Examination. *3rd ed. St. Louis: Mosby; 1995.)*

Box 8-1
Do's and Don'ts for Managing Inverted, Pseudoinverted Nipples

Do	*Don't*
• Tickle the baby's lip (with either finger or breast) until the infant opens *wide*. Look carefully; the infant can almost always open wider! This is probably the *most important* intervention for helping the infant to latch on to an inverted or pseudoinverted nipple.	• Allow the infant to latch on in increments (i.e., have his mouth only partly open, then gradually take more of the tissue into his mouth). This will only make the mother's nipple sore.
• Suggest that the infant breastfeed on the inverted side first. Infants are more hungry when they first go to the breast and may be more likely to take whatever is offered. After a few days, the nipple is frequently less inverted or less dimpled.	• Use a syringe to "pull out" the nipple. This technique was reported anecdotally,[19] but it has no basis in scientific research. The worst case of sore nipples I have ever seen was created using this technique.
• Assist the mother to roll her nipple and gently pull it out before offering the infant the breast.	• Recommend Hoffman's technique. This technique, which manipulates the nipple vertically and horizontally, has never been proved (by anyone except Hoffman, several decades ago) to be effective. One study showed that it was clearly ineffective.This technique may damage nipple tissue, making the overall breastfeeding experience even more difficult.
• Help the mother to hold her nipple so that it protrudes. Sometimes, a scissors hold (rather than a C-hold) is all that is needed to accomplish this.	
• Try any "tricks" to entice the infant to suckle. For example, express a little colostrum onto the nipple so that the infant can taste it first.	• Use ice to get the nipple to protrude. Admittedly, ice will indeed cause the nipple to protrude, but it causes another problem, too. Ice interferes with the signals to the brain that create the milk-ejection reflex. If the woman is engorged, ice may be applied to relieve *breast distention after* the feeding but should never be applied to *nipples before* feeding.
• Suggest wearing a breast shell between feedings.	
• Try applying the electric pump for a few seconds.	

Some nipples are not truly inverted; they appear inverted, but when compressed they readily evert; these are sometimes called *umbilicated* nipples.[6] In these nipples there is adequate ductal "length" but a deficiency of the underlying connective tissue; hence, the nipples at rest do not protrude from the base but can be everted with the hand or by the suckling infant.

The inverted nipple—if it is a lifelong problem—is usually a unilateral condition. If it occurs during pregnancy, it is unlikely that the nipple will be inverted at term. If palpation reveals an inverted nipple, determine the woman's parity and length of gestation before interpreting the meaning of these data. Nulliparas are likely to have nipples that invert early in the pregnancy but evert later.[7] Regardless of parity, nipples that were everted during the first trimester may become inverted during the third trimester. For this reason, assess the breasts at least once during the first trimester (or the first visit) and during the last trimester. Reassure the first-trimester gravida that the inverted nipple may evert later in pregnancy; no intervention is required at this time. If the problem has not

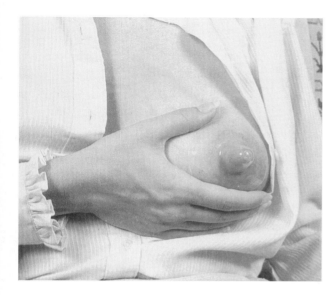

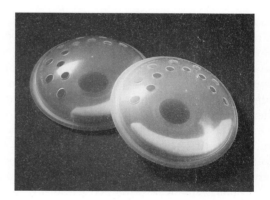

Fig. 8-8 Nipple shields. *(Courtesy Medela, Inc.)*

Fig. 8-9 Breast shells. *(Courtesy Medela, Inc.)*

resolved by the third trimester, some interventions may be helpful during either the antepartum or postpartum periods.

IMPACT OF INVERTED NIPPLES ON BREASTFEEDING AND RECOMMENDATIONS

It is entirely possible for the mother to breastfeed when she has an inverted nipple. Getting the infant to latch on to an inverted nipple, however, can be a thorny problem. Some effective and ineffective solutions are listed in Box 8-1.

If an inverted nipple persists until late in the third trimester, consider recommending breast shells. Not to be confused with nipple *shields* (shown in Figure 8-8), breast *shells* (shown in Figure 8-9) are designed to evert, not cover up, the inverted nipple. Table 8-3 shows the difference between breast shells and nipple shields. The shells are designed to exert pressure on the nipple and help it protrude from the base by gentle suction.

Opponents of breast shells question both their influence on the woman's decision to breastfeed and their effectiveness. Research suggests that some women who wore shells prenatally were less likely to initiate breastfeeding; they complained that the shells cause discomfort, embarrassment, sweating, rash, and milk leakage.[8] For women who were highly motivated, however, these factors did not seem to be a deterrent to breastfeeding.

TABLE 8-3
COMPARISON OF NIPPLE SHIELDS AND BREAST SHELLS

	Nipple Shields	Breast Shells
Primary reason for using	Inverted nipple	Inverted nipple
Description	Shaped similar to rubber nipple	Plastic dome-shaped device
When worn	During feeding	Between feedings
Disadvantages	Abrade nipple tissue, prevent nipple from getting adequate stimulation (hence, milk supply decreases), and frequently an infant who has breastfed with a shield refuses to nurse without it; multiple studies have documented the detrimental effects of nipple shields	Usually none; can be too "tight"; this can be relieved by using a bra extender
Effectiveness	Not effective in solving the problem; only offers a band-aid for the problem	Helps nipple to evert
Comments	Should be used only as a last-resort management strategy	Initiated prenatally if the woman has inverted or flat nipples but can be used postpartum if they were not used prenatally

Modifed from Biancuzzo M. *Breastfeeding the Healthy Newborn.* White Plains, NY: March of Dimes Foundation; 1994.

The effectiveness of prenatal breast shells has been disputed.[8,9] However, the careful consumer of research will note that these studies were done in the United Kingdom. One should hesitate to generalize the results to the U.S. population, where differences in product structure or use and different social norms may influence results. Furthermore, these studies addressed *prenatal* use of the shells, and *postpartum* use has never been studied. Until research proves that these devices do not work, they are worth trying if the inconveniences associated with them (e.g., discomfort and embarrassment as listed above) do not seem to be deterrents for mothers.

At the risk of denying research results, several colleagues and I have often recommended shells and have noted dramatically better clinical results. Shells appear to work best when they are worn prenatally, but postpartum mothers have noticed good results when these are worn between feedings. This is an area that requires further research.

Frequently, mothers are given nipple shields because the mother has flat or inverted nipples. This intervention must be seriously reconsidered, however. In nearly all cases, infants can latch on without the use of the shield. Beyond the issue of flat or inverted nipples, Lawrence asserts that "there are no medical problems where a shield is a good solution"[2(p245)] Rather than being a good solution, it is entirely possible that shields could create more problems than they solve.

Nipple shields have been associated with numerous problems. Some recent reports have suggested that shields are safe and effective,[10-12] but these studies are unconvincing when scrutinized carefully. For example, one recent study[13] suggested that shields were safe and effective, but the small sample size, lack of rigorous control, retrospective data, and self-selection of the subjects made the results of this study questionable. Slightly less than half of the subjects were considered "successful" (breastfeeding until at least 6 weeks of age) with apparently no measure of weight gain or milk transfer and no indication if the data were statistically significant. However, well-controlled studies have demonstrated adverse effects from these devices. The older shields, which were thick and made of latex rubber ("Mexican Hat" style), dramatically reduced

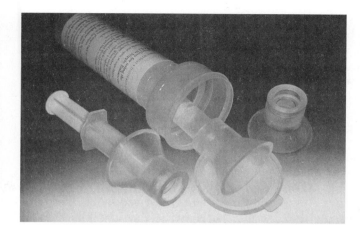

Fig. 8-10 Evert-It. *(Courtesy Maternal Concepts, Inc.)*

milk supply and made the infant vulnerable to altered sucking patterns.[14] The newer type, made of thin silicone, can worsen nipple pain and damage.[15] One well-controlled study clearly showed that even the newer silicone nipple shields are associated with insufficient milk supply and all of its resultant problems, including failure to thrive.[16]

Mothers who use shields are vulnerable to nipple skin abrasion because the shield rubs as the infant is suckling. Furthermore, it is difficult to get the infant to accept the bare breast after he has become accustomed to using the shield. Some nurses try to wean the infant from the shield by using a scissors to cut the opening of the shield a little more each day. This method does little to alleviate this problem, but it is better to achieve good latch-on in the first place rather than try to "wean" the infant from the shield. Suggesting a makeshift nipple shield—using the latex rubber nipple from a bottle—should absolutely never be done. These seriously impede milk transfer and are likely to abrade the skin both because they were not designed to fit on humans and because they are made from latex.

Do not recommend Hoffman's exercises. These exercises, which require the woman to stretch her nipples in both the horizontal and the vertical direction, were designed to stretch and break the fibers that "tie" the inverted nipple. In 1953, Hoffman showed good results in the two cases he described.[17] However, no research study since has shown any benefit from these exercises, and one study has shown detrimental effects.[8]

Other "exercises" for the breast may not be useful and may only dissuade the woman from initiating breastfeeding. Nipple rolling, for example, involves grasping the nipple with the thumb and forefinger, pulling the nipple out to the point of discomfort, then releasing it. This practice has been associated with preterm uterine contractions and has not been associated with improved breastfeeding success.[18]

An anecdotal report recommended a cutoff syringe.[19] This practice is potentially harmful. I have never used this technique, but I once saw a mother who had had this technique performed by an experienced breastfeeding specialist. Hers was the worst case of a damaged nipple I have ever seen. The nipple had a deep fissure, and narcotic analgesics were required to manage the pain. Furthermore, the woman's overall impression of breastfeeding was marred by this experience. It is also important to recognize that using a piece of equipment for other than its intended purpose invites litigation.

Some new devices have been manufactured that are designed to evert the inverted nipple: the Evert-It (Figure 8-10) and the Niplette™ (Figure

8-11). To date, no well-controlled scientific studies have shown either of these devices to be helpful or harmful. The Evert-It is designed to be used in the postpartum period to evert the nipple just prior to latch-on. The Niplette, designed by a plastic surgeon, is designed to permanently correct inverted nipples while the woman is not pregnant, or through the seventh month of pregnancy. (The Niplette can also be used postpartum to facilitate latch-on.) The Niplette has limited use during pregnancy because nipples that are inverted early in pregnancy frequently evert later in pregnancy, and the manufacturer's instructions prohibit use of the device in later pregnancy.

Surgical correction of inverted nipples is possible and was recorded as early as 1873.[20] Recent studies have questioned how to best perform the procedure in order to preserve the woman's ability to breastfeed.[6]

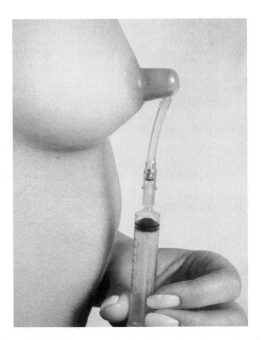

Fig. 8-11 Niplette by Avent. *(Courtesy Avent America, Addison, Ill.)*

A summary of points for physical assessment of the breasts is provided in Table 8-4.

PREEXISTING BREAST/NIPPLE PROBLEMS

Problems with the breasts or nipples can be identified by subjective and objective data. Good interview techniques (described in Chapter 4) and simple physical assessment techniques will be helpful in identifying those conditions that have existed prior to lactation and may influence the breastfeeding experience.

Breast Pathology

Fibrocystic Disease

Fibrocystic disease is a benign condition in which cysts form within enlarged ducts. Typically, the woman reports tenderness that increases just before menses. On physical examination, multiple, round, mobile nodules can be palpated bilaterally; borders are well defined, and the consistency is soft to firm.[21] While these nodules may become somewhat more tender and noticeable during lactation, they do not preclude breastfeeding.

Suspicious Lumps, Breast Cancer, Radiation Therapy

No woman should wait for her routine medical examination to discover a lump. Lumps are usually apparent to women themselves or to their partners. The American Cancer Society and all health care providers continually emphasize to women the importance of performing breast self-examination to promote early detection. The woman who has never performed breast self-examination, however, will find it more difficult to learn during lactation, since there will be mul-

PHYSICAL ASSESSMENT OF THE BREASTS AND AXILLAE

	Observations	Deviations and Clinical Implications
Inspect Both Breasts While the Patient's Arms Are Hanging Loosely at Her Sides, and Compare the Following		
Size	Breasts may be small, moderate, or large but should enlarge during pregnancy and lactation	Size of breasts prior to pregnancy does not affect ability to produce milk or to breastfeed; the key is for both breasts to enlarge from their pre-pregnant state
Symmetry	Breasts and nipples should be symmetrical	Asymmetrical breasts may be due to • Inadequate glandular tissue and failure to enlarge during pregnancy; determine if mother can completely lactate from that breast • Uneven stimulation of breasts; infant has preferred side, or mother is suckling multiple infants with differing needs • Pathology
Contour	Describe as • Conical • Convex • Pendulous • Large pendulous	Women with various contours are able to successfully breastfeed
Retractions or dimpling	Retraction or dimpling is abnormal	Retraction or dimpling of the breast skin indicates pathology; refer to physician
Skin color, texture, and general appearance	Skin should not appear shiny	• Skin may appear stretched if engorged, but should not appear shiny • Presence of red streaking is pathological, and requires referral • Peau d'orange is pathological and requires immediate referral
	Striae may be present during pregnancy and lactation	These are harmless
Venous patterns	Dilated subcutaneous veins during pregnancy and lactation are readily visible	
Lesions	Any number of lesions may be present on the breast; these may be unremarkable or may be pathological	Common lesions include eczema, herpes, and various others; unlike eczema, which does not preclude breastfeeding and is bilateral, Paget's disease appears as a crusty lesion on the breast, but it is unilateral; except for herpes lesions, breastfeeding can continue uninterrupted when lesions are covered
Supernumerary nipples	These may be found anywhere along the milk line, prior to or during lactation	These do not preclude breastfeeding, but they may "drip" while the infant is being fed
Inspect Both Areolae and Nipples While the Patient's Arms Are Hanging Loosely at Her Sides, and Compare the Following		
Size, shape, and symmetry	Nipples and areola should look the same	Unilateral deviation usually suggests presence of pathology
Location	Nipples should be centered on the areola	Slightly off-center nipple not problematic but requires mother to be more careful about centering the infant on the areola
Color	Areola will darken during pregnancy and lactation Color should appear even	Darkening is normal • Horizontal white stripes • Vertical white stripes

Continued

T A B L E 8-4
PHYSICAL ASSESSMENT OF THE BREASTS AND AXILLAE—cont'd

	Observations	Deviations and Clinical Implications
Intactness	Nipple/areola skin should be intact	• Cracking • Bleeding • Fissures
Size	Varies	Varies
Protractility	Most nipples are everted	• Inverted • Flat • Dimpled
Discharge	• Delineate *secretion* from *discharge* (see text) • Describe characteristics of discharge	Most nipple discharges are benign in nature but should be referred to physician because they may be malignant

tiple nodules, normally associated with lactation, and she may be unable to differentiate normal from worrisome signs until she learns the landscape of her nonlactating breasts.

Throughout her life, the woman must lose no time in identifying any suspicious lump and seeking prompt follow-up. However, women are especially vulnerable to delaying follow-up during pregnancy and lactation.[22] In an attempt to attribute the problem to their lactation status, serious problems can be overlooked.

Women who require radiation while lactating should wean. Occasionally, however, women undergo treatment for radiation prior to childbearing. The radiation therapy causes fibrosis and massive destruction of the lobules.[1] The effects of radiation on lactation have not been well documented, so it is difficult to provide the woman with any realistic expectation of what will happen in relation to future breastfeeding experiences.

There are a few cases in which lactation following radiation therapy was successful, but most attempts have been unsuccessful. Unfortunately, nearly all published reports lack a definition of "successful" lactation. Most reports are anecdotal, with few controlled studies, so it is difficult to reach any substantive conclusions.

Two cases were reported by Rodger and colleagues. In one case, the woman lactated from both the irradiated and the untreated breast; in the other case, the woman lactated only from the untreated breast.[23] In one study the majority of patients were unable to lactate from the treated breast, and only one patient "successfully" lactated from the treated breast for 4 months.[24] Another study reported that a woman will lactate from the affected side in only about 25% of cases.[25] One woman was able to fully lactate from the untreated breast but produced only small amounts of colostrum and milk from the previously irradiated breast for about 2 months, while the untreated breast lactated normally.[26] In another case, the treated breast showed no characteristic changes in size and did not lactate.[27] The effects of radiation are poorly understood. One expert has suggested that success or failure of lactation may be dose-related.[28]

Breast Surgery

In many respects, caring for the woman who is undergoing breast surgery is similar to caring for any other person undergoing surgery. Preoperative management should focus on advocating for informed consent, providing options and anticipatory guidance, carrying out actions that maintain homeostasis during the immediate recovery period, and implementing a teaching plan designed to optimize full physical and psychological recovery. In this sense, an operation on the mammary gland bears many similarities to an operation on the thyroid gland. There are, however, some unique aspects to caring for the woman who is undergoing breast surgery. In this culture the breast is more than a mammary gland; it in some way helps the woman to define herself as a woman and a mother. The nurse bears much responsibility for helping the woman to mobilize her emotional resources to deal with this procedure, which invades not only her body but her privacy and her self-concept. This text does not intend to replicate the comprehensive directives for breast surgery outlined in more general textbooks.

Nowadays, it is not uncommon for women of childbearing age to have had prior therapeutic or cosmetic breast surgery. Often, however, women receive little encouragement or practical information from their surgeons about the implications for lactation. Two situations may emerge. In one, the woman wants to breastfeed long after the time when the surgery was performed; in this case, the surgery may have been performed for either therapeutic or cosmetic reasons. In the other situation, the woman needs breast surgery while she is lactating; this is a less common occurrence, but for therapeutic reasons it does occasionally arise. Either situation has clear implications for those providing care, with less clear indications for how lactation will actually progress.

Surgery Prior to Initiation of Lactation

Surgery that is performed on the breast prior to lactation may or may not have a significant impact on lactation. Multiple factors influence the woman's ability to lactate after surgery, but generally speaking her success or failure is related to whether and to what degree the following structures were affected: (1) tissue—the amount of tissue removed, and the extent and character of resulting scar tissue or contractures, and the interruption of the nipple/areolar complex; (2) ducts—whether the lactiferous ducts are intact after the surgical procedure; (3) blood supply—whether it is interrupted; and (4) nerves—whether they are intact. Simply stated, the more intact the structures, the better the chances for successful lactation, which will depend largely on the procedure performed and the type of incision the surgeon used.

Generally, five different incisions can be used when performing breast surgery. These include periareolar, infra-submammary, axillary, pedicle (transposition), free nipple (autotransplantation). Upon inspection, it is fairly easy to determine which type of incision was performed. Figure 8-12 shows the location of the incisions.

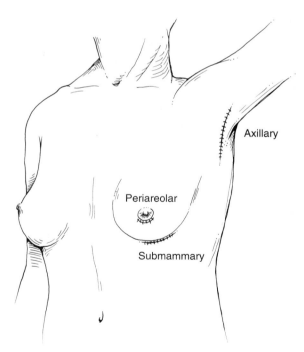

Fig. 8-12 Types of incisions used for breast surgery.

Types of Incisions

The *periareolar* incision is a half circle around the lower border of the areola. The advantage of this type of incision is that it is less visible. It carries several disadvantages, however, including possible loss of sensation. This incision, compared with other types, may make the woman more vulnerable to lactation failure.[29,30] Damage to the lactiferous ducts is likely with a periareolar incision, and although engorgement may uniformly occur, milk production and emptying occur only in the areas where the ducts are intact.[1] Usually, the periareolar technique is used for biopsies or for augmentation mammaplasty.

The *infra-submammary* is located mostly beneath the mammary gland. An advantage to this type of incision is that breastfeeding is possible. A disadvantage, however, is that it is located close to the edge of the bra, which may interfere with wound healing in the beginning or cause irritation later on. Another possible disadvantage is that the scar tissue is visible. This technique is used for augmentation.

The *axillary* incision is located at the axilla. It provides a clear advantage because it is practically invisible, unless the woman raises her arm. Relatively little has been written about this type of incision, but it appears that lactation is likely to be successful following its use. A disadvantage is that the axillary incision may result in contractures of the skin, and that breast cancer detection is more difficult. This technique can be used for augmentation or, occasionally, biopsy.

With the *pedicle*, or *transposition*, technique, the nipple/areola complex remains attached to the underlying parenchyma; this "stem" of tissue remains intact, while wedges of excess tissue are excised from the sides and undersides of the stem. This type of incision is used frequently and enables the surgeon to leave the skin of the nipple/areola complex, lactiferous ducts, blood supply, and some nerves intact. One study showed that 72% of patients who had this incision were able to lactate,[31] and another study's results suggest that most will lactate.[30]

The *free nipple* technique is seldom used nowadays. Usually, it is indicated when the woman has extremely large breasts. Because this technique disrupts the nipple/areola complex and severs lactiferous ducts, subsequent lactation is unlikely. Also, women with this type of incision tend to have decreased nipple sensation.[32]

Surgical Procedure

Aside from the type of incision used, multiple factors affect breastfeeding and lactation. As for all mothers, breastfeeding is more likely to be successful if the mother receives accurate information and ongoing support for her decision. The information she receives prior to the procedure will result in her realistic or unrealistic expectations of how breastfeeding is likely to proceed; receiving information prior to and during the breastfeeding experience will help her to consider some alternatives, including unilateral breastfeeding. The woman's self-image and her feelings of comfort or guilt about having the surgery should be considered. The procedure used, the indication for the surgery in the first place, and the use of prostheses are all factors that contribute to the breastfeeding experience.

There are really four central questions to explore when the mother has had prior breast surgery: (1) Are there reassuring signs of milk production? (2) Is there evidence of milk ejection and drainage? (3) What are the woman's concerns, anxieties, and goals? and (4) What is the effect on the infant (i.e., is he making adequate weight gains)? Answers vary, depending on the individual woman and on the surgery performed. Overall, women with prior breast surgery are more likely to have decreased milk supply than those who have not had surgery.[30]

BREAST REDUCTION

Women may elect to have their breasts reduced for a variety of physical and psychological reasons. Especially large breasts, called *macromastia*, can cause a variety of physical discomforts—posture problems, "back trouble," and other discomforts. Such large breasts, which tend to be familial, also interfere with the woman's self-image; her breasts are usually disproportionate to the rest of her body, and she may feel very self-conscious. Typically, women who seek reduction surgery are very young—often in their late teens. They may not value breastfeeding as something they would later wish to do, or may not recognize how the surgery could limit their feeding options. Complications, including infections and galactorrhea, have been reported,[33,34] in addition to the impact on milk supply as described earlier.

Usually, the pedicle technique is used for reduction mammaplasty, as shown in Figure 8-13. Because most of the ducts, blood supply, and nerves remain intact, breastfeeding is usually possible after this type of surgery. One case report describes a mother who had one breast reduced, using the pedicle technique. Both breasts became fully engorged by 84 hours postpartum, but milk yield from the reduced breast was noticeably less than that from the other breast.[35] Other patients have reported a slight delay in engorgement.[36] Most women who have undergone reduction using this technique have reportedly experienced "normal lactation and breastfeeding," but the authors had no objective criteria by which to measure "normal."[37] Other authors offer similar conclusions—that is, women have "sufficient milk," but they make no mention of measure of milk yield or infant test-weighings.[38] In one study only 35% of women who had had sugery using the pedicle technique initiated and continued breastfeeding, but again, there was little evidence of how "successful" the experience was.[39] Neifert reports that she has encountered women who can produce and deliver a full supply of milk after reduction surgery using the pedicle technique, but she cautions that in most cases supplementation with artificial milk is required for the infant to make adequate weight gains.[1]

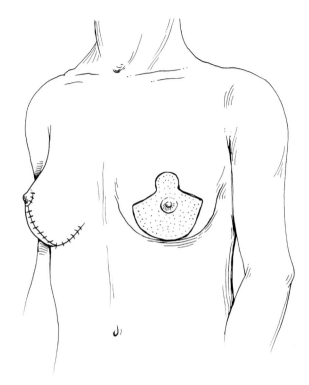

Fig. 8-13 Reduction surgery: pedicle technique.

Reduction surgery is also accomplished through the free nipple (autotransplantation) technique. If the woman is unable to lactate successfully afterward she is likely to blame herself for seeking reduction surgery. In the real world, whether or not the surgery ruined her chances of lactating is a moot point; the surgery has been done and cannot be undone. She may find it comforting to know that some women with macromastia are never able to fully lactate because the extraordinary amount of adipose tissue crowds the lactiferous ducts, rendering them less functional.

BREAST AUGMENTATION
Breast augmentation is usually done using the periareolar technique, which clearly carries a risk

of lactation failure. Lactation has reportedly occurred following breast augmentation.[40] However, there is no acknowledgment of quantity of milk or the infant's well-being as a yardstick for success. In controlled studies, lactation insufficiency is more likely in augmented than in non-augmented women; more specifically, the periareolar approach was most significantly associated with lactation insufficiency.[29,30]

The implants used for augmentation raise another issue. Even if lactation is possible, the question becomes: Is breastfeeding safe? Two types of implants are used for augmentation: saline and silicone. Many women raise questions about the safety of the silicone, fearing that it will "leak" into their milk. The silicone itself is inert and it does not break down; it also is found in over-the-counter products like Di-gel. Other products in the implant do break down, but whether they present a safety hazard is not well understood. The other products are toluenediisocyanate (TDI) and toluenediaminene (TDA), which have been implicated as carcinogenic in industry (e.g., in seat covers), but their safety has not been described in the lactation literature. It is possible, however, to test a pregnant women's urine for breakdown products; if they are present, it is likely that they also will be present in the milk postpartum. The testing can be done by the National Medical Services (800-522-6671).

SURGICAL BIOPSY

If a simple biopsy procedure is used, there apparently is no effect on subsequent lactation. However, if a periareolar incision is used, lactation is seriously hampered. One woman, who had successfully breastfed her first infant prior to the biopsy, was later unable to successfully lactate from the affected breast for a second infant. The woman experienced bilateral engorgement, but normal milk flow from the affected breast was impeded. She tried the usual interventions to increase stimulation and enhance the milk-ejection reflex—warm packs, oxytocin nasal

spray, and starting the feeding on the affected side—but after 6 weeks she realized that her efforts had failed to produce any meaningful change. However, she was able to produce enough milk with the unaffected breast; soon the infant ceased nursing on the affected side, and the breast involuted.[41]

MASTOPLEXY

A mastoplexy is a breast "lift." The skin from the submammary area is involved, and the resulting scar looks similar to that following reduction surgery. Lactation is likely to be unaffected because only the skin is involved, but this has not been studied.

LUMPECTOMY

A lumpectomy is performed to remove a lump in the breast. Lumpectomies may be performed during lactation, or the woman may be required to wean her infant prior to the surgery, since the lactating breast is very vascular. The effects on lactation are not well described. One woman who had a lumpectomy, axillary node dissection, and whole-breast external radiation therapy produced only drops of milk from the treated breast, but she breastfed successfully from the untreated breast.[42]

MASTECTOMY

A mastectomy is the surgical removal of the breast. If a woman has had only one breast removed, it is entirely possible to breastfeed using the other breast.

Breast Surgery While Lactating

Elective surgery involving the breast should be postponed as long as possible. Encourage the woman to explore this option if she has not already done so. Even a short delay would provide her with more options, for example, time to collect and store milk if she chooses to do so. In nonelective situations, however, it is entirely possible that the need for the surgery outweighs the infant's need to breastfeed. A few guiding principles will help to organize care for this woman.

Preoperative Nursing Care of the Lactating Woman

Ask, or suggest that the mother ask, when breastfeeding can resume. This is undoubtedly a question that is on her mind, so it is best to address it before the surgery rather than after. If it is anticipated that breastfeeding cannot resume for a very long time, the woman should be so informed; she may choose to wean. However, the definition of "too long" should be her definition; the health care team should not discourage her from maintaining lactation until the infant can return to the breast, unless that is contraindicated.

The location of the woman's incision may determine whether she can continue breastfeeding. The infant's mouth, which generally harbors bacteria, should not touch a new incision. Where the mother will be hospitalized may present some logistic problems with the breastfeeding experience. If she is admitted to the general surgical floor—which is likely—there may be restrictions on the presence of infants. Some hospitals are more relaxed about this, and permit the infant to room in if the mother accepts full responsibility for his care. Depending on the extent of her surgery, she may or may not be able to do this. Help her to gather objective information so that she can choose options that best fit her needs and those of her infant.

Identify any equipment or resources that the mother may need during her period of separation from the infant (see Chapter 10). It is always wise to review the anticipated length of separation, and her financial and emotional resources to cope with prolonged milk expression. Suggest that she consider expressing and saving her milk unless her physician feels this would be contraindicated. If her milk is only temporarily unsafe, instruct her to "pump and dump" until the circumstances change.

Postoperative Care of the Lactating Woman

Postoperative care of the lactating woman is in many ways similar to postoperative care for a nonlactating woman. There are, however, some specific areas that need to be addressed.

NURSING ASSESSMENTS AND ACTIONS

Check the mother's breasts. It is likely that a separation from the infant, even for a short time, will result in milk stasis. At a minimum, this is uncomfortable. At worst, it can trigger a host of other problems associated with lack of drainage, including extreme engorgement, which would impede wound healing. Ideally, bring the infant for suckling. If this is not possible, encourage the mother to express milk from her breasts. Offer comfort measures, such as ice to the breasts, and a mild analgesic as ordered.

Perform the usual assessments for a postoperative patient, with some minor modifications. Note the location and extent of the incision; reevaluate whether the infant should go to the breast if his mouth will be on or very near to the incision, since the infant's mouth has bacteria that would impede wound healing. Check the incision for drainage and note the color of the drainage. Note the woman's intake and output; count suckled or expressed milk as output!

CONSIDER IMPACT OF MEDICATIONS

Safe administration is always part of the nurse's responsibility, but in this case the drug must be safe for both the mother and the infant. Be certain the prescriber knows the woman is lactating. If several analgesics are ordered for postoperative pain, offer the one that is least likely to have adverse effects on the infant (see Chapter 9). It is, however, unethical to expect a woman to forfeit analgesics if she really needs pain control. Breastfeeding is less likely to succeed if the mother's pain is not managed.

OPTIMIZE BREASTFEEDING AND LACTATION EFFORTS

Be creative in finding ways to optimize the breast-feeding experience. For example, if breastfeeding from the operative breast is contraindicated, suggest that the woman feed from the unaffected side until the affected side is ready for breastfeeding again. Even if she is using both breasts, the stress and separation may diminish her milk supply. Help her to understand that supply can be reestablished relatively quickly, assuming that the separation is minimal and that she is making an uneventful recovery.

HELP HER DEAL WITH PSYCHOLOGICAL IMPACT

Help the mother to deal with her sense of loss and separation. She may feel that she is depriving the baby of her milk or guilty that she does not feel well enough to feed him. Reassure her that she must take care of herself before she can take care of her infant. If previously expressed milk is unavailable, providing artificial milk for the infant is not a disaster, particularly when lactation has already been well established.

The Lactating Woman's Infant: Implications for Care

If the infant is separated from the mother for a substantial length of time, the infant is vulnerable to dehydration or failure to thrive. Collaboration with the pediatrician and thorough follow-up are essential to ensure adequate food and fluids for the infant.

COMMON BREAST PROBLEMS RELATED TO LACTATION

The mother may experience several problems during the course of lactation. Most of these problems can be prevented or alleviated by the nurse; others require the nurse's swift recognition and referral to the primary care provider.

"Sore Nipples"

For at least a half century, lactating mothers have been complaining about "sore nipples."[43] Unfortunately, the word *complaint* has a negative connotation, but a "complaint" about painful nipples does not make the mother a "complainer." The mother's complaint is legitimate; indeed, many mothers do experience painful nipples—which they describe as "sore nipples"—and complaining about their pain or discomfort is the first step in resolving the problem. Sore nipples may include nipple pain, nipple damage, or both.[44]

Nipple Pain

When a person experiences pain, it is the body's way of alerting the brain that something is wrong; ignoring the soreness will lead to increased soreness accompanied by nipple damage, including cracks and fissures. Sometimes pain exists when visible damage cannot be observed, but the mother's complaint is the first signal for prompt identification of the problem and corrective actions. Ask questions designed to elicit information about the cause of pain, adapting them to fit the breastfeeding situation, as described in Box 8-2.

It is imperative to understand and to explain to the mother that sore nipples are not an expected consequence of breastfeeding. Breastfeeding is not meant to be painful; if it were, the species would not have survived. Nipple pain or discomfort is a signal for help, not a cause for discontinuing breastfeeding.

Nipple Damage

If the underlying problem is not corrected, nipple pain will eventually progress to nipple damage. Once the nipple skin is no longer intact, a cascade of deleterious physical and psychological effects follow. By this time the mother has endured the adverse physical and psychological effects.

Box 8-2
Questions to Ask About Nipple Pain

- Where is the soreness?
- When did it begin?
- Is it present just at the beginning of the feeding or throughout the feeding? Or does it persist after the completion of the feeding?
- Describe the characteristics of the pain. Is it dull, shooting, or hot?
- Describe the intensity of the pain on a scale of 1 to 10, with 1 being mild discomfort and 10 being exquisite pain.
- Ask for phrases to describe the pain, to elicit responses such as "like there was broken glass in my nipple" or "like it was liquid fire."

The nurse needs to assess the damage and generate an appropriate plan of action. At the center of this plan is patient education and support.

Nipple damage may range from a slightly imperceptible white compression stripe to a gaping fissure. Damage to the nipple may include erythema, edema, fissures, blisters, inflamed areas, eschar, white patches, dark patches, yellow patches, peeling, pus, and ecchymosis.[45] Note and describe the lesion as well and as completely as possible, and initiate follow-up evaluation.

Causes of Nipple Pain and/or Damage

For over a half century, experts have tried to find the causes and treatments for sore nipples,[46,47] and the insights of these experts are still well worth reading. The most frequent cause of sore nipples is poor positioning. The underlying reason for sore nipples during the first few days may not be a cause for concern, if good latch-on has been achieved. During the first few days, the milk ducts are not yet filled with milk, and this may cause discomfort. Also the mother is unaccustomed to having an infant suckle at the breast; peak intraoral pressures can reach as high as 135 mm Hg.[48] Other reasons for sore nipples are worrisome and must be investigated and corrected immediately.

Simple Mismanagement

The most frequent cause of sore nipples is inflammation and/or abrasions and bruising of the nipple that occurs as a result of poor positioning. If the subjective reports of pain are not accompanied by objective data that suggest other problems, observe the feeding session and be especially alert to poor latch-on. Question the mother about the location of her pain. Pain that is perceived on top of the nipple is likely to be caused by poor latch-on and/or tongue thrusting. To correct the problem, observe the feeding. If the infant does not demonstrate good latch-on as described in Chapter 5, initiate corrective actions. If the infant is thrusting his tongue, try inserting a gloved finger and holding the infant's tongue down for about 30 seconds before latching on. This is not always helpful, but it is worth a try.

Pain that is perceived on the underside of the nipple is more likely caused by the nipple being tipped upward when the mother offers the breast. It is acceptable—perhaps even advisable—to tip the breast slightly upward so that the infant can readily latch on, chin first. However, the mother must quickly stop tipping the breast as soon as the infant has an adequate grasp of the nipple/areola or else soreness and bruising are likely to result. Use of the palmar grasp makes the mother particularly vulnerable to tipping the nipple upward during the feeding, since she may exert more pressure on the underside of her breast when she uses this position. To avoid this problem, alert the mother to stop tipping the breast as soon as the infant latches on.

Obviously, pain due to mismanagement is best relieved by determining the cause of the pain and correcting the underlying problem. By observing

Historical Highlight

Sore Nipples

A descriptive study was conducted on a total of 114 primiparas and multiparas from their 1st to 11th postpartum day. All were healthy and had average-weight, healthy newborns. Dr. Gunther identified two types of lesions that differed in nature, position, and time of incidence: the petechial (erosive) lesion and the ulcerative lesion (i.e., fissure). About 62% had the erosive type of lesion, and about 4% had the ulcerative type of lesion; three women had both types.

Gunther described four grades of soreness: (1) soreness but no visible change; (2) edema of papillae visible; (3) petechiae, separated; (4) petechiae, merged to form a transverse crescent. The petechial lesions were small and almost always preceded by translucent edema. The most extensive petechiae merged to form a red, crescent-shaped lesion across the nipple. Erosion of the epithelium from a ruptured blister was also noted. Gunther emphasized that the line of merged petechiae across the nipple corresponded to where the infant exerted the most pressure. Unlike the erosive type, the onset of ulcerative lesions was noted after a few days.

Gunther further explained that nipple soreness was related to lack of swallowing and that soreness was not reported as frequently when the infant could be heard swallowing. Negative pressure was measured, and it was shown that the infant exerted greater negative pressures on the breast when there was very little milk to be obtained (either because it was shortly after birth, or at the end of feeding when very little milk was left). The infant used high continuous negative pressure, but the pressure was relieved when the infant swallowed.

Infants in this study were limited in the amount of time they suckled. Obviously, this did not prevent the sore nipples. Further, there was no attempt to correct their positioning at the breast, and one might wonder if negative pressure would have been so high if the infants had been positioned differently. Nonetheless, today's nurse has much to learn from this study in terms of points to look for in assessing the breasts, the futility of limiting suckling time in an attempt to prevent sore nipples, and the need to evaluate milk transfer as evidenced by audible swallowing.

From Gunther M. Sore nipples: causes and prevention. *Lancet* 1945;249:590-593.

the feeding, one can usually determine the cause of the problem.

Anatomic Variations

The common myth that fair-skinned women are more vulnerable to nipple soreness than darker-skinned women is without substance. While those of us in clinical practice have seen this many times and may be skeptical about the research results, there are, to date, no controlled studies that support casual observations.[49]

Inverted nipples may cause discomfort when the mother puts the infant to the breast. As discussed earlier, often the best treatment for inverted nipples is suckling at the breast.

At least temporarily, engorgement results in

an alteration of the contour of the nipple. The nipple/areola complex shortens in the presence of engorgement, making it more difficult for the infant to achieve good latch-on. Instruct the mother to express a little milk by hand until the nipple/areola softens enough so that the infant can achieve a proper grasp. This should alleviate the problem.

If there is any alteration of the infant's orofacial structure, the mother may experience sore nipples. I am aware of one case where the mother complained of exquisitely sore nipples. A smacking sound could be heard when the infant nursed, so everyone's first inclination was to presume that there was poor positioning. After adjusting the infant's position, however, the mother still com-

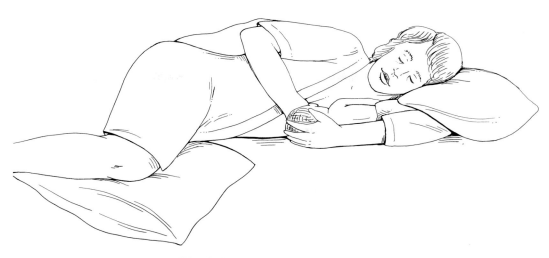

Fig. 8-14 Modified side-lying position.

plained of sore nipples. As it turned out, no one had given the infant a complete digital examination of the oral cavity. When that occurred, the likely cause of the sore nipples was identified. The infant had a cleft of the soft palate. Similarly, mothers whose infants have a short frenulum are likely to complain of sore nipples. However, do not assume that the cause of the mother's sore nipples is the infant's anatomy. One mother complained of very sore nipples and blamed her infant's cleft lip. When I observed the dyad breastfeeding, however, it immediately became evident that the cause of the sore nipples was a poor latch-on. When the infant opened wide and latched on, the problem of sore nipples almost immediately disappeared.

Unrelieved Negative Pressure
Nipples can become sore when they are exposed to unrelieved negative pressure, such as occurs during prolonged nonnutritive suckling, improper use of a breast pump, a delayed let-down, or not breaking the suction before removing the infant from the breast. Explain these possibilities to

the mother and offer corrective strategies (see Chapter 5).

Sometimes mothers of infants who are true barracudas, as described in Chapter 5, will experience nipple soreness. This discomfort is particularly remarkable during the first few days. Assuming that the discomfort is due to this aggressive suckling style, not improper positioning at the breast, a few recommendations may be helpful. First, reassure the mother that this discomfort will not last forever; it should disappear after a few weeks. In the meantime, suggest that she offer the least-sore breast first because the infant's suck is more vigorous on the first side. Also, suggest using different positions. At one feeding use the cradle position; at the next feeding use the side-lying position; at the next feeding use the football hold. A modified side-lying position, as shown in Figure 8-14, is a fourth alternative. Using different positions alternates where the pressure points occur and should lessen the discomfort.

Use and Misuse of Products
Sometimes sore nipples are iatrogenic; they occur as the result of using some products. An electric

breast pump that is used improperly will cause problems, for example, if the user turns the suction on too high and leaves it there. Nipple shields, wet breast pads, creams or ointments that produce allergic reactions, and using or abusing various other products will result in sore nipples.

Prolonged exposure to wet nursing pads or to moisture build-up in poorly vented breast shells may result in tissue breakdown and hence cracked nipples. Using plastic-lined breast pads, or not replacing moist pads also creates tissue breakdown. Drying the nipples by simply keeping the bra flaps down and exposing the nipples to air is perhaps the best remedy. A hairdryer, adjusted to the low setting and fanned about 6 to 8 inches from the breast, works well to dry the nipples.

Other Causes

Other causes of nipple pain may be more pathological, and the root of the pain, usually poor positioning, leads to cracks and fissures. (See Chapter 5 for a discussion of proper positioning.)

Clinical Management Priorities

Sore nipples usually can be prevented. Over the years, several recommendations have been given for preventing and/or treating sore nipples. Some of these treatments have been shown to be ineffective; others appear to be effective. A summary of a few helpful strategies is found in Box 8-3.

Correct the Underlying Problem

To resolve the problems, it is helpful to first understand the normal structure and function of the nipple skin and the event that results in soreness. Usually, the skin protects the body against loss of fluids from within and from invasion of substances from without. When the nipple skin is no longer intact, the whole organism becomes more vulnerable to infection and pain.

Box 8-3

Tips for Managing Sore Nipples

1. Determine the root of the problem. Otherwise, interventions may cause more harm than good.

2. Instruct the mother to discontinue using practices or products that are likely to cause or exacerbate sore nipples. This includes rubbing the nipples with a towel, using soap or alcohol products, using creams or ointments that she may be allergic to, not changing wet breast pads promptly, and using nipple shields.

3. Correct poor positioning. An asymmetrical latch-on, incremental latch-on, "dragging" on a large breast (use rolled-up towel under the breast to alleviate drag), and sucking the nipple instead of the areola all contribute to sore nipples.

4. Reduce pressure on the sore spot. Feed on the less-sore side first, since the infant's suck is most vigorous when he starts. Alternating positions for a few days (e.g., cradle hold at this feeding, side-lying hold at next feeding, football hold at next feeding) may be helpful.

5. Enhance milk-ejection reflex. Warm compresses or massaging before feeding or while the infant pauses during feeding helps an eager infant to obtain milk without excessive sucks prior to let-down.

The nurse has a vital role to play in identifying the underlying physical problem that is causing or contributing to the sore nipples. Using physical assessment skills and good interview techniques will elicit data that help determine the root of the problem. Using another intervention to "cover up" the problem is counterproductive.

Offer Interim Comfort Measures

Assuming that a corrective action has been initiated, the question still remains: What should we do in the meantime? Starting on the less-sore side first and eliciting a milk-ejection reflex helps.

It may be helpful to alternate positions; use cradle hold for the first feeding, side lying for the next feeding, and football hold for the following feeding. This helps to reduce the pressure on the same spot.

Recognize and Respond to Emotional Impact
For over half a century, "sore nipples" have been reported as the reason for early weaning.[44,50-55] Help women to understand that sore nipples are not an expected consequence of breastfeeding, and that the situation is only temporary.

Use Effective Treatment Strategies
The following treatments are helpful if the woman has nipple pain, nipple damage, or both.

GOOD LATCH-ON
Good latch-on is the key to preventing sore nipples. See Chapter 5 for a discussion of how to achieve good latch-on.

APPLICATION OF MILK OR COLOSTRUM
Whether or not human milk is effective in treating traumatized nipples has yet to be completely proved. One research study showed no difference,[56] while expert clinicians are staunch defenders of this practice.[2] In some cultures human milk is used for many skin irritations. There appear to be no harmful effects, and therefore no reason to not recommend this practice, which clinical experience has shown to be beneficial.

Causes, goals, and strategies for dealing with sore nipples are described in Table 8-5.

Discourage Ineffective or Harmful Treatments
"PREPARING" THE NIPPLES
Several decades ago, pregnant women were instructed to "prepare" for breastfeeding by rubbing their nipples vigorously with a bath towel. This action may create rather than prevent or resolve a problem. Rubbing the nipples vigorously with a towel removes the protective epithelial cells. Furthermore, such stimulation to the breasts may stimulate uterine contractions, causing preterm labor.

TOPICAL CREAMS AND OINTMENTS
Over the years, a variety of topical creams and ointments have been recommended as a panacea for sore nipples. These include A&D ointment, bag balm, lanolin (unprocessed lanolin, made from sheep's wool), and modified lanolin (lanolin that has been processed). None have been proved effective in scientific studies, as shown in the Research Highlight. If the mother is allergic to creams and ointments, she will experience sore nipples. In these and similar cases, recommend discontinuation of the product and concentrate on proper positioning at the breast. Topical medications prescribed for situations where visible nipple skin damage exists are a different matter (see later discussion).

LIMITING SUCKLING TIME
Limitation of suckling time has been recommended for decades as a way to prevent nipple soreness, but it has never been proved effective.[57]

Evaluate Corrective Strategy
All too often a reasonable strategy is recommended to resolve the problem, but the problem does not resolve. Make no assumptions. Continue physical assessment and observe the feeding. Most important, ask the mother. If she continues to report sore nipples, pursue the root of the problem and initiate corrective strategies.

Engorgement

Engorgement is the distention of body tissue. The emphasis here is on *tissue* distention; it is a *sign* of milk production, but the term *engorgement* is not equivalent to milk production or milk volume.

TABLE 8-5
CAUSES AND CLINICAL STRATEGIES FOR SORE NIPPLES

Causes	Possible Contributing Factors	Prevention and Goals	Clinical Strategies
Simple mismanagement of breastfeeding	Improper positioning and latch-on	Achieve proper latch-on	As described in Chapter 5
	Unrelieved negative pressure when milk is not yet abundant	Minimize unrelieved negative pressure	Encourage use of both breasts at each feeding to minimize unrelieved negative pressure
	Not breaking suction before removing infant from breast		Teach mother to break suction by using her finger if she needs to take the infant off the breast
Deviations from normal	Flat or retracted nipples	Achieve good latch-on	Listen for audible swallowing
	Pathological engorgement	Prevent milk stasis	Avoid pathological engorgement by early, frequent, and effective feeding (i.e., milk transfer)
	Breast infections	Prevent milk stasis	Assess for breast infections and initiate treatment if indicated
Improper use of apparatus/products	Improper use of breast pumps	Demonstrate and explain proper use of equipment	Decrease intensity of suction and increase number of suction cycles
	Prolonged exposure to moist breast pads	Allow air to circulate to nipple	Change pads frequently
			Use no pads or disposable pads if infection is present (e.g., candidiasis), since this provides medium for growth
	Allergies to creams and ointments	Avoid contact with potential allergens	Discontinue use
	Use of nipple shields	Avoid trauma to nipple tissue	Discontinue use
	Use of cutoff syringe to evert nipples	Avoid trauma to nipple tissue	Use devices designed for everting nipples

Newton and Newton[58] assert that engorgement begins when milk is retained in the alveoli; the alveoli become distended and compress the surrounding ducts (see Box 8-4). Engorgement involves two elements: (1) congestion and increased vascularity, and (2) accumulation of milk[2] (see Historical Highlight).

Types of Engorgement

There are two types of engorgement: physiological and pathological. It is important to differentiate the two in terms of clinical recognition and management.

Physiological Engorgement
The breasts begin to fill with milk around the second postpartum day, depending on how early and how frequently the infant has gone to the breast. Some degree of engorgement is physiological, and its absence should be considered a red flag for further follow-up.

Unfortunately, the word *engorgement* has often carried a negative connotation. Help the new

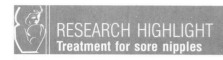

Citation
Pugh LC, Buchko BL, Bishop BA, Cochran JF, Smith LR, Lerew DJ. A comparison of topical agents to relieve nipple pain and enhance breastfeeding. *Birth* 1996;23:88-93.

Purpose
To examine the effectiveness of three topical agents—USP-modified lanolin, warm water compresses, and expressed breast milk with air drying—in relieving nipple pain and to determine if there were any early predictors of breastfeeding 6 weeks postpartum.

Design/Population/Sample
Experimental design: 177 women who were over age 18; primapara; vaginal delivery; low-risk pregnancy, labor, and delivery; gestational age more than 37 weeks; English speaking; telephone in the home; and singleton birth with no newborn complications.

Methods
All women were given breastfeeding instruction per hospital guidelines and telephone contact information to accommodate postdischarge questions. Subjects were randomly assigned to experimental or control group. There were four groups: (1) USP-modified lanolin, (2) warm compresses only, (3) expressed breast milk massaged into the nipples and areolae with air drying, and (4) education only. Self-report of pain was assessed at postpartum days 4, 7, and 14, and the McGill pain questionnaire was used for a validity check. A follow-up call was made at 6 weeks to determine if the mother was still breastfeeding at that time.

Results
There were no differences among groups in terms of the intensity of pain reported or number of weeks that breastfeeding continued. Continuation of breastfeeding beyond 6 weeks was more likely when mothers were fully, rather than partially, breastfeeding.

Critical Comment and Clinical Application
The results of this study support earlier findings that topical agents were no more effective than education only. Clinicians should discontinue recommending creams and ointments, since these have not been proved to be effective in relieving pain and may only present an unnecessary nuisance and expense for the mother.

Historical Highlight

Postpartum Engorgement of the Breast
A study was conducted on 47 women at the Hospital of Pennsylvania. The women were first seen within 24 hours of delivery, then seen again to determine the amount of engorgement at a mean of 67 hours (range 38-100 hours) after delivery. The engorgement was rated as 0, +1, +2, +3 or +4; a rating of 0 was given if there was no engorgement, and +4 was given to describe very hard, lumpy, tense breast tissue.

The reseachers measured the amount of milk obtained in these women by weighing the infant before and after the feeding, and by measuring the amount of milk obtained by the pump. Today, we know these measures would have been somewhat inaccurate because pumps were not as efficient then as now, and test-weighing on the balance scales—which were used at that time—would have been inaccurate measure of milk obtained from the breast.

However, the authors draw some important conclusions that have implications for today's care. They state: "Our conception of engorgement is that it begins with retention of milk in the alveoli. The alveoli become distended and compress surrounding milk ducts. This leads to obstruction of the outflow of milk, further distention of the alveoli, and increased obstruction. If unrelieved this may lead to secondary vascular and lymphatic statis. Increasing pressure in the obstructed portion of the breast gradually causes cessation of secretion [of milk] and eventually it is probably that milk is reasorbed" (p. 666). To date, no research has refuted this statement.

The authors emphasize that there are three main reasons why milk is retained in the alveoli: (1) failure of the milk-ejection reflex, (2) mothers may allow insufficient suckling, and similarly (3) hospital protocols do not allow for sufficient infant suckling in terms of frequency of feedings or duration at the breast.

From Newton M, Newton NR. Postpartum engorgement of the breast. *Am J Obstet Gynecol* 1951;61:664-667.

mother to recognize the signs and symptoms of physiological engorgement as positive; the tissue distention heralds the "coming-in" of her milk supply. Most of all, impress upon her that when the tissue distention goes away, it does not mean that the milk goes away. She may assume that she already has an oversupply of milk and therefore may deny the infant access to the breast, thinking that more stimulation will only exacerbate the situation. Instruct her to continue breastfeeding, since the degree of tissue distention is not equivalent to the degree of milk supply. To the contrary, not having the infant drain the breasts will only worsen the problem because milk stasis invites pathological engorgement.

Pathological Engorgement

Pathological engorgement occurs when the amount of tissue distention is preventable, extreme, or the result of some unphysiological cause. In most circumstances, pathological engorgement is preventable. The woman who is experiencing pathological engorgement is likely to have many factors that can be or should have been modified, including early initiation of the first feeding(s), frequency of feedings, feeding duration, and supplementation.[59] To the extent possible, encourage the mother to breastfeed the infant for the first half year to year of life and for more than eight feedings per day. Instruct the woman to leave the infant at the breast until milk has been completely transferred from both sides, and to avoid supplementation. This should prevent most episodes of pathological engorgement.

Clinical Manifestations

Always include the breasts as part of the overall postpartum assessment, and ask the woman about her sensations of fullness. Some women report that they feel a sudden, unmistakable "coming-in" of milk, while others report a more gradual onset and are less aware of the "coming-in." Engorgement happens sooner and more severely in second-time breastfeeding mothers than in those who have never lactated before.[60] When the milk does become abundant, the woman may have a slight fever and general malaise. She may become tearful. Warn the woman well ahead of time that the sensation she will experience around day 3 is due to swelling of the *tissue*; the swelling will go away, but that will not mean that the *milk* has gone away!

There are several signs and symptoms of engorgement. Some of those associated with pathological engorgement are present with physiological engorgement, but to a greater degree. The signs and symptoms of engorgement may involve only the areola, only the body of the breast (peripheral engorgement), or both. Box 8-4 compares and contrasts clinical manifestations.

Areolar Engorgement

Areolar engorgement is distention of the areolar tissue only. It is not uncommon for the areola to become distended to the extent that the nipple is shortened and may virtually disappear. From a practical standpoint, this creates a snowballing problem; the infant is unable to latch on and effectively empty the breast, milk accumulates, and the engorgement becomes more severe and more painful.

Peripheral Engorgement

Peripheral engorgement is likely to occur in the presence of areolar engorgement. Peripheral engorgement includes the "body" of the breast and is more likely to be a sign of pathological rather than physiological engorgement.

Treatments and Recommendations

Engorgement can and should be prevented. Avoid practices that make the woman vulnerable

Box 8-4
Engorgement

Areolar Engorgement

Obliterates nipple; difficult for infant to properly grasp areola. Collecting ducts will not be milked and therefore do not empty.

May occur alone or in conjunction with peripheral engorgement.

More likely to occur during physiological engorgement. Treatment:

- Hand expression to soften the areola so that the infant can get a good grasp of the nipple and areola.

Peripheral Engorgement

Initially, engorgement is vascular; therefore pumping is not productive and may be traumatic. Breasts are full, hard, tender; swelling starts at the clavicle and goes to the lower ribcage and from the midaxillary line to the midsternum. Most likely to occur with areolar engorgement.

More likely to occur during pathological engorgement. Treatment:

- Frequent breastfeeding around the clock! Relief is based on establishment of milk flow.
- Wear supportive bra 24 hours a day.
- Warm showers and warm packs help to release accumulation of milk.
- Cold packs *after* breastfeeding to decrease congestion.
- If ordered, administer analgesic immediately before breastfeeding; drug will not reach milk for at least 1/2 hour (aspirin, acetaminophen, codeine, short-acting barbiturates).
- Manual expression and massage.

Data derived from Lawrence RA. *Breastfeeding: A Guide for the Medical Profession.* 4th ed. St. Louis: Mosby; 1994.

to pathological engorgement—scheduled feedings, supplementing with formula or water, nipple shields, and other practices that upset the natural supply-and-demand phenomenon.

The aim of treatment is to decrease the overdistention of the ducts. Any intervention that achieves this aim is desirable, since the infant himself provides the best relief for engorgement. Ductal distention will be minimized if accumulation of milk can be reduced, or if vascular congestion can be reduced. Recommend warm showers, warm compresses, or leaning over a basin of warm water to reduce the accumulation of milk in the ducts. Suggest applying cold packs after breastfeeding to cause vasoconstriction, thereby reducing vasocongestion. (Cold packs on or near the nipples *before* feedings can interfere with the milk-ejection

reflex.) Perhaps the most convenient and accessible cold pack is a bag of frozen vegetables. Frozen peas work especially well because their shape and size allow the bag to be flexible. Ice packs are certainly acceptable, but they are more rigid when frozen, and they make a watery mess as they melt. Frozen gel packs are soft and flexible but somewhat expensive.

Hand expression is the treatment of choice for areolar engorgement. (It may give some relief for peripheral engorgement as well.) Assist the mother to express a little milk—just enough to soften the nipple/areola complex. Softening usually can be accomplished by expressing less than 15 ml. This enables the infant to attach properly and will be the start of problem resolution. Avoid using an electric breast pump because the negative pressure exerted and pump's flange are more likely to cause trauma to tissue that is already taut and distended.

If the degree of engorgement is already causing the mother pain, however, initiate measures to reduce the pain and solve the problem. Usually a variety of analgesics are ordered for the discomforts associated with the postpartum recovery. In general, start by offering the most mild analgesic ordered (such as acetaminophen), since this usually is sufficient to relieve the discomfort associated with breast engorgement.

Cool cabbage leaves have been used to relieve engorgement. Most of the reports on their effectiveness are anecdotal, with few research studies to demonstrate beneficial effects. One study suggested that maternal confidence and reassurance seemed to be as effective as the cabbage leaves, and another showed that the cabbage leaves were no more effective than cold gel packs.[61]

Plugged Duct

Description and Etiology

A plugged duct is a duct that has, for whatever reason, not drained well. Frequently, it is due to inadequate emptying of the breast—for example, when an infant has an inadequate suck. It could also be the result of other causes, such as a bra that is too tight or a cream that has been used on the nipple. The plugged duct is not a problem per se, but it can result in mastitis if it is not corrected.

Clinical Manifestations

Typically, the woman who presents with a plugged duct will complain of a tender, sore lump that is not accompanied by a fever or other signs of infection. It may feel hot to the touch.

Treatments and Recommendations

Instruct the woman to continue frequent nursing, alternating the position of the infant (cradle, side-lying, football). If the infant is unable to suckle, suggest a pump, or better still teach hand expression (see Chapter 10). Hand expression works well because it enables the woman to "milk" the spot with her fingers. Warm, moist heat also helps. Ideally, recommend that the woman express milk by hand while she leans over a basin of warm water. In this way, her fingers can "milk" the ducts, while the heat causes vasodilation and the leaning over allows gravity to enhance drainage.

Mastitis

Description and Etiology

Mastitis is an infection of the breast's ductal system. Milk stasis and nipple trauma predispose the ductal system to bacterial contamination. The nipple damage is the portal of entry for the invading bacteria, which are usually *Staphylococcus aureus*, but sometimes *Escherichia coli* and more rarely *Streptococcus*. Any mother with milk stasis is at high risk for a plugged duct, engorgement, mastitis, or all three. (Table 8-6 compares and contrasts these conditions.) The mother who has sore nipples is at risk for developing mastitis because she has not allowed the infant to adequately remove the milk. Tight bras, a missed feeding, or plugged ducts are contributing factors. Additionally, mothers who have been exposed to the organism, or those with lowered body defenses or extreme fatigue, are vulnerable. The highest incidence of mastitis occurs around 5 to 6 weeks postpartum.[62]

Clinical Manifestations

Generalized and localized signs and symptoms occur soon after the invading organism appears.

Since the condition rarely occurs in the hospital, the mother usually calls and reports systemic symptoms associated with infection: aching, flulike symptoms, chills, and general malaise. She will also describe localized signs, including a swollen, hot, often hard breast with red streaking. The redness is usually confined to one quadrant, as shown in Figure 8-15. Frequently, it is the upper outer quadrant, since this is the location of the largest amount of glandular tissue. Be sure to ask the mother if these localized signs appear in only one breast because this may help to determine the urgency of the problem. Engorgement and mastitis share some common signs, but engorgement is always bilateral and mastitis is almost always unilateral. Also, note whether the mother has any lumps, since plugged ducts frequently contribute to mastitis.

Treatments and Recommendations

Advise the woman who has signs and symptoms of mastitis to seek medical help immediately.

T A B L E 8-6

COMPARISON OF FINDINGS OF ENGORGEMENT, PLUGGED DUCT, AND MASTITIS

Characteristics	Engorgement	Plugged Duct	Mastitis
Onset	Gradual, immediately postpartum	Gradual, after feedings	Sudden, after 10 days
Site	Bilateral	Unilateral	Usually unilateral
Swelling and heat	Generalized	May shift a little or no heat	Localized, red, hot, and swollen
Pain	Generalized	Mild but localized	Intense but localized
Body temperature	<38.4° C	<38.4° C	>38.4° C
Systemic symptoms	Feels well	Feels well	Flulike symptoms

From Lawrence RA. *Breastfeeding: a guide for the medical profession.* 4th ed. St. Louis: Mosby; 1994.

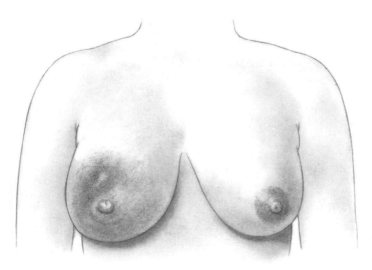

Fig. 8-15 Mastitis. *(From Lawrence RA. Breastfeeding: A Guide for the Medical Profession. 4th ed. St. Louis: Mosby; 1994.)*

Usually, antibiotic therapy results in rapid relief. Impress upon her that she must continue breastfeeding while she is experiencing mastitis! Explain that discontinuation of breastfeeding will only worsen the situation. The milk will become "backed up" in the ducts, and milk stasis provides food for the invading organism. Other priorities for care are listed in Box 8-5.

Box 8-5
Priorities for Care: Mastitis

- Identify patients who are at risk for developing mastitis and initiate patient teaching to reduce its likelihood.
- Use inspection, palpation, and good interview skills to recognize the presence of an invading organism; refer to physician immediately.
- Encourage frequent, regular breastfeeding with adequate drainage of each breast! If the infant is unable to completely empty the breast, initiate pumping.
- Instruct the mother to start the infant on the unaffected side first. When the infant comes to the affected side, his suck will be less vigorous, and she will have already experienced a milk ejection, thereby making the experience less painful.
- Initiate patient teaching: review steps to overcome any infection, including increasing fluids, maintaining bed rest, and taking prescribed antibiotics on time and for the full course.
- Reassure the mother that the prescribed antibiotic is compatible with breastfeeding (see Chapter 9).
- Suggest comfort measures: warm packs will promote drainage of the ductal system, but ice packs will cause vasoconstriction and increase comfort. Either may be used. A bra may be worn to promote comfort, but be cautious in this recommendation; sometimes the bra the mother owns is too tight and has caused the problem in the first place. If a mild analgesic, such as aspirin or acetaminophen, has been prescribed, encourage her to take it. Otherwise, her pain level may cause her to discontinue the feeding before the infant can remove the milk, and milk stasis therefore worsens.

The most likely cause for recurrent mastitis is that the mother did not finish the prescribed round of antibiotics. Or she may not have had enough rest to fortify her body's natural defenses. Occasionally, however, the mother may have a chronic bacterial infection, a secondary fungal infection (e.g., *Candida albicans*), or some more serious underlying disease. Insist that she seek medical help immediately, since she may be somewhat cavalier about this situation or just assume it will improve, which it will not.

The most important teaching points about mastitis are related to stress and fatigue.[63] Suggest to the woman that she take the infant to bed with her and discourage well-meaning visitors who deprive her of rest. Encourage her to seek help from friends or relatives who would be willing to perform household chores so that she can take care of herself and her infant.

Candidiasis/Thrush

Description and Etiology

Candida is a fungal organism that normally inhabits the mouth, vagina, and intestines. An overgrowth of *Candida* can occur, however, leading to the infection known as *candidiasis*, more commonly known as "thrush" or "yeast" (and formerly called "monilia"). Candidiasis can occur on the lactating woman's nipples and the inside of her infant's mouth (oral thrush), as well as the infant's diaper area (diaper rash) and the mother's vagina. The discussion here will be limited to oral thrush (the mother's nipples and infant's mouth). When the infection is present at one site, however, there is a high likelihood that it will affect another as well.

Women who breastfeed are at risk for developing candidiasis because, like other fungi, *Candida albicans* typically thrives on carbohydrates, so the lactose in milk provides the ideal food for the organism's growth. As described earlier, having mastitis predisposes the woman to future candidiasis infections. Other factors have been identified as risk factors for developing breast candidiasis: vaginal candidiasis, nipple trauma, and previous antibiotic use.[64] Antibiotics destroy the normal flora that would otherwise oppose the overgrowth of *Candida*. Having prior nipple damage makes the nipple vulnerable to growth of *Candida*. Using pacifiers contaminated with *Candida* can contribute to the problem. Diabetics, with suppressed immune systems, and anemic women are at increased risk for candidiasis.

Clinical Manifestations

Physical assessment may reveal one or more signs and symptoms in the infant, the mother, or the mother's partner. Clinical experts have clearly delineated the signs and symptoms for the lactating mother, breastfeeding infant, and the mother's partner, which are summarized and augmented here.[65] Typically, the infant will have white patches in the mouth, which are easily mistaken for milk. If a white patch clings to the infant's tongue when rubbed with a clean finger or cotton-tipped swab, it is likely to be thrush; rubbing a white patch leaves a red or bleeding spot. In addition, the oral sign is frequently accompanied by a bright red rash extending from the infant's anus outward. The infant may be feeding poorly or may refuse to eat. He may also be restless and irritable.

Inspect the color of the mother's nipples; they may be bright red or purple. Sometimes the bright red nipples are in sharp contrast to the paler areola—the nipple looks almost like a raspberry atop the areola. Inspect for lesions; on rare occasions, the white plaque can be seen, but in most cases it cannot. Even if it is visible, it may be dismissed on the assumption that it is only milk on the nipple. Frequently, the woman's partner is asymptomatic, but if he has engaged in any oral contact with her breast, he may have white patches in his mouth. He also may have a red rash on his penis, and may complain of itching and burning.

The mother is likely to complain of pain. Ask her to use a phrase to describe the pain. She may complain of a severe burning sensation or may say it feels like her milk is on fire. Others will say that their nipple feels like it has broken glass in it. Some report a shooting pain.[66] All of these descriptions require further follow-up.

Treatments and Recommendations

When either the mother or the infant exhibits signs of candidiasis, refer both for prompt treatment. If the mother is breastfeeding more than one infant, the entire group must be treated. Candidiasis is easily passed back and forth from the infant's mouth to the mother's breast, and therefore can be extremely difficult to eradicate without prompt, thorough treatment of all the involved parties, including the partner.

Treatment for candidiasis is best carried out with a simple understanding of how yeast thrives. Yeast flourishes in a warm, moist, dark place such as inside the vagina, bra, bra pads, folds of the skin, and the diaper; therefore, these are likely environments for growth. (Re-used breast pads will promote the growth of *Candida*; if they are used, breast pads should be disposable.) Once the diagnosis of candidiasis has been established, initiate some simple measures and reinforce the prescribed treatment regimen.

A few simple suggestions can help solve the problem. Explain to the woman that the warm, moist, dark environment is created when the lactating nipples are constantly inside of the bra. In addition, the fungus thrives on the milk. Suggest that she rinse her nipples and air dry them after feeding, and encourage her to spend at least a few minutes during the day with the bra flaps down and the nipples exposed to the light. If the mother expresses her milk while she is experiencing candidiasis, explain that she may feed it to the infant during that time but should not freeze it for later use. Boil for 20 minutes all parts of the breast pump that come in contact with the milk, as well as nipples or pacifiers, at least once a day. Discourage pacifiers, since these become just one more medium that can transfer the organism.

Medications may be prescribed for the mother, the infant, or the mother's partner; which drug is prescribed usually depends on the severity of the infection and whether the candidiasis is primarily oral, genital, or gastrointestinal. The discussion here will be limited to those drugs used for oral candidiasis.

Topical treatments are usually used for oral thrush. These generally fall into two categories: corticosteroids and antifungal (or antiinfective) drugs. A nonsystemic (topical) antifungal agent, such as nystatin, is the recommended therapy for oral thrush. Several agents are listed in Table 8-7. Some preparations are combination products, containing both an antifungal (e.g., nystatin) and triamcinolone (a corticosteroid). Frequently, combination products (e.g., Mycolog II, Myconel, Mytrex F) are recommended during the first 3 days or so when the pain is most severe. After the pain has subsided, the woman and her infant complete the 14-day treatment with the noncortisone preparation (e.g., nystatin only). Clotrimazole has also been used successfully.[67] Emphasize to the woman the importance of completing the treatment for herself and her infant, even after the symptoms have diminished or disappeared.

Instruct the mother to apply topical agents to the nipple and areola and to the infant's oral area as described in Table 8-7. It is not necessary to remove the cream before breastfeeding. Antifungals or antiinfective creams (or lotions) are not absorbed through the mucous membranes. Furthermore, these same drugs are safe for and prescribed for infants. Corticosteroid preparations may be slightly absorbed, but these do not need to be removed before feeding, either. Advise the mother that she may apply an antifungal cream to the infant's diaper area with her fingers after each diaper change. She must, however, wash her hands well after touching the infected area.

In the United States, a less common but increasingly popular treatment is gentian violet, a purple dye that can be applied using a cotton swab to "paint" the inside of the infant's mouth and the nipple/areola complex. Suggest that the mother use a bib when applying this to the infant's mouth, since it will stain clothing.

Systemic treatments, such as fluconazole (Diflucan) are generally prescribed when candidiasis has been resistant to topical medications. Although the safety of the concentration of this drug in the milk has been questioned,[68] the dosage that the infant would receive from the mother's milk is less than what would be prescribed for the infant.

Do not assume that the problem is resolved just because the therapy has begun; all parties must be reevaluated to make sure that signs and symptoms do not persist. Sometimes, a medication that was initially effective, or that was effective during the first episode, loses its effectiveness with subsequent episodes. The goal is to conquer the fungus by prompt, simultaneous treatment of all parties involved.

Breast Abscess

Description and Etiology

An abscess can occur anywhere on the body. Typically, it is a pus-filled cavity that is surrounded by inflamed tissue. The inflammation is a localized infection, usually staphylococcal. Less frequently, it may be caused by *Streptococcus*.[69]

COMMON TREATMENTS FOR CANDIDIASIS ASSOCIATED WITH BREASTFEEDING*

Drug	How Supplied	Dosage Range and/or Frequency	Drug Administration and Teaching Responsibilities
Gentian violet	Solution	Mother: use 0.5% or 1% solution Infant: use 0.5% or 1% solution	Caution that using a solution stronger than 1% or too frequent applications can irritate or ulcerate the infant's oral mucosa or the mother's nipple/areolar skin Stains skin and clothing Suggest disposable breast pads to avoid clothing stains
Nystatin (Nilstat)	Oral suspension	Infant: apply as directed, usually qid	Apply oral suspensions to infant's cheeks, gum line, and tongue Hold infant snugly while applying medicine, since it creates initial discomfort in the oral mucosa Use one cotton-tipped applicator for one side of the mouth; do not reinsert the applicator into the bottle; use a clean applicator to apply the medication to the other side
Nystatin (Mycostatin)	Cream	Mother: apply liberally to nipple/areolar area bid after breastfeeding	Instruct mother to apply this liberally to her nipple/areolar area after breastfeeding Wait 10 minutes before replacing bra It is not necessary to remove this cream from nipples before the infant breastfeeds
Clotrimazole (Lotrimin)	Cream, lotion, topical solution	Mother: 1%; apply to nipple/areolar area liberally bid after breastfeeding	Emphasize importance of continuing this antifungal treatment for a total of 14 days; reassess mother and infant after 4 weeks Instruct mother to apply cream liberally to her nipple/areolar area It is not necessary to remove this cream from nipples before the infant breastfeeds
Myconazole (Monistat-Derm)	Cream	Mother: apply to nipple/areolar area liberally bid after breastfeeding	Emphasize importance of continuing this antifungal treatment for the prescribed treatment period Instruct mother to apply cream liberally to her nipple/areolar area after breastfeeding It is not necessary to remove this cream from nipples before the infant breastfeeds
Nystatin and triamcinolone (Mycolog II)	Cream	Mother: apply to nipple/areolar area liberally bid or tid after breastfeeding	Indicated for severe pain; this product is usually used for about 3 days; the therapy continues with nystatin only (14 days total) Instruct mother to apply cream liberally to her nipple/areolar area after each breastfeeding It is not necessary to remove this cream from nipples before the infant breastfeeds
Clotrimazole and betamethasone (Lotrisone)	Cream	Mother: apply liberally to nipple/areolar area bid after breastfeeding	Indicated for severe pain; this product is usually used for the first 3 days; the therapy continues with clotrimazole only (14 days total) Instruct mother to apply cream liberally to her nipple/areolar area It is not necessary to remove this cream from nipples before the infant breastfeeds
Fluconazole (Diflucan)	Tablet	As directed	This drug does pass into mother's milk, but the amount in milk is still less than what would be prescribed for an infant Emphasize to the mother that she should tell the pediatrician if she is taking fluconazole so that he can adjust the infant dosage accordingly
Fluconazole (Diflucan)	Oral suspension	6 mg/kg first day; 3 mg/kg thereafter for at least 2 weeks	May be given to the infant via dropper

*If the mother is also suffering from a vaginal yeast infection, she will need to see her primary caregiver for treatment.

Clinical Manifestation

Upon inspection, there is redness due to the blood accumulation at the site where the inflammatory process occurs. Swelling occurs due to formation of the pus. When interviewing the woman, ask about pain that she is experiencing, since the abscess is painful because of the pressure of the pus against the nerve tissue.

Treatments and Recommendations

For healing to occur, the abscess must drain. Encourage the woman to continue breastfeeding frequently, since emptying the ducts expedites the drainage. The milk is "clean" unless the abscess ruptures into the ducts.[2] Watch for signs and symptoms of infection in the infant, and refer him for medical treatment if indicated.

In most cases, antibiotics (see Chapter 9) are prescribed for the woman (and for the infant, if indicated). Other interventions may be needed as well. Sometimes a surgical drain is put in to get adequate drainage. In that case, breastfeeding can probably continue. The caveat here is that the drain must be far enough away so that it is not involved in the feeding process. Whether or not the infant breastfeeds, the important thing is to drain the ductal system as completely as possible when the breasts feel full.

If the physician orders cultures of the mother's milk, instruct her on the correct way to obtain a midstream "clean-catch" specimen. This process is fairly simple, with steps similar to those used to obtain a "clean-catch" specimen of urine. Instruct the woman to wash her hands vigorously with soap and water, then to rinse her breasts with plain water. She should initiate hand expression, then discard the first 3 to 5 ml of milk. A small sample should be expressed into a sterile container. Emphasize to her the importance of keeping her nipple well away from the cup so that sterility can be maintained. The specimen should then be capped (touching only the outside of the cap), labeled, and taken to the laboratory immediately.

Galactocele

A galactocele is a closed sac in or under the skin that is lined with epithelium and contains fluid or semisolid material. These are fairly uncommon and are believed to be caused by the blockage of a milk duct.[2] Inspection reveals a smooth, rounded, raised area; compressing the sac produces some milky fluid. The exact cause of a galactocele is unknown, but sometimes it can follow breast reduction surgery.[70]

Blisters

Blisters on the nipple are caused by poor positioning. These should be recognized early, and the infant assisted to open wide and achieve adequate latch-on.

PREEXISTING HEALTH PROBLEMS AND THEIR RELATIONSHIP TO BREASTFEEDING

Maternal Infections

Breastfeeding usually can be initiated and continue uninterrupted for most cases, as shown on Table 8-8. In most of these cases, recommendations in relation to breastfeeding and/or isolation are based on Lawrence[71] and the American Academy of Pediatrics' Red Book.[72] These directives should be incorporated into the hospital's infection control policy and/or unit policy or protocol. When these issues are addressed in a written document, the mother is more likely to have uninterrupted experiences of breastfeeding.

There are five classes of infectious organisms: (1) bacteria, (2) viruses, (3) fungi, (4) protozoa, and (5) helminths. Common infections and their relationship to the perinatal period are outlined briefly in the following sections.

T A B L E 8-8
TYPES OF INFECTIONS AND BREASTFEEDING SAFETY RECOMMENDATIONS

Type of Infection	Example/Problem	OK to Breastfeed in the U.S.?	Conditions/Comments
Bacterial	Acute infectious process, including: premature rupture of membranes; longer than 24 hours without fever and delivery of full-term or preterm infant	Yes	Respiratory, reproductive, gastrointestinal infections
	Maternal fever greater than 38° C twice, 4 hr apart, 24 hr before to 24 hr after delivery, or endometriosis; full-term or preterm infant	Yes	Infant should be treated with antibiotics
	Salmonella infection	Yes	Infant should be treated with antibiotics
	Shigella	Yes	If culture is negative
	Tuberculosis		
	• Mother with inactive disease	Yes	
	• Mother with active disease	No	No *until treatment is established*
Viral	HIV	No	Recommendation from Centers for Disease Control and Prevention and American Academy of Pediatrics
	Hepatitis		
	• Hepatitis A	Yes	As soon as mother receives gamma globulin
	• Hepatitis B	Yes	After infant receives HBIG, first dose of hepatitis B vaccine should be given before hospital discharge
	• Hepatitis C	Yes	If no co-infections (e.g., HIV)
	Venereal warts	Yes	Venereal warts have not been reported to occur on the breast; genital warts do not contraindicate breastfeeding
	Herpes viruses		
	• Cytomegalovirus	Yes	Passively transferred maternal antibodies in human milk make breastfeeding safe
	• Herpes simplex	Yes	Except if lesion is on breast
	• Varicella zoster (chicken pox)	Yes	As soon as mother becomes noninfectious
	• Epstein-Barr	Yes	
	Human T-cell leukemia virus type I	No	
Fungus	Candidiasis	Yes	Treatment for all parties is imperative
Protozoa	Toxoplasmosis	Yes	

Adapted from Lawrence RA. *A Review of Medical Benefits and Contraindications to Breastfeeding in the United States (Maternal and Child Health Technical Information Bulletin).* Arlington, VA: National Center for Education in Maternal and Child Health; 1997.

Bacteria

Staphylococcal and streptococcal infections are very common during the perinatal period. In general, staphylococcal and streptococcal infections do not preclude breastfeeding. Mothers whose membranes have been ruptured for more than 24 hours are especially vulnerable to infection. However, their infants should begin breastfeeding and continue uninterrupted.

Signs and symptoms of bacterial infections should be noted promptly. When assessing the mother for signs and symptoms of infection during the first few days after delivery, however, the nurse must recognize that an otherwise unexplained low-grade fever is not necessarily due to an infection; it may be associated with physiological engorgement. If maternal fever is greater than 38° C twice, artificially fed infants should be isolated from the mother, but breastfed infants should be with their mothers and should initiate and continue breastfeeding.

If a bacterial infection is confirmed, antibiotic therapy is started. Some hospital policies may require that the mother have therapeutic serum levels of the drug for at least 12 hours before the infant is allowed to go to the breast. Policies that require a greater number of hours are based on the needs of artificially fed infants, who do not have the advantage of immunities from their mothers as do the breastfed infants. Even if the severity of the infection is such that the mother needs to be isolated from other patients, she and her infant can usually remain together.

E. coli are usually the culprit in urinary tract infections, which are common in perinatal patients. These infections are self-contained; breastfeeding should be initiated and continue uninterrupted. Usually antibiotics that are safe for pediatric use are prescribed for the mother. Antibiotics for the mother work well but may cause diarrhea in the breastfeeding infant. Encouraging fluids, while important with any patient who has a urinary tract infection, is especially important with the lactating mother, since maternal fluids are lost through breastfeeding. Offering cranberry juice to the mother to acidify her urine is particularly helpful.

It is also important to remember that not all staphylococcal bacteria are pathogenic; staph is frequently found on the nipples.

Streptococcal infections can occur in postoperative wounds. Drainage or red streaking on the incision is likely to indicate a streptococcal infection, which requires medical management. Generally, these mothers are treated with antibiotics, and isolation from the infant is not indicated. However, strict hand washing by health care personnel and the mother is imperative.

Group B streptococcus (GBS) can occur in maternal endometritis, amnionitis, and urinary tract infection. Generally, penicillin is the recommended therapy. If the infant becomes infected, cultures of the milk are ordered; collect a sample using the technique described previously.

Viruses

Herpes

There are four types of herpes viruses: cytomegalovirus (CMV), herpes simplex virus (HSV), herpes varicella zoster virus (VZV), and Epstein-Barr virus. Implications related to breastfeeding are found on Table 8-8.

Hepatitis

There are several types of hepatitis; all are viral, but they differ in route of transmission, clinical course, and treatment. The three most common types are hepatitis A, B, and C. Hepatitis D and E have been recognized more recently and are less well understood.

HEPATITIS A

Hepatitis A is rarely transmitted vertically. (*Vertical transmission* means transfer from one generation to the next, through either the mother's milk or the placenta; *horizontal transmission* is the spread of infection by contact from one person to another, usually through contact with contaminated material.) Hepatitis A has a short incubation period, and in most cases requires little special care for the infant. Breastfeeding should be initiated and continue uninterrupted.

HEPATITIS B

Hepatitis B is transmitted vertically. If a woman has active hepatitis during the third trimester or at delivery, her infant should immediately receive HBIG at delivery. Rooming-in is in the best interest of all the patients on the unit, since this mother should not visit the nursery. She may, however, breastfeed the infant after he has been immunized with HBIG.

HEPATITIS C, D, AND E

These forms of hepatitis are not as well understood as hepatitis A and B. Currently, most experts recommend that infants with hepatitis C may breastfeed[72]; infants infected with hepatitis D and E should not.

Fungi

The main fungal infection that is encountered in breastfeeding mothers is candidiasis. Oral candidiasis—an overgrowth of *Candida* in the infant's mouth or on the mother's nipples—was discussed earlier in this chapter because of its direct link to breastfeeding. There is no need to isolate the infant from the mother; she may initiate and continue breastfeeding uninterrupted.

Protozoa

Toxoplasmosis is the most common protozoan affecting pregnant women. There is no need to isolate the infant from the mother; she may initiate and continue breastfeeding uninterrupted.

Alterations in Endocrine and Metabolic Function

Hormones play a significant role during both pregnancy and lactation. (See Chapter 3 for a more complete discussion.) Therefore, alterations in endocrine and metabolic function usually become more evident during those times. The readiness of the mammary gland is controlled largely by placental lactogen and prolactin.

Diabetes Mellitus

Diabetes mellitus does not preclude breastfeeding. While breastfeeding is usually initiated because of its benefits to the infant, this is an excellent example of how it also is beneficial to the mother. Prolactin maintains mammary gland insulin receptors to ensure anabolism—metabolism that converts simple substances into more complex compounds. Apparently, this hormone enhances the anabolic processes to bring about better diabetic control during lactation.

Studies have shown that breastfeeding is beneficial for both insulin-dependent diabetic mothers (IDDM) and gestational diabetic mothers. Insulin-dependent diabetic mothers who breastfeed exclusively have lower fasting glucose levels at 6 weeks postpartum (82 +/− 40 mg/dl) than do women who began but later stopped breastfeeding (145 +/− 37 mg/dl) or IDDM mothers who initially chose to bottle feed (120 +/− 30 mg/dl).[73] Gestational diabetics have improved glucose metabolism while breastfeeding (during the 4- to 12-week period), and fasting blood glucose levels are significantly lowered (93 +/− 13 vs. 98 +/− 17 mg/dl; $p = .0001$).[74] Furthermore, breastfeeding helps reduce or delay the onset of diabetes in subsequent pregnancies.[74]

There are differences in milk composition in women with IDDM, but this does not preclude breastfeeding. In IDDM, milk production and composition are altered by many factors, including method of delivery, feeding frequency, fetal condition, gestational age, mastitis incidence, metabolic control, and maternal dietary intake.[75] Good control of the woman's glucose status is important not only for her general well-being but also for lactation. It appears that poor metabolic control results in a delay of lactogenesis.[76]

Thyroid Disease

If the mother has hypothyroid disease, she may breastfeed. Usually, however, these women are taking thyroid replacement tablets at home, and they frequently forget to bring them along to the hospital or to tell the nurse during the excitement of childbearing. Women who are hypothyroid should be reminded to take their thyroid replacement tablet; otherwise, their milk production may be insufficient.

If the mother has hyperthyroid disease, she can breastfeed if the infant is monitored biochemically while the mother is taking thyroid preparations. Methimazole (Tapazole) and Thiouracil BF are contraindicated during breastfeeding. A minimal amount of propylthiouracil (PTU) reaches the milk because it is ionized and protein-bound.[77] Therefore, encourage breastfeeding but monitor the infant's T-4 and TSH levels.

Pituitary Dysfunction

Sheehan's syndrome can occur after severe postpartum hemorrhage. The hemorrhage causes necrosis of the pituitary and hypopituitarism. The pituitary gland, which secretes hormones associated with lactation, including prolactin, is particularly vulnerable to decreased vascular flow, and this results in mammary involution and lactation failure. Sheehan's syndrome occurs in about 0.01% to 0.02% of postpartum women and results in lactation failure.[2]

Galactorrhea means lactation not associated with childbirth or breastfeeding. The condition is sometimes a symptom of a pituitary gland dysfunction. It can also occur after reduction mammaplasty.[78]

Other Conditions

Eclampsia

Breastfeeding is not initiated when seizure precautions are in effect, when the maternal dose of phenobarbital is >360 mg/day, or until the case is reviewed by the physician. The mother may express her milk during this time. Whether the milk should be saved and given to the infant or discarded depends on the dosage of drugs that the mother is receiving and the discretion of the physician.

Diarrhea

If the newborn has diarrhea, it is best managed by breastfeeding. If the mother has diarrhea, breastfeeding may continue uninterrupted.

MAINTAINING ADEQUATE MILK SUPPLY

As a general rule, supply is generated in response to demand. It is important to recognize, however, that "demand" is more related to removing the milk than to frequency of simply being at the breast. (See Chapter 5 for complete explanation.) Only occasionally, it is difficult or impossible to achieve and maintain an adequate milk supply.

Primary Lactation Failure

This text uses the term *lactation failure*, in sharp contrast to *insufficient milk supply*. The former term is used to describe a situation whereby lactation is not possible because of some serious irreversible factor. The latter is used to describe some situation in which, with better breastfeeding management, milk supply could improve.

Insufficient glandular development is one possibility for lactation failure.[79] The three case studies presented show that there can be a primary, physiological basis for why some women cannot breastfeed. This condition, however, is thought to be extremely rare. It might be predicted by absence of prenatal breast changes or the absence of postpartum engorgement. Either or both of these findings warrant further investigation. If this diagnosis is made, help the woman to understand that the inability to lactate is not her "fault." Keep the focus on the mammary gland, not the breast, and help the woman to recognize that certain deficiencies occur in certain individuals—just as one woman may be born without a fully functioning pancreas, another can be born without a fully functioning mammary gland.

Placental retention is another cause of lactation failure. From early in their education, nurses are taught to observe for hemorrhage as a sign of placental retention. However, hemorrhage may not be the first sign of placental retention in all cases. Neifert and colleagues[80] showed that the first sign of retained placenta was related to lactation status. In the three cases reported, women did not experience breast engorgement and leaking of milk. I once took care of a 15-year-old primipara who had had a cesarean delivery for cephalopelvic disproportion. She had not chosen to breastfeed, so no one was paying much attention to her lactation status. On the third day postpartum, she passed a piece of placenta about the size of a small lemon. Retained placenta had occurred without the presence of hemorrhage. In both the documented and the anecdotal cases, there is a clear lesson to be learned: do not assume that hemorrhage is the only or first indicator of retained placenta. Include the woman's breasts as part of the overall assessment whether or not she is breastfeeding; they may provide useful information about her overall well-being.

Some other primary causes of lactation failure may exist. The impact of anemia on lactation is poorly understood, but some data suggest an association between anemia and milk supply.[81] Similarly, the role of sodium content in the milk is incompletely understood, but it appears that when elevated levels of sodium persist, lactogenesis is impaired and there is a high risk of failure.[82] Unilateral lactation failure after breast biopsy has been reported.[41]

INSUFFICIENT MILK SUPPLY

The phenomenon of insufficient milk supply is difficult to understand. Experts have generated frameworks based largely on the premise that physiological or emotional conditions or events contribute to insufficient milk supply.[2,83,84] These frameworks, while well researched and technically correct, have limited usefulness for the practicing nurse who continually hears mothers say that they "don't have enough milk." It is easy to take the mother's comment at face value, but this may or may not be the case. In clinical practice, it has become readily apparent that sometimes there is an *actual* insufficient milk supply (i.e., production of milk is insufficient), or the milk-ejection reflex is not functioning optimally. In most cases, however, mothers have a *perceived* insufficient milk supply; that is, lack of maternal motivation or understanding of basic lactation physiology leads them to believe that their supply is inadequate.[83]

The academic literature offers little to illuminate the clues that distinguish actual insufficient milk supply from perceived insufficient milk supply. This is an important distinction for the clinical nurse who is gathering both subjective and objective data from the mother. Clinical experience and research studies consistently substantiate that "not enough milk" is the primary concern of primiparas[85] and the reason for discontinuing breastfeeding.[86-91]

Actual and perceived insufficient milk supply are certainly interrelated. For purposes of clarity, however, this text will discuss them separately.

Insufficient Milk Supply: Actual

Hill and Humenick[84] describe insufficient milk supply in terms of potential determinants and indicators. They use the words *determinant* to mean a factor that is likely to lead to insufficient milk supply and *indicators* to mean those factors that can be observed and quantified. Potential determinants include both indirect and direct influences on milk production. Indicators include such factors as decreased infant weight gain and the need for increased supplementation. The framework, shown on Figure 8-16, reflects inad-

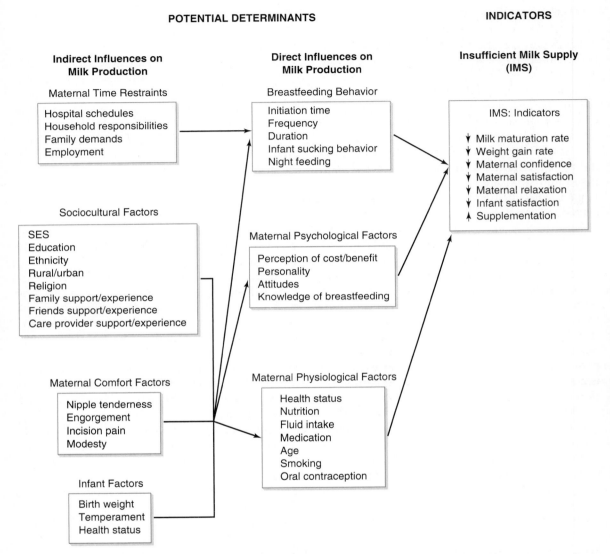

Fig. 8-16 Insufficient milk supply: potential determinants and indicators. *(From Hill PD, Humenick SS.* Insufficient milk supply. *Image J Nurs Sch 1989;21:145-148.)*

equate production, while a suboptimal milk-ejection reflex is dimly implied. Mothers are especially at risk for insufficient milk supply when they have low-birth-weight infants.[92]

Insufficient Milk Supply: Perceived

Two teams have delineated some important concepts about women's perceptions of having insufficient milk. Segura-Millan, Dewey, and Perez-Escamilla compiled several potential risk factors for perceived insufficient milk.[83] Theirs is a useful list, but many of the factors listed—such as hormonal contraceptives—are not necessarily limited to a perceived situation; these can indeed result in *actual* poor production.

Refining their earlier work, Hill and Aldag[93] described both determinant factors and potential indicator factors for "reported" insufficient milk supply. While the authors do not specify the possibility of perception, it is apparent that at least three out of five "determinants" in their study are closely linked to perceptions that mothers might have. Potential determinant factors were identified as maternal confidence, paternal support, maternal health, mother-in-law disapproval, and infant birth weight. Potential indicators included infant behavior factors (fussy, refused, poor feeder, poor weight gain), solid food factors, and formula factors (whether or not artificial milk was used and, if so, the pattern—"topping off" a feeding or completely replacing a feeding with artificial milk).

Insufficient Milk Supply, Actual or Perceived: A Management Strategy

Unfortunately, insufficient milk supply that is at first only perceived can rapidly turn into a real insufficient milk supply. This happens because mothers interpret their infants' behaviors (short sleep times or fussiness after eating) as a sign that they need more milk. To compensate, they introduce artificial milk. (Some mothers introduce sol-

ids before 8 weeks as well.) When the infant has artificial milk, he will suckle less frequently at the mother's breast, and, according to the law of supply and demand, her milk will indeed become insufficient.

Priorities for care are listed in Box 8-6. It is difficult to prioritize these, since the order of priority will be different depending on whether the problem is actual or perceived. Furthermore, how each mother reacts to the situation will also determine the priority order.

Instill Confidence in the Mother

In one study, 80% of the mothers expressed concern that they had an insufficient supply of milk.[83] Underlying these words are a number of self-doubts: Is my body capable of providing enough milk for my baby? Am I starving my baby? Is my milk good enough/rich enough for my baby? Can I really do this? Whether or not these doubts

---

Box 8-6

Priorities for Care: Insufficient Milk Supply

- Instill confidence in the mother.
- Determine whether problem is real or perceived.
- Identify associated nonreassuring signs.
- Initiate strategies to increase milk production.
- Enhance milk-ejection reflex, if indicated.
- Correct mismanagement of breastfeeding.
- Verify or initiate measures to achieve audible swallowing.
- Develop plan to overcome deviations noted on physical assessment.
- Note pathological conditions and refer the woman for medical help as appropriate.
- Help mother develop realistic expectations about infant's needs and behavior.
- Set a target date; contract with mother to continue breastfeeding until that date.
- Identify multiple sources of support.
- Counter negative messages.

C L I N I C A L   S C E N A R I O

Insufficient Milk Supply

At change-of-shift report, you hear that Mrs. H., G5 P5, had a spontaneous delivery about 36 hours ago, and has four breastfed children ranging in age from 2 to 12 at home. However, Mrs. H. is bottle feeding this newborn. You find it strange that she is bottle feeding after breastfeeding four other infants. What would you do, if anything?

Possible Strategy

Explore the situation further. Introduce yourself to Mrs. H., establish rapport with her, and when the time seems right, explore the issue with her. Use open-ended questions, such as: "Mrs. H., I see from your medical record that you have breastfed your other four children, and I was a little puzzled because I can remember very few mothers who bottle feed after they have breastfed their other babies. Are our records correct?" After this question, Mrs. H. will probably tell you that, indeed, she has elected to artificially feed this infant. If she does not elaborate, ask another open-ended question, for example, "Can you tell me a little about your last experience breastfeeding?" At this point, Mrs. H. will probably tell you her story. Each time she was pregnant, she made up her mind to breastfeed, but each time she had to give up after only a few days because the baby "wasn't getting enough milk." You are silently thinking that it is likely that a few days signals trouble—maybe milk transfer never happened. Rather than dwell on Mrs. H.'s past "mistakes," you try to capitalize on her commitment and give her confidence that this time can be different. It might be helpful to offer a response something like this: "Mrs. H., you are a very experienced mother, and I can see you really wanted to breastfeed each time that you had a baby. There are many ways to build an abundant supply of milk, and no better time to start than right now. See how your baby is sucking on his fist and turning his head toward you? I'll bet Jason would take your breast right now, and I'd be willing to show you some ways to get started building a good milk supply if you'd like to breastfeed."

Outcome

Like other examples in this book, Mrs. H. is real person. She eagerly agreed to put Jason to her breast, and in the process we talked about signs that indicated that milk transfer was occurring. She quickly observed, "I didn't know all those things last time, and wasn't sure I was doing it right." Mrs. H. gained confidence because she had more ways to reassure herself that it was going well; indeed, Jason suckled enthusiastically. His mother exclusively breastfed him for more than 6 months.

are verbalized, it is important to recognize that the mother needs self-confidence to succeed not only with breastfeeding but also with mothering. Mothers are more likely to have perceived insufficient milk supply if they have ambivalent feelings about breastfeeding.[86] Provide continuous, positive feedback to the woman about reassuring, objective signs that lactation is going well when it is. If it is not going well, reassure her that she has done the right thing by coming for help and that most breastfeeding problems are transient and solvable.

Determine If Problem Is Actual or Perceived

Having an actual problem means that physiological factors such as inadequate production, inad-equate ejection, or poor milk transfer are present. An "actual" insufficient milk supply is either physiological or functional. Physiological means that the infant's needs are greater than the amount of milk synthesized by the mammary gland—this is rare. Functional problems are usually related to milk transfer; the amount of milk synthesized would be adequate for the infant's needs, but it is not being transferred.

Identify Nonreassuring Signs

If the supply is truly insufficient, it will be accompanied by signs of insufficient production or suboptimal milk ejection. For example, a physiological problem exists when enlargement of the breasts during pregnancy has not been noted and engorgement in the postpartum period has not occurred. These women have *primary lactation failure*. Mothers may have some, but not enough, milk for their infants. Mothers who do not have signs of a functioning milk-ejection reflex or whose infants are not making adequate weight gains or do not have adequate output are likely to have an insufficient milk supply, due mostly to inadequate *milk transfer*. A physiological problem also exists when the infant's needs are great or capabilities are few; this would include infants who cannot suckle well or those with increased basal needs (see Chapters 6 and 7). These statements are rather generalized, but all are objective, quantifiable signs that, when absent, constitute an actual, not perceived, problem.

Initiate Strategies to Increase Milk Production
Strategies to increase milk production are many and varied, depending on the cause. Mothers whose infants have a weak or inadequate suck may need to express milk after feedings to adequately empty their breasts. Offering the breast to the infant more frequently may or may not help to increase supply. It will help only if the infant is swallowing; that is, if milk is not transferred, the mere presence of the infant is insufficient. Sometimes, mothers of multiples will have a low milk supply because one or more infants are not suckling at the breast for all feedings. The best strategy in this case is to get all of the infants to the breast for each feeding. If this is not possible, increase the frequency of hand or pump expression.

Enhance Milk-Ejection Reflex
Several strategies will help elicit a better milk-ejection reflex. Warm packs or warm showers before the breastfeeding session, massaging the breasts prior to feeding, or relaxation techniques (quiet room, imagery, soft music) are often effective.

Correct Mismanagement of Breastfeeding
The strategy that is most often needed is to correct general mismanagement of breastfeeding. Various forms of mismanagement have contributed to insufficient milk supply. For the newborn, feeding intervals of greater than 2 or 3 hours, taking the infant off the breast before he has completely finished, switch-nursing (rapid switching of the infant from one breast to the other during one feeding), and using nipple shields are prime contributors to the problem. Absence of audible swallowing and skipping night feedings are among the most frequent mismanagement occurrences.

Similarly, women are often given recommendations to increase their milk supply that are useless. The most common recommendation is to drink more fluids. However, merely increasing maternal fluids does not increase milk volume.[94,95] (See Figure 4-2.) A variety of galactogues—substances that are thought to increase milk supply, such as beer or brewer's yeast—may help a little.

Verify or Initiate Measures to Achieve Swallowing
The concept of audible swallowing cannot be overemphasized! Hearing the infant swallow is an objective, reassuring sign that milk is being produced, milk is being ejected, and milk is being transferred into the infant's digestive tract. Not being able to verify audible swallowing is always a worrisome sign; the woman has or will have an insufficient milk supply. (The converse is not true, however. The mother may be synthesizing plenty of milk, her ejection reflex may be vigorous, and the infant may be swallowing milk, but if he has a high need, the mother's supply may indeed be insufficient to meet his need.)

Develop Plan to Overcome Deviations
While performing physical assessment of the breasts, note problems that may impede breastfeeding success. These are discussed at length earlier in the chapter.

Note Maternal Health and Health Habits
Maternal health and health habits can influence milk supply. Anemia has been implicated as a

possible cause of insufficient milk supply.[81] Increased stress, fatigue, and infection are possible causes. Smoking also decreases milk supply, and smokers are more likely to report an insufficient supply of milk than nonsmokers.[96]

Help Mother Develop Realistic Expectations

Frequently, mothers cite infant fussiness as the reason they think they do not have enough milk, or as the reason they introduce artificial milk or even solids. Review with the mother the normal sleep-wake cycles, the stomach capacity of the infant, and the signs and symptoms of hunger and satiety (see Chapter 6).

Set a Target Date

It is often helpful to refocus the mother so that she can see the proverbial light at the end of the tunnel. Many mothers can't see themselves reaching their 6-month goal. Therefore, I often suggest that they circle a day on the calendar about 2 or 3 weeks from the time they call. Toward the end of the conversation, I say, "Circle Day X on your calendar. Do not allow yourself to quit until then. Also write some reward for yourself on the calendar for Day X—a date with your husband, a new outfit, or a new gadget for your kitchen—some treat you would enjoy. If you feel tempted to stop breastfeeding before that date, call me; if you make it to that date, give yourself that reward. Celebrate!" This approach has worked for several mothers. It gives them an opportunity to achieve a short-term goal, and it reassures them that support is available. My part of the contract is to provide continuous reassurance during that time. Their part of the contract is to continue breastfeeding. This is not equivalent to saying that I want them to breastfeed for only a short time. It simply helps them to overcome the urge to stop in the short run; in the long run, all of those with whom I have used this technique have continued to breastfeed for many months. The key is to get them over an obstacle when their confidence and determination are low.

Identify Multiple Sources of Support

A good strategy when talking with mothers about breastfeeding problems in general, and this one in particular, is to get them to identify at least three sources of support. (The more, the better.) One support person, however committed, is not enough. Even the most supportive person can be unavailable for various reasons. Therefore, the mother needs to quickly identify another she can call for support when she needs it.

Counter Negative Messages

Mothers encounter negative messages at the individual and cultural level. Nurses cannot control the behavior of others; they can only control their own behaviors and responses. Therefore, give multiple, clear, positive messages about breastfeeding in general. Respect the cultural beliefs of the woman and her family, but avoid negative messages and reiterate reassuring messages about the woman's capabilities in terms of providing enough milk for her infant.

Oversupply

Occasionally, mothers can have an oversupply of milk.[97] While this would be a happy situation for most, some mothers seem baffled by it. The mother with an oversupply of milk is particularly vulnerable to milk stasis. Therefore, observe her for signs and symptoms of inflammation or infection. Advise her to breastfeed with the infant somewhat above the nipple because this will slow down a quick flow of milk. Refer her to a donor milk bank if she wishes to donate unused milk (see Chapter 11).

Relactation/Induced Lactation

In most cases, lactation commences immediately after the birth of the infant. Sometimes, however, this is not the case. A woman may wish to lactate for a child whom she has not borne; lactation is then induced. In other situations, the woman may have been unwilling or unable to initiate lactation immediately after the birth of the infant. In either case, some guiding principles provide a foundation of care.

Explore the Mother's Desire to Breastfeed

Open a dialogue with the woman about why she wants to breastfeed. Asking the "why" question, however, must be done in such a way that she does not feel she needs to defend her position. It would be more useful to say, "You seem excited about adopting a baby, and just as excited about the possibility of breastfeeding. Tell me a little about how you heard about breastfeeding adopted babies and what you found most appealing about it." Or, if the woman recently gave birth but did not initiate breastfeeding immediately thereafter, one approach might be: "I'm delighted to hear you'd like to breastfeed Sara. It would be helpful to me if you could tell me a little about how she was fed right after birth, and how you felt about that." In this way, it is easier to determine if breastfeeding was started and stopped, or if it was never started at all. If it was never started, in recounting the details of what happened, the woman will give some indications about whether the infant was not breastfed because she chose not to do so or because circumstances were such that she was unable to.

Like any other breastfeeding mother, this mother will need to be confident and committed in order for breastfeeding to be successful. Explore with her the capabilities and limitations related to the potential breastfeeding experience. Her capabilities and limitations, as well as those of the infant, need careful consideration. The younger the infant, the more likely the success. One of my former patients had a 52-day-old infant when she decided to breastfeed. This can be done, but this woman will have to put forth more effort and wait longer to realize success than the woman who decides to start lactating for a 7-day-old infant. As a general rule, the time it takes to establish lactation is about the same as the hiatus between the time of delivery and the time stimulation is initiated.

The mother also has capabilities and limitations in this situation. The nullipara is less likely to be successful than the woman who has lactated before.[98] The mother who can devote a fair amount of time to stimulating her breasts, either with suckling the infant or using the electric breast pump (or both), is more likely to be successful than one who has time constraints.

Help the Mother to Establish Realistic Expectations

In exploring the woman's motives for breastfeeding, it is also important to understand her goals. The motive, really, is why she wants to breastfeed (i.e., a reflection of her decision-making *process*). The goal is the *outcome* she hopes to obtain from the decision. The woman who hopes to obtain a warm, close relationship with her infant will surely be rewarded. Women who focus on the relationship, rather than on the volume of milk produced, are more likely to evaluate their experience positively.[99] The woman who wishes for her infant to have nothing except her milk—for whatever reason—may be in for a disappointment.

Some literature has been encouraging; in one study, 89% of the women who had not given birth to the infant they were breastfeeding were successful.[100] In many cases, however, this may not happen. The mother may not be able to lactate well enough to provide for her infant without the help of banked donor milk or artificial milk.

Determine the Infant's Prior Experience

When interviewing the mother, the infant's prior experience will soon become evident. Any infant who has been fed with bottles only may indeed have difficulty trying to breastfeed.

Initiate Strategies to Increase Milk Supply

First, it is imperative that the woman have a basic understanding of the lactation process, the same as any other mother. She also will need to initiate strategies to increase her milk supply. The strategies listed in Box 8-5 should be helpful.

Seek Support From Family and Health Care Team

More than other women, this woman's family must provide strong support for her decision to breastfeed. The entire health care team must support her decision as well. The nurse is in an ideal position to coordinate these efforts. Not everyone will agree with the mother's decision or her rationale; they may need some help in realizing that feeding is part of mothering and that this value in some way drives the woman's desire to breastfeed.

Teach Mother Signs of Adequate Infant Intake

The infant who is breastfed under these circumstances is vulnerable to dehydration and/or failure to thrive. Provide the mother with a list of reassuring and nonreassuring signs, as found in Chapter 5.

CONTRAINDICATIONS TO BREASTFEEDING AND LACTATION

Usually, breastfeeding is best for both the mother and the infant. In relatively few circumstances the primary health care provider may determine that breastfeeding is contraindicated because it poses a safety threat for the infant. Even in those cases where breastfeeding is contraindicated, it may be contraindicated for only a temporary period, rather than indefinitely. See Box 8-7 for a

Box 8-7

Priorities for Care When Breastfeeding Is Contraindicated or Temporarily Halted

- When in doubt, allow the infant to suckle, at least until the condition in question is confirmed as a strict contraindication to breastfeeding.
- Clarify any misunderstandings between the patient, her physician, and the staff about whether breastfeeding is truly contraindicated.
- In very few circumstances, breastfeeding is strictly prohibited. (See Table 8-8.) In most situations, cessation of breastfeeding, if ordered, is only temporary.
- Explain to the mother, in simple terms, why breastfeeding is contraindicated at this time. Focus on the safety of her infant and avoid any implication that her milk is "dirty" or that she has done something "bad."
- Initiate and update information about when breastfeeding may resume.
- Advocate rooming-in. Isolation of the mother or the infant is seldom indicated, and should be based on current research that supports the agency's infection control policy.
- Collaborate with the mother and the physician to develop a plan for adequate infant nutrition for both the long and the short term; in most cases, expressed milk is best (mother's own milk or banked donor milk), while in a few cases artificial milk may be required.

description of priorities for care when breastfeeding is contraindicated. Usually, breastfeeding is contraindicated because of some infectious diseases or because of certain medications the mother is ingesting.

Infectious Diseases

Whether or not infectious disease contraindicates breastfeeding depends on two factors: transmission and associated medication. In some cases, breastfeeding is absolutely contraindicated; in other cases, it is only temporarily contraindi-

Box 8-8
Practical Recommendations for HIV and Human Milk

- Discourage women in the United States from breastfeeding if HIV has been *confirmed*.
- If HIV has been confirmed, explain benefits of donor milk for these infants (see Chapter 11).
- Refer to your agency's infection control manual to gain more information on "body fluids."
- Human milk is not on the OSHA list of "body fluids" that transmit HIV.
- Gloves are not *required* when in contact with women's nipples, but gloves are *recommended* to prevent transmission of microorganisms from patient to patient.
- Gloves are not required when handling human milk (e.g., pouring human milk from one container to another).
- Washing hands, before and after patient contact, is the most important infection control action.

cated. Table 8-8 describes cases that will guide clinical management. Women in the United States who are HIV-positive should not be encouraged to breastfeed.[101] However, health care workers have questions about the safety of human milk that may be contaminated with HIV. Some practical recommendations are given in Box 8-8.

Drugs

There are few prescription drugs that are strictly prohibited during lactation. Illicit drugs are prohibited during breastfeeding (see Chapter 9). In most cases, it is safe to administer the first dose of a drug to the mother and allow the infant to breastfeed while simultaneously checking with the physician to get the go-ahead for breastfeeding. In some situations, however, even one dose of the medication strictly prohibits breastfeeding. See Chapter 9 for a more detailed discussion.

Other

Some environmental conditions also prohibit breastfeeding. Environmental contaminants such as herbicides and pesticides usually do not preclude breastfeeding. Heavy metals and radionuclides are contraindicated.[71]

SUMMARY

Assessment of the mother's physical well-being is essential for good breastfeeding management. Preexisting problems affecting either the breast itself or the woman's overall health can influence the breastfeeding experience. Problems can also develop while the woman is lactating. In either case, special strategies can be used to help the woman breastfeed for as along as she wishes. Insufficient milk supply and sore nipples are the most frequently mentioned concerns; neither should be a consequence of breastfeeding, and both are usually temporary and solvable. Furthermore, there are very few situations where breastfeeding is contraindicated. In most cases, then, the nurse can provide sensitive counseling and special strategies to help the woman attain her goals related to breastfeeding.

References

1. Neifert M. Breastfeeding after breast surgical procedure or breast cancer. *NAACOGS Clin Issu Perinat Womens Health Nurs* 1992;3:673-682.
2. Lawrence RA. *Breastfeeding: A Guide for the Medical Profession.* 4th ed. St. Louis: Mosby; 1994.
3. Thompson J, Wilson S. *Health Assessment for Nursing Practice.* St. Louis: Mosby; 1996.
4. Neifert MR, Seacat JM. Medical management of successful breast-feeding. *Pediatr Clin North Am* 1986;33:743-762.

5. Hunt MJ, Salisbury EL, Grace J, Armati R. Black breast milk due to minocycline therapy. *Br J Dermatol* 1996;134:943-944.

6. Terrill PJ, Stapleton MJ. The inverted nipple: to cut the ducts or not? *Br J Plast Surg* 1991;44:372-377.

7. Hytten FE. Clinical and chemical studies in human lactation. *Br Med J* 1954:175-182.

8. Alexander JM, Grant AM, Campbell MJ. Randomised controlled trial of breast shells and Hoffman's exercises for inverted and non-protractile nipples. *Br Med J* 1992;304(6833):1030-1032.

9. The MAIN Trial Collaborative Group. Preparing for breast feeding: treatment of inverted and non-protractile nipples in pregnancy. *Midwifery* 1994;10:200-214.

10. Clum D, Primomo J. Use of silicone nipple shield with premature infants. *J Hum Lact* 1996;12:287.

11. Brigham M. Mothers' reports of the outcome of nipple shield use. *J Hum Lact* 1996;12:291.

12. Bodley V, Powers D. Long-term nipple shield use: a positive perspective. *J Hum Lact* 1996;12:301.

13. Wilson-Clay B. Clinical use of silicone nipple shields. *J Hum Lact* 1996;12:279.

14. Woolridge MW, Baum JD, Drewett RF. Effect of a traditional and of a new nipple shield on sucking patterns and milk flow. *Early Hum Dev* 1980;4:357-364.

15. Jackson DA, Woolridge MW, Imong SM, et al. The automatic sampling shield: a device for sampling suckled breast milk. *Early Hum Dev* 1987;15:295-306.

16. Auerbach KG. The effect of nipple shields on maternal milk volume. *J Obstet Gynecol Neonatal Nurs* 1990;19:419-427.

17. Hoffman JB. A suggested treatment for inverted nipples. *Am J Obstet Gynecol* 1953;66:346-348.

18. Bremme K, Eneroth P, Kindahl H. 15-Keto-13, 14-dihydroprostaglandin F_{2a}, and prostaglandin E_2 or oxytocin therapy for labor induction. *J Perinat Med* 1987;15:143-151.

19. Kesaree N, Banapurmath CR, Banapurmath S, Shamanur K. Treatment of inverted nipples using a disposable syringe. *J Hum Lact* 1993;9:27-29.

20. Skoog T. Surgical correction of inverted nipples. *J Am Med Wom Assoc* 1965;20:931-935.

21. Seidel HM, Ball JW, Dains JE, Benedict GW. *Mosby's Guide to Physical Examination*. 3rd ed. St. Louis: Mosby; 1995.

22. Canter JW, Oliver GC, Zaloudek CJ. Surgical diseases of the breast during pregnancy. *Clin Obstet Gynecol* 1983;26:853-864.

23. Rodger A, Corbett PJ, Chetty U. Lactation after breast-conserving therapy, including radiation therapy, for early breast cancer. *Radiother Oncol* 1989;15:243-244.

24. Higgins S, Haffty BG. Pregnancy and lactation after breast-conserving therapy for early stage breast cancer. *Cancer* 1994;73:2175-2180.

25. Tralins AH. Lactation after conservative breast surgery combined with radiation therapy. *Am J Clin Oncol* 1995;18:40-43.

26. Varsos G, Yahalom J. Lactation following conservation surgery and radiotherapy for breast cancer. *J Surg Oncol* 1991;46:141-144.

27. Ulmer HU. Lactation after conserving therapy of breast cancer? *Int J Radiat Oncol Biol Phys* 1988;15:512-513.

28. Rostom AY. Failure of lactation following radiotherapy for breast cancer. *Int J Radiat Oncol Biol Phys* 1988;15:511.

29. Hurst NM. Lactation after augmentation mammoplasty. *Obstet Gynecol* 1996;87:30-34.

30. Neifert M, DeMarzo S, Seacat J, Young D, Leff M, Orleans M. The influence of breast surgery, breast appearance, and pregnancy-induced breast changes on lactation sufficiency as measured by infant weight gain. *Birth* 1990;17:31-38.

31. Mandrekas AD, Zambacos GJ, Anastasopoulos A, Hapsas DA. Reduction mammaplasty with the inferior pedicle technique: early and late complications in 371 patients. *Br J Plast Surg* 1996;49:442-446.

32. Townsend PL. Nipple sensation following breast reduction and free nipple transplantation. *Br J Plast Surg* 1974;27:308-310.

33. DeCholnoky T. Augmentation mammaplasty: survey of complications in 10,941 patients by 265 surgeons. *Plast Reconstr Surg* 1970;45:573-577.

34. Song IC, Hunter JG. Galactorrhea after reduction mammaplasty. *Plast Reconstr Surg* 1989;84:857.

35. Schoch RM. Breast feeding after reduction mammoplasty. *J Nurse Midwifery* 1985;30:240.

36. Hughes V, Owen J. Is breast-feeding possible after breast surgery? *MCN Am J Matern Child Nurs* 1993;18:213-217.

37. Aboudib JH, de Castro CC, Coelho RS, Cupello AM. Analysis of late results in postpregnancy mammoplasty. *Ann Plast Surg* 1991;26:111-116.

38. Hatton M, Keleher KC. Breastfeeding after breast reduction mammoplasty. *J Nurse Midwifery* 1983;28:19-22.

39. Harris L, Morris SF, Freiberg A. Is breast feeding possible after reduction mammaplasty? *Plast Reconstr Surg* 1992;89:836-839.

40. Hugill JV. Lactation following breast augmentation: a third case. *Plast Reconstr Surg* 1991; 87:806-807.

41. Day TW. Unilateral failure of lactation after breast biopsy. *J Fam Pract* 1986;23:161-162.

42. Findlay PA, Gorrell CR, d'Angelo T, Glatstein E. Lactation after breast radiation. *Int J Radiat Oncol Biol Phys* 1988;15:511-512.

43. Newton NR, Newton M. Relationship of ability to breastfeed and maternal attitudes toward breast feeding. *Pediatrics* 1950;5:869-875.

44. Newton N. Nipple pain and nipple damage. *J Pediat* 1952;4:411-423.

45. Ziemer MM, Pigeon JG. Skin changes and pain in the nipple during the 1st week of lactation. *J Obstet Gynecol Neonatal Nurs* 1993;22:247-256.

46. Woolridge MW. Aetiology of sore nipples. *Midwifery* 1986;2:172-176.

47. Gunther M. Sore nipples: causes and prevention. *Lancet* 1945;249:590-593.

48. Medoff-Cooper B, Weininger S, Zukowsky K. Neonatal sucking and clinical assessment tool: preliminary findings. *Nurs Res* 1989;38:162-165.

49. Hewat RJ, Ellis DJ. A comparison of the effectiveness of two methods of nipple care. *Birth* 1987;14:41-45.

50. Ziemer MM, Paone JP, Schupay J, Cole E. Methods to prevent and manage nipple pain in breastfeeding women. *West J Nurs Res* 1990;12:732-743.

51. deCarvalho M, Robertson S, Klaus MH. Does the duration and frequency of early breastfeeding affect nipple pain? *Birth* 1984;11:81-84.

52. Gosha JL, Tichy AM. Effect of a breast shell on postpartum nipple pain: an exploratory study. *J Nurse Midwifery* 1988;33:74-77.

53. Kearney MH, Cronenwett LR, Barrett JA. Breast-feeding problems in the first week postpartum. *Nurs Res* 1990;39:90-95.

54. L'Esperance C. Pain or pleasure: the dilemma of early breastfeeding. *Birth Fam J* 1980;7:21-25.

55. Storr GB. Prevention of nipple tenderness and breast engorement in the postpartal period. *J Obstet Gynecol Neonatal Nurs* 1988;17:203-209.

56. Pugh LC, Buchko BL, Bishop BA, Cochran JF, Smith LR, Lerew DJ. A comparison of topical agents to relieve nipple pain and enhance breastfeeding. *Birth* 1996;23:88-93.

57. L'Esperance C, Frantz K. Time limitation for early breastfeeding. *J Obstet Gynecol Neonatal Nurs* 1985;14:114-118.

58. Newton M, Newton N. Postpartum engorement of the breast. *Am J Obstet Gynecol* 1951;61:664-667.

59. Moon JL, Humenick SS. Breast engorgement: contributing variables and variables amenable to nursing intervention. *J Obstet Gynecol Neonatal Nurs* 1989;18:309-315.

60. Hill PD, Humenick SS. The occurrence of breast engorgement. *J Hum Lact* 1994;10:79-86.

61. Nikodem VC, Danziger D, Gebka N, Gulmezoglu AM, Hofmeyr GJ. Do cabbage leaves prevent breast engorgement? a randomized, controlled study. *Birth* 1993;20:61-64.

62. Devereux WP. Acute puerperal mastitis: evaluation of its management. *Am J Obstet Gynecol* 1970;108:78-81.

63. Riordan JM, Nichols FH. A descriptive study of lactation mastitis in long-term breastfeeding women. *J Hum Lact* 1990;6:53-58.

64. Tanguay KE, McBean MR, Jain E. Nipple candidiasis among breastfeeding mothers: case-control study of predisposing factors. *Can Fam Physician* 1994;40:1407-1413.

65. Hancock KF, Spangler AK. There's a fungus among us! *J Hum Lact* 1993;9:179-180.

66. Amir LH. *Candida* and the lactating breast: predisposing factors. *J Hum Lact* 1991;7:177-181.

67. Johnstone HA, Marcinak JF. Candidiasis in the breastfeeding mother and infant. *J Obstet Gynecol Neonatal Nurs* 1990;19:171-173.

68. Force RW. Fluconazole concentrations in breast milk. *Pediatr Infect Dis J* 1995;14:235-236.

69. Rench MA, Baker CJ. Group B streptococcal breast abscess in a mother and mastitis in her infant. *Obstet Gynecol* 1989;73(5, pt 2):875-877.

70. Bronson DL. Galactorrhea after reduction mammaplasty. *Plast Reconstr Surg* 1989;83:580.

71. Lawrence RA. *A Review of the Medical Benefits and Contraindications to Breastfeeding in the United States (Maternal and Child Health Technical Information Bulletin)*. Arlington, VA: National Center for Education in Maternal and Child Health; 1997.

72. AAP Committee on Infectious Disease. *Red Book*. Elk Grove Village, IL: American Academy of Pediatrics; 1994.

73. Ferris AM, Dalidowitz CK, Ingardia CM, et al. Lactation outcome in insulin-dependent diabetic women. *J Am Diet Assoc* 1988;88:317-322.

74. Kjos SL, Henry O, Lee RM, Buchanan TA, Mishell DR, Jr. The effect of lactation on glucose and lipid metabolism in women with recent gestational diabetes. *Obstet Gynecol* 1993;82:451-455.

75. Neubauer SH. Lactation in insulin-dependent diabetes. *Prog Food Nutr Sci* 1990;14:333-370.

76. Neubauer SH, Ferris AM, Chase CG, et al. Delayed lactogenesis in women with insulin-dependent diabetes mellitus. *Am J Clin Nutr* 1993;58:54-60.

77. Kampmann JP, Johansen K, Hansen JM, Helweg J. Propylthiouracil in human milk: revision of a dogma. *Lancet* 1980;1:736-737.

78. Bruck JC. Galactorrhea: a rare complication following reduction mammaplasty. *Ann Plast Surg* 1987;19:384-385.

79. Neifert MR, Seacat JM, Jobe WE. Lactation failure due to insufficient glandular development of the breast. *Pediatrics* 1985;76:823-828.

80. Neifert MR, McDonough SL, Neville MC. Failure of lactogenesis associated with placental retention. *Am J Obstet Gynecol* 1981;140:477-478.

81. Henly SJ, Anderson CM, Avery MD, Hills Bonczyk SG, Potter S, Duckett LJ. Anemia and insufficient milk in first-time mothers. *Birth* 1995;22:86-92.

82. Morton JA. The clinical usefulness of breast milk sodium in the assessment of lactogenesis. *Pediatrics* 1994;93:802-806.

83. Segura-Millan S, Dewey KG, Perez-Escamilla R. Factors associated with perceived insufficient milk in a low-income urban population in Mexico. *J Nutr* 1994;124:202-212.

84. Hill PD, Humenick SS. Insufficient milk supply. *Image J Nurs Sch* 1989;21:145-148.

85. Mogan J. A study of mothers' breastfeeding concerns. *Birth* 1986;13:104-108.

86. Hillervik-Lindquist C. Studies on perceived breast milk insufficiency: a prospective study in a group of Swedish women. *Acta Paediatr Scand Suppl* 1991;376:1-27.

87. Bevan ML, Mosley D, Solimano GR. Factors influencing breast feeding in an urban WIC program. *J Am Diet Assoc* 1984;84:563-567.

88. Gunn TR. The incidence of breast feeding and reasons for weaning. *N Z Med J* 1984;97:360-363.

89. Hawkins LM, Nichols FH, Tanner JL. Predictors of the duration of breastfeeding in low-income women. *Birth* 1987;14:204-209.

90. Hill PD. Effects of education on breastfeeding success. *Matern Child Nurs J* 1987;16:145-156.

91. Holt GM, Wolkind SN. Early abandonment of breast feeding: causes and effects. *Child Care Health Dev* 1983;9:349-355.

92. Hill PD, Hanson KS, Mefford AL. Mothers of low birthweight infants: breastfeeding patterns and problems. *J Hum Lact* 1994;10:169-176.

93. Hill PD, Aldag J. Potential indicators of insufficient milk supply syndrome. *Res Nurs Health* 1991;14:11-19.

94. Dusdieker LB, Booth BM, Stumbo PJ, Eichenberger JM. Effect of supplemental fluids on human milk production. *J Pediatr* 1985;106:207-211.

95. Dusdieker LB, Stumbo PJ, Booth BM, Wilmoth RN. Prolonged maternal fluid supplementation in breast-feeding. *Pediatrics* 1990;86:737-740.

96. Hill PD, Aldag JC. Smoking and breastfeeding status. *Res Nurs Health* 1996;19:125-132.

97. Livingstone V. Too much of a good thing: Maternal and infant hyperlactation syndromes. *Can Fam Physician* 1996;42:89-99.

98. Auerbach KG, Avery JL. Induced lactation: a study of adoptive nursing by 240 women. *Am J Dis Child* 1981;135:340-343.

99. Auerbach KG, Avery JL. Relactation: a study of 366 cases. *Pediatrics* 1980;65:236-242.

100. Nemba K. Induced lactation: a study of 37 non-puerperal mothers. *J Trop Pediatr* 1994;40:240-242.

101. American Academy of Pediatrics Committee on Pediatric AIDS. Human milk, breastfeeding, and transmission of human immunodeficiency virus in the United States. *Pediatrics* 1995;96:977-979.

9

The Nurse's Role in Drug Therapy During Breastfeeding and Lactation

Very frequently, discussions about the use of drugs while breastfeeding focus on the safety of the drug. Yet only those who have prescriptive privileges—physicians, nurse-practitioners, or others—can make the final determination of safety. In most situations the nurse must have confidence that the clinician prescribing the drug determined that the benefits outweigh the risks. But the nurse is then faced with such questions as: When should I question the safety of a drug that has been prescribed? What side effects should I anticipate and observe for? When is the best time to administer the drug? How can I become a patient advocate and facilitate patient education? What strategies can I use to minimize drug risk and exposure?

The purpose of this chapter is to help the nurse who does not have prescriptive privileges to assume appropriate responsibility with respect to drug administration for the lactating mother and her infant. Those who have prescriptive privileges should refer to the medical reference books listed in the resources section at the end of this chapter.

NURSE'S ROLE

Over the years, the role of the nurse has changed dramatically. However, medication administration has been and continues to be one of the most common responsibilities that the nurse must assume. Unfortunately, however, the nurse's role with respect to administering medication to the breastfeeding mother-infant dyad has been omitted from most nursing school curricula. As a result, nurses can be easily confused by what they are supposed to do about a lactating mother and her breastfed infant.

The nurse's responsibility to the lactating mother and her breastfed infant is in some respects not unlike her responsibility to nonlactating women, or to artificially fed infants. The nurse's primary responsibility for drugs focuses on patient teaching, patient advocacy, and ensuring safety by administering the drug in a way that achieves optimal therapeutic and minimal adverse effects.

Patient Advocacy

Frequently, one of two situations exists where the nurse needs to become an advocate for the breastfeeding mother. The first is the situation where a drug that will interfere with breastfeeding or cause potential harm for the infant has been or may be prescribed for the lactating mother. This is likely to occur in major medical centers where multiple specialists may be involved in the woman's care, and some may be unaware that she is breastfeeding. In this case, the nurse needs to coordinate communication and become an advocate for the patient's safety. Ideally, the situation can be avoided by noting in a conspicuous place—for example, on the front of her medical record—that the woman is breastfeeding.

More commonly, however, the reverse situation occurs. Very frequently, drugs are withheld or breastfeeding is interrupted by some member of the interdisciplinary team who is well intentioned but ill informed. In this case, the nurse needs to provide data that show that the drug can be safely given during breastfeeding and lactation. The common approach of "the drug might be harmful so let's stop breastfeeding" is unacceptable, since it perpetuates the erroneous notion that the benefits of artificial milk outweigh the benefits of human milk. As the next section explains, very few drugs are actually contraindicated during breastfeeding. In this case, therefore, the nurse needs to become an advocate for helping the woman to get the medication she needs and continue breastfeeding until it has been shown that the risk outweighs the benefit, which in most cases it does not.

Patient Teaching Responsibilities

Perhaps the first and foremost teaching responsibility is to assure lactating mothers that a drug has not been prescribed without careful thought and consideration of the risks and benefits involved. Furthermore, it is helpful to abolish the myth that the breast is like a sieve. Although nearly all drugs enter the milk, the quantity is usually very small. Hence, there may be little, if any, adverse effect on the infant. Although this is not true in all cases, it may be reassuring for the mother to know that the number of drugs generally recognized as safe during lactation far outnumbers those that are dangerous or absolutely contraindicated.

Beyond this, however, the mother needs to be informed of the drug's effects on her milk production and her infant. She also needs to be aware of the effect of substances such as caffeine and nicotine, as well as over-the-counter drugs.

Effects of the Drug on Milk Production

Although some drugs may not be "harmful" to the infant, they may cause the mother's milk to decrease in volume. If the mother takes these drugs during lactation, the infant should be carefully monitored for sufficient weight gain.

Smoking has been listed as a contraindication to breastfeeding by the American Academy of Pediatrics (AAP).[1] Smoking reduces milk volume but also has other harmful effects on both the mother and the infant. Counseling during the prenatal period should be aimed at helping the mother to quit smoking while she is still pregnant. Chapter 4 also discusses smoking during breastfeeding.

Lactating women may wish to resume their use of artificial birth control. For the most part, artificial birth control methods do not affect milk supply. (See section later in this chapter on commonly prescribed drugs.) Traditional birth control pills should *not* be used while lactating, but the "mini" pill has not been shown to have any ill effects on lactation.

Some drugs decrease prolactin levels and therefore decrease milk production. Examples include alcohol (in excessive amounts), antihistamines, barbiturates, bromocriptine, estrogens, and others. If these or other prolactin-inhibiting drugs are prescribed, inform the mother of their effects. Help her to realize that her supply may be so severely curtailed that she may be forced to stop breastfeeding earlier than she had planned.

Adverse Effects on the Infant

Frequently, women who are pregnant or just delivered ask the nurse whether drugs that are prescribed for medical or obstetrical conditions are harmful to the infant. Ideally, this question would be answered by the physician, but frequently it is not. In most cases, however, reassure the woman that drugs used for conditions that occur during pregnancy or parturition do not preclude breastfeeding. For example, magnesium sulfate, which may be given to arrest preterm labor or for maternal hypertension during pregnancy, delivery, or immediately postpartum, is generally recognized as safe for breastfeeding infants.[2] The drug is nearly always given intravenously to the mother, but it is poorly absorbed in the infant's gastrointestinal tract, and hence safety is not an issue. The drug may, however, have undesirable effects on the newborn. Anecdotally, I have noted that some newborns—if their mothers have been treated with the drug for a substantial time—have diminished reflexes, including a less than vigorous suck reflex immediately after birth. Terbutaline, also used recently to arrest preterm labor or more classically for maternal respiratory difficulty, is also considered compatible with breastfeeding[1] and has no significant effect on the breastfed infant.[3]

The effects of intrapartum analgesia and anesthesia on breastfeeding continue to be a controversial issue. In particular, there are numerous reports but no consensus about whether epidural anesthesia contributes to poor breastfeeding. Until data are clearer, advise patients to seek nonpharmacological methods of pain relief during labor.

Very frequently postpartum patients raise questions about whether prescribed analgesics are harmful to the infant. In most cases, they are not. Ibuprofen is perhaps the most commonly prescribed analgesic for the postpartum woman, and its use has not been shown to be detrimental[4,5]; it is considered compatible with breastfeeding by the AAP. Another drug that frequently is given for postpartum pain is oxycodone with acetaminophen (Percocet). Quoting Marx et al., one source[6] reports that this medication has no apparent effects on the breastfeeding newborn, and peak milk concentrations occur 1½ to 2 hours after the first dose and are variable thereafter. The AAP does not give guidelines with respect to this drug. Similarly, ½ grain (30 mg) of codeine and acetaminophen (Tylenol #3) is frequently prescribed for postpartum pain. Acetaminophen is compatible with breastfeeding, as described later in this chapter, and codeine has been shown to have no significant effects on infants in studies conducted as early as 1947[7] and later.[8] Therefore, give Tylenol #3 with confidence that it will adequately relieve the mother's pain without detrimental effects to the newborn.

Advise the mother of any potential side effects for the infant as a result of drugs that have been prescribed for her (Box 9-1). For example, behavioral changes in the infant may be seen after the administration of a narcotic anal-

Box 9-1
Signs and Symptoms of Infant Response to Drug

Behavioral Changes
- Alertness
- Neuromuscular irritability/flaccidity
- Sleep patterns

Gastrointestinal Alterations
- Feeding behaviors
- Diarrhea, constipation

Skin Rashes

gesic, or gastrointestinal symptoms may be seen after the mother has ingested antibiotics. Skin rashes can also be observed after the mother has taken antibiotics.

After women are discharged from the hospital, questions about drugs other than therapeutic medicines arise. Mothers often ask about alcohol. Alcohol is not contraindicated for lactating mothers, but it should be consumed in moderation. The Subcommittee on Nutrition[9] has determined that consumption of more than 0.5 g of alcohol per kilogram of maternal body weight may impair the milk-ejection reflex. (For a woman weighing 132 pounds, this translates to approximately 2 to 2.5 oz of liquor, 8 oz of table wine, or 2 cans of beer per day.) While this may seem surprising to some, the aversion to alcohol for breastfeeding mothers is culturally biased. In other cultures, women regularly consume this amount of alcohol—frequently in the form of wine—and no deleterious effects have been shown.

Caffeine may cause infants to be wakeful and cranky. Consumption should be limited to 1 to 2 cups of caffeinated beverages per day. While most mothers usually associate caffeine with coffee, remind them that it is also contained in soft drinks, chocolate, tea, and other products. Emphasize that caffeine is a drug; like other drugs, it should be consumed with caution.

Alternatives to OTC Drug Therapy

Ideally, all women would check with their physician or other primary health care provider before taking over-the-counter (OTC) medications. When this does not happen, however, the nurse may find herself in a situation where she is giving the advice. In today's society, it is often difficult to give advice about OTC and other medications. On one hand, telling women to never take any OTC products while lactating may only be a deterrent to breastfeeding. On the other hand, women should not be medicating themselves unless they understand that the drug may have an impact on their ability to produce milk or their infant's safety. The nurse, then, may find herself facing some practical questions about OTC drugs.

There are about 3000 OTC products in the United States today but only about 700 active ingredients in those products. This is because the active ingredients are found in many different combination products. An important clinical consideration, therefore, is: Does the woman really need the combination product, or would a single-entity product provide the relief she needs? Advise the woman that, whenever possible, she should not take a combination product. Similarly, sometimes nonpharmacological remedies relieve the woman of her symptoms, and these should be used whenever possible (see discussion later in this chapter).

Administration Responsibilities

This next section explains how the prescriber decides whether a drug is safe. However, the nurse must make several determinations after the drug has been prescribed: (1) Is the drug contraindicated during lactation? (2) Who should recommend cessation of breastfeeding, and under what circumstances? (3) When should the dose be given? and (4) Which drug should be offered to the woman when several prn drugs are ordered?

RESEARCH HIGHLIGHT
Short-term use of commonly prescribed medications poses little risk to breastfed infants

Citation
Ito S, Blajchman A, Stephenson M, Eliopoulos C, Koren G. Prospective follow-up of adverse reactions in breast-fed infants exposed to maternal medication. *Am J Obstet Gynecol* 1993;168:1393-1399.

Focus
This prospective study was designed to identify adverse effects of groups of medications—antibiotics, analgesics, antihistamines, sedatives, antidepressants, and antiepileptics—on healthy infants. A total of 838 breastfed infants were observed for adverse effects when their mothers took at least one medication.

Results
Of the 838 subjects, only 94 women (11%) reported minor adverse effects in their infants that were associated with the drug therapy: antibiotics, 19.3% (32/166); analgesics or narcotics, 11.2% (22/196); antihistamines, 9.4% (8/85); antidepressants or antiepileptics, 7.1% (3/42). Most commonly, antibiotics caused diarrhea, analgesics caused drowsiness, antihistamines caused irritability, and antidepressants and antiepileptics caused drowsiness. However, none of the adverse drug reactions was severe enough to require medical attention.

Strengths, Limitations of the Study
The large sample size and the prospective design strengthen the findings of this study. Some limitations include the fact that data were collected from mothers' self-reports, and the fact that they were counseled to look for the anticipated side effects. The time of the drug administration was not noted in relation to the time the infant fed or the observation of symptoms, and hence may influence the results.

Clinical Application
These data add to what has been reported anecdotally in many published single-case reports and in clinical practice, as well as some controlled studies. The small number of infants who reportedly experienced an adverse effect and the mild nature of the effects should help clinicians to encourage continuation of breastfeeding and give anticipatory guidance about possible adverse effects. The short-term effects of maternal medication on breastfed infants pose little risk for infants, and breastfeeding should be continued unless data show that the risks of maternal medication passed to the infant outweigh the benefits of continued breastfeeding.

Is the Drug Contraindicated During Lactation?

Contrary to popular myth, very few drugs are strictly contraindicated during lactation. As a general rule, any drug that is prescribed for infants is not contraindicated during breastfeeding. More specifically, the AAP position statement[1] includes seven tables, which classify medication and other chemicals based on their compatibility with breastfeeding, as shown in Box 9-2. According to the AAP, only 14 drugs are strictly contraindicated during breastfeeding, as shown in Table 9-1 and Table 9-2. Some require temporary cessation of breastfeeding.

Who Should Recommend Cessation of Breastfeeding?

Breastfeeding should not be automatically discontinued just because a woman has started to receive a drug that the nurse thinks may be unsafe. Except for radioactive metabolites, however, it is not harmful to give one dose of a prescribed drug while pursuing its safety with the prescriber.[10] Therefore, administer the dose prescribed and discuss with the prescriber any concerns that might arise about the safety of the drug given during lactation. If the drug is contraindicated, of course, it should be immediately discontinued.

T A B L E 9-1

DRUGS THAT ARE CONTRAINDICATED DURING BREASTFEEDING

Drug	Reason for Concern, Reported Sign or Symptom in Infant, or Effect on Lactation
Bromocriptine	Suppresses lactation; may be hazardous to the mother
Cocaine	Cocaine intoxication
Cyclophosphamide	Possible immune suppression; unknown effect on growth or association with carcinogenesis; neutropenia
Cyclosporine	Possible immune suppression; unknown effect on growth or association with carcinogenesis
Doxorubicin*	Possible immune suppression; unknown effect on growth or association with carcinogenesis
Ergotamine	Vomiting, diarrhea, convulsions (doses used in migraine medications)
Lithium	One-third to one-half therapeutic blood concentration in infants
Methotrexate	Possible immune suppression; unknown effect on growth or association with carcinogenesis; neutropenia
Phencyclidine (PCP)	Potent hallucinogen
Phenindione	Anticoagulant: increased prothrombin and partial thromboplastin time in one infant; not used in United States

*Drug is concentrated in human milk.

From American Academy of Pediatrics. The transfer of drugs and other chemicals into human milk. *Pediatrics* 1993;93:137-150.

Box 9-2

AAP Tables Describing the Transfer of Drugs and Other Chemicals Into Human Milk

Table 1	Drugs that are contraindicated during breast-feeding
Table 2	Drugs of abuse: contraindicated during breast-feeding
Table 3	Radioactive compounds that require temporary cessation of breastfeeding
Table 4	Drugs whose effects on nursing infants are unknown but may be of concern
Table 5	Drugs that have been associated with significant effects on some nursing infants and should be given to nursing mothers with caution
Table 6	Maternal medication usually compatible with breastfeeding
Table 7	Food and environmental agents: effect on breastfeeding

From American Academy of Pediatrics Committee on Drugs. The transfer of drugs and other chemicals into human milk. *Pediatrics* 1994;93:137-150.

T A B L E 9-2

DRUGS OF ABUSE: CONTRAINDICATED DURING BREAST-FEEDING*

Drug Reference	Reported Effect or Reasons for Concern
Amphetamine†	Irritability, poor sleeping pattern
Cocaine	Cocaine intoxication
Heroin	Tremors, restlessness, vomiting, poor feeding
Marijuana	Only one report in literature; no effect mentioned
Nicotine (smoking)	Shock, vomiting, diarrhea, rapid heart rate, restlessness; decreased milk production
Phencyclidine	Potent hallucinogen

*The Committee on Drugs strongly believes that nursing mothers should not ingest any compounds listed in Table 9-2. Not only are they hazardous to the nursing infant, but they are also detrimental to the physical and emotional health of the mother. This list is obviously not complete; no drug of abuse should be ingested by nursing mothers even though adverse reports are not in the literature.

†Drug is concentrated in human milk.

From American Academy of Pediatrics. The transfer of drugs and other chemicals into human milk. *Pediatrics* 1994;93:137-150.

Box 9-3
Scheduling Doses of Medication for Lactating Mothers

General Guidelines
- Whenever possible, give the dose of medication immediately after the infant has breastfed. In this way, the peak serum concentration of the drug in the breast milk should be lowest at the time of the next feeding.
- Check the *Physician's Desk Reference* to determine the onset and peak of action. If possible, schedule the dose so that the peak concentration occurs when the infant is not at the breast.

PRN Analgesics
- If it is being used to relieve postpartum cramps, give the drug approximately 30 minutes before the feeding so that the onset of the drug coincides with the increased uterine cramps that often accompany the feeding.
- In other cases, give the dose immediately after the infant has breastfed.

Daily Medications
- The dose should be given just before the woman goes to bed (or at the beginning of the longest feeding interval).

Box 9-4
Priorities of Care for the Breastfeeding Dyad During Drug Therapy

- Work collaboratively with the mother and the entire health care team to minimize risk and maximize benefits of therapeutic medications.
- Communicate to the entire health care team that the woman is breastfeeding; encourage her to tell *all* of her health care providers.
- Teach the woman to observe for adverse effects of the drug on her ability to lactate or possible responses the infant may exhibit.
- Never make a unilateral decision to discontinue the drug or breastfeeding.
- Be an advocate; suggest that the mother get a second opinion when one health care provider takes a "let's discontinue breastfeeding just to be safe" approach. Remind her that artificial feeding may cause a host of other problems for her and her infant.
- Question an order if the AAP clearly identifies the drug as strictly contraindicated.
- Reassure the mother that the drug that has been prescribed for her is generally recognized as safe for the breastfeeding infant, if indeed that is the case.
- When possible, coordinate administration time of the drug so that peak levels reach the milk when the infant is unlikely to breastfeed.

Sometimes, overzealous staff members mistakenly forbid breastfeeding for drugs that require only a temporary cessation of breastfeeding, such as metronidazole (Flagyl) and radiopharmaceuticals. In this case, the nurse needs to be an advocate, assuring both the staff and the mother that this situation requires a temporary interruption of breastfeeding but is not a reason to wean. Furthermore, the nurse will need to initiate a "pump and dump" routine with the mother, as described in Chapter 10.

Ultimately, the person who prescribes the drug assesses its risk and benefits during breastfeeding. The mother makes the final decision about ingesting a drug and continuing breastfeeding. As a patient educator and advocate, the nurse can fa-

cilitate communication between health care providers that ultimately assures safety.

When Should the Dose Be Taken?

Very frequently, nurses find themselves in the position of scheduling the dose if the woman is hospitalized, or recommending to the woman when she should take her medications. Although there is no one-size-fits-all solution, a few guidelines can be used when determining the optimal time for administration, as shown in Box 9-3. Ideally,

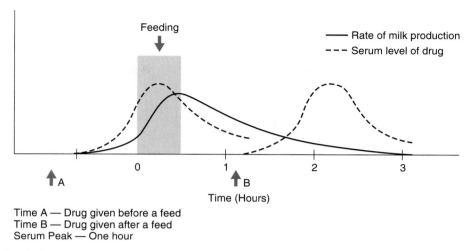

Fig. 9-1 Peak serum level of drug at various times relative to a single feeding. *(From National Center for Education in Maternal and Child Health.* The Art and Science of Breastfeeding. *Arlington, VA: 1986.)*

the drug should be given so that its serum peak does not coincide with the time of maximal milk secretion. Of course, maximal milk secretion occurs during and right after a feeding. Therefore, it is usually, although not always, best to administer the drug toward the end of or immediately after the feeding so that in most cases the peak serum level will be reached before the next feeding (peak milk secretion time) occurs. Figure 9-1 shows the peak serum level of drug at various times relative to a single feeding.

What Determinations Should Be Made About PRN Doses?

Frequently, more than one analgesic is ordered for the postpartum woman. When determining which drug to offer, first assess the extent of her discomfort. A woman who has a forceps delivery today may require acetaminophen with codeine (Tylenol #3), whereas tomorrow she may get adequate relief with 650 mg of acetaminophen (Tylenol) only. In other cases, more than one nar-

cotic analgesic may be ordered; choose the one that has most consistently been generally recognized as safe for lactating women.

It is important to keep in mind that the new mother is taking medications because she herself is experiencing a difficulty. Therefore, her efforts to breastfeed should be reinforced and applauded. Priorities for care when the mother is breastfeeding are identified in Box 9-4.

DETERMINING DRUG SAFETY

Only the health care provider who has prescriptive privileges can make the final recommendation about the compatibility of a drug with breastfeeding. To safely administer the drug, support or question the medication order, or reassure the mother of the safety of the drug, the nurse should have a fundamental understanding of how the drug is determined to be safe during breastfeeding (Box 9-5).

Box 9-5
Key Terms

Term	Definition
Absorption	The process by which a medication moves from its site of administration (extravascular) to the systemic circulation (intravascular).
Distribution	The movement of a medication from the systemic circulation to different tissue sites.
Excretion	Elimination of metabolites of drugs and, in some cases, the active drug itself.
Extravascular	Outside a blood vessel. Extravascular routes of drug administration do not involve direct administration into the blood compartment. Common *extravascular* routes of administration include the oral, dermal, ocular, nasal, intramuscular, intradermal, subcutaneous, rectal, vaginal, intrathecal, and endotracheal routes.
First-pass effect	The fraction of the oral dose that never reaches the systemic circulation because of hepatic metabolism during absorption; it is responsible for incomplete bioavailability.
Intravascular	Inside a blood vessel. Intravascular routes of drug administration involve direct administration of medication into the blood compartment or systemic circulation. This includes intravenous (IV) and intraarterial routes.
Half-life	The time it takes for the concentration of a medication to decrease by 50%.
Metabolism	The process by which the body inactivates the drug; also called *biotransformation*.
Metabolite	A substance produced by metabolic action. Metabolites may or may not be pharmacologically active.
M:P ratio	The ratio of the concentration of a substance in the milk to the ratio of the same substance in the plasma.
Peak plasma concentration	A commonly used indicator for determining the *extent* of the absorption.
Pharmacokinetic	Pharmacokinetic characteristics describe the *rates* at which medications are absorbed, distributed, metabolized in, and eliminated from the body.
Routes of administration	There are two routes of administration; intravascular and extravascular. *Intravascular* administration involves direct administration of a medication into the blood compartment or systemic circulation. This includes intravenous and intraarterial administration.
Toxic	Of, or pertaining to, a poison.

Drug Pharmacokinetics

Pharmacokinetic characteristics describe the *rates* at which medications are absorbed, distributed, metabolized in, and excreted from the body. Specific pharmacokinetic characteristics differ from medication to medication, although similarities may exist among groups of medications. Further, these characteristics vary for different patient populations. For example, infants may have very different rates of drug metabolism in the liver compared with older children and adults.

When these pharmacokinetic characteristics are applied to specific patients and the medications they are receiving, we refer to this as *clinical pharmacokinetics*. The clinical pharmacokinetics of a specific medication is considered for both the lactating mother and her infant.

Absorption

Absorption is the process by which a medication moves from its site of administration (extravascular) to the systemic circulation (intravascular). Absorption is dependent on the specific extravascular route used, the size of the medication molecule, and the dosage form.

Medications that are administered intravascularly—most commonly through the intravenous route—do not go through an absorption phase because they are introduced directly into the systemic circulation and therefore are 100% absorbed. Conversely, medications that are administered extravascularly (orally, rectally, etc.) need to be absorbed into the systemic circulation. Drugs cannot enter the mother's milk until they are in the systemic circulation. When one is choosing an appropriate route of drug administration for the lactating woman, the primary considerations are the *extent* and the *rate* of absorption.

Peak plasma concentration is a commonly used indicator for determining the *extent* of the absorption. As an example, after a 500-mg dose of acetaminophen (Tylenol), a peak plasma concentration of 2 micrograms per milliliter is expected within 60 minutes after administering the dose.

Time to peak plasma concentration is an indicator of the *rate* of absorption. Rates of absorption vary for different medications and for different routes of administration. For example, a medication that can be administered orally or intramuscularly must go through an absorption phase before it can move to the systemic circulation. The rate of absorption following oral administration may differ significantly from the intramuscular absorption rate. Furthermore, intramuscular absorption rates can vary, depending on the size of the muscle used for medication administration and the amount of blood flow to the muscle. Rates of absorption also depend on the dosage form that is used for medication delivery. Sustained-release oral, transdermal, and intramuscular dosage forms exist. The sustained-release nature of these forms dictates that their absorption will be prolonged.

Rate and extent of absorption are considered when determining if a medication can be used safely during breastfeeding. These absorption characteristics apply to both the mother and the infant. If a medication is not absorbed following oral administration to the mother, it will not appear in her milk. If a mother has received an intravenous medication that is not orally absorbed, that medication will not be absorbed in her infant's gastrointestinal tract, even though it may be present in the milk.

Vancomycin can be used to illustrate several of these points. Vancomycin is a large molecule that has minimal systemic absorption following oral administration. If a woman is taking oral vancomycin, very little, if any, of the medication would be found in her milk, since it is not absorbed orally. However, if the woman is taking vancomycin intravenously, the drug would be found in her milk. However, because the drug is not absorbed orally, her infant—who would ingest it orally—will have little systemic exposure to it.

Distribution

Distribution is the movement of a medication from the systemic circulation to different tissue sites. When determining the risk-benefit ratio of a medication during breastfeeding, several factors are considered, including lipophilic or hydrophilic characteristics, molecular weight, plasma protein binding, ionization, and volume of distribution. Each of these factors can have a significant impact on the presence of a medication in human milk.

Lipophilic or Hydrophilic Characteristics

Medications that are lipophilic are more soluble in fat than they are in water. Conversely, hydrophilic medications are more soluble in water than in fat. Therefore, more lipophilic medications are more likely to be well distributed to tissue sites in the body, including the breast. This is because the alveolar epithelium of the breast is a lipid layer. Subsequently, lipophilic medications are more likely than hydrophilic medications to be concentrated in human milk. Small amounts of hydrophilic medications can be distributed into the milk via pores in the basement membranes and intercellular spaces.

In full-term infants, body fat accounts for approximately 12% of body weight. In the preterm infant, the body fat concentration may be as low as 3%. In the preterm infant with less body fat, larger amounts of lipophilic medications may be distributed to the brain when compared to full-term infants. Therefore, lipophilic medications that have sedating effects on the central nervous system will have more profound effects on preterm infants.

The fat content of milk itself must also be considered. This may be difficult because, as Chapter 3 explains, fat is the most variable component of milk. It is especially important to note that the fat content of the milk is greatest at the end of the feed.

Molecular Weight

Molecular weight was discussed early in regard to absorption. Similar to absorption, distribution of medications to human milk is limited by the molecular weight of the medication. More simply stated, the size of a drug influences its distribution. Medications with molecular weights greater than 100 daltons may not be distributed into human milk. Common examples of drugs with molecular weights too large to cross the membrane include insulin and heparin.

Plasma Protein Binding

Medications in the plasma can be either free or bound to protein, and the degree of protein binding ranges from minimal to extensive. The percentage of the drug that is bound to protein is not freely available, and diffusion across the cell membrane is unlikely for the protein-bound percentage, as shown in Figure 9-2. Therefore, there is no pharmacological effect from this protein-bound portion. Warfarin, for example, which is over 97% plasma protein bound, is not found in human milk in significant amounts. Conversely, the percentage of drug that is free (not protein bound) can easily diffuse across the cell membrane and is then distributed in human milk. Lithium, for example, is not bound at all to plasma proteins and is found in human milk, which explains why it is contraindicated during breastfeeding.

The same principles regarding protein binding can be applied to the breastfeeding infant. In newborns, protein accounts for 12% of body weight. In the preterm infant with a significantly lower birth weight, the total amount of available protein will also be significantly lower. If total protein is decreased, the number of protein binding sites will also be decreased. As a result, more medication that is not bound to plasma protein will be available for both pharmacological and toxicological effects.

Drugs that have high protein binding can

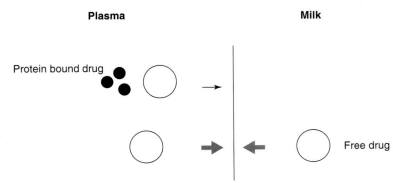

Fig. 9-2 Diffusion of a protein-bound drug. *(From National Center for Education in Maternal and Child Health.* The Art and Science of Breastfeeding. *Arlington, VA: 1986.)*

have significant effects on the infant during the first 7 days of life. Bilirubin is bound to plasma proteins, and thus medications that are also bound to plasma proteins can displace bilirubin. The result is an increase in free bilirubin and possible kernicterus in the newborn whose serum bilirubin levels are considerably less than 20 mg/dl.

Ionization

Substances that are ionized have an electrical charge, and ionization is a pH-dependent characteristic. The pH of a medication or body fluid indicates whether it is an acid or base; a pH of 7 is considered basic. The pH of human plasma is 7.4 (i.e., slightly basic). The pH of human milk ranges from 6.8 to 7.3 (i.e., slightly acidic).

When an acidic medication appears in an acidic body fluid, the medication is un-ionized. An un-ionized medication is readily distributed to tissue. However, if that same medication is found in a more basic body fluid, it will be ionized. Ionized medications, which have an electrical charge, are not well distributed to tissue. Different molecules are ionized at different pH levels. The molecules may be ionized in the blood or in the milk, but if a medication is ionized in the bloodstream, it tends to stay ionized in the bloodstream; hence, it diffuses more slowly across the membrane, as shown in Figure 9-3.

Drugs that are weak acids have higher concentrations in plasma than in milk. Drugs that are weak bases have equal or higher concentrations in milk when compared with plasma. For example, amphetamine, which is a weak base, is un-ionized in the basic pH of plasma and is found in high concentrations in human milk.

Volume of Distribution

Following absorption, medications are distributed from the plasma compartment to tissue sites. The degree of distribution is often described as the *volume of distribution*. Medications with volumes of distribution less than 1 L/kg are described as having a low volume of distribution. A good example is caffeine, which has a volume distribution of

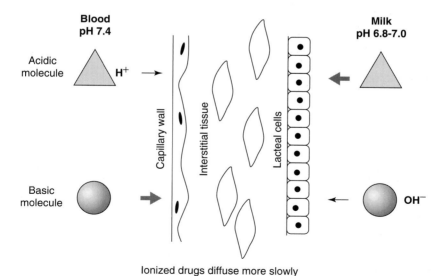

Fig. 9-3 Diffusion of ionized molecules. *(From National Center for Education in Maternal and Child Health.* The Art and Science of Breastfeeding. *Arlington, VA: 1986.)*

about 0.5, and easily passes into the milk. Conversely, volumes of distribution above 3 L/kg are considered high. A good example is digoxin, which has a volume distribution of about 5.0 L/kg, and little gets into the milk.

Metabolism

Metabolism, also called *biotransformation*, is the process by which the body inactivates the drug. Metabolism of medications occurs primarily in the liver, but it can also occur in other areas, including the blood, kidneys, and stomach. Metabolites, produced as a result of metabolism, may have pharmacological and toxicological effects. The mother's and the infant's ability to metabolize the drug influences the drug's effect during breastfeeding.

The antidepressant imipramine is an example of how metabolism influences breastfeeding. Imipramine is metabolized in the liver to the antidepressant desipramine. Both imipramine and desipramine can be found in human milk. Subsequently, the infant who is breastfeeding could experience some of the central nervous system effects of these antidepressants.

Acetaminophen is generally recognized as safe during lactation. Figure 9-4 shows how an adult metabolizes and excretes the drug. About 90% of acetaminophen is conjugated with sulfate and glucuronide in the liver. Approximately 4% of acetaminophen is metabolized via the hepatic P-450 system to a toxic intermediate, NAPQI. Following therapeutic doses of acetaminophen, however, this toxic metabolite is quickly detoxified by hepatic glutathione. (The metabolite of a

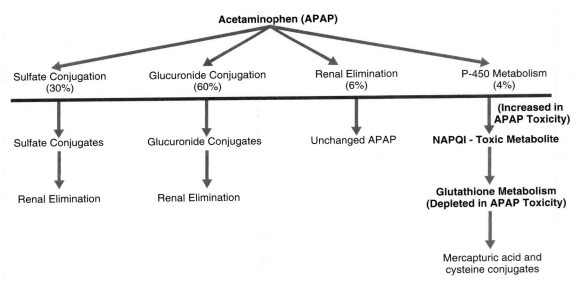

Fig. 9-4 Metabolism and elimination of acetaminophen. Acetaminophen is known to be safe during lactation. This diagram shows how an adult metabolizes the drug and excretes it. Notice that there are several pathways by which to break it down and that the metabolites are excreted in the urine. The infant also handles acetaminophen well but differently via the sulfate conjugation pathway, which does not lead to toxic metabolites. This elaborate diagram illustrates the complexity of pharmacokinetics and is a reminder that the question of drugs in human milk is not a simple one.

drug may or may not be pharmacologically active.)

Excretion

After a drug is metabolized, it must be excreted. It may be excreted as a metabolite or as active drug. Excretion occurs primarily through the kidneys and the gastrointestinal tract following hepatic metabolism. Renal clearance of unchanged medications and of metabolites of medications is a major route of medication elimination from the body. In preterm infants, renal clearance will probably be prolonged. Cocaine, for example, is metabolized in the plasma and the liver. Both unchanged cocaine and its metabolites are then excreted into the urine. Cocaine is distributed to human milk, and it can be absorbed, to some degree, in the breastfed infant's gastrointestinal tract. The infant's urine analysis will reveal cocaine and its metabolites after this exposure during breastfeeding.

Elimination of the drug is accomplished by metabolism and excretion. Half-life, which is the time it takes for the concentration of a medication to decrease by 50%, is used to characterize the rate of elimination of medications from the body. For example, the medication theophylline has a mean half-life of 8 hours in a healthy adult patient. If the patient has a therapeutic plasma concentration of 16 mcg/ml at noon, she will have a plasma concentration of 8 mcg/ml at 8 PM based on an 8-hour half-life. After 4 to 5 half-lives, a medication will have been virtually eliminated from the body.

The concept of half-life forms the basis for the AAP's recommendation to take a dose of medication immediately after breastfeeding. If the drug has a relatively short half-life, a significant amount or possibly all of it will have been eliminated by the time of the next feeding.

Drugs with a particularly short half-life are preferable to those with a relatively long half-life.

For example, Keflex, which may be given for postpartum infections, and ibuprofen, which is very frequently given for postpartum "cramps" and other discomforts, have short half-lives.

Maternal and Infant Health and Physiology

Maternal

As mentioned earlier, the mother's ability to metabolize and excrete the drug is important. Therefore, the nurse should be alert to any maternal history of renal or hepatic insufficiency, or to any clinical signs that suggest this might be a problem.

As explained earlier, drugs enter the circulation as either protein-bound or free. Usually, more drug will be found in the plasma than in the milk because only a small free fraction of drug can cross the biological membrane. During the first 5 to 7 days of lactation, however, the free fraction increases. Therefore, some drugs such as salicylates, phenytoin, and diazepam more readily cross into the milk.[10] Furthermore, the spaces between alveolar cells are more "open" at delivery and gradually "tighten" after the first few days. Hence, the amount of drug that passes into the milk is greater during the first few days. On the other hand, there is a relatively small amount of milk present for the infant to consume on those first few days, so this should not present a problem in most cases.

Infant

A complete and interesting explanation of the infant's health in relation to his ability to metabolize and excrete the drug is presented by Lawrence.[10] Briefly, the infant's ability to metabolize and excrete the drug is of paramount importance. The age of the infant is also especially important;

preterm infants have more immature systems and have less ability to adequately detoxify and excrete the drug.

The Breast: A Selective Organ

As described earlier, the breast is not a sieve; through pharmacokinetics, the amount of drug that reaches the mother's systemic circulation is considerably less than what she initially ingested. Further, all of the drug that is in the mother's bloodstream does not necessarily go into the milk. The parenchyma (organ tissue) is separated from the blood, and this prevents or slows the passage of drug from the maternal circulation to the milk. The milk, of course, is secreted by the lacteal cells in the alveoli. The question then becomes, How does the drug pass from the maternal circulation into the cells?

Drugs can pass into the alveoli by one of several processes: passive diffusion (from an area of higher concentration to an area of lower concentration), facilitated diffusion (from an area of higher concentration to an area of lower concentration), and active diffusion (from an area of lower concentration to an area of higher concentration). Not unlike the way drugs cross membranes in other parts of the body, many drugs cross the alveolar membrane primarily by passive diffusion. With passive diffusion, small molecules are excreted through the cytoplasm of the lacteal cells, but they can also enter the alveolus through the intercellular spaces prior to the closing of the tight junctions in the first few days postpartum. The concentration of the drug in the milk will depend not only on the concentration gradient but also on the lipid solubility, degree of ionization, protein-binding, and other factors. Drugs that are acidic are not attracted to human milk, which is also acidic. Drugs bound to albumin in the plasma are not available to pass into milk.

The milk-to-plasma ratio is an important consideration; it is the ratio of the concentration of a substance in the milk to the concentration of the same substance in the plasma at the same time. However, drugs move back and forth between the maternal systemic circulation and the milk. When milk is being actively produced during a feeding, the drug in the plasma at that time is available to pass into the milk. That is why the level in plasma during a feeding is significant. A milk-to-plasma measurement is also related to time after dosing and peak plasma time. If passive diffusion occurred continuously, unrestrained by binding and other factors over an indefinite period of time, the milk-to-plasma ratio would be 1. However, because the properties of the drug slow down the diffusion process, the milk-to-plasma ratio is usually much less than 1. A typical milk-to-plasma ratio for many drugs of medium molecular size is .005 to .05.

There is an important distinction between the milk-to-plasma ratio and the total amount passed into milk. For example, if the milk-to-plasma ratio is .03, that does not mean that 3% of the drug is passed into the milk. The total amount passed into milk depends on the pharmacokinetics described earlier, as well as the rate of milk secretion. Furthermore, the mother's blood volume is about 10 times greater than the volume of milk she secretes, so in general the percentage of drug passed into the milk is much lower.

DRUGS COMMONLY USED DURING BREASTFEEDING

Table 9-3 shows groups of medications that are commonly used during breastfeeding. The tables include the generic and brand names of the medication, the milk-to-plasma ratio, AAP recommendations, and additional comments on the use of these medications. The reader should keep in mind, however, that like other tables and lists,

Text continued on p. 304

MEDICATIONS COMMONLY USED DURING LACTATION

Antibiotics and Other Antiinfectives

Generic Name	Trade Name(s)	Milk:Plasma	AAP Designation	Comments
Acyclovir	Zovirax	0.6-4.1	6	Compatible with breastfeeding.
Amoxicillin	Amoxil, Trimox, Wymox	0.014-0.043	6	Compatible with breastfeeding.
Amphotericin B	Amphocin, Fungizone	Not available	Not available	This medication is used in infants.
Ampicillin	Omnipen, Totacillin	0.2	Not available	This medication is used in infants.
Aztreonam	Azactam	0.005-0.009	6	Compatible with breastfeeding
Carbenicillin	Geocillin	0.02	Not available	This medication is used in infants. Not well absorbed from the GI tract.
Cefadroxil	Duricef	0.009-0.019	6	Compatible with breastfeeding.
Cefazolin	Ancef, Kefzol	0.02	6	Compatible with breastfeeding.
Cefonicid	Monocid	0.02	Not available	This medication is excreted in low concentrations into milk.
Cefotetan	Cefotan	0.05-0.07	Not available	This medication is excreted in low concentrations into milk.
Cefoxitin	Mefoxin	Not available	6	Excretion into milk varies among women.
Ceftizoxime	Cefizox	Not available	Not available	This medication is used in infants.
Ceftriaxone	Rocephin	0.03-0.04	6	This medication is used in infants.
Cephalexin	Keflex, Keftab	0.008-0.014	Not available	Has very short half-life.
Cephalothin	Keflin	0.073-0.500	Not available	This medication is used in children.
Chloramphenicol	Chloromycetin	0.05-0.73	4	The AAP advises caution in breastfeeding given the potential for idiosyncratic bone marrow suppression.
Ciprofloxacin	Cipro	0.85-2.14	Not available	Not recommended in breastfeeding due to the risk for arthropathy.
Clarithromycin	Biaxin	Not available	Not available	This medication is used in children older than 6 months. This medication is distributed to milk in animals.
Clindamycin	Cleocin	0.1-3.0	6	This medication is used in infants.
Erythromycin	ERYC, PCE Dispertab, E-Mycin, Ery-Tab	0.02-1.60	6	An increased risk of jaundice exists in newborns if they are already jaundiced.
Fluconazole	Diflucan	Not available	Not available	Two published cases exist in which this medication has been used safely in infants.
Gentamicin	Garamycin, Jenamicin	0.4-2.1	Not available	Increases in free bilirubin may be seen. The medication is used in infants.
Isoniazid		0.5-3.0	6	This medication is used in children.
Ketoconazole	Nizoral	Not available	Not available	This medication is not used in children less than 2 years old.
Methicillin	Staphcillin	Not available	Not available	This medication is used in infants.
Metronidazole	Flagyl, Metric 21, Prostat, Metro IV	0.45-1.80	4	This medication may be mutagenic. When used as a one-time dose for trichomoniasis, breastfeeding can be resumed after 12-24 hours to allow for medication excretion. The mother needs to "pump and dump."

Adapted from Lawrence RA. *Breastfeeding: A Guide for the Medical Profession.* 5th ed. St. Louis: Mosby; 1999.

Continued

MEDICATIONS COMMONLY USED DURING LACTATION—cont'd

Antibiotics and Other Antiinfectives

Generic Name	Trade Name(s)	Milk : Plasma	AAP Designation	Comments
Nafcillin	Nallpen, Unipen	Not available	Not available	This medication is used in infants.
Nitrofurantoin	Macrodantin, Macrobid, Furadantin	0.3-2.0	6	Hemolytic anemia may occur in G_6PD-deficient children.
Norfloxacin	Noroxin	Not available	Not available	In one case report this medication was excreted in milk.
Nystatin	Mycostatin, Nilstat, Nystat Rx, Nystex	Not available	Not available	This medication is poorly absorbed. It is used in infants.
Ofloxacin	Floxin	0.98-1.66	Not available	Not recommended in breastfeeding due to the risk for arthropathy.
Oxacillin	Bactocill	Not available	Not available	Excreted in low concentrations in milk. Increases in free bilirubin may be seen.
Penicillin G	Pfizerpen	0.016-0.370	Not available	This medication is used in infants.
Penicillin V	Beepen, Ledercillin, Pen-Vee K, Veetids	0.016-0.130	Not available	This medication is used in infants.
Rifampin	Rifadin	0.19-0.60	6	This medication is excreted in milk. It is used in infants. It may cause milk to turn orange.
Streptomycin		0.12-1.00	6	This medication is excreted in milk. It is not orally absorbed.
Sulfamethoxazole	Bactrim (with trimethoprim), Gantanol, Septra (with trimethoprim)	0.06	6	Increases in free bilirubin may be seen. Contraindicated in children with G_6PD deficiency.
Tetracycline	Achromycin, Panmycin, Sumycin	0.2-1.5	6	This medication is excreted in low concentrations in milk. It is not well absorbed in the infant.
Vancomycin	Vancocin, Vancoled	1	Not available	This medication is excreted in milk. Oral absorption in the infant is poor.

Anticonvulsants

Generic Name	Trade Name(s)	Milk : Plasma	AAP Designation	Comments
Carbamazepine	Tegretol, Epitol	0.24-0.69	6	Although this medication is found in milk, plasma concentrations in the infant are low.
Clonazepam	Klonopin	0.33	Not available	In neonates, elimination of this medication may be prolonged.
Phenobarbital		0.2-1.0	5	In infants, elimination of this medication may be prolonged. Accumulation may occur with chronic use.
Phenytoin	Dilantin	0.13-2.00	6	If the maternal plasma concentration is within the therapeutic range, this medication is safe during breastfeeding.
Valproate	Depakene, Depakote (Divalproex)	0.10-0.42	6	This medication is excreted in low concentrations in milk.

Adapted from Lawrence RA. *Breastfeeding: A Guide for the Medical Profession.* 5th ed. St. Louis: Mosby; 1999.

MEDICATIONS COMMONLY USED DURING LACTATION—cont'd

Antidepressants

Generic Name	Trade Name(s)	Milk : Plasma	AAP Designation	Comments
Amitriptyline	Elavil, Endep	0.50-1.69	4	Although this medication and its metabolite are excreted into milk, it has not been detected in infant plasma.
Amoxapine	Asendin	0.21	4	This medication and its metabolite are excreted into milk. Appreciable concentrations of both have been measured in infant plasma.
Desipramine	Norpramin, Pertofrane	0.4-1.6	4	This medication and its metabolite are excreted into milk.
Doxepin	Adapin, Sinequan	0.30-2.39	4	This medication and its metabolite are excreted into milk. One case exists of an infant who experienced major adverse effects from this medication.
Fluoxetine	Prozac	0.21-0.29	4	This medication and its metabolite are excreted into milk.
Imipramine	Tofranil, Janimine	0.08-1.00	4	This medication and its metabolite are excreted into milk in low concentrations.
Lithium	Eskalith, Lithane, Lithobid, Lithotabs	0.24-0.66	1	This medication is excreted into milk in high concentrations. Infant plasma concentrations reflect milk concentrations. Significant risk for lithium toxicity exists.
Sertraline	Zoloft	Not available	Not available	The AAP designates a related antidepressant, fluoxetine, as a medication whose effects are unknown but may be of concern.

Antihistamines

Generic Name	Trade Name(s)	Milk : Plasma	AAP Designation	Comments
Chlorphenira-mine	Aller-Chlor, Chlortri-meton, Efidac; *this medication exists in many combination products*	Not available	Not available	This medication is excreted into milk.
Clemastine	Tavist	0.25-5.00	4	
Diphenhydra-mine	Benadryl, Compoz, Diphenhist, Gena-hist, Sleepinal, Unisom; *this medication exists in many combination products*	Not available	Not available	This medication is excreted into milk.
Loratadine	Claritin	1.2	Not available	This medication and its metabolite may be excreted into milk.

Continued

MEDICATIONS COMMONLY USED DURING LACTATION—cont'd

Artificial Birth Control Substances

Generic Name	Trade Name(s)	Milk:Plasma	AAP Designation	Comments
Ethinyl estradiol	Estinyl; *this medication exists in many combination products*	0.250		Undergoes first-pass metabolism. May interfere with lactation. There may be a decrease in the quality and quantity of milk. Infants receive natural estradiol from mother not taking the drug. Amount depends on what part of cycle mother is in.
Levonorgestrel	Norplant, Levlen, Triphasil	0.072-0.365	6	Norplant does not undergo first-pass effect or affect milk production.
Medroxyprogesterone	Depo-Provera, Amen, Cycrin	0.8-1.0	6	Increased prolactin level before and after sucking. When 3-month injection given, no decrease in amount of milk produced; 6-month injection had a strong negative effect.
Norgestrel	Ovette; *this medication exists in many combination products, including Lo/Ovral*	0.1-0.2	No data	In milk: peak 2 hr; if taken alone, below detection level by 4 hr; if taken with norethisterone, high level in milk for 24 hr.

Drugs of Abuse

Generic Name	Milk:Plasma	AAP Designation	Comments
Cocaine	Not available	2	This drug is excreted into milk in large concentrations. The child is at risk for toxicity and dependence.
Ethanol	0.78-1.40	6	This drug is excreted into milk in high concentrations. The child is at risk for toxicity and dependence.
Heroin	2.1	2	The infant is at risk for toxicity and dependence.
LSD	Not available	Not available	This drug may be excreted into milk.
Marijuana	>1	2	This drug and its metabolites are excreted into milk.

Non-Opiate Analgesics

Generic Name	Trade Name(s)	Milk:Plasma	AAP Designation	Comments
Acetaminophen	Feverall, Genapap, Panadol, Tylenol; *this medication exists in many combination products*	0.2-1.9	6	This medication is excreted into milk in low concentrations. This medication is used in children.
Aspirin	*This medication exists in many combination products*	0.03-1.00	5	This medication is excreted into milk in low concentrations. The child could be at risk for adverse effects and toxicity.
Diflunisal	Dolobid	0.02-0.07	Not available	This medication is excreted into milk in low concentrations.
Fenoprofen	Nalfon	0.02	Not available	This medication is excreted into milk in low concentrations.

Adapted from Lawrence RA. *Breastfeeding: A Guide for the Medical Profession.* 5th ed. St. Louis: Mosby; 1999.

MEDICATIONS COMMONLY USED DURING LACTATION—cont'd

			Non-Opiate Analgesics—cont'd	
Generic Name	Trade Name(s)	Milk:Plasma	AAP Designation	Comments
Ibuprofen	Advil, Haltran, Menadol, Motrin, Nuprin	0.01	6	This medication is excreted into milk in very low concentrations.
Indomethacin	Indocin	0.06-1.48	6	One case of potential indomethacin-induced seizures has been reported. Despite this report, the AAP considers indomethacin to be compatible with breastfeeding.
Ketorolac	Toradol	0.02-0.04	6	
Naproxen	Aleve, Anaprox, Naproxen	0.01	Not available	This medication is excreted into milk in very low concentrations.
Piroxicam	Feldene	0.01-0.03	6	This medication is excreted into milk in very low concentrations. This medication is not found in the child's plasma in appreciable concentrations
Tolmetin	Tolectin	0.01	6	

			Opiate Analgesics	
Generic Name	Trade Name(s)	Milk:Plasma	AAP Designation	Comments
Codeine	*This medication also exists in many combination products*	1.3-2.5	6	This medication is excreted into milk in low concentrations.
Fentanyl	Duragesic, Sublimaze	2.1	6	
Meperidine	Demerol	1.0-1.4	Not available	Although this medication is excreted into milk, adverse effects have not been reported.
Methadone	Dolophine	0.3-1.5	6	No adverse effects have been reported when the mother is taking 20 mg or less per day.
Morphine	*This medication exists in multiple generic forms*	0.23-5.07	6	

			Sedative Hypnotics	
Generic Name	Trade Name(s)	Milk:Plasma	AAP Designation	Comments
Alprazolam	Xanax	Not available	Not available	This medication is excreted into milk.
Chloral Hydrate	Aquachloral Supprettes	0.09-3.00	6	This medication and its metabolites are excreted into milk. This medication is used in children.
Chlordiazepoxide	Libitabs, Librium	Not available	Not available	Increases in free bilirubin may occur.
Diazepam	Valium	0.1-2.7	4	
Lorazepam	Ativan	0.15-0.26	4	Elimination of this medication is prolonged in neonates.
Oxazepam	Serax	0.10-0.33	Not available	
Temazepam	Restoril	0.09-0.63	4	
Triazolam	Halcion	Not available	Not available	This medication is excreted into milk.

this one should not be used as the sole resource or criterion for determining the risk-benefit-ratio of a specific drug.

STRATEGIES TO MINIMIZE DRUG EXPOSURE AND RISK DURING BREASTFEEDING

Wellstart International has developed strategies that are designed to minimize the harmful effects of drug therapy during breastfeeding and lactation. Based on Wellstart's principles,[11] a series of questions follows. Although the person prescribing the medication assumes the greatest amount of responsibility, there are clear implications for the nurse, particularly the hospital staff nurse or visiting nurse who cares for the mother and newborn.

Is Medication Essential?

Very often, drugs are used when other remedies may work just as well. This is especially true with OTC products. For example, if the woman is tempted to buy an OTC expectorant, suggest that she drink quantities of water. Water is an excellent expectorant and often works better than the commonly used OTC product guiafenisin. Similarly, the woman who complains of sinus congestion may be tempted to self-medicate. Instead, suggest that she use a humidifier, which is very effective in relieving head congestion.

Dissuade the woman from using combination OTC products, as mentioned earlier. Similarly, suggest a topical product rather than a systemic product if that is a reasonable alternative. For example, Neo-synephrine nose drops are a better choice than pseudoepinephrine tablets.

Can Therapy Be Delayed?

Sometimes drug administration or therapy that may result in drug administration can be delayed. For example, hormonal birth control pills can be used, but it is better if the woman can delay using the progestin-only oral contraceptive until around 6 weeks. In this way, breastfeeding can be well established before the hormone is used. Meanwhile, suggest alternative methods of birth control.

Similarly, help the woman to determine if an elective surgery that will require postoperative drug administration can be delayed. The same may hold true for complicated dental procedures.

Should Breastfeeding Be Temporarily Delayed?

Sometimes a drug that provides a needed benefit for the mother poses a potential risk to the infant. If so, plan for the interruption and use the strategies suggested in Chapter 10 to facilitate breastfeeding when the mother and infant are separated.

Can Only Drugs With Established History Be Used?

For some drugs—especially new drugs—there is little or no information available in terms of their effect on lactation or the breastfeeding infant. If possible, persuade the mother and her physicians to explore other choices.

Can Only Drugs With Known Poor Passage Into Milk Be Used?

Drugs that do not pass readily into mothers' milk are preferable to those that do. In the hospital setting, it may be helpful to make a list of drugs that are commonly prescribed on the unit, separating them into columns: those that easily pass into milk and those that do not. While this should not provide the sole criteria for whether the drug can be prescribed, it should help nurses to feel safe administering drugs that do not readily pass into milk.

Can Alternative Routes of Administration Be Used?

Using a different route of administration may decrease the amount of drug in the mother's milk. Of course, the nurse cannot change the route of administration without a written order, but she can become an advocate for the woman. For example, an inhaled bronchodilator would be preferable to an oral agent for asthma because the inhaled drug would minimize the amount of the drug that gets into the milk.

SUMMARY

While safety is of critical importance to the breastfeeding mother and her infant, the nurse has many other responsibilities with respect to drugs and breastfeeding. Educating the woman about the effects of the drug, becoming her advocate, and administering the drug so that adverse effects on the infant are minimized requires some planning, but it can be done. In most cases, breastfeeding and drug therapy are not mutually exclusive. Through pharmacokinetics, very little of drug ingested actually reaches the infant, and very few drugs are strictly contraindicated during lactation. However, health care providers and consumers can never be cavalier about drug therapy; they should use strategies to minimize the risk of any possible adverse effects.

SUGGESTED RESOURCES

American Academy of Pediatrics Committee on Drugs. The transfer of drugs and other chemicals into human milk. *Pediatrics* 1994;93:137-150.

The American Academy of Pediatrics Committee on Drugs periodically updates this statement, which divides drugs into four categories such as those shown in Box 9-2. The list is not meant to be all-inclusive, but it is an excellent source of information.

Briggs GG, Freeman RK, Yaffe SJ. *Drugs in Pregnancy and Lactation.* 5th ed. Baltimore: Williams and Wilkins; 1998.

This textbook is an excellent resource that classifies drugs into five categories (A, B, C, D, and X), ranging from those that have shown no evidence of harm to human subjects to those that are contraindicated.

Lawrence RA. *Breastfeeding: A Guide for the Medical Profession.* 5th ed. St. Louis: Mosby; 1999.

This book has become the international standard for breastfeeding management. It has an excellent chapter on drugs and breastfeeding, along with an appendix describing pertinent information on multiple drugs. The appendix was based on more than 750 references.

Hale T. *Medications and Mothers' Milk.* 7th ed. Amarillo, TX: Pharmasoft Publishing; 1998.

This book is a companion for the clinician who interacts with lactating mothers. Common drugs are listed, with concise comments about the half-life of the drug, milk-to-plasma ratio, AAP listing, and other pertinent data.

References

1. American Academy of Pediatrics Committee on Drugs. The transfer of drugs and other chemicals into human milk. *Pediatrics* 1994;93:137-150.

2. Cruikshank DP, Varner MW, Pitkin RM. Breast milk magnesium and calcium concentrations following magnesium sulfate treatment. *Am J Obstet Gynecol* 1982;143:685-688.

3. Lindberg C, Boreus LO, de Chateau P, Lindstrom B, Lonnerholm G, Nyberg L. Transfer of terbutaline into breast milk. *Eur J Respir Dis Suppl* 1984;134:87-91.

4. Townsend RJ, Benedetti TJ, Erickson SH, et al. Excretion of ibuprofen into breast milk. *Am J Obstet Gynecol* 1984;149:184-186.

5. Nation RL, Hackett LP, Dusci LJ, Ilett KF. Excretion of hydroxychloroquine in human milk. *Br J Clin Pharmacol* 1984;17:368-369.

6. Briggs GG, Freeman RK, Yaffe SJ. *Drugs in Pregnancy and Lactation.* 5th ed. Baltimore: Williams and Wilkins; 1998.

7. Sapeika N. The excretion of drugs in human milk: a review. *J Obstet Gyneacol Br Commonw* 1947;54:426.

8. Findlay JW, DeAngelis RL, Kearney MF, Welch RM, Findlay JM. Analgesic drugs in breast milk and plasma. *Clin Pharmacol Ther* 1981;29:625-633.

9. Institute of Medicine Subcommittee on Nutrition. *Nutrition During Lactation.* Washington, DC: National Academy Press; 1991.

10. Lawrence RA. *Breastfeeding: A Guide for the Medical Profession.* 4th ed. St. Louis: Mosby; 1994.

11. Woodward-Lopez G, Creer AE, eds. *Lactational Management Curriculum: A Faculty Guide for Schools of Medicine, Nursing and Nutrition.* San Diego, CA: Wellstart International; 1994.

4

Choices: Sources
of Nutrition and
Delivery Techniques

10

$\mathcal{P}$roviding Human Milk When Mother and Infant Are Separated

$\mathcal{I}$deally, the breastfeeding mother and her infant are together 24 hours a day. This situation, allowing the infant unlimited access to his mother's breasts, best facilitates breastfeeding and lactation. Sometimes, however, planned or unplanned circumstances make this impossible or impractical, and separation occurs. Although breastfeeding can be initiated or continued throughout the separation period, the mother may need counseling and support to overcome some barriers that interfere with the breastfeeding relationship.

SEPARATION

The lactating mother may experience a range of emotions if she is separated from her infant. Depending on the reason for the separation, the new mother may experience any emotion from being mildly bothered—for example, if she is going out for the evening—to feeling profound grief, for example, when the infant is critically ill. Often, mothers will report breastfeeding "problems," but this is a misnomer; such "problems" may be manifestations of her inconvenience, frustration, feelings of inadequacy, or grief.

How greatly the separation affects breastfeeding depends on where in the lactation process the separation occurs, the frequency and duration of the separation, and whether the separation was planned or unplanned. If an infant has been breastfeeding vigorously for at least 1 month, lactation is likely to be well established, and the mother usually has relatively little difficulty getting the infant back to the breast and producing enough milk to satisfy his needs when the two are reunited. Being separated prior to this time, however, is counterproductive to breastfeeding efforts, and it may be relatively difficult to achieve good latch-on and adequate milk production after the separation. This interferes with the natural supply and demand principle; unless the mother is expressing milk, supply will become diminished. During the first week, even a few days of separation between the mother and the term infant can result in breastfeeding attrition.[1] "Weaning" begins as soon as the infant has access to anything other than his mother's breasts. For the compromised infant who has never gone to the breast, this critical biological and psychological period is gone forever and some barriers may arise, but unless the infant has a permanently disabling condition, initiation of breastfeeding is entirely possible at any time.

The frequency and duration of the separation, as well as the circumstances, can influence the breastfeeding experience. For example, the mother who wishes to attend her elementary school child's annual concert may be gone for only one feeding on one particular night. A woman who is hospitalized for a cholecystectomy will be unavailable for several consecutive feedings, but after a few days the separation ceases. Other times, the separation continues for many days and occurs on a fairly regular basis, for example, if the woman is employed. If the infant is hospitalized for a critical illness, the separation may be for 24 hours a day and may continue for months. In all of these situations, the key is to identify the possible barriers to breastfeeding while separated so that helpful strategies can be initiated early on. Multiple problems and concerns arise regardless of the circumstances. These may include inconvenience, negative reactions from others, self-doubts, and keeping up a sufficient milk supply. These potential barriers, along with possible responses, are noted in Table 10-1.

T A B L E 10-1

BREASTFEEDING WHILE SEPARATED: LIKELY BARRIERS AND RESPONSES

Possible Barrier for Mother	Basis for Response
Unnecessary/Unwanted Separation Breastfeeding in public is not an acceptable cultural norm.	Women may feel forced to leave infants at home while they run errands, attend events, and so forth. Help them find ways to breastfeed discretely.
Inconvenience Not having the infant at the breast is an inconvenience. The woman must express, collect, and store her milk. When carrying out these activities, she may find herself changing her clothing, hauling equipment, and struggling to find privacy.	Help the mother to recognize that feeding the infant artificial milk imposes a different set of inconveniences, so she may find that breastfeeding is, in the long run, better for her as well as for her infant.
Negative Reactions From Others Well-meaning relatives, friends, or supervisors may challenge the woman's decision to breastfeed while she is separated from her infant.	Help the woman to see that the decision to provide her own milk is a personal decision, and one that is driven by values. Give her an opportunity to talk about the reactions of others. Praise her for her choice to give the valuable gift of human milk, which cannot be duplicated in artificial milk. Remind her that artificial milk is not completely hassle-free.
Self-Doubts There are many moments when the woman herself questions, "Why am I doing this?" when artificial milk looks so simple, safe, and convenient.	Reinforce to the woman that only she can provide mother's milk, and that she is capable of doing so. Emphasize that artificial milk is not equivalent to human milk.
Keeping Up Milk Supply This is a primary concern for all mothers, and it is magnified when the infant is not at the breast, or is at the breast only minimally.	General suggestions listed in Chapter 8 as well as some specific strategies listed later in this chapter will help in establishing and maintaining a milk supply when mother is separated from her infant.

When mothers are separated from their infants, they may need to overcome some or all of the barriers noted here. It is the nurse's role to provide education and support that will help to establish and maintain breastfeeding and lactation under both planned and unplanned circumstances.

Planned Separations

Planned separations are easiest to deal with from an emotional and logistic standpoint. The mother can take control of the situation and put into place mechanisms that will enhance rather than thwart her breastfeeding efforts. The two most common situations are going out and being employed.

"Going Out" Situations

When mothers say they are going out, this usually means that they plan to be away for a short interval of time, and that the event happens irregularly or intermittently. Breastfeeding mothers can and should go out; otherwise, the myth that breastfeeding "ties you down" becomes a reality. Mothers who are going out for a short time—perhaps 2 or 3 hours to run errands, attend events, and so forth—have some simple options.

In many circumstances, the mother can take the infant with her. If the woman is feeling torn between her need to get out and her need to be with her infant, encourage her to bring the infant to a movie theater for her first outing. She may be pleasantly surprised that she can comfortably breastfeed in a public place, and having the first experience in a darkened environment may help her to gain the confidence to do it elsewhere.

If she needs to or chooses to be separated from her infant, she must consider the impact of the separation on the breastfeeding experience. The impact on breastfeeding varies from situation to situation. For example, there is little impact for the mother who goes out to do errands for a few hours. She can leave her infant with a reliable caregiver and breastfeed just prior to leaving and just after returning home. This is unlikely to create a problem with breastfeeding.

The mother who is going out to a party for the evening may experience a more dramatic impact. The idea of going to a party begs the question of whether the mother intends to consume alcoholic beverages. Mature mothers are likely to consume only a small amount of alcohol, and this will not hurt the infant. (See Chapter 4 for a discussion of safe amounts.) Sometimes mothers, especially teenage mothers, blatantly tell the nurse that they intend to get drunk. Lecturing these young women on the hazards of alcohol is unlikely to result in their changing their minds. A better approach is to deal with the reality of the situation and help them to avoid any harmful effects to the infant. Counsel these mothers to express and discard their milk at least until they are no longer feeling the influence of the alcohol.

Maternal Employment

More than half of the women in the United States are employed. Employment does not preclude breastfeeding, but the separation requires some adjustments. The key to successful breastfeeding after returning to the workplace depends largely on the education and planning that occur in the prenatal period, immediate postnatal period, and before returning to work.

Prenatal Period
As with all mothers, breastfeeding education for the employed mother must begin during the prenatal period. During pregnancy, the focus should be on motivation and decision making, not the how-to of breastfeeding in the work setting.

Motivation—or the lack thereof—and *misconceptions* are two common reasons that influence a woman's intention to breastfeed. An early study found that the intention to work was associated with a decision not to breastfeed,[2] but a later study showed no such association.[3]

Women may lack motivation because it seems inconvenient or simply unrealistic to breastfeed while holding a job. The woman may say, "I can't breastfeed because I want to [or need to] go back to work," which is tantamount to saying, "It's too difficult for me to combine working with breastfeeding." To explore this further, acknowledge the conflict between work and mothering, and ask open-ended questions that facilitate a discussion about the woman's needs and values. A good response to this statement might be, "Being a mom and an employee can make some difficult demands on us. What do you think would be the hardest thing for you to deal with if you were both working and breastfeeding?" Suggesting ways to overcome the barrier she identifies may motivate her to breastfeed.

Similarly, the woman's decision to breastfeed may be initially colored by misperceptions that breastfeeding is incompatible with employment. Unlike the barriers that are discussed in the next sections—barriers that are likely to occur—these misconceptions are usually based more on myth than on reality. She may rethink the breastfeeding decision if the situation is reframed.

Help the woman to see that breastfeeding is a benefit to the beleaguered employee. Feeding an infant takes time. The mother may find suckling or pumping is often less time-consuming than purchasing, shelving, preparing, and storing artificial milk, cleaning bottles, and recycling containers. Furthermore, if she is working outside the home because of economic need, the cost of buying artificial milk and medications for a frequently sick infant may seriously gouge her net income. Remind her that breastfed infants have fewer ear infections, upper respiratory infections, and diarrhea—illnesses that are frequent causes of mothers losing time from work. The idea is to motivate the mother by highlighting what is in it for *her*. Table 10-2 shows verbatim quotes that the mother is likely to express, and a basis for reframing the discussion.

Listening to the perceived barriers and reframing the basic concepts may help the woman

TABLE 10-2

OBJECTIONS AND MISCONCEPTIONS ABOUT BREASTFEEDING WHILE EMPLOYED

Possible Objection or Misconception	Reframing: Basis for Discussion
"Breastfeeding takes too long."	Breastfeeding may actually take less time.
"Breastfeeding is too much trouble."	Breastfeeding may be more convenient.
"I have a very demanding job."	Women who breastfeed have fewer absences from work than mothers who artificially feed.
"I have a very stressful job; I'll be too nervous to breastfeed."	Breastfeeding provides a connection with the baby and a time for relaxation after work.
"I have too many other things to do."	Money that would be spent on artificial milk could instead be used for household services. Artificial milk costs around $1200 the first year.

to choose breastfeeding. However, the woman's needs, goals, and choices—not the nurse's agenda—should drive her decision. An informed decision can be reached by helping the woman to explore perceived barriers or conflicts, and discussing options that may minimize or overcome real or perceived barriers.

IDENTIFYING PERCEIVED BARRIERS

The expectant mother may be reluctant to choose breastfeeding because she feels the conflict between work responsibilities and mothering responsibilities, and assumes that breastfeeding will intensify that conflict. However, *role conflict*—not breastfeeding per se—is usually the problem. And, although contemporary fathers are often willing to help, the mother is usually the primary caregiver. The woman will be more likely to choose breastfeeding if she can more fully grasp the salient issues.

Help her to understand that returning to her place of employment will add to her workload, and that she will frequently feel the push and pull

Box 10-1
Mother's Instructions to Caregiver

- Do not underfeed; human milk is easily and quickly digested; the baby will be hungry about every 2 or 3 hours.
- Do not microwave the milk. Put it in a basin of warm water to thaw.
- Hold the baby during feedings; do not prop the bottle.
- Do not overfeed when mother is expected within the hour; give enough milk to satisfy the baby until mother returns.

between the demands on her time as an employee and the demands on her time as a mother. Breastfeeding does not necessarily reduce or intensify the difficulties of balancing motherhood and career responsibilities. And these difficulties are magnified for the professional woman, whose employment responsibilities often continue after she leaves the office.

Pregnant mothers may worry about *logistical barriers* that may not actually exist postpartally; other barriers may indeed exist, but the mother may be able to plan for or modify the factors so that breastfeeding becomes a realistic option. For example, one potential problem is finding a caregiver who will support the mother's breastfeeding efforts. A caregiver who does not value the breastfeeding relationship or does not feed the infant in a way that maximizes the mother's efforts will be a deterrent to successful breastfeeding. The pregnant woman needs to begin seeking a caregiver who both values the breastfeeding relationship and understands the basic biological and psychological mechanics of supply and demand. Suggest that the mother provide the caregiver with a card that has specific, written instructions that support breastfeeding, as shown in Box 10-1.

Other problems are more related to the *work setting*. In general, problems are related to lack of administrative or peer support, lack of a room furnished with essential equipment, and lack of privacy.[4] Women are likely to experience opposition

in the workplace if supervisors or peers cannot see how breastfeeding benefits employee productivity or the company's bottom line. This potential barrier can be minimized with some advanced planning. Encourage the woman to be honest with her supervisor about her plans to breastfeed or express milk during the workday. Arm her with facts that show that doing so will improve her comfort (and hence concentration) during the workday, and is likely to result in fewer absences from work to care for a sick child.

A historical and ongoing problem is a lack of a room at the work site where the woman may express her milk; women have had to use the bathroom to express milk because it has frequently been the only place where they can find privacy. This is unfortunate, since the bathroom is a place for excretions, not secretions—such as human milk. Ideally, a readily accessible site for expressing milk would include comfortable furnishings, running water and a sink, a small table to hold the pump, another small table to hold related paraphernalia, and an electric pump.

Even with a designated room for mothers, lack of privacy can be a problem. Having a room with essential equipment available does not necessarily ensure privacy. For example, it is entirely likely that the door—which may open to a busy corridor—will suddenly swing open. Anxiety about an intrusion will inhibit the woman's milk ejection reflex. This may be an unspoken fear that the woman does not immediately reveal. Elicit from the woman what her friends may have told her about intrusions. Reassure her that portable screens, shawls, or other cover-ups can be used to minimize her exposure.

OVERCOMING PERCEIVED BARRIERS,
EXPLORING OPTIONS

Even when the gravida recognizes the benefits of initiating breastfeeding, she may think that breastfeeding and being employed are all-or-nothing situations. Part-time breastfeeding is better than no breastfeeding, and part-time employment may be an option to full-time employment.

There are two issues where the mother has several options; the first relates to flexibility within the employment situation, and the second relates to flexibility within the breastfeeding relationship.

During the antepartum period, suggest that the woman set realistic goals within the limitations of her employment responsibilities. Help her to sort through her options, including how long she can be on maternity leave, and whether she can return on a part-time or flextime basis until gradually resuming full-time employment (if full-time employment is a goal). Suggest that she explore such options as job sharing or contracting with her supervisor to use phone, facsimile, and other telecommunications technology to complete work at home. Emphasize that any amount of breastfeeding is beneficial; initiating breastfeeding, but discontinuing after returning to the workplace is not a failure. If the woman wishes to resume work full time, recommend that she negotiate for a gradual return to a full-time position. Focus on breastfeeding as the best choice and a realistic option.

Part-time breastfeeding is a realistic option. Until the antepartum woman is motivated to breastfeed, and sees it as a realistic option within her employment situation, efforts to preach the "how-to" of breastfeeding will fall on deaf ears. Several realistic options can be implemented postpartum but should be discussed as possible options during the antepartum period. These include the following.

Feed the infant at the breast on demand. It is entirely possible for the mother to put the infant to the breast on demand during the workday. This option is ideal for the self-employed woman, but it can work for others as well. This option is feasible if the mother can reasonably travel from her workplace to the caregiver's location, or if the caregiver can bring the infant to her. This is less feasible for a woman who does not have flexible break times or does not work close to the caregiver, or if her employer objects. The advantage of this system is that breastfeeding can continue with little difference between the stay-at-home situation and the back-to-work situation. Maintaining an adequate milk supply is best facilitated with this plan. The disadvantage is that it can result in unscheduled interruptions that may interfere with the mother's work responsibilities.

Express milk while separated from the infant. Expressing milk during work hours is an option frequently chosen by mothers who work outside the home. This works best when the mother can express milk more or less on demand, and at times when the infant would normally be suckling. The advantage of this option is that the woman is more comfortable after expressing, and therefore more able to concentrate on her work. Within this model, she has two other options: she may store and save the milk, or she may discard it. Most women prefer to save it, but some do not. One woman I worked with would stand over a sink and quickly hand express, letting the milk flow into the sink. She worked only part-time, boasted of a plentiful supply, and didn't feel any particular need to save and store the milk.

Breastfeed only when with the infant. This is a theme with distinct variations. Most frequently, it entails breastfeeding after work in patterns known as bunch feeding or cluster feeding. This means that the mother offers numerous feedings to the infant when she is present, in the evening and/or during the weekend. Another variation is reverse-cycle feeding, which entails sleeping with the infant and letting him breastfeed as often as he pleases during the night. This may be counterproductive for most employed mothers, however, because they may feel completely exhausted in the morning, and fatigue will affect their milk supply. For others, it may work fine.

Avoid the temptation to teach everything about breastfeeding during the antepartum period, since this approach is probably counterproductive. Women do generate a series of questions about the mechanics of pumping and saving, but one must wonder if they are really asking for how-to instructions or for reassurance that breastfeeding is a realistic option. A general answer is probably better than a detailed discourse, since principles of adult education suggest that adults are most likely to retain and use information that is time-sensitive.[5] So keep the focus on *choosing* breastfeeding. The woman is more likely to retain the how-to information when it is presented in the later postpartum period.

Immediate Postnatal Period

Unless the woman perceives the initial breast-feeding experience as pleasurable and satisfying, continuation of breastfeeding after returning to work is a moot point. During the immediate postpartum period, she needs to establish lactation and receive support for her choice to initiate and continue breastfeeding.

Presumably, the woman has already considered alternative ways to combine breastfeeding with working. If she made determinations earlier, however, she may have had a change of heart after the birth of her infant. Sometimes, a pregnant woman who is firmly determined to return full-time to the workplace makes a complete turnaround after the infant is born; she may decide to be a full-time mother instead. If this becomes the case, help the woman to reevaluate the options so that she can confirm a strategy that will best fit her needs and goals.

Before Returning to Work

Before returning to employment, the woman should confirm plans to resume work on a full-time, part-time, or flextime basis. She must also continue to be motivated and receive support for her decision to continue breastfeeding. Motivation is the most important element in combining breastfeeding and employment.[6] Motivation to continue breastfeeding after returning to work is most likely when early breastfeeding was satisfying, and when the woman has adequate information and support for continuation (Table 10-3). Support must come from all factions: from family, coworkers, employer, and the health care team.

Such support should help the woman with the following tasks.

COPING WITH PROBLEMS OF SEPARATION

Separation is difficult whether or not the woman is lactating. Counsel the woman about the emotional responses of leaving the infant as well as the practical aspects of breastfeeding while being employed. Leaving her infant on the first day back at work will be traumatic; the added responsibility of providing milk for her infant may seem like an insurmountable task. Strongly encourage her to negotiate for a return date of Thursday or Friday; a mother is most anxious during the first week back at work, and this allows her to look forward to a weekend that is only a day or two away.[7]

OVERCOMING OTHERS' OBJECTIONS

The woman's efforts and motivation may erode with negative responses from others. Help her to give up the idea of "converting" relatives, coworkers, or supervisors who are negative about breastfeeding. Rather, suggest that she enlist the support of a few colleagues at work or others who have successfully breastfed. Their encouragement and support will probably outweigh the negative messages given by the naysayers.

MASTERING ACTIVITIES THAT PROMOTE SUCCESS

The woman needs to be well rehearsed and fairly skilled at expressing her milk before she returns to the work setting so that she can accomplish the task in as little time as possible. This is particularly important if the woman has a fixed and relatively short time for a break.

Expressing is a skill to be mastered; teach her this skill by using active learning techniques. Then require a return demonstration and encourage her to push herself to perform the skill a little faster each day so that she is maximally efficient by the time she returns to work. Also, encourage her to set up as much of the equipment as possible before she starts work in the morning, if that is possible.

T A B L E   10-3

SUGGESTED TEACHING PLAN FOR EMPLOYED MOTHER

	Focus	Content/Activities

Prenatal	Motivate mother to *choose* breastfeeding	**I. Goals of care**
		A. Recognize benefits of breastfeeding for herself and her infant
		B. Recognize that breastfeeding and outside employment are not mutually exclusive
		
		II. Nursing approach
		A. Discuss barriers and facilitators
		   1. How breastfeeding fits with personal and professional needs and values
		   2. Perceived barriers to initiating and continuing breastfeeding while employed
		B. Focus on mother's needs, goals, and choices, not on nurse's agenda or values
		
		III. Options
		A. Explore possible options for continuing breastfeeding after returning to the workplace
		   1. Breastfeeding is not necessarily an all-or-nothing endeavor after returning to work
		   2. When, whether, and how much to return to work; discuss all possible alternatives
		B. Identify value of breastfeeding for employer

Birth to 4 weeks	Provide support for mother's choice to *initiate* breastfeeding and information to help her gain skills and confidence	**I. Goals of Care (Woman)** A. Achieve affective and psychomotor objectives to carry out effective breastfeeding B. Perceive initial breastfeeding experience as successful and enjoyable **II. Nursing Approach** A. Focus on establishing breastfeeding; avoid the temptation to teach everything the woman ever needs to know about breastfeeding while working; focus on breastfeeding only B. Reinforce and praise choice to breastfeed; bolster confidence that breastfeeding is the right choice C. Focus on mother's needs, goals, and choices, not on nurse's agenda or values **III. Options** A. Reevaluate how or if to continue breastfeeding after returning to work B. Revisit expressing and saving as one possibility that is not an all-or-nothing alternative

ACTIVATING A TRANSITION PLAN

Continuation of breastfeeding after returning to work is best accomplished when a transition plan has been developed and initiated before the first day back at work. The nurse has a critical role to play in helping the woman to develop a transition plan that includes issues related to supplementation, expressing milk, leaving the infant, and developing an overabundant supply of milk.

When, how, and how often to offer supplementation. Remind the mother that bottles are not the only alternative for delivering milk (see Chapter 12), but they are the most widely accepted among caregivers and may be offered to the infant before the mother returns to work. However, timing is critical. Giving a bottle before lactation is well established undermines breastfeeding efforts; giving a bottle at 2 weeks—if all is going well—

T A B L E 10-3

SUGGESTED TEACHING PLAN FOR EMPLOYED MOTHER—cont'd

	Focus	Content/Activities

After 1 month	Facilitate a practical plan to help mother continue breastfeeding in the employment setting	**I. Goals of care**
		A. Determine best option
		  1. Whether, how much, and when to return to work
		  2. Begin addressing pertinent points of transition plan
		B. Devise a plan that minimizes barriers and maximizes facilitators
		
		II. Nursing approach
		A. Focus on mother's needs, goals, and choices, not on nurse's agenda or values; complete success, by the mother's definition, may never happen, so praise efforts
		B. Discuss concerns (general; talk about impact, not how-to)
		  1. Fatigue, role overload
		  2. Separation, reluctance to leave infant
		  3. Anxiety about caregivers or day care
		C. Identify potential barriers and possible solutions if woman wishes to maintain lactation after returning to the workplace
		  1. Insufficient milk supply
		    a. Rest—prioritize, and
		    b. Allow infant to suckle as often as possible
		      • Breastfeeding infant at midday is an option (mother commutes to place where infant is, or someone brings infant to her)
		      • In contrast, some mothers do reverse cycle feeding
		      • Lots of weekend breastfeeding
		      • Strategies to increase milk supply (as described in Chapter 8)
		    c. Express (mimic time infant is at breast)
		  2. Lack of support from employer/coworkers/family/caregivers
		    a. Talk to employer
		    b. Talk to coworkers
		    c. Caregivers—give practical directives (e.g., when to feed infant)
		  3. Time to express milk in the work setting
		  4. Difficulty getting infant to take bottle
		D. Suggest possible facilitators
		  1. Join support group
		  2. Introduce bottle no sooner than 1 month (rationale)
		  3. Offer bottle once a week thereafter (rationale: builds parent's confidence that infant will do this) and leave infant—ideally ask someone other than mother to give bottle
		  4. Start expressing milk at least 2 weeks ahead (rationale: builds supply and confidence)
		  5. Develop an overabundant supply
		
		III. Options
		  Implement transition plan as desired

may be acceptable, but waiting until 4 weeks is preferable. Thereafter, a bottle may be given once a week. If the first bottle contains warm breast milk, the infant is more likely to accept it because it contains the sweet milk he is accustomed to.

Furthermore, the bottle is more likely to be accepted when it is offered by someone other than the mother; if the infant smells milk in the mother's breasts and the bottle, he will prefer the breasts. Seeing her infant accept the bottle from someone else builds the mother's confidence that he will continue to do so in her absence.

Discourage waiting until 3 months to offer a bottle, since the infant is likely to reject the bottle at this time.[8] By this developmental stage, an infant's sucking is more conscious than reflexive, and it may be difficult, if not impossible, to get him to accept the bottle. A cup, dropper, syringe, or another method other than an artificial nipple may be more helpful at this time, as discussed in Chapter 12.

Expressing milk. Explore with the mother various options for expressing milk. Milk may be expressed by hand (hand expression) or by using a pump (manual, battery, or electric); these are discussed later in the chapter. The type of expression the employed mother uses is often a matter of personal preference and what meets the needs of her situation.

Encourage the mother to start expressing her milk at least 14 days prior to returning to work. This will accomplish two objectives. First, it will help her to develop her own stockpile of frozen milk to be used in her absence; second, it will help to minimize the problem of a dwindling supply, which frequently occurs as soon as the woman returns to work.

Leaving infant for a period of time. Suggest to the mother that she leave her infant with a trusted caregiver for a brief period prior to returning to work. This does not necessarily need to be the person who will be the full-time caregiver after she returns to work. The purpose of this first outing is for the mother to have a feeling of confidence that the infant will be safe and content in her absence. Otherwise, her first day back at work may result in multiple panicked phone calls and little ability to concentrate on her work.

Developing an overabundant supply of milk. Strongly encourage the mother to develop an overabundant supply of milk prior to returning to work. This will accomplish two things. Typically, the milk supply is reduced after the mother returns to work, so if this overabundant supply is reduced, it is likely that the mother will have an adequate amount later. The extra can be put in the freezer in case the infant needs it. Second, it will give the mother confidence that she has plenty of milk, or that she can rely on the freezer supply if her own supply dwindles.

After Returning to Work

If the woman chooses to breastfeed after she returns to work, make every effort to assist her in her endeavors. Breastfeeding attrition can and does occur, however. Studies show that despite intentions to the contrary, once women actually return to the workplace weaning happens as early as 2 or 3 months postpartum, even after adjusting for demographic variables.[3] Multiple factors, many of which are beyond the woman's control, including travel schedules, result in cessation, even though the woman had originally intended otherwise.[9] Women in professional roles are likely to breastfeed longer than those in clerical positions, most probably because they have greater time flexibility[10] and more control over their work environments.

The two factors that probably are most relevant to whether women continue breastfeeding are the timing of the return and the number of hours worked. Those factors that are associated with cessation include full-time (rather than part-time) employment[11] and earlier return to the workplace.[12] Women who return to work before 2 months generally experience more problems and discontinue breastfeeding sooner than those who return after 2 months.[13] Those who are most likely to succeed in their endeavors to combine breastfeeding with working return to work on a part-time basis, delay returning to work for at least 4 months, or both.[7]

Several problems have been identified for the employed breastfeeding mother.[6] Few of these problems are specific to the employment situation; most may be experienced by other breastfeeding mothers, particularly those who are separated from their infants. The following common problems can be minimized through good counseling.

FATIGUE

Fatigue is the most significant problem reported by working mothers.[6] Fatigue is really more a symptom of parenting than of breastfeeding, and it can be minimized by reducing factors that contribute to role overload. Help mothers to set realistic standards for themselves (continue to do the same activities but with a less perfectionist approach) and to reprioritize others. There are no easy answers here, and talking with the woman about her needs, goals, and values will help her to develop a routine that is workable for her and her family.

FINDING TIME TO EXPRESS

Finding enough time to express milk at work can be a real challenge. This problem can be at least partially prevented if the mother masters the skill before returning to work so that she does not waste any time learning the skill on the job.

CLOTHING AND MODESTY

Expressing milk at work can leave clothes looking soggy and disheveled. To minimize this problem, suggest that the woman choose printed designs and washable clothing, and that she wear a camisole (to camouflage some of the leaking).[14] Discourage dresses that zip up the back because they wrinkle when the woman is expressing.

MAINTAINING MILK SUPPLY

While most mothers worry that they have an insufficient supply of milk, the worry escalates for the working mother who does not have the continuous stimulation of her infant. The most important strategy is to develop an overabundant supply prior to returning to work. Suggest other strategies that have built-in success features specific to the working mother. These include the following:

- *Express milk.* Ideally, the working woman should express milk at the times when her infant would normally be hungry.

- *Breastfeed frequently.* Each weekend, the mother should put the infant to the breast very frequently. This will help her to have an overabundant supply each Monday so that if her supply dwindles during the week, she still has enough to satisfy the infant. Breastfeeding frequently during the after-work hours will help, too.

- *Rest and relax.* Finding rest or relaxation might be very difficult for the woman who faces the pressures of both job and family. Using relaxation techniques during the times she pumps may be helpful (suggest listening to soft music on a portable tape player). A picture of the infant or something that smells like the infant may also be helpful. Privacy in the workplace is essential to relaxation.

- Many other strategies for increasing milk supply are discussed in Chapter 8.

The barriers to breastfeeding while employed are many and varied, but so are the potential solutions. The woman must be prepared to overcome the individual, interpersonal, and system problems that occur. A patient education program that focuses on motivation, generating options, and anticipatory guidance will help her to overcome many of these problems. The nurse needs to set goals and priorities in accordance with the time line of the birth as shown in Box 10-2. The vast majority of women who successfully combine work and breastfeeding overwhelmingly agree that it is "worth it."[15]

Box 10-2
Goals for the Employed Breastfeeding Mother

Prenatal (Nursing Focus: Intentions and Perceptions)
- Choose to initiate breastfeeding.
- Identify perceived barriers and explore possible options for combining work and breastfeeding, including how and when to return to work. Ideally, devise a plan to return as late as possible.
- Seek caregiver who values breastfeeding relationship.
- Consider/explore strategies to deal with realities of breastfeeding after returning to work.

Immediate Postnatal (Nursing Focus: Successful Initiation)
- Perceive initial breastfeeding experience as successful and enjoyable.
- Achieve affective and psychomotor objectives to carry out effective breastfeeding.
- Establish full milk supply.
- Establish strong support system.
- Consider/explore/confirm strategies to deal with realities of returning to work.

Before Returning to Work (Nursing Focus: Anticipating Realities of the Challenge)
- Develop a clear plan to overcome logistical problems of separation, including plan for expressing milk in the work setting (time/location) if appropriate.
- Display confidence to overcome others' objections (legal right, short maternity leave, talk to employer about his advantages, talk to coworkers).
- Engage in activities that promote cognitive, affective, and psychomotor learning.
- Successfully implement a transition plan.

After Returning to Work (Nursing Focus: Overcoming Barriers)
- Review preprinted "how-to" card.
- Identify specific problems encountered and seek appropriate help.
- Muster professional and peer support.

Unplanned Separations

Sometimes, unplanned separations occur early in the newborn period. For example, occasionally a postpartum mother may be unable to put the infant to the breast because she is critically ill. The mother may be too weak, or even unconscious, and the nurse may need to be a true advocate for both establishing and maintaining the mother's wish to lactate. In this case, the nurse will need to determine whether the woman intended to breastfeed and then proceed accordingly.

During the newborn period, however, separation usually occurs because the infant is ill. This is usually an unplanned event—most mothers expect a healthy infant who will be able to immediately go to the breast—but a plan to deal with the separation must quickly be developed and implemented. Breastfeeding efforts for ill newborns generally constitute a five-step process,[16] includ-

ing initial education, initiating nonnutritive time at the breast, progress toward nonnutritive sucking, progress toward nutritive sucking, and transition to breastfeeding. Expanding on that framework, the nurse's responsibility centers around initiating, continuing, and, if necessary, discontinuing breastfeeding efforts.

Initial Education and Maternal Care

No assumptions should be made about the mother's original decision about feeding method, since this decision may be altered if a newborn is very sick or preterm. Mothers whose infants are less than 33 weeks' gestation are less likely to pursue their initial decision to breastfeed.[17] Therefore, the initial counseling session should have both an affective and a psychomotor focus.

Begin with an affective focus. Convey to the mother your awareness of her infant's condition,

CLINICAL SCENARIO

Employed Mother, Reduced Milk Supply

Your colleague Pat calls and says that she is 5 weeks postpartum and returned to work 2 weeks ago. Now, she says, she thinks she does not have enough milk for her daughter. She is expressing her milk at work, saving it, and bringing it home, but during the day a caregiver provides artificial milk for the baby. The infant "takes it like a champ" but always seems dissatisfied after feeding at the breast. Furthermore, Pat says that she doesn't feel her breasts are very full.

How would you respond to Pat?

Possible Strategies

First, it is safe to presume that Pat is dissatisfied with the situation as it is, or she wouldn't be calling in the first place. However, it is important to get a clearer picture about what Pat's main objective is and what her life has been like. Since she delivered the newborn, she has taken off only a very short time from work. Some open-ended questions would be good for starters, for example:

"Well, you know, Pat, earlier this morning I was thinking that life gets pretty hairy in this hospital even on quiet days. I really can't imagine how it must be to face a pile of work that's been accumulating for 3 weeks while you're on maternity leave, and then trying to express your milk and take care of your daughter. Seems to me it might be stressful and fatiguing, and often moms don't have as much milk if they're tired or fatigued. Tell me a little about how your day goes, and when you breastfeed Jennifer, and how often you express your milk."

Pat will relate a story of feeding Jennifer when she rises, then getting ready for work and feeding her again just before she leaves. She gets to work around 8 AM; then uses a pump to express around 11:00. She expresses her milk again around 2:00 PM, then picks up Jennifer at the sitter's around 5:00, and sometimes she is not hungry when Pat arrives. She feeds her again around 7:00 and again before they go to bed, and her husband gives the baby a bottle at night. She says she feeds Jennifer about every 3 to 4 hours on the weekend.

Do not skip over the basics. Ask Pat how the feedings go with Jennifer. What signs are reassuring that milk transfer is actually happening? (See Chapter 5.)

Stop her when she says she is using a pump. Inquire what kind of pump she is using and how the session goes—is she able to relax and get plenty of milk? Ask open-ended and closed-ended questions to obtain more information. You will discover several points:

- Pat is using a pump that does not have optimal cycles or suction. Suggest that she rent a large-motor, self-cycling electric pump.

- She finds it difficult to let down to the pump. Suggest that she bring relaxation audiotapes to her office, use warm compresses, or look at a picture of Jennifer to help.

- She has not heard of cluster feedings. Point out that cluster feedings—feeding several times in a short period—may be especially helpful on the weekends.

- She has not identified sleeping with Jennifer as an option. Explore her feelings about night feedings and explain that breastfeeding at night may or may not help—it provides more stimulation to her breasts but may cause her to be more tired in the morning. Sleeping in close proximity to Jennifer (with Jennifer in bed with her mother or in the same room) helps mother and infant synchronize their sleep cycles, and mothers often report feeling more rested.

- Help her to revisit the possibility of part-time employment as an option.

Outcome

The most helpful strategy for Pat was finding ways to relax at work, increasing the frequency of breastfeeding after work and on the weekends, and using a more efficient pump at work. She was able to exclusively breastfeed Jennifer for several months, and partially breastfeed thereafter.

and give her an opportunity to talk about her feelings, anxieties, and questions. Open a dialogue with her by using open-ended questions. For example, it might be appropriate to say, "Mrs. X., I see from the record that you planned to breastfeed Michael. It will probably be several weeks before he is big enough and strong enough to nurse at your breast, but in the meantime, his health could be improved by having your milk fed to him through his tube. Is that something you'd like more information about?"

If the mother decides to lactate for her infant, praise her choice and convey confidence in her ability to express her milk. The mother, who may think that only the doctors and hospital staff can care for her critically ill newborn, should be helped to realize that her milk is as important to the infant's well-being or even survival as the technological advances in the neonatal intensive care unit (NICU). Capitalize on the idea that only she can provide the most life-sustaining nutrients, the first "immunization" and the first "antibiotic." Women are frequently intimidated by the technical aspects of the NICU[18] and need to recognize the miraculous power of human milk. The greatest priority at the initial counseling session is to convey confidence in the woman's ability to provide the most important component of her infant's well-being.

Mothers need to hear a clear and consistent message that they are "doing a good job" with expressing their milk. Frequently, there is very little volume in the collection device, and this can be discouraging. To overcome this, downplay volume as an indicator of success and consider using a small syringe to hold the milk that is expressed; it looks like more when it is in a smaller container.

Second, teach the psychomotor skills involved in expressing. Expressing milk with an electric pump is the preferred method when the infant is very ill and expression is expected to continue over many days or even months. Media, including videotapes and pamphlets, are helpful for reinforcement (see Appendix B), but there is

no substitute for individualized help when the woman first learns. Return demonstrations are ideal, since they promote active learning and therefore better knowledge retention.

The initial pumping session should not be delayed, although it frequently is. Less than half of mothers of low-birth-weight infants do not pump until 24 hours after giving birth, and nearly a quarter delay past 96 hours.[19] This delay should be avoided, primarily because the mother needs early stimulation but also because a delay in initiating pumping increases the bacterial count of the milk.[20] If the mother wishes to breastfeed, instruct her to initiate pumping within 6 hours after birth. There should be a clear, written standard of care that reflects this.

Documentation is essential for comprehensive care of the lactating woman and her newborn. Frequently, the only thing that is noted on the medical record or kardex is "patient pumping." This notation does not adequately describe the care required or given by the health care team. Note when pumping started, how often pumping is needed, amounts obtained (this counts as output on a critically ill mother's intake-output record), the status of the woman's breasts (soft, filling, firm, engorged), and any problems with painful or damaged nipples. There should also be a clear message on the kardex about how much, if any, assistance the mother requires in order to pump.

After the initial counseling session, education and support should continue to reinforce the woman's choice to breastfeed and her efforts to pump. A strong social support system improves breastfeeding duration.[21] Discharge planning should begin early; mothers themselves have identified the need for additional information after discharge.[22]

Nonnutritive Sucking

Nonnutritive time at the breast is nipple nuzzling and/or skin-to-skin contact without milk transfer. Nonnutritive time is often a precursor to breast-

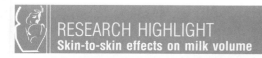

RESEARCH HIGHLIGHT
Skin-to-skin effects on milk volume

Citation
Hurst NM, Valentine CJ, Renfro L, Burns P, Ferlic L. Skin-to-skin holding in the neonatal intensive care unit influences maternal milk volume. *J Perinatol* 1997;17:213-217.

Purpose
This study sought to evaluate the effects of skin-to-skin contact on maternal 24-hour milk volume in mothers of preterm infants.

Design and Methods
This retrospective study involved 23 mothers (8 in experimental group and 15 in control group). Mothers initiated pumping within 48 hours using a hospital-grade electric breast pump every 3 hours for at least 15 minutes for a total of six sessions per day. The mean age of the infants was 27.7 weeks gestation. The skin-to-skin contact began 8 to 26 days after birth (mean 15 days after birth). The mothers pumped and the volume of milk was measured at one (baseline), two, three, and four weeks.

Results
The average volume for the 24-hour period was 499 ml in the experimental group, compared with 218 ml in the control group. During 2 weeks, the study group had a strong linear increase in milk volume, in contrast to no substantial change in the control group. The number of mothers who quit pumping before discharge was similar in both the study group and the control group. However, of the 6 who dropped out of the control group, *all* had low milk volume (range 90-360 ml/24 hours), and all expressed feelings of inadequacy that they were unable to provide 100% of their infant's milk.

Critical Comment and Clinical Application
Skin-to-skin contact has many physiological and psychological benefits as documented in the literature over the last two decades. This simple intervention has no apparent disadvantage and costs nothing. The results of this study should be replicated with larger samples, since it appears to help mothers of preterm infants attain milk volumes more similar to those found in term infants.

feeding and is usually used for ill or preterm newborns. Although many professionals use the term *skin-to-skin contact* interchangeably with *kangaroo care*, there is a technical difference. With kangaroo care the mother "holds her diaper-clad premature infant against her skin beneath her clothing" in a way that permits the newborn to have unrestricted access to his mother's breast for breastfeeding, or simply nipple nuzzling.[23] Skin-to-skin contact suggests that the infant is held skin-to-skin on his mother's (or father's) chest for a preplanned period of 2 hours a day. (From a clinical standpoint the difference in these terms is only slight, but research studies may use the more or less restricted practice in the methodology.) There are multiple benefits to this practice. Skin-to-skin contact reduces maternal anxiety,[24] and mothers who use this method lactate up to 4 weeks longer than those who do not.[25] Skin-to-skin contact has also been associated with in-

creased milk volume, as described in the Research Highlight.[26]

Progress Toward Nonnutritive Sucking

Nonnutritive sucking—sucking on an "empty" breast—is the next logical step. While having skin-to-skin contact with the mother, the infant can be encouraged to suck on the mother's breast, and whether he obtains milk is not the goal. When newborns are at this stage, they may have their mouth on the breast but not latch on or suckle; if they do, they may swallow once or twice, and they frequently fall asleep at the breast.[16] At this point gastric feeding and maternal pumping continue, but the parents should be taught to observe for infant hunger cues. Nutritive sucking, or direct breastfeeding in which the infant both sucks and swallows, is the next step in the progression.

CLINICAL SCENARIO

Handicapped Mother, Preterm Newborn

The wait for the elevator was longer than usual, so I used the stairs. This was not my idea of how to start out a Monday morning, but I walked from the third floor to the eighth floor and found Jeanne, 23 weeks pregnant, in the intensive care unit. Not only was she in respiratory failure, she was legally blind, and very frightened for herself and her fetus. This had been a long-awaited pregnancy.

I don't remember why I was called for her case that morning—probably to assess her fetus's heart rate. What I remember much more distinctly is climbing and descending many, many flights of stairs between Jeanne's 23rd and 31st week of gestation to respond to complex obstetric concerns. She went from the ICU to the medical unit to the high-risk antepartum unit to the psychiatric unit back to the high-risk antepartum unit to the labor floor and back again. Doctors told her she was risking her life for her fetus; she said she didn't care.

Jeanne finally had a cesarean delivery, and her newborn was admitted to the neonatal intensive care unit. We got her started expressing milk by electric pump within 6 hours of her delivery. This was no small task, since Jeanne could scarcely see what she was doing, and she was fragile both physically and emotionally. However, she soon built a good milk supply. She had a slow recovery from her surgery and still suffered many respiratory difficulties.

Eventually, her infant was strong enough to suckle. Jeanne was delighted, and the feeding sessions went well. Jeanne relied completely on how it "felt" when the infant was at the breast. She never experienced sore nipples, and her infant made good weight gains.

Jeanne repeatedly said how important breastfeeding was for her—that she had waited so long to conceive and had had such a difficult pregnancy. She had multiple challenges to overcome for both herself and her infant, but she emphasized that breastfeeding was "the most wonderful, exhilarating experience." She continued exclusive breastfeeding for about 5 months and did not wean for some time thereafter.

Progress Towards Nutritive Sucking

At some point the infant will be more able to successfully latch onto and suckle the breast. His skill in suckling effectively is usually inconsistent in the beginning. When the newborn does effectively coordinate suck-swallow-breathe, however, the first goal is to have one direct breastfeeding per day. Then gradually increase the number until direct breastfeeding is achieved for all feedings. Ideally, this occurs prior to discharge, although it frequently does not.

Direct Breastfeeding; Nutritive Sucking

Delaying direct breastfeeding until the infant has attained a certain weight or gestational age is counterproductive. And the infant should not be required to demonstrate successful bottle feeding before he goes to the breast. Rather, when the infant can coordinate suck, swallow, and breathe, he is ready to start direct breastfeeding. Typically this occurs around 34 weeks (corrected) age,* although it is possible for it to occur sooner or later.

How often the infant feeds depends on his circumstances. An infant who is at or near term but did not have direct breastfeeding immediately following birth because of illness may feed on demand. Preterm infants are another case. Typically, orders are written for preterm infants to feed about every 2 or 3 hours. Such a schedule works well at first because the infants are frequently in a semidrowsy state and need to be awakened for feedings. It is important, however, to observe and record when the infant starts to exhibit feeding cues. Ideally, the infant should move to cue-based rather than scheduled feedings before discharge.

---

*Corrected age means the number of weeks of intrauterine plus extrauterine life. If an infant was born after 30 weeks' gestation and is now 4 weeks after birth, the infant is said to be 34 weeks corrected age.

Discontinuing Lactation, If Necessary

Sometimes a mother may say that she no longer wants to express milk for her compromised newborn. This is not at all uncommon. The nurse's reaction to this decision is critical. On one hand, there must not be a message that implies the nurse is indifferent or unwilling to help the mother succeed with pumping. On the other hand, the woman's statement should not be interpreted as a final decision. When a mother says that she is unwilling to continue, respond with an acknowledgment of her feelings and decision, and an open-ended question about what drove the decision. One appropriate example might be: "Oh gosh. I was thinking that things were going very well with your pumping. I'm wondering if you have truly made a final decision, or if maybe you are having some difficulties and need more help and support from the staff and your family." In this way, if she has truly made up her mind, she can gracefully say, "No, I've really made up my mind." If, on the other hand, she is discouraged at the moment, she has the option to reveal what she thinks is not going well or what kind of support she needs. If she needs more help, provide it. If she has truly made up her mind, respond by reassuring her that revisiting her prior decision is okay, and that you are still there to help her. Acknowledge that she is the best judge of her own feelings and capabilities, and that you are confident that she is a good mother. Help her to verbalize any feelings of failure, but focus on all of the strategies that she has used to succeed and reinforce the goodness of any amount of human milk that the infant has received. Optimize her interaction with the infant and teach her good bottle-feeding skills.

Sometimes a mother needs to discontinue her efforts to breastfeed because her infant dies. This is very traumatic, because the milk she has expressed for her infant was done in the hopes that he would survive. All of the physical feelings of nourishing an infant are still present in her breasts, but there is no infant in her arms. Some mothers want to donate their milk to other infants; this is best accomplished by contacting the Human Milk Banking Association of North America (see Appendix A). Donating to a milk bank may make the bereaved mother feel as though she has at least helped another child. (Discourage any informal sharing of milk between individual mothers, since this can be a liability issue.) Above all, praise the mother for her commitment to breastfeeding, empathize with her loss, and be present to her not as a breastfeeding expert but as a caring professional.

Meanwhile, the physical discomforts of overdistention are difficult. The woman may be tempted to use the pump to relieve her feeling of fullness, so it is important to explain that continued use of the pump will not help her to stop lactating. Instruct the woman to gradually wean herself from the pump by decreasing first the duration of pumping episodes and then the frequency. To relieve her feelings of fullness, suggest that she stand in the shower to allow the milk to escape, then use ice to reduce the congestion.

EXPRESSING HUMAN MILK

The word *expression* is often used to connote obtaining milk from the breasts using the hands. Technically, however, the term *expression* means using one's hands or a pump to obtain the milk. Expressing is indicated for both maternal and infant reasons. Likely indications include (1) when the mother needs to stimulate her breasts to initiate or increase her supply, (2) when the infant is unable to adequately suckle at the breast and the mother needs more stimulation, and (3) when the infant is separated from the mother.

Women who are separated from their infants have many options. They can (1) express and discard their milk (sometimes called "pump and dump"); (2) express, collect, and store; or (3) express, discarding sometimes and saving other times. The option a woman chooses depends on the infant's needs and health status, her own time constraints, and the situation that is causing the separation. For example, a working mother may have a very short break and prefer to pump and dump her milk. The disadvantage of this, of course, is that her infant will probably need to receive artificial milk in her absence. Other women prefer to express their milk and feed it to their infants later. The obvious advantage is that the infant will reap the benefits of human milk, whether he is sick or well. Milk that has dripped from one breast while the infant feeds at the other, called *drip milk*, is lower in calories, may become contaminated, and should not be collected for later use.[27,28]

There are two basic methods of expression: hand expression and mechanical expression (pumping). Both have advantages and disadvantages; ideally, lactating women will be taught to use both methods.

Hand Expression

In this text the term *hand expression* is synonymous with *manual expression,* although some people use manual expression to mean using a manual pump as opposed to an electric or battery-operated one. Hand expression should be in every lactating woman's repertoire of skills. A woman may have inadvertently left her manual pump at her sister's house across town, or a power failure

---

T A B L E   10-4

PROCEDURE FOR HAND EXPRESSION

Purpose/Rationale
Hand expression can be used whenever the mother needs to express milk from her breast. Milk expressed by hand has relatively few bacteria, and the procedure is easy to learn. Hand expression can be used in place of or in conjunction with a pump.

Equipment
- Warm compresses (towel or diaper wet with warm water and wrung out works well)
- Collection container (sterile or clean container, depending on age and health status of infant)
- Nursing funnel if available or preferred

Procedure	Rationale/Key Points
Instruct the mother to thoroughly wash her hands	Hand washing is the single most effective means of preventing infection
Apply warm compresses to the breast	Increases vascularity; this stimulation may result in milk-ejection reflex
Massage breast; in each quadrant, start with gentle tactile stimulation until fully massaging tissue; repeat in other quadrants	Tactile stimulation facilitates milk-ejection reflex
Place thumb and forefingers in direct opposition to each other (e.g., 12 o'clock and 6 o'clock), about 1 to 1½ inch behind the nipple	Note that 1 to 1½ inch behind the nipple may or may not be at the outer edge of the areola
Push straight against the chest wall (for large breasts, first lift and then push into chest wall)	Mimic peristaltic motion of the infant's tongue
Lean over and direct sprays of milk into container (or funnel, if preferred and available)	To save milk that sprays
Occasionally, massage distal areas	To drain distal lobules
Repeat above sequences at different position (e.g., 9 o'clock and 3 o'clock)	All quadrants of breast should be drained
Store collected milk per hospital policy	To give to infant

may render her electric pump useless, but hands are always readily available! Contrary to popular belief, hand expression is not necessarily time-consuming; it is a skill that simply needs to be acquired. Once she has mastered it the woman who hand expresses may be every bit as speedy obtaining milk as her pump-toting contemporaries.

Hand expression costs nothing and is a skill that can be mastered with only a little practice. A procedure for hand expression is found in Table 10-4. Mothers who are reluctant to try hand expression because previous attempts have been unsuccessful usually have had inadequate instruction. There are two good strategies to overcome this. First, teach hand expression when success is most likely—when the woman is engorged or when the infant is feeding on the contralateral breast. She will quickly see the results of her efforts! Otherwise, suggest that the woman sit in a bathtub of warm water, leaning forward. Both the warmth and the force of gravity will aid in her efforts. Teach the woman to massage her breasts

and hand express just prior to using a pump; doing so aids in milk ejection. Troubleshoot for the reason hand expression did not work. The correct technique for hand expression is shown in Figure 10-1. Typically, women fail to push inward toward the chest, and place their fingers somewhere other than over the lactiferous sinuses. Check for these two problems. Also, provide patient education media; several are listed in Appendix B. The pamphlet by Marmet and the videotape by Frantz are superb.

Hand expression works well in several situations. Suggest hand expression to soften an engorged nipple/areola complex before the infant latches on; it is much less complicated than teaching a woman to use a pump for only a few milliliters of milk. Reassure the mother of a preterm infant that hand expression is *safe* for her infant because it harbors relatively few bacteria,[29,30] but it is not *efficient* if the mother and infant will be separated for a substantial time. Remind the mother that hand expression can be

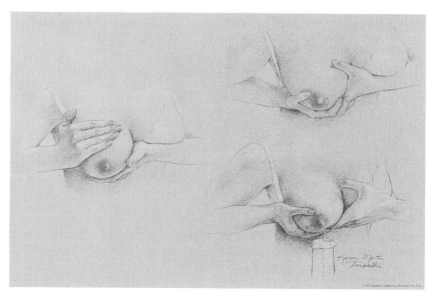

Fig. 10-1 Hand massage (left) expression (right). *(Courtesy Karen Martin [artist] and Childbirth Graphics [publisher].)*

Box 10-3
The Ideal Breast Pump

Efficiency

- Removes milk as rapidly as 75 ml/10 minutes with fat part of milk retained.
- Container accommodates at least 4 oz (120 ml).
- Pump adapts and/or converts to infant nurser.

Comfort

Pressure Control

Amount and length of vacuum is selected by mother and automated to provide suction equivalent to healthy term infant. Infants apply suction for less than 1 second at a time with a mean *negative pressure* of −50 to −155 mm Hg at a rate of 42 to 60 times per minute.* Initial suction would be at least −200 mm Hg to stimulate milk flow.

Pressure Exertion

Pressure exertion is −50 to −155 mm Hg, with a maximum of −240 mm Hg to stimulate milk flow.

Size and Shape of Flange ("Breast Cup")

A flange that fits properly surrounds the areola so that the nipple can move back and forth easily during pumping. The nipple should have room to be drawn out, and the flange should be adequate to transmit pressure or milking action to the collecting ampulae under the areola. The smaller the flange, the greater the pressure exerted directly on the mother's nipple tip. Conversely, the larger and deeper the flange, the greater the stimulation of the alveolar region of the breast, which may contribute to activation of the let-down reflex during pumping. Ideal range is:

68-72 mm of the outer diameter
35-40 mm depth of the flange

Flange Is Flexible

Flexibility is thought to provide more stimulation to lactiferous sinuses through areolar compression.

Cycling

A pump that cyles, rather than maintains constant negative pressure, is less likely to cause trauma to the nipple or areola.

Convenience

- Readily available; mother can purchase or rent at local drugstore or company can ship pump and/or accessories within 24 hours. Spare parts easily available.
- Easy to assemble, having as few parts as possible.
- Portable.
- Easy to handle.
- Provides visual feedback to mother: can she see the amount of milk in the collecting chamber?
- Attaches to bottle with universal thread so that milk can be expressed directly into the container and capped with a tight-fitting lid.

Sterility/Cleanliness

- Sterility should be easily maintained with less than 1400 colonies/ml. This can be accomplished when all the parts of the pump that are in contact with the milk can be safely boiled or put into an electric dishwasher, or by using disposable parts.
- Avoid pumps that have several small nooks and crannies that are difficult to reach when cleaning.
- Closed systems do not allow ambient air into the milk, which could potentially introduce bacteria into the system, thereby reducing cross-contamination from one user to the other.

Other

- Pump should be appropriate to circumstances surrounding pumping. For example, most mothers who pump on a regular basis for several months for an ill infant usually benefit most from an electric pump rather than a hand pump.
- Good instructions provided. The instructions should show importance of hand washing, how to assemble, how to sterilize, and how to use. Instructions should use simple language and give graphic or pictorial illustrations.
- Can mother afford this pump, or will insurance or Medicaid or WIC give assistance with the pump?

*Asquith MT, Pedrotti PW, Stevenson DK, et al. Clinical uses, collection and banking of human milk. *Clin Perinatol* 1987;14:173-185.

used as an adjunct to pumping when the pump is unavailable or out of commission.

Breast Pumps

Pumping can be used in place of or in addition to hand expression. Consumer education should be aimed at helping the mother to both choose and use a pump. The following sections are intended to compare the different types of pumps available and to give tips for using the pump.

Breast pumps are a wonderful invention, but they are clearly second-rate compared with the infant. This is an important perspective; in a world where technology is highly revered, it is easy to forget that the infant provides many more advantages than the pump.

There are some fundamental differences between pumps and infants. The main difference lies in which type of pressure is primarily used—negative pressure or mechanical pressure (negative pressure is like a vacuum cleaner; mechanical pressure is like sweeping with a broom). At the breast, the infant obtains milk primarily through mechanical pressure (i.e., the oral musculature does the "work" of stripping milk from the lactiferous sinuses); negative pressure is used primarily to hold the nipple/areola in place. In contrast, a pump relies primarily on negative pressure, while having little, if any, mechanical pressure.

Similarities between the pump and the infant are desirable. There is no ideal pump, but features that are important to consider include efficiency, comfort, convenience, sterility, and miscellaneous other factors.[31] Features of the "ideal" pump are described in Box 10-3. Actually, the ideal pump is one that most closely mimics the action of the infant. Specific information describing the capabilities and limitations of nearly every pump currently on the market is available.[32]

Mothers frequently ask nurses which pump is best. There is no easy answer to this question.

Some pumps are better under a certain set of circumstances, or for a certain woman. Each type of pump has advantages and disadvantages. The nurse needs to assist the mother to choose a pump that offers the most advantages for her circumstances; what might work well for a mother who suckles a well infant may not work for a mother with a critically ill infant. The two best questions to use in helping the mother to determine what is best for her circumstances are: (1) How frequently and for how long will she use the pump? and (2) How much time does she have to complete the pumping session? (This is probably a greater issue for the working mother.) Pumps can be described in terms of two general categories: manual and motor-driven.

Manual Pumps

Manual pumps are those that are not automated in any way. There are three categories of manual pumps: bulb pumps, cylinder pumps, and trigger pumps. Bulb pumps are not efficient and have only a 5-ml collecting chamber that needs to be emptied frequently. More important, they harbor bacteria even when boiled. Do not recommend these pumps for any mother in any circumstance.[33] Trigger pumps create a vacuum by using the trigger handle, as seen in Figure 10-2. Cylinder pumps consist of two cylinders, as shown in Figure 10-3. The inner one fits inside of the outer one, and they create a vacuum when the mother pulls the outer cylinder down. The outer cylinder collects milk; later a nipple can be screwed on, and the outer cylinder doubles as a feeding device. Except for the gasket, which must be removed for cleaning, no part of the cylinder pump harbors bacteria, and all parts can be easily disassembled and cleaned. Popular brands include the Kaneson, Evenflo, Gerber, and Medela Manualectric.

Manual pumps typically have less suction power than automated pumps. The mother controls the number of "suck cycles" by the number

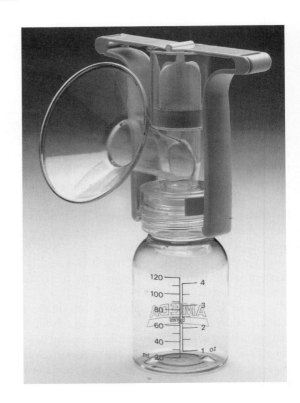

Fig. 10-2 Hand-operated pump—trigger style. *(Courtesy Hollister and Ameda-Egnell, Inc.)*

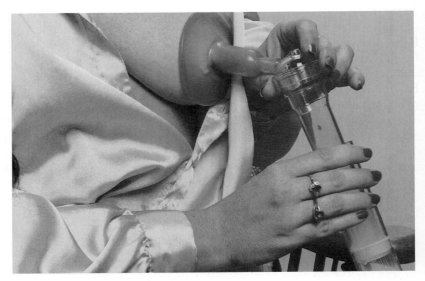

Fig. 10-3 Hand-operated pump—cylinder style. *(Courtesy White River, Inc.)*

of times she pulls the outer cylinder (of a cylinder pump) and the distance she pulls it. The amount of suction exerted will increase, however, as the cylinder fills. Manual pumps do offer several advantages. They are less expensive than other types of pumps—usually under $30. They are also lightweight and easily portable. Recommend a manual pump for a fully lactating mother with an abundant supply who occasionally needs a pump for a full-term, healthy infant who also suckles on a regular basis. For example, mothers who are going out for the evening are good candidates for a hand pump. Mothers who pump only occasionally may have difficulty with their milk-ejection reflex, but this is not the fault of the pump.

Motor-Driven Pumps

Motor-driven pumps can be categorized as small motor, moderate-size motor, or large motor. They are either battery-operated or electric. The size of the motor generally determines the suction power, cycles per minute, and suck/release. Small-motor pumps have limited suction power, and the suck/release interval is fairly long—about 10 to 20 per minute.

Battery-Operated Pumps

Generally, smaller or moderately sized motor-driven pumps are battery-operated, as shown in Figure 10-4. Battery-operated pumps are designed to be used with a battery, but they may be equipped with a power adapter. Battery-operated pumps vary tremendously from one brand to another, from those that exert little negative pressure and are very inefficient to those that are nearly as efficient as electric pumps, so it is difficult to categorize the advantages and disadvantages in terms of their efficiency. However, there are a few commonalties. Many battery-operated pumps convert or attach to a nurser, they are lightweight and clean, and cost under $100. A possible disadvantage, however, is that the pump may be noisy, and a woman may hesitate to use it in a room where she does not want to be noticed.

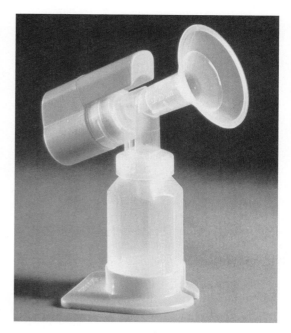

Fig. 10-4 Battery-operated pump. *(Courtesy Medela, Inc.)*

The batteries are fairly expensive and wear down quickly, so this may be a disadvantage for some mothers. Recommend a battery-operated pump for a fully lactating mother who needs the pump on a semiregular basis and has a full-term, healthy infant who also suckles.

Electric Pumps

Hospital-grade, full-size electric pumps are the gold standard for pumps. Generally, the maternity floor has at least one that is wheeled from room to room, such as the one shown in Figure 10-5; more recently, hospitals have purchased wall-mounted units for individual patient rooms, as shown in Figure 10-6. Hospital-grade pumps are most efficient, since the motor—not the mother—applies the mechanical effort. Electric pumps yield a greater volume of fat than hand-held pumps,[34] which is especially beneficial for critically ill infants. Currently, some smaller versions of hospital-grade pumps are nearly as efficient, such

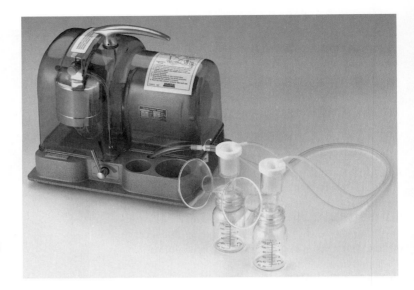

Fig. 10-5 Electric pump, hospital-grade. This pump can be placed on a bedside stand or a portable stand and wheeled from room to room. *(Courtesy Hollister's Ameda Egnell.)*

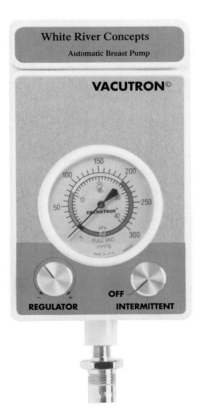

Fig. 10-6 Electric pump, hospital-grade, with wall mount. *(Courtesy White River, Inc.)*

as that shown in Figure 10-7. Some anecdotal reports have suggested that some smaller versions are less efficient, but research has not confirmed this.

Electric pumps and some battery-operated pumps can be fitted with a bilateral accessory kit; that is, there are two flanges, and the machine pumps both breasts at the same time (also called *double pumping*), as shown in Figure 10-8. The electric pump with a double accessory kit appears to result in higher prolactin levels and thus higher volumes of milk than other methods of pumping,[35-37] and it takes less time than the single accessory kit.[38]

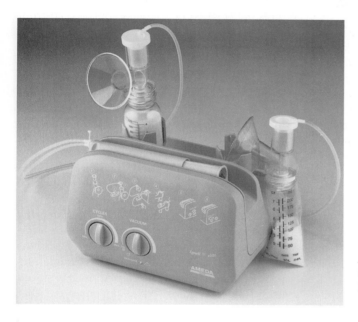

Fig. 10-7 Electric pump, hospital-grade, but lightweight for portability. Can be used with battery or built-in rechargeable battery. *(Courtesy Hollister's Ameda Egnell.)*

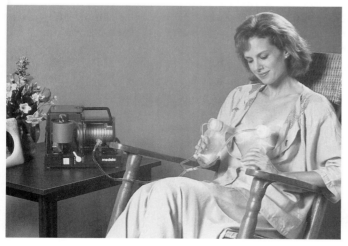

Fig. 10-8 Woman expressing milk with a hospital-grade electric pump fitted with a double accessory kit. *(Courtesy Medela, Inc.)*

Although electric pumps seem to have only advantages because they most closely simulate the suckling infant, a disadvantage is the cost for the accessory kit and related paraphernalia. The accessory kit for the mother costs from about $25 to $50, depending on whether she uses the unilateral or the bilateral kit. Most women would be unable to purchase a hospital-grade pump, since they cost several hundred dollars. They can rent a hospital-grade pump, however, and sometimes insurance will pay for the rental. Typically, renting for 3 months or less costs about $2.50 per day; if the mother wishes to rent for 6 months or more, the fee is about $1 per day. The local Women, Infants and Children (WIC) office sometimes has pumps available for WIC participants, and most pump depots have a program available for mothers who would otherwise be unable to pay for using the pump.

Recommend a hospital-grade pump for mothers of seriously compromised infants who are not expected to feed directly at the breast for some time. Otherwise, be sensitive to the cost involved and recommend a less-expensive type if another pump would be adequate for the task.

How to Express Using a Pump

Show the mother how to operate the pump. To reinforce teaching, provide her with written instructions or videotapes specific to the particular pump she is using. Ideally, the mother should do a return demonstration.

There has been much controversy over whether it is necessary or advisable to discard the first 5 ml of milk that is expressed. The original rationale for this practice was to decrease the bacteria that accumulate just inside the nipple. Although Meier and Wilks[39] recommended this technique, there is no further evidence that it is beneficial. The Human Milk Banking Association of North America (HMBANA) has determined that discarding the first 5 ml of milk is unnecessary if the milk is being given to the mother's own infant; donor milk is another matter.[33] Their recommendation came after a thorough analysis of the existing research. Furthermore, there is a practical side to this question: the mother of a preterm infant may have expressed only a few milliliters immediately after birth. Whatever benefit there may be to decreasing bacteria is outweighed by the value of the colostrum itself.[40]

There is no set rule for how long to express milk on each side. Mothers of well infants should express whenever the infant would usually be at the breast (and their breasts feel full). Recommend that they express until the sprays diminish on one side, and then switch to the other side (if using a single set-up.) Then repeat the process until the breast is "emptied."

If the infant cannot go to the breast for a prolonged period (i.e., the infant is unable to suckle), the goal is to achieve a minimum of 100 minutes of pumping per day during at least five pumping sessions.[41] (In other words, the interval is less important than the minimum number of sessions and the total time achieved.) These guidelines represent the *minimum*; more pumping is always better. Older studies have documented that mothers who delivered between 28 and 37 weeks' gestation can expect to pump about 342 ml ±229 ml per 24 hours.[42] The lower end of this range is considerably less than the amount produced by the fully lactating mother (i.e., the mother who has an infant suckling at the breast), who produces an average of nearly 700 ml per day during the first month,[43,44] but it is likely that nowadays, with better pumps and better support, women would be able to pump more than these amounts.

Problems With Expressing Milk

Even with the best pumps, mothers can and do encounter problems. The most common problems include the following.

Difficulty Letting Down to the Pump

Regardless of the type of pump used, some mothers may encounter problems. Help the mother to remember "great results with stimulation," or gravity, relaxation, warmth, and stimulation. The following are some ideas that may help to elicit the milk-ejection reflex:

- *Gravity:* Lean forward to maximize the use of gravity.
- *Warmth:* Apply warm compresses. Or start by leaning forward while using a hand pump in a warm shower.
- *Relaxation:* Dim the lights and play soft music. When mothers of low-birth-weight or very-low-birth-weight infants listened to a 20-minute audiotape designed to promote relaxation, they could pump up to 121% more than those who did not.[45] Also, keep a picture of the baby nearby. Have skin-to-skin contact as often as possible.
- *Stimulation:* Gently hand massage; this aids in ejection of milk already stored in acini.[46]

Discouragement

Women who express their milk often have feelings of frustration, futility, and discouragement. Even with excellent education, the first few times expressing often do not go as well as mothers had hoped, and they often stop pumping milk, citing "insufficient milk" and "too time-consuming" as reasons for quitting.[22] It is important to realize that expressing is a skill to be mastered, and it may take four or five times before the woman is able to do it with relative ease and confidence. Furthermore, women may perceive a pump as messy and mechanical, with resulting feelings of embarrassment and awkwardness.[47]

These feelings can be frustrating and are best managed through sensitivity and anticipatory guidance. Help the woman to overcome some of these feelings by doing the following: (1) warn her ahead of time that she may obtain only drops the first few days after delivering, and anything more should be considered a bonus; (2) accentuate feelings of relaxation and confidence by presenting expression as easy and manageable; and (3) store milk in small containers, which will make it look like a greater volume.

Sore Breasts/Sore Nipples

Assuming that there is no direct breastfeeding, sore nipples or sore breasts are caused by improper use of the pump. They require prompt intervention. A simple but frequently overlooked cause is that the mother has removed the pump from her breast with the suction still applied. If this is the case, instruct her to shut the suction off first, or to break the suction with her hand. A cracked nipple or an excoriated areola can also be due to unrelieved or excessive negative pressure, or to improper positioning of the flange. Start problem solving by making sure that the mother is using the pump as directed. Turning the pressure volume up too high (or too soon) can be the root of the problem. Failing to center the flange over the nipple is another possibility. After the problem is corrected, it may take a few days for the soreness to disappear. In the meantime, recommend warmth, hand massage, and some hand expression prior to using the pump so that less negative pressure will be needed to begin expressing. Sometimes a plugged duct will occur when a woman is pumping; this happens because one of the milk ducts is not being properly drained. A good remedy is hand massage and hand expression.

Insufficient Milk Supply

All of the strategies listed earlier for increasing milk supply should be used. Additionally, it is especially important for mothers of preterm infants to understand that not having enough milk may be the result of their stress, which can impede milk production and milk ejection. These mothers may benefit from skin-to-skin contact. Additionally, women who smoke and have preterm infants are particularly at risk for decreased milk volume.[48]

COLLECTING AND COLLECTION DEVICES

Collecting and storing milk for well infants has few rules or regulations. Well newborns can better tolerate a loss of nutrients or the presence of pathogens. Collecting and storing milk for ill infants, however, requires more thought. Milk should be thought of as "white gold," and each drop should be saved and put in a container that preserves it best. Typically, mothers obtain very little milk the first day. A few tips are useful in preserving both the milk and the mother's positive perception:

- Hold a medicine cup to just beneath the nipple when removing the flange. This will help to preserve those drops of colostrum or milk that would otherwise be lost when the flange is removed from the breast.
- Use a large-bore needle (18-gauge or larger) to get drops of milk out of the bottom of the collection container.
- Save colostrum into a 3-ml or 5-ml syringe. Seeing a syringe full or nearly full is much more encouraging to a mother than seeing a 4-oz bottle with only a tiny film on the bottom.

Choosing the Right Container

No one container is perfect for all circumstances; instead, a variety of containers have specific advantages and disadvantages for a particular set of circumstances. Ideally, the container would accommodate the amount of milk that the infant would consume at one feeding, would not harbor bacteria, and would preserve the protein, carbohydrate, fat, micronutrients, macronutrients, and other components of the milk.

Size

The container should hold about as much milk as the infant will consume at one feeding. Therefore, this will vary with the age and health of the infant. During the first few days after birth, the mother of a critically ill infant will want to start expressing milk but may burst into tears when she sees how little colostrum or milk she has obtained. She will be more encouraged by seeing her milk nearly filling a 3-ml syringe than seeing it lost in a 4-oz bottle.

Materials

Containers for human milk are made of either glass or plastic. Plastic containers can generally be categorized as polycarbonate, polystyrene, polypropylene, and polyethylene; a comparison is found in Table 10-5. Clear, hard plastic bottles—so clear they resemble glass—are made of *polycarbonate*; an example is the Evenflo bottle. Dull or cloudy hard plastic bottles are either *polystyrene* or *polypropylene*. An example of polystyrene is the Volu-feed bottle.* Using these as containers for storage eliminates the need for pouring milk from another container to feed infants whose intake is less than 60 ml and must be precisely measured. An example of the *polypropylene* container is the storage bottle by Medela. The plastic bags specially designed for holding human milk are made out of *polyethylene*.

Some NICUs purchase 50-ml plastic centrifuge tubes for milk storage. The tubes are available from a number of manufacturers. Corning

---

*Manufactured by Ross Laboratories.

T A B L E 10-5

COMPARISON OF MATERIALS USED FOR HUMAN MILK STORAGE CONTAINERS

Plastic	Looks Like	Examples	Comments
Polystyrene	Cloudy plastic	Volufeed® (Ross)	When frozen milk becomes heated, polymers are unstable Very little research available to determine effects on milk
Polypropylene	Milky white plastic	Accufeed® (Wyeth)	Freezing in this container decreases lysozyme and lactoferrin[51] Some loss (29%) of vitamin C, but this is not statistically significant[76]
Polyethylene	Clear plastic	Bags from Medela Bags from Egnell Bags from Playtex	Bags can puncture easily; they are not designed for freezing Not all are alike; some brands have nylon between the polyethylene layers which prevents puncture and adherence Loss of fat is significant Does not interact with water- and fat-soluble nutrients such as vitamin A, zinc, iron, copper, sodium, and protein nitrogen Up to 60% lower secretory IgA antibodies (specific for *E. coli* polysaccharides) are lost; these adhere to the polyethylene[51]
Polycarbonate	Sturdy; clear plastic; looks just like glass	Cherubs bottle (Playtex) Clear storage bottles by Evenflo Ameda Hygenikit	Very little research available to determine effects on milk Can be autoclaved
Glass	Clear	Pyrex	Leukocytes are destroyed when frozen milk is reheated; this is due to the freezing/thawing, *not* the glass Does not interact with water- and fat-soluble nutrients[51,80] Storage results in adherence of cells with plastics and with glass, but more cells are "released" and become functional when milk is stored in glass[51,81] Colostral cells do not adhere to glass[80]

Modified from Biancuzzo M. Comparison of Materials Used for Human Milk Storage Containers. Conference *Promoting Successful Breastfeeding for the Premature Neonate*, Rochester, NY; 1992. Used with permission.

Co-Star manufactures several types; the most convenient ones for human milk storage are the *polypropylene*, presterilized centrifuge tubes with pointed bottoms that stand upright in a rack. These rigid, opaque tubes have tight-fitting lids, and their small size is convenient for storing small amounts of milk.

Any discussion of collection and collecting devices somewhat overlaps with a discussion about storage, because collection and storage both affect the preservation of milk components and the pathogens that may enter the milk. Three factors influence preservation of milk components: container material, temperature, and time. (Temperature and time will be addressed in the section on storage.) The effects of the container, temperature, and length of storage on milk components and potential pathogens are summarized in Table 10-6. Consider the advantages and disadvantages of glass and plastic, as well as the health of the infant who will be receiving the milk (i.e., a well infant can better tolerate fewer optimal conditions).

Even though there are distinct advantages and disadvantages, in general milk may be safely stored in either glass or *hard* plastic. Leukocytes stick to the *glass*, but their phagocytic ability is unaffected.[49] A recent study in India has reconfirmed the benefit of glass containers.[50] The authors examined cells in terms of total cell count, the viability of cells, and whether they adhere to the container. Their findings showed that milk

T A B L E   10-6

EFFECTS OF CONTAINER TYPE, TEMPERATURE, AND TIME ON MILK COMPONENTS AND POTENTIAL PATHOGENS

		Comments/Findings
Components of milk	Cellular components	Lymphocytes were decreased[30]
	Fats	Losses occur with gavage feedings[68,69]
		Altered when frozen or refrigerated, rather than fresh[70-72]
		Decreases when stored in polyethylene bags
		Hospital-grade pump with automatic cycling best maintains the fat content of the milk[29,30,34,72,73]
	Proteins	
	• Lactalbumin	No changes reported
	• Lactoferrin	Decreases if milk is in polyethylene bags[51]
		Decreases across time[51]
	• Lysozyme	Decreases if milk is in polyethylene bags[51]
		Decreases across time[74]
		Activity reduced 97% after boiling[75]
		Decreases if milk is thawed in microwave[66]
	• sIgA	Decreases with heat treatment[75]
	• sIgA specific to E. coli	Decreases when milk is stored in polyethylene bags[51]
		Decreases significantly when milk is thawed in microwave[66]
	Carbohydrates	No changes reported
	Vitamins	
	• Fat soluble	Decrease if amount of fat decreases
	• Water soluble	About 65% of vitamin C lost when milk is stored at excessive temperatures (37° C)[72]
		Vitamin C reduced; folacin and vitamin B_6 significantly reduced when milk is pasteurized[76]
	Minerals	
	• Major	No significant changes reported
	• Micro	No significant changes reported
Pathogens in milk	Bacterial	Storing beyond 4 hr at room temperature (approximately 72° F or 22° C) increases likelihood of bacterial contamination; study designs vary and this is a conservative interpretation[54,55,57-59,61]
		Milk stored in refrigerator beyond 48 hr can increase risk of bacterial growth[77,78]
		Delaying milk expression after delivery of the infant has been associated with higher bacterial counts in early milk[20,41]
		Most organisms in milk are normal flora[55]
	Viral	CMV and HIV can be destroyed with pasteurization[79]

and colostrum stored in glass containers yielded a desirable percentage of free-living cells in suspension.

Polyethylene

Commercial breast milk bags, shown in Figure 10-9, are made primarily of *polyethylene*. The practical disadvantage of these containers is that they leak or puncture easily. A relatively simple solution is to double-bag, or put the filled bags into a rigid container during storage. However, a more important disadvantage is that secretory IgA specific to *E. coli* polysaccharides adheres to the polyethylene bags and is reduced by as much as 60%, so these bags are less than optimal for the preterm infant.[51]

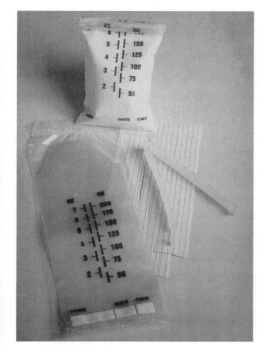

Fig. 10-9 Plastic bags for storing milk.

Polycarbonate

Studies have not investigated the effects of polycarbonate bottles, but there are no documented adverse effects from using them in clinical practice.

Polystyrene

Polystyrene was not designed to store human milk, and its effect on breast milk storage has not been studied.

How to Collect Milk

First, choose a container that best fits the needs of the situation, based on information in the previous section. Whether the container needs to be sterile is a matter for debate. The Human Milk Banking Association of North America recommends storing milk in *sterile* containers for *ill or preterm* infants. Data have suggested that pathogens found in milk are not significantly different whether or not the container is sterile.[52] Therefore, it is acceptable to store milk for *well* infants in *clean* containers. Although some hospital protocols specify using sterile containers for infants who are critically ill, this is unnecessary given that the flange, tubing, and other apparatus are only rinsed between pumping sessions. Milk that goes to a full-term healthy newborn is acceptable in a clean container.

Whether milk can be "layered" depends on the circumstance. If the infant is hospitalized, avoid adding a layer of milk to a previously frozen sample.[33] The layering itself is not the problem; rather, opening and closing the container each time creates the possibility of contamination. If the infant is at home, however, this practice is probably acceptable, but teach the mother to chill the latest addition before she adds the fresh milk to the frozen sample. This will reduce the possibility of bacterial growth.

The collected milk should be capped tightly; it should not be stored with only the nipple atop the container, since this provides an entry for pathogens[53] and, more important, leads to oxidation of milk components—a deleterious effect. The container should be labeled with the infant's name and the date it was collected. (Stamping labels ahead of time with the patient's identifying data is a good way to label the containers.) Then milk should be used in the order it was collected. There is no need to routinely culture mother's own milk. (Donor milk is another matter; it is discussed in Chapter 11.)

SAVING AND STORING

A simple checklist, intended for consumers, that describes the how-to of collecting, pumping, storing, using, and reheating is shown in Box 10-4. A

Box 10-4

Guidelines for Consumer Education: Collecting, Pumping, Storing, Using, Reheating

Assembling the Equipment
- ❏ Washcloth, towels, or diapers.
- ❏ Clean or sterile plastic or glass container.
- ❏ Pump and related equipment (flange, tubing, etc.).

Preparing the Breasts
- ❏ Wash hands.
- ❏ Put a washcloth, towel, or diaper under very warm running water until it is thoroughly soaked. Squeeze out water. Put on breast.
- ❏ Massage breasts: begin with gentle finger stimulation and gradually increase to stroking and then massage.
- ❏ Begin at outer edges of each breast quadrant and move toward the nipple.
- ❏ Hand express a few drops, just to get the milk flowing.

Pumping the Breasts
- ❏ Follow manufacturer's directions for operating pump.
- ❏ Follow manufacturer's directions for cleaning. For most, this involves simply cleaning the flange and tubing with soapy water and rinsing thoroughly after each use (or wash and rinse in electric dishwasher).

Storing in Refrigerator
- ❏ Put in refrigerator immediately.
- ❏ Refrigerator temperature should be ≤39° F (5.5° C).
- ❏ Use within 48–72 hours; otherwise transfer to freezer.
- ❏ Previously frozen breast milk may be refrigerated for up to 24 hours.

Storing in Freezer
- ❏ Use within 2–4 weeks if in freezer compartment in a refrigerator (old-fashioned type).
- ❏ Use within 3 months if in freezer section of refrigerator at less than −20° C (−4° F) (judge by hardness of ice cream).
- ❏ Use within 6 months if in deep freezer.

Using/Thawing/Rewarming
- ❏ Use oldest milk first.
- ❏ Thaw in refrigerator or in bowl of lukewarm water.
- ❏ Warm in basin of water.

---

more detailed list, outlined in Box 10-5, highlights key instruction points for implementing a teaching plan for mothers. These key points apply to all mothers regardless of their circumstances. Recommendations for expressing and storing human milk are different for full-term, healthy neonates than for those who are sick. A comparison is found in Table 10-7.

Mother's own milk that is saved or stored is often incorrectly referred to as *banked milk*. This term should be used only when referring to donor milk. In this chapter the focus is on storing the mother's own milk (i.e., the woman who saves and stores the milk for her own infant). In saving and storing mother's own milk, three things must

be considered: (1) *temperature* (refrigerating, freezing), (2) *processing* (heat-treating or freezing the milk), and (3) *material* of the container. Table 10-6 highlights the effects of temperature, processing, and container material on milk components and possible pathogens.

Whereas the container material primarily affects the *components of milk*, as discussed previously, storage temperature and processing are more likely to affect *pathogens*. The titer of secretory IgA for *E. coli* polysaccharides occurs because it adheres to the side of some polyethylene bags; this is clinically important. Expert authors and clinicians have differing opinions about using these bags to store milk for compromised infants,

Box 10-5
Providing Human Milk for All Infants: Key Instruction Points

General
- Once a day, rinse your breasts with water while bathing or showering. It is not necessary to wash breast or nipples before each pumping session.
- Wash your hands well with soap and water each time before you express your milk. Use a nail brush to clean under fingernails once a day, or if hands are especially soiled or nails especially long.

Expressing Milk
- Use a method of expression that is appropriate to your circumstances.
- Express milk into a container.
- Thoroughly wash pump parts that are removable and those parts that have touched the milk. Use hot, soapy water and rinse well, place parts on a clean towel, cover them with another clean towel, and allow them to air dry. You may also dry them with a clean towel or put all of the removable parts through the dishwasher cycle.

Collecting
- Select a container that is appropriate, depending on how you express and your infant's circumstances.
- Package milk in amounts that the infant takes at one feeding.
- Pour the milk only once to decrease risk of contamination.
- Label the milk.

Storing
- Store the milk in the back of the refrigerator or the freezer, not in the door.
- Storage recommendations differ according to whether the infant is well or sick. See accompanying recommendations.
- Make sure the lid is solid, not a nipple with a hole.

Transporting
- Milk can be transported in an insulated bag or chest.

Thawing/Reheating
- Place in the refrigerator for a day.
- For a quick thaw, hold the frozen milk container under cool or lukewarm running tap water or place it in a bowl of lukewarm water.
- Gently rotate the milk container. The cream part will be separated from the rest of the milk, and rotating the container mixes it together. Do not shake vigorously.
- Never microwave. Hot spots can develop because heating is uneven. Additionally, this reduces the levels of IgA, decreases the activity of lysozyme, and encourages growth of *E. coli*.

Source: Human Milk Banking Association of North America. *Recommendations for Collection, Storage and Handling of a Mother's Milk for Her Own Infant in the Hospital Setting.* West Hartford, CT: HMBANA; 1993.

but the Human Milk Banking Association of North America strongly recommends not using them for this purpose.[33]

Bacterial contamination can happen at any time during pumping, collecting, or storing milk. And "there is no consensus about the bacteriological criteria for untreated human milk fed to babies in neonatal units."[54] However, most of the organisms that have been found in human milk are normal flora.[55,56]

Room Temperature

Whether or not milk may be stored at room temperature is largely dependent on the infant who is going to receive it. Early research suggested that mature milk can stand at room temperature for up to 6 hours[57,58] before being given to a well infant. This directive has been further refined; milk may stand at room temperature for up to 4 hours if the room temperature is no warmer than

T A B L E   10-7

PROVIDING MOTHER'S MILK FOR WELL OR SICK INFANTS: A COMPARISON

		Full-Term Healthy Infant	Infant in Intensive Care Unit
Pumping	Initiation	• Put full-term, healthy newborn, not pump, to breast	• Pump early (within first 6 hr) to increase milk production and reduce bacteria
	Frequency	• Pump as often as the infant would breast-feed	• Pump at least 5 times per day
	Duration	• Pump until the sprays diminish and the breast feels soft (usually 10-15 minutes)	• Pump at least 100 min per 24 hr with an *electric* pump
	Method	• Short-term, doesn't matter	• Electric hospital-grade pump
Collecting	Routine screening for bacteria	• Not necessary	• Not necessary
	Discarding first few milliliters	• Not necessary	• Not necessary
	Containers	• Any clean container is acceptable	• Small, sterile containers; centrifuge containers (50 ml) work best for tiny infants; use glass or hard-sided plastic
	Labeling	• If infant is at home, label with date	• Label with date, time, infant's name, and nursery location, ID number, other pertinent identifying data
	Quantity	• Put into one container only what infant is likely to consume in one feeding; for infants less than 1 month old this will be about 2-3 oz	• Put into one container only what infant is likely to consume in one feeding; the amount will vary dramatically from one infant to the other, depending on health status; consult with staff
	Layering	• Probably okay	• Not advised; bacterial contamination is more likely
Storing	Room temperature	• Store up to 4 hr	• Not advised
	Refrigerator <4° C (39° F)	• Store up to 72 hr	• Store up to 48 hr
	Freezer compartment <−20° C (−4° F)	• Store up to 3 mo	• Store up to 3 mo
	Deep freezer < −20° C (−4° F)	• Store up to 6 mo	• Store up to 3 mo; preferable to use out-dated human milk rather than artificial milk
Transporting	Refrigerated milk	• In its own container	• In insulated box or chest
	Frozen milk	• In insulated box or chest, no ice	• In insulated box or chest, no ice
Delivery	Thawing	• Thaw in refrigerator for 24 hr; for quick thaw, run under lukewarm tap water	• Thaw in refrigerator for 24 hr; for quick thaw, run under tap water
	Pasteurizing	• Not recommended for mother's own milk	• Not recommended for mother's own milk
	Continuous gavage	• Does not apply	• Change tubing every 4 hr
			• Shorten feeding tube (see text)

Source: Human Milk Banking Association of North America. *Recommendations for Collection, Storage and Handling of a Mother's Milk for Her Own Infant in the Hospital Setting.* West Hartford, CT: HMBANA; 1993.

25° C (77° F) or up to 24 hours if the room is no warmer than 15° C (59° F).[59] Colostrum may stand without likelihood of contamination for up to 24 hours,[58] presumably because of its large amount of antiinfective properties. Apart from concerns about pathogens, milk may also stand at room temperature of 15° to 25° C (59° to 77° F) without a decrease in the important digestive enzymes lipase and amylase.[60]

Refrigeration

There is no significant bacterial colonization of milk that has been stored in the refrigerator for up to 48 hours.[61] Milk should be stored at temperatures colder than 4° C (39° F)[62] for up to 24[59] to 48 hours,[63] since there is no significant bacterial colonization of milk before then.[61] Storage in glass containers at 4° C (39° F) for 48 hours causes a decrease in the viability of the cells and in macrophage and neutrophil concentration. Lymphocyte concentration is not affected.[64]

Freezing

Storing and feeding from the same bottle decreases possible contamination when the milk is poured from the storage container to the feeding bottle, so this approach is frequently used. It is best to collect milk into hard-sided containers—either glass or plastic—instead of bags because they are not susceptible to puncturing. (Other disadvantages of plastic bags have been discussed earlier in the chapter.)

Freezing destroys living cells such as antimicrobial factors.[54] Therefore, milk should be given fresh whenever possible. If it is not practical to provide fresh milk, milk may be safely stored in the freezer for different amounts of time, depending on the type of freezer. Milk can be safely stored in old-fashioned freezers—the type with the freezing compartment inside the refrigera-

tor—for up to 1 month. Most households, however, have a separate freezing compartment above, below, or beside the refrigerator section. Milk can be safely stored in these freezers for up to 3 months. The freezer should be kept at approximately −20° C (−4° F) or cooler. Milk may be safely stored in deep freezers for up to 6 months. These times are optimal, but until a year has elapsed, it is better to use "outdated" human milk than artificial milk.

TRANSPORTING

Milk may be transported in the collection container, and the container put into an insulated chest or carrying case; adding ice to frozen milk is unnecessary. On a long trip it may be wise to add ice packs to the container to transport refrigerated milk. The more expensive chests that hold six-packs work well, but disposable Styrofoam carriers are adequate.

THAWING AND REHEATING

It is always best to give the milk fresh.[54] If that is not possible, however, freeze it and thaw it in amounts that the infant is likely to consume at one feeding. For tiny preterm newborns, this may be only a few milliliters. Healthy, term infants will consume less than 3 oz per feeding during the first month of life.

Milk can be thawed in one of two ways. The preferred method is to thaw it in the refrigerator overnight because secretory IgA is best preserved through this method.[65] If this is not possible, put the container of milk under lukewarm water (<44 to 49° C; 111 to 120° F) until it has thawed.[65]

Milk or other foods for infants should never be microwaved. Microwaving at high temperatures decreases the amount of antiinfective factors present, and the safety of microwaving at lower temperatures has not been established.[66] Case reports show that infants have been severely burned by food that has been "warmed" in the microwave.[67]

SUMMARY

Separation often can and does occur and may be either planned or unplanned. The key to an optimal experience for both the mother and her infant is to develop a plan to maintain lactation. For the well infant who is away from his mother intermittently, the mother can devise a plan well ahead of time to ensure that lactation continues as planned. For the compromised infant, the nurse often needs to initiate a plan to help the mother get started lactating and then, along with the mother, develop a more precise plan about how to express, save, store, transport, and collect her milk. Above all, the nurse must help the woman to see that expressing and storing her milk is a realistic and rewarding alternative.

References

1. Elander G, Lindberg T. Short mother-infant separation during first week of life influences the duration of breastfeeding. *Acta Paediatr Scand* 1984; 73:237-240.
2. Scrimshaw SC, Engle PL, Arnold L, Haynes K. Factors affecting breastfeeding among women of Mexican origin or descent in Los Angeles. *Am J Public Health* 1987;77:467-470.
3. Gielen AC, Faden RR, O'Campo P, Brown CH, Paige DM. Maternal employment during the early postpartum period: effects on initiation and continuation of breast-feeding. *Pediatrics* 1991;87:298-305.
4. Katcher AL, Lanese MG. Breast-feeding by employed mothers: a reasonable accommodation in the work place. *Pediatrics* 1985;75:644-647.
5. Knowles M. *The Modern Practice of Adult Education.* New York: Associated Press; 1980.
6. Auerbach KG. Employed breastfeeding mothers: problems they encounter. *Birth* 1984;11:17-20.
7. Auerbach KG. Assisting the employed breastfeeding mother. *J Nurse Midwifery* 1990;35:26-34.
8. Frederick IB, Auerbach KG. Maternal-infant separation and breast-feeding: the return to work or school. *J Reprod Med* 1985;30:523-526.
9. Moore JF, Jansa N. A survey of policies and practices in support of breastfeeding mothers in the workplace. *Birth* 1987;14:191-195.
10. Kurinij N, Shiono PH, Ezrine SF, Rhoads GG. Does maternal employment affect breast-feeding? *Am J Public Health* 1989;79:1247-1250.
11. Ryan AS, Martinez GA. Breast-feeding and the working mother: a profile. *Pediatrics* 1989;83:524-531.
12. Auerbach KG, Guss E. Maternal employment and breastfeeding: a study of 567 women's experiences. *Am J Dis Child* 1984;138:958-960.
13. Kearney MH, Cronenwett L. Breastfeeding and employment. *J Obstet Gynecol Neonatal Nurs* 1991;20:471-480.
14. Greenberg CS, Smith K. Anticipatory guidance for the employed breast-feeding mother. *J Pediatr Health Care* 1991;5:204-209.
15. Hills-Bonczyk SG, Avery MD, Savik K, Potter S, Duckett LJ. Women's experiences with combining breast-feeding and employment. *J Nurse Midwifery* 1993;38:257-266.
16. Bell EH, Geyer J, Jones L. A structured intervention improves breastfeeding success for ill or preterm infants. *MCN Am J Matern Child Nurs* 1995;20:309-314.
17. Hunkeler B, Aebi C, Minder CE, Bossi E. Incidence and duration of breast-feeding of ill newborns. *J Pediatr Gastroenterol Nutr* 1994;18:37-40.
18. Cohen SP. High tech-soft touch: breastfeeding issues. *Clin Perinatol* 1987;14:187-196.

19. Hill PD, Brown LP, Harker TL. Initiation and frequency of breast expression in breastfeeding mothers of LBW and VLBW infants. *Nurs Res* 1995; 44:352-355.

20. Asquith MT, Pedrotti PW, Harrod JR, Stevenson DK, Sunshine P. The bacterial content of breast milk after the early initiation of expression using a standard technique. *J Pediatr Gastroenterol Nutr* 1984;3:104-107.

21. Kaufman KJ, Hall LA. Influences of the social network on choice and duration of breast-feeding in mothers of preterm infants. *Res Nurs Health* 1989;12:149-159.

22. Forte A, Mayberry LJ, Ferketich S. Breast milk collection and storage practices among mothers of hospitalized neonates. *J Perinatol* 1987;7:35-39.

23. Anderson GC. Current knowledge about skin-to-skin (kangaroo) care for preterm infants. *J Perinatol* 1991;11:216-226.

24. Affonso D, Hurst I, Mayberry L, Haller L, Yost K, Lynch M. Stressors reported by mothers of hospitalized premature infants. *Neonatal Netw* 1992; 11:63-70.

25. Whitelaw A, Heisterkamp G, Sleath K, Acolet D, Richards M. Skin to skin contact for very low birthweight infants and their mothers. *Arch Dis Child* 1988;63:1377-1381.

26. Hurst NM, Valentine CJ, Renfro L, Burns P, Ferlic L. Skin-to-skin holding in the neonatal intensive care unit influences maternal milk volume. *J Perinatol* 1997;17:213-217.

27. Gibbs JH, Fisher C, Bhattacharya S, Goddard P, Baum JD. Drip breast milk: its composition, collection and pasteurization. *Early Hum Dev* 1977; 1:227-245.

28. Lucas A, Gibbs JA, Baum JD. The biology of human drip breast milk. *Early Hum Dev* 1978;2:351-361.

29. Tyson JE, Edwards WH, Rosenfeld AM, Beer AE. Collection methods and contamination of bank milk. *Arch Dis Child* 1982;57:396-398.

30. Liebhaber M, Lewiston NJ, Asquith MT, Sunshine P. Comparison of bacterial contamination with two methods of human milk collection. *J Pediatr* 1978;92:236-267.

31. Johnson CA. An evaluation of breast pumps currently available on the American market. *Clin Pediatr (Phila)* 1983;22:40-45.

32. Frantz K. *Breastfeeding Product Guide 1994.* Sunland, CA: Geddes Productions; 1993.

33. Arnold LDW, ed. *Recommendations for Collection, Storage, and Handling of a Mother's Milk for Her Own Infant in the Hospital Setting.* West Hartford, CT: Human Milk Banking Association of North America; 1993.

34. Green D, Moye L, Schreiner RL, Lemons JA. The relative efficacy of four methods of human milk expression. *Early Hum Dev* 1982;6:153-159.

35. Zinaman MJ, Hughes V, Queenan JT, Labbok MH, Albertson B. Acute prolactin and oxytocin responses and milk yield to infant suckling and artificial methods of expression in lactating women. *Pediatrics* 1992;89:437-440.

36. Auerbach KG. Sequential and simultaneous breast pumping: a comparison. *Int J Nurs Stud* 1990; 27:257-265.

37. Hill PD, Aldag JC, Chatterton RT. The effect of sequential and simultaneous breast pumping on milk volume and prolactin levels: a pilot study. *J Hum Lact* 1996;12:193-199.

38. Groh-Wargo S, Toth A, Mahoney K, Simonian S, Wasser T, Rose S. The utility of a bilateral breast pumping system for mothers of premature infants. *Neonatal Netw* 1995;14:31-36.

39. Meier P, Wilks S. The bacteria in expressed mothers' milk. *MCN Am J Matern Child Nurs* 1987; 12:420-423.

40. Carroll L, Osman M, Davies DP. Does discarding the first few millilitres of breast milk improve the bacteriological quality of bank breast milk? *Arch Dis Child* 1980;55:898-899.

41. Hopkinson JM, Schanler RJ, Garza C. Milk production by mothers of premature infants. *Pediatrics* 1988;81:815-820.

42. DeCarvalho M, Anderson DM, Giangreco A, Pittard WB III. Frequency of milk expression and milk production by mothers of nonnursing premature neonates. *Am J Dis Child* 1985;139:483-485.

43. Lonnerdal B, Forsum E, Hambraeus L. A longitudinal study of the protein, nitrogen, and lactose contents of human milk from Swedish well-nourished mothers. *Am J Clin Nutr* 1976;29:1127-1133.

44. DeCarvalho M, Robertson S, Merkatz R, Klaus M. Milk intake and frequency of feeding in breast fed infants. *Early Hum Dev* 1982;7:155-163.

45. Feher SD, Berger LR, Johnson JD, Wilde JB. Increasing breast milk production for premature infants with a relaxation/imagery audiotape. *Pediatrics* 1989;83:57-60.

46. Yokoyama Y, Ueda T, Irahara M, Aono T. Releases of oxytocin and prolactin during breast massage and suckling in puerperal women. *Eur J Obstet Gynecol Reprod Biol* 1994;53:17-20.

47. Morse JM, Bottorff JL. The emotional experience of breast expression. *J Nurse Midwifery* 1988; 33:165-170.

48. Hopkinson JM, Schanler RJ, Fraley JK, Garza C. Milk production by mothers of premature infants: influence of cigarette smoking. *Pediatrics* 1992; 90:934-938.

49. Paxson CL Jr, Cress CC. Survival of human milk leukocytes. *J Pediatr* 1979;94:61-64.

50. Williamson MT, Murti PK. Effects of storage, time, temperature, and composition of containers on biologic components of human milk. *J Hum Lact* 1996;12:31-35.

51. Goldblum RM, Garza C, Johnson C, Harrist R, Nichols BL, Goldman AS. Effects of container upon immunologic factors in mature milk. *Nutr Res* 1981;1:449-459.

52. Pittard WB III, Geddes KM, Brown S, Mintz S, Hulsey TC. Bacterial contamination of human milk: container type and method of expression. *Am J Perinatol* 1991;8:25-27.

53. Wilks S, Meier P. Helping mothers express milk suitable for preterm and high-risk infant feeding. *MCN Am J Matern Child Nurs* 1988;13:121-123.

54. Pardou A, Serruys E, Mascart Lemone F, Dramaix M, Vis HL. Human milk banking: influence of storage processes and of bacterial contamination on some milk constituents. *Biol Neonate* 1994; 65:302-309.

55. Sosa R, Barness L. Bacterial growth in refrigerated human milk. *Am J Dis Child* 1987;141:111-112.

56. Law BJ, Urias BA, Lertzman J, Robson D, Romance L. Is ingestion of milk-associated bacteria by premature infants fed raw human milk controlled by routine bacteriologic screening? *J Clin Microbiol* 1989;27:1560-1566.

57. Nwankwo MU, Offor E, Okolo AA, Omene JA. Bacterial growth in expressed breast-milk. *Ann Trop Paediatr* 1988;8:92-95.

58. Pittard WR, Anderson DM, Cerutti ER, Boxerbaum B. Bacteriostatic qualities of human milk. *J Pediat* 1985;107:240-243.

59. Hamosh M, Ellis LA, Pollock DR, Henderson TR, Hamosh P. Breastfeeding and the working mother: effect of time and temperature of short-term storage on proteolysis, lipolysis, and bacterial growth in milk. *Pediatrics* 1996;97:492-498.

60. Hamosh M, Henderson TR, Ellis LA, Mao JI, Hamosh P. Digestive enzymes in human milk: stability at suboptimal storage temperatures. *J Pediatr Gastroenterol Nutr* 1997;24:38-43.

61. Larson E, Zuill R, Zier V, Berg B. Storage of human breast milk. *Infect Control* 1984;5:127-130.

62. Lavine M, Clark RM. The effect of short-term refrigeration of milk and addition of breast milk fortifier on the delivery of lipids during tube feeding. *J Pediatr Gastroenterol Nutr* 1989;8:496-499.

63. Lemons PM, Miller K, Eitzen H, Strodtbeck F, Lemons JA. Bacterial growth in human milk during continuous feeding. *Am J Perinatol* 1983;1:76-80.

64. Pittard WB III, Bill K. Human milk banking: effect of refrigeration on cellular components. *Clin Pediatr (Phila)* 1981;20:31-33.

65. Sigman M, Burke KI, Swarner OW, Shavlik GW. Effects of microwaving human milk: changes in IgA content and bacterial count. *J Am Diet Assoc* 1989;89:690-692.

66. Quan R, Yang C, Rubinstein S, et al. Effects of microwave radiation on anti-infective factors in human milk. *Pediatrics* 1992;89(4, pt 1):667-669.

67. Hibbard RA, Blevins R. Palatal burn due to bottle warming in a microwave oven. *Pediatrics* 1989; 82:382-384.

6

d-
ıg
i-
r

69

_f

.... during tube feeding. *Arch Dis Child* 1985;60:164-166.

70. Bitman J, Wood DL, Mehta NR, Hamosh P, Hamosh M. Lipolysis of triglycerides of human milk during storage at low temperatures: a note of caution. *J Pediatr Gastroenterol Nutr* 1983;2:521-524.

71. Friend BA, Shahani KM, Long CA, Vaughn LA. The effect of processing and storage on key enzymes, B vitamins, and lipids of mature human milk. I. Evaluation of fresh samples and effects of freezing and frozen storage. *Pediatr Res* 1983;17:61-64.

72. Garza C, Johnson CA, Harrist R, Nichols BL. Effects of methods of collection and storage on nutrients in human milk. *Early Hum Dev* 1982;6:295-303.

73. Minder W, Roten H, Zurbrugg RP, Gehriger G, Lebek G, Nagel G. Quality of breast milk: its control and preservation. *Helv Paediatr Acta* 1982; 37:115-137.

74. Garza C, Nichols BL. Studies of human milk relevant to milk banking. *J Am Coll Nutr* 1984;3:123-129.

75. Welsh JK, May JT. Anti-infective properties of breast milk. *J Pediatr* 1979;94:1-9.

76. VanZoeren-Grobben D, Schrijver J, Van den Berg H, Berger HM. Human milk vitamin content after pasteurisation, storage, or tube feeding. *Arch Dis Child* 1987;62:161-165.

77. Berkow SE, Freed LM, Hamosh M, Bitman J, Wood DL, Happ B et al. Lipases and lipids in human milk: effect of freeze-thawing and storage. *Pediatr Res* 1984;18:1257-1262.

78. Jensen RG, Jensen GL. Specialty lipids for infant nutrition. I. Milks and formulas. *J Pediatr Gastroenterol Nutr* 1992;15:232-245.

79. Dworsky M, Stagno S, Pass RF, Cassady G, Alford C. Persistence of cytomegalovirus in human milk after storage. *J Pediatr* 1982;101:440-443.

80. Garza C, Butte NF. Energy concentration of human milk estimated for 24-h pools and various abbreviated sampling schemes. *J Pediatr Gastroenterol Nutr* 1986;5:943-948.

81. Williamson MT, Murti PK. Effects of storage, time, temperature, and composition of containers on biologic components of human milk. *J Hum Lact* 1996;12:31-35.

11

Nutritional Sources for Newborns

Throughout this text, there has been a clear emphasis on the idea that direct, exclusive breastfeeding is the ideal source of nutrition for newborns, older infants, and older children whether they are well or compromised. When the newborn is not feeding directly at the breast or when supplementation is medically indicated, other alternatives must be explored.

The aim of this chapter is to describe the indications, advantages, and limitations of four basic sources of nutrition for the infant who is not breastfeeding directly: (1) fresh mother's milk—either modified or unmodified; (2) previously stored mother's milk—modified or unmodified; (3) donor milk; and (4) artificial milk. A basic understanding of these nutritional sources will enable the nurse to provide better consumer education and to advocate for human milk as the ideal source for maintaining homeostasis in the infant.

These four sources are available for both healthy and compromised infants. If the infant is healthy and direct breastfeeding is interrupted—for example, the mother is employed outside the home—the mother should be strongly urged to use her own previously stored milk. If the infant is critically ill, the nurse should have a thorough understanding of the prescribed source of nutrition, educating and explaining to families why other sources of nutrition may be ordered in addition to the mother's own milk. If the infant is healthy and direct breastfeeding is not possible, the nurse needs to advocate human milk—the mother's own milk or donor milk—as the best source of nutrition for the infant. Artificial milk is only one—and the least desirable—of the available alternatives.

HUMAN MILK

Human milk is unquestionably the gold standard for infant nutrition in all cases.[1] Ideally, the full-term, healthy infant experiences direct, exclusive breastfeeding; the milk itself and the act of feeding provide many advantages, as outlined in previous chapters.

When direct breastfeeding is not possible—for whatever reason—fresh milk or previously stored mother's milk is the next best choice, as described in Chapter 10. Expressed milk varies in the amount of benefits it provides for the infant. Freshly expressed mother's own milk offers the most benefit, followed by previously stored mother's own milk, and then donor milk. Artificial milk ("formula") is always inferior to human milk.

Mother's Own Milk: Fresh

Fresh milk comes from the infant's own mother and is given immediately or almost immediately—without processing or storing—to the infant. By definition, fresh milk is from the mother, never from donors. Milk from the infant's own mother, or mother's own milk ("MOM," or expressed mother's milk ["EMM"]) is best when given fresh to the infant (as opposed to refrigerated or frozen). Of course, the infant gets fresh milk when feeding directly at the breast (direct breastfeeding), but he may also receive fresh milk if the mother expresses the milk and gives it to him to consume via some other method, as described in Chapter 12. More than milk that has been processed or stored, fresh milk has the greatest nutritional value for the infant.

During the early days of breastfeeding, full-term, healthy newborns should be given mother's milk only. Artificial milk supplements should be given only when medically indicated. Acceptable medical reasons for supplementing full-term, healthy newborns are outlined by the U.S. Committee for UNICEF and are found in Box 5-2.

Mother's Own Milk: Previously Stored

When mother's own milk is not given to the infant immediately (or almost immediately), it is stored, usually in a container in either the refrigerator or the freezer. Previously stored milk may be more practical to use in some situations. For example, the employed mother may wish to leave milk in the refrigerator for her infant, or the mother of a critically ill infant may live many miles from a tertiary care center and may need to leave her milk for the infant to consume later. Previously stored milk can be used for either well or compromised newborns. It is important to remember, however, that the requirements for saving and storing are more rigorous for compromised infants than for well infants, as described in Chapter 10.

As Chapter 10 explains, however, temperature, the type of container, and the length of storage influence the milk. Milk that is not promptly fed to infants may be altered in one of two ways. First, some of the components of the milk may be diminished during storage. Even if milk is not exposed to extremes in temperature, exposing it to light results, within 3 hours, in a 50% reduction in riboflavin content and 70% loss of vitamin A.[2] Second, pathogens may enter stored milk. The operative word here is *may* because stored milk, although it *may* be vulnerable to these limitations, is an excellent alternative to fresh milk.

Modified Mother's Own Milk

The American Academy of Pediatrics states, "Human milk is the preferred feeding for all infants, including premature and sick newborns, with rare exception."[1] However, a compromised newborn who is unable to breastfeed directly may need to have his mother's milk "modified" in some way; for example, he may need expressed milk with an added fortifier. The fortifier may be added to either fresh or previously stored milk.

Parents of preterm, low-birth-weight (LBW) or very low-birth-weight (VLBW) infants may seem bewildered when suddenly the slogan "breast is best" has been replaced with a message that seemingly says "breast alone is inadequate." The nurse may find that at one moment she is emphasizing the superiority of human milk for the compromised infant, including its antiinfective properties, biospecificity, easy digestibility and absorption, presence of enzymes, and low renal solute load as discussed in Chapter 7. In the next moment she may need to explain why artificial milk or human milk fortifier has been ordered. It is important that parents not receive a seemingly conflicting message. Human milk *is* best for these infants. If the infant could consume an adequate volume of human milk, indeed he could receive enough proteins, fats, carbohydrates, and calories without modification or artificial supplementation. (Calcium and phosphorus would still be insufficient.) However, the compromised infant may have a very small stomach capacity, a limited ability to suckle, a high metabolic rate, or all of these or other factors. Therefore, human milk alone may not meet his nutritional needs in some circumstances.

Fortified Milk

If the infant's needs are so great that he is unable to consume sufficient quantities of human milk to support growth and development, human milk can be fortified. Table 11-1 shows the volume of human milk, with and without fortification, that the newborn would need to consume to meet the suggested daily requirements.

Generally, fortifiers are indicated when the infant's birth weight is less than 1500 g (or 1800 g, depending on the hospital's protocol). These VLBW infants cannot thrive on their mother's milk only. Consuming human milk only, without fortifier, has been associated with poor growth rates and unmet nutritional needs during hospitalization and thereafter.[3-11] They are also at risk

for osteopenia and rickets of prematurity. (Refer to Chapter 7 for a more complete discussion of preterm needs.)

Commercially prepared products can be added to mother's own milk to fortify it with extra nutrients, especially calcium, phosphorus and protein, as well as carbohydrate, sodium, potassium, and magnesium. Some contain zinc, copper, and vitamins. To date, no studies have compared the efficacy of different brands of fortifiers.

There are two types of fortifiers: powdered and liquid. Both add energy and other nutrients to human milk. When a preterm, VLBW infant can tolerate human milk at greater than 100 ml/kg/day, supplementation using a human milk fortifier is started[12] and continues until the infant is taking all feedings from the breast directly or weighs 1800 to 2000 g, depending on the nursery protocol. Usually, the fortifier is added gradually until the ideal "dose" is achieved, often referred to as *full fortification*. Full fortification is a 1:1 concentration for the liquid product, and 4 packets of the powdered product per deciliter (100 ml). The goal is to achieve a weight gain of approximately 15 g/kg/day.[13]

Powdered fortifier (Enfamil Human Milk Fortifier) is likely to be ordered when a sufficient volume of mother's milk is available, but the infant needs more calories and other nutrients than what he consumes from the human milk. Similarly, if volume needs to be restricted, the powder is preferable because more human milk can be given.

To administer a feeding using the *powdered* fortifier, dissolve the powder in the mother's milk. Check the order to be sure the amount is within acceptable limits. A typical order might start with adding one or two packets per 100 ml of mother's milk, then progress to 2 packets, 3 packets, and then 4 packets. The 4 packets per 100 ml of milk (or 1 packet per 25 ml of milk) provide approximately 82 kcal/100 ml (24 kcal/ounce) to the infant; this is usually the maximum amount ordered. To dissolve the powder, first run the milk under water until it reaches about 37° C (98° F).

TABLE 11-1

VOLUME (ML) NEEDED TO MEET ESTIMATED DAILY NUTRIENT REQUIREMENTS PER KILOGRAM OF INFANT BODY MASS

This table shows the volume of human milk that would meet estimated daily nutrient requirements per kilogram of infant body mass. For example, the infant would need to consume 176 ml of human milk per kilogram per day in order to obtain a requirement of 120 kcal/kg/day. In some situations, this is not possible. By fortifying the milk, however, the infant could consume less volume (e.g., 146 or 160 ml) and meet the requirement. (Values based on manufacturer's product information leaflet.)

Nutrient	Estimated Daily Requirements per Kilogram	Human Milk Only	Human Milk Plus 4 Packets of HMF/100 ml	Human Milk Fortified With Natural Care (1:1 Dilution)
Kilocalories	120 kcal	176ml	146	160
Protein	≥3 g	286	171	184
Calcium	200 mg	714	169	201
Phosphorus	100 mg	714	169	202
Sodium	2 mEq	256	183	174
Potassium	2 mEq	149	114	99

Add the fortifier and shake (avoid overshaking). Warming the milk helps, but the fortifier can be difficult to dissolve.

Liquid fortifier (Similac Natural Care) is most likely to be used when the mother does not have a sufficient volume of milk. It provides volume as well as nutrients. Also, fortified milk has a lower osmolarity (and therefore lower renal solute load) in the liquid, rather than the powdered, form. However, the liquid fortifier provides a lesser amount of calories, calcium, and phosphorus than the powdered fortifier, as shown in Table 11-2.

Before administering a feeding using the liquid fortifier, check the order to make sure it is within acceptable limits. A typical order might start with adding 1 part liquid fortifier to 2 parts human milk; if the infant can tolerate this for at least 24 hours, he can advance to "full fortification" (i.e., 1 part liquid fortifier to 1 part human milk). When human milk is in a 1:1 ratio with the Natural Care, however, it provides about 22 kcal per ounce. Some nursery protocols may allow a little powdered fortifier to be added after the mother's milk is diluted 1:1 with the liquid fortifier to increase the calories and nutrients without further diluting the human milk.

Until recently, newborns were not discharged to home using fortifier. Discharge nutrition is a controversial issue at this point, with some centers discharging infants to home while still using the fortifier. One possible rationale for using liquid fortifier at home is if the mother has especially low milk volume. If the neonatal team determines that there are substantial benefits to this practice, the newborn may be discharged with an order to continue fortification of his mother's milk. If this is the case, discharge planning needs to include specific instructions about how to combine the fortifier with human milk. A possible rationale for using powdered fortifier is that the mother has plenty of her own milk frozen and wishes to give a "relief" bottle. The cost of the fortifier should be considered, however, as well as its availability. Frequently these products are both cost-prohibitive and difficult to obtain. Furthermore, the extra expense is borne by the parents, not by their health insurance company.

Fortified human milk is more advantageous than artificial milk. In one study, infants who

T A B L E 11-2

NUTRIENTS PROVIDED BY SIMILAC NATURAL CARE (NC) AND ENFAMIL HUMAN MILK FORTIFIER (HMF), PER 100 ML

This table shows the amount of nutrient provided by human milk alone and when it is combined with fortifier. For example, when 1 packet of human milk fortifier is added to 1 dl (100 ml) of human milk it provides 0.72 kcal per ml (approximately 22 kcal per ounce). NB: The recommended dilution is 1:1 for Natural Care; more concentrated feedings are not recommended except in unusual circumstances. The recommended dilution for Human Milk Fortifier is 4 packets/dl (100 ml). Values based on manufacturer's product information leaflet.

	Natural Care Only	Human Milk with Similac Natural Care				Human Milk	Human Milk With Enfamil Human Milk Fortifier			
Ratio	Alone	1:3	1:2	1:1	2:1	Alone	1 pkt/dl	2 pkt/dl	3 pkt/dl	4 pkt/dl
kcal	81	78	77	75	72	68	72	75	79	82
CHO (g)	8.61	8.26	8.14	7.91	7.67	7.2	7.88	8.55	9.23	9.9
Protein (g)	2.2	1.91	1.82	1.63	1.43	1.05	1.23	1.4	1.58	1.75
Fat (g)	4.41	4.28	4.24	4.16	4.07	3.9	<3.93	<3.95	<3.98	<4
Ca (mg)	171	135.3	123.3	99.5	75.7	28	50.5	73	95.5	118
P (mg)	85	67.3	61.3	49.5	37.7	14	25.3	36.5	47.8	59
Na (mEq)	1.52	1.34	1.27	1.15	1.03	.78	0.86	0.93	1.01	1.09
K (mEq)	2.69	2.36	2.24	2.02	1.79	1.34	1.45	1.55	1.65	1.75
Vitamin D (IU)	122	92	82	62	42	2	54.5	107	159.5	212

◄———— Increasing Concentrations ————   ———— Increasing Concentrations ————►

were fed fortified human milk and supplemented with preterm artificial milk when maternal milk supply was inadequate made weight gains about the same as cohorts who were fed only artificial milk. The important factor here is how much human milk the infant receives; with adequate maternal supply, those fed *mostly* human milk made better weight gains than those who were exclusively formula-fed.[14]

Hindmilk Only

It is often difficult for compromised newborns to get the hindmilk while at the breast, particularly if they tire easily. Expressing milk and giving hindmilk only is one strategy for providing extra fat and calories. This is a relatively new concept, and little research has been done on the efficacy of this practice. However, recently, LBW infants made significantly greater weight gains when given hindmilk only.[15]

Donor Milk: Human Milk Banking

Definition

Donor milk is milk that has been expressed by a lactating mother for an infant other than her own. She donates this milk to a donor milk bank, and it is distributed to infants whose mothers cannot provide human milk. Donor milk is processed, whereas mother's own milk is not. This is important because processing human milk—usually through heat-treating—affects the components and potential pathogens of human milk. Donor milk is frequently "pooled," meaning that it may have come from several different women.

Indications

If the mother's own milk is unavailable—the mother is unable or unwilling to lactate—donor milk, while less desirable than mother's own milk, is preferable to artificial milk. However, banked donor milk must be prescribed. A frequent reason for prescribing it is prematurity. Preterm infants who are fed pasteurized donor milk have better outcomes than those who are fed artificial milk.[16] However, multiple other reasons have been reported for using donor milk, as described in Box 11-1.

Limitations and Considerations

Although donor milk has many nutritional benefits, other factors may be potential deterrents to using it. The fee for human milk varies from bank to bank but is usually about $2.50 per ounce. Usually, but not always, this processing fee is covered by the parents' health care insurance, Medicaid, or the Women, Infants and Children (WIC) program if an order has been written for the milk. Also, donor milk has become less popular since the unsubstantiated fear of disease transmission has become greater.

Donor milk is processed. Technically, refrigerating, freezing, and thawing are ways of processing human milk, but here the discussion will be limited to the more detrimental processing that typically occurs with donor milk, namely, pasteurization and lyophilization. (These processes are never recommended for mother's own milk.) Subjecting milk to pasteurization or lyophilization alters three basic factors: (1) immune factors—immunoglobulins,[17] antibodies to *E. coli*, lactoferrin,[18] and viable lymphocytes[19]; (2) antiviral (CMV, HIV); and (3) bacteria.

Pasteurization

Pasteurization is a heating process whereby organisms in milk are destroyed. The Human Milk Banking Association of North America (HMBANA) standard is to pasteurize human milk at a

Box 11-1
Clinical Uses of Donor Milk

Nutritional Uses

Prematurity
Failure to thrive
Malabsorption syndromes
Short-gut syndrome
Renal failure
Feeding intolerance
Inborn errors of metabolism
Postsurgical nutrition
Cardiac problems
Bronchopulmonary dysplasia
Pediatric burn cases

Medicinal/Therapeutic Uses

Treatment for infectious diseases (intractable diarrhea, gastroenteritis, infantile botulism, sepsis, pneumonia, hemorrhagic conjunctivitis)
Postsurgical healing (omphalocele, gastroschisis, intestinal obstruction/bowel fistula, colostomy repair)
Immunodeficiency diseases (severe allergies, IgA deficiencies, HIV)
Inborn errors of metabolism
Solid organ transplants (including adults)
Noninfectious intestinal disorders (ulcerative colitis, irritable bowel syndrome)
Topical burn treatment

Preventive Uses

Necrotizing enterocolitis
Crohn's disease
Colitis
Allergies to bovine and soy milks/feeding intolerance
During immune suppression therapy

From the Human Milk Banking Association of North America, 1998.

temperature of 62.5° C for 30 minutes. Pasteurizing milk destroys its cellular content, including lymphocytes,[20] and the immunoglobulin and antiinfective properties are decreased.

Lyophilization

Lyophilization is the "rapid freezing and dehydration of the frozen product under high-vacuum freeze drying."[21] This process is undertaken to destroy pathogens, but it results in some destruction of cells as well. Lyophilization is never used in the

United States, but it is sometimes used in other countries.

Donor Milk Banks

The term *human milk bank* refers to those hospitals that operate and staff a formal donor milk bank and accept milk not only from mothers of hospitalized infants but from donors as well. (The term *banked milk*, which appears frequently in research studies, can be misleading; it may correctly refer to donor milk or incorrectly to mother's own milk that has simply been stored.) This terminology is important because donor milk is processed, as shown in Figure 11-1, whereas mother's own milk usually is not.

HMBANA has defined the characteristics of a donor human milk bank; the definition and those in North America who meet it are listed in Appendix A. Donor milk banks belong to the HMBANA. Among other goals, this organization develops standards for milk banking practices and reviews those guidelines annually to see that they conform with current research.

For recipients, the benefits of donor human milk are many, and the risks are negligible. Only expressed breast milk is suitable for donation. Dripped milk—milk that drips from the contralateral breast while the infant is feeding at the other breast—is unacceptable because the energy value is low[22] and contamination is likely.[23,24] Further, milk is accepted only from healthy lactating women who meet the criteria to become donors. (Sometimes, potential donors are excluded only temporarily, for example, if they are receiving short-term medication therapy.) Working closely with the Centers for Disease Control and Prevention and the Food and Drug Administration, HMBANA has established four screening processes to prevent contaminated milk from being dispensed: (1) a thorough health history is obtained from the potential donor, (2) volunteer donors undergo serological testing, (3) donated milk is pasteurized, and (4) donated milk is tested for bacteria both before and after pasteurization, and milk is not dispensed unless its bacterial count is at zero.

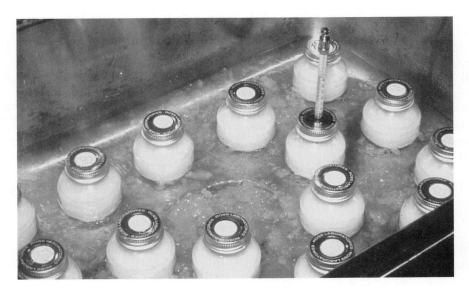

Fig. 11-1 Processing donor milk at human milk bank. Note water bath with bottle containing monitoring thermometer.

Milk banks provide benefits for donors, also. Typically, mothers make one-time donations when they have an unused supply in storage. This may happen when an older infant is consuming more solids than milk. The mother finds many containers of her milk occupying the freezer space but can't bring herself to discard the milk; donating the milk overcomes both obstacles. Sometimes, the mother of a critically ill infant has expressed and saved many ounces of milk for her own infant who later dies. She may gain some sense of consolation by donating her milk with the hope that it will help another to survive. Occasionally, a woman volunteers to express milk for the milk bank on a regular basis. In this case, the woman is producing more milk than her infant wants or needs to suckle; she therefore donates the oversupply to the bank. As advocates, we can help donors and recipients to reap the benefits of donor milk banks as described in Box 11-2.

Box 11-2
How Can We Help Potential Donors and Recipients?

- Approach the physician in charge of the patient's care and urge him to consider ordering donor human milk. If he agrees, he should then contact the HMBANA office (see Appendix A). Office personnel will direct the physician or other prescriber to the milk bank that is either geographically closest, or the bank that has the best supply of donor milk on hand. The physician must then write a prescription for the milk. Prescriptions may be faxed and followed with a hard-copy to the milk bank.

- Help the prescriber to gather pertinent details before sending the prescription to the milk bank. For example, the prescription must note the condition for which the donor milk is being prescribed, and the number of ounces required per day. Generally, the milk is shipped in batches for a 1 to 2 week supply.

- Oppose anyone who says that donor milk is not an option because the milk bank is too far away from the recipient. The milk can be shipped anywhere in the country. Multiple methods of transport have been used; if there is a substantial distance involved, the milk is usually shipped frozen with dry ice by overnight delivery service.

- Encourage women to become donors if their infants cannot use all of their milk. Refer women who wish to become donors to the HMBANA to see if they meet the eligibility criteria for becoming donors.

- Reassure potential donors that getting their milk to a milk bank is a realistic option. If the mother lives near a milk bank, she or a family member can drive the milk to the bank, or the bank sometimes has a volunteer pick up milk from local residents. If the mother does not live near a milk bank, however, she should consider donating to a milk bank that accepts out-of-state donations. Whether or not banks accept milk from out-of-state donors depends on their supply, which can vary dramatically from month to month. These banks nearly always pay for shipping the milk and for the cost of donor serological screening. If the donor has had blood drawn at her local hospital, she should ship a sample with the milk in order to spare the bank the cost.

- Persuade policy-makers to make donor milk the social norm. For example, encourage physicians to order a "stock" supply of donor milk. The physician can order a certain number of ounces of donor milk for the inpatient facility rather than for an individual patient. In this way, the donor milk is immediately available, and it deters staff from giving artificial milk.

- Become involved in legislation modeled after the New York State law that entitles all infants access to human milk. The public health law says, ". . . any and all infants requiring human breast milk be assured access to sufficient quantities of wholesome human breast milk, donated by concerned lactating mothers on a continual and systematic basis." (See Appendix D-3 for full text and citation.)

- Incorporate the topic of donor milk into childbirth classes. When parents become aware of this alternative, they will begin to ask their health care providers to prescribe it. Similarly, mothers who have unused milk are likely to consider donating it if they recognize how their gift could be a lifesaver for another. Both the supply and demand could increase if only there was more awareness of donor human milk banks.

Modified from Biancuzzo M. Using banked donor milk: A realistic option. *Childbirth Instructor* September/October 1998.

ARTIFICIAL MILK AND OTHER SUPPLEMENTS

Artificial milk differs significantly from human milk, as described in earlier chapters. The *standard* formula differs, particularly with respect to concentrations of phosphorus and calcium, and renal solute load, summarized in Table 11-3.

Standard "Formula"

Standard "formulas" are designed for full-term, healthy newborns. Although some purport to be like mother's milk, none are; all artificial milk is inferior to human milk. These artificial substitutes may be either (1) milk protein based (casein predominant or whey predominant); (2) soy protein based; or (3) protein hydrolysate based.

Milk-Based Artificial Milk

The standard product provides 20 calories per ounce. The source of protein differs, depending on whether the formula is casein predominant or whey predominant. Carbohydrate is provided in the form of lactose from fat-free cow's milk. Fat is usually provided from vegetable sources. The formulas also contain minerals, vitamins, taurine, inositol, choline, and one or more stabilizers or

TABLE 11-3
COMPOSITION OF HUMAN MILK AND STANDARD ARTIFICIAL MILKS*

	Milk Based				Protein Hydrolysate Based	
	Mature Human Milk	Casein Predominant†	Whey Predominant‡	Isolated Soy Protein Based§	Casein=	Whey¶
Energy (kcal)	700	667	667	667	667	667
Protein or protein equivalent (g)	10.5	14.5	15 to 15.2	16.5 to 21	18.6 to 19	16
Fat (g)	39	36	36 to 38	36 to 36.9	27 to 37.5	34
Fatty acids (g)						
Polyunsaturated	4.8	13	4.9 to 11	4.7 to 14	12.8 to 15.8	4.4
Saturated	17.4	16	15 to 19.1	14.9 to 18.1	3.5 to 18.2	14.5
Monounsaturated	14.9	6	5.4 to 14	5.1 to 14.2	2.6 to 7	15.1
Linoleic	3.9	8.8	3.3 to 8.8	3.3 to 8.8	10.8 to 13.6	4.3
Carbohydrate (g)	72	72	69 to 72	68 to 69	68.9 to 91	74

*Data apply to formulas marketed in 1997. Values are units per liter at standard dilution (667 kcal).
†Similac, Gerber Baby Formula.
‡Enfamil, SMA.
§Isomil, Prosobee, Nursoy, Gerber Soy Baby Formula.
=Nutramigen, Alimentum.
¶Good Start.
#Also available with 1 mg of iron per liter.
Modified from Foman SJ. Composition of Feedings for Infants and Young Children. In Foman SJ. *Nutrition of Normal Infants.* St. Louis: Mosby, 1993. Data on human milk based on American Academy of Pediatrics. *Pediatric Nutrition Handbook.* 4th ed. Elk Grove Village, IL: American Academy of Pediatrics, 1998.

T A B L E 11-3

COMPOSITION OF HUMAN MILK AND STANDARD ARTIFICIAL MILKS—cont'd

	Milk Based				Protein Hydrolysate Based	
	Mature Human Milk	Casein Predominant†	Whey Predominant‡	Isolated Soy Protein Based§	Casein=	Whey¶
Minerals						
Calcium (mg)	280	492	420 to 470	600 to 710	640 to 710	430
Phosphorus (mg)	140	380	280 to 320	420 to 510	430 to 510	240
Magnesium (mg)	35	41	45 to 53	51 to 74	51 to 74	45
Iron (mg)	0.3	12#	12 to 12.8#	11.5 to 12.8	12 to 12.8	10
Zinc (mg)	1.2	5.1	5 to 5.3	5 to 5.3	5.1 to 5.3	—
Manganese (μg)	6	34	100 to 106	170 to 200	200 to 210	—
Copper (μg)	252	610	470 to 640	470 to 640	510 to 640	—
Iodine (μg)	110	94.6	60 to 69	60 to 100	48 to 100	—
Selenium (μg)	15	15	12	7 to 15.6	15.6 to 19	—
Sodium (mg)	180	183	150 to 184	200 to 300	300 to 320	160
Potassium (mg)	525	710	560 to 730	700 to 830	730 to 740	660
Chloride (mg)	420	433	375 to 430	375 to 560	540 to 580	390
Vitamins						
Vitamin A (IU)	2230	2030	2000 to 2100	2000 to 2100	2030 to 2100	3000
Vitamin D (IU)	22	410	400 to 430	400 to 430	305 to 430	600
Vitamin E (IU)	2.3	20	9.5 to 21	9.5 to 21	20 to 21	12
Vitamin K (μg)	2.1	54	55 to 58	100 to 106	100 to 106	82
Thiamin (μg)	210	680	530 to 670	410 to 670	410 to 530	600
Riboflavin (μg)	350	1010	100 to 1060	610 to 1000	610 to 640	1350
Niacin (μg)	1500	7100	5000 to 8500	5000 to 9130	8500 to 9130	7500
Vitamin B$_6$ (μg)	205	410	420 to 430	410 to 430	410 to 530	750
Folate (μg)	50	100	50 to 106	100 to 106	100 to 106	90
Vitamin B$_{12}$ (μg)	0.5	1.7	1.3 to 1.6	2 to 2.1	2.1 to 3	2.2
Pantothenic acid (μg)	1800	3040	2100 to 3200	3000 to 3170	3200 to 5070	4500
Biotin (μg)	4	30	15 to 15.6	35 to 64	30 to 53	22
Vitamin C (mg)	40	60	55	55 to 81	55 to 60	80
Other nutrients						
Cholesterol	150	11	33	0	<10	<11
Taurine (mg)	540	45	40	40 to 45	40 to 45	—
Choline (mg)	92	108	100 to 106	81 to 85	54 to 90	120
Inositol (mg)	149	32	32	27 to 68	32 to 34	61
Potential renal solute load (mosm)‡	75	133	127 to 136	163 to 181	171 to 172	134

RESEARCH HIGHLIGHT
Delayed gastric emptying in formula-fed preterm infants

Citation

Ewer AK, Durbin GM, Morgan ME, Booth IW. Gastric emptying in preterm infants. *Arch Dis Child* 1994;71:F24-F27.

Focus

This experimental study was conducted to determine the effects of whey-based artificial milk versus human milk on gastric emptying time. Fourteen Australian infants with a median gestational age of 33 weeks and mean birth weight of 1650 g were studied between day 4 and day 26. The infants served as their own controls during 46 nasogastric feedings of at least 150 ml/kg/day, with an interval of at least 2 hours between feedings. The type of feeding alternated; for example, the infant would be given human milk at one feeding and a whey-based artificial milk (60% whey, 40% casein) at the next.

Results

The gastric emptying time was about twice as fast for human milk as for artificial milk ($p < .0001$).

Strengths, Limitations of the Study

The investigator was blind to the method of feeding in this study, and the infants served as their own controls. The study is also convincing because of the high level of significance; the probability of this difference occurring by chance alone is only 1 in 10,000. These findings, however, may not be generalizable to later oral feedings (as opposed to gastric feedings in this study).

Clinical Application

These findings are consistent with the findings of Cavell's 1979 study. The results of the current study have clear implications for the nurse. First, parents should be informed of the benefits of human milk for preterm infants. Second, the nurse must advocate for hospital protocols that recognize human milk as the preferred source of nutrition for low-birth-weight and very-low-birth-weight infants. The nurse must also assess for signs of feeding intolerance and be aware of the influence of potential problems associated with artificial products, especially with early gastric feedings.

---

emulsifiers.[25] All formulas contain some iron, but those with at least 1 mg/100 kcal are referred to as *iron fortified*.

The most widely available casein-predominant formula in the United States is Similac. The ratio of whey to casein, while recently improved, still falls short of the low casein ratio found in human milk. Until recently, three whey-predominant formulas were available in the United States: Enfamil (Mead Johnson/Bristol-Myers Squibb), SMA (Wyeth), and Similac PM 60/40 (Ross Laboratories). However, SMA is no longer available in the United States.

If human milk is unavailable, milk protein-based formulas are safe for newborns, although they do have various consequences as discussed in previous chapters. Infants should be supplemented with artificial milk only if it is medically indicated.

Soy-Based Artificial Milk

Isolated soy protein–based artificial milks are free of cow's milk protein and lactose. They provide 20 kcal per ounce. The protein is supplemented with l-methionine (improves nitrogen balance, weight gain, urea nitrogen excretion, and albumin synthesis); l-carnitine (optimizes mitochondrial oxidation of long-chain fatty acids); and taurine (functions as an antioxidant and, along with glycine, is a major conjugate of bile acids in early infancy).[26] The carbohydrate component is lactose-free, and instead is corn starch or other saccharides. The fat is vegetable-based, rather than cholesterol-based. (For a discussion of the importance of cholesterol, see Chapters 3 and 7.)

In most cases, milk-based artificial milks are preferred when human milk is unavailable. Soy-based artificial milks are indicated for infants with galactosemia and hereditary lactase deficiency. Artificial milks that are soy-based are not designed or recommended for preterm infants who weigh less than 1800 g.[26] The aluminum content is at least 20 times greater than that in human milk, and because aluminum competes with calcium for absorption, the preterm infant becomes even more at risk for decreased skeletal bone mineralization. The presence of phytoestrogens in soy formulas, while very high in rodents, is currently under investigation in human subjects.

The mother who is breastfeeding may have heard myths that soy-based artificial milks are better for breastfed infants than milk-based formulas. This is simply untrue. A few points, noted from the official position of the American Academy of Pediatrics,[26] provide a sound basis for answering questions raised by breastfeeding mothers:

- Isolated soy protein–based formula has no advantage over cow's milk protein–based formula as a supplement for the breastfed infant.
- The routine use of isolated soy protein–based formula has no proven value in the prevention or management of infantile colic.
- The routine use of isolated soy protein–based formula has no proven value in the prevention of atopic disease in healthy or high-risk infants.

Protein Hydrolysate–Based Formulas

Protein hydrolysate–based formulas, such as Alimentum, Nutramigen, and Progestimil, contain nitrogen in the form of enzymatically hydrolyzed protein. Parents sometimes erroneously assume these are better substitutes for human milk than milk protein–based formulas. To the contrary, these formulas were not designed for routine use. They were intended for infants with specific problems, including food protein–induced enterocolitis and atopic reactions to milk or isolated soy proteins.[25]

"Special Formula"

Preterm "formula" (e.g., Similac Special Care 20 and Similac Special Care 24, Enfamil Premature Formula 20 and Enfamil Premature Formula 24, and Preemie SMA) is designed for preterm or low-birth-weight newborns. Those labeled "20" provide 20 kcal per ounce, and those labeled 24 have 24 kcal per ounce. Table 11-4 compares nutrients of Similac Special Care 24, Enfamil Premature Formula 24, and Preemie SMA.

Formulas designed for preterm infants support bone accretion rates when the infant is fed at least 120 kcal per kilogram per day. Preterm formula is designed for feeding preterm infants who weigh less than 2000 g and who are rapidly growing. Sometimes, however, this special preterm formula is given to infants who are well over 2000 g and who may not have such rapid growth (i.e., they are closer to discharge than to birth). More recently, other special formulas (e.g., Neocare) have been designed for those infants who were born at low birth weight and have been started on the preterm formula, but who are no longer experiencing the rapid growth that occurs directly after birth and are approaching hospital discharge.

It is permissible and even desirable to "inoculate" artificial milk with a "dose" of colostrum. It may be impractical to give such a small amount of colostrum to the infant, especially if it needs to go through a feeding tube. By "inoculating" the feeding, one provides the antiinfective and immune benefits of the colostrum to the infant. This practice, once more prevalent, has recently fallen out of favor because some clinicians have

T A B L E 11-4

FORMULAS FOR LOW-BIRTH-WEIGHT AND PREMATURELY BORN INFANTS (24 CAL/OZ; 81 CAL/DL) PER LITER

	"Preemie"* SMA 24 Liquid (Wyeth, Philadelphia, Pa)	Similac Special Care 24 Liquid (Ross, Columbus, Ohio)	Enfamil Premature 24 Liquid (Mead Johnson, Evansville, Ind)
Energy, kcal	810	812	810
Protein, g	20†	22‡	24‡
Fat, g	44§	44.1‖	41¶
Polyunsaturated, g	6.4	8.4	10.3
Monounsaturated, g	14.7	4.8	4.6
Saturated, g	20.3	25.2	26.2#
Linoleic acid, g	4.0	5.7	8.6
Carbohydrate, g	86**	86.1**	90††
Minerals			
Calcium, mg	750	1460	1340
Phosphorus, mg	400	730	670
Magnesium, mg	70	100	55
Iron, mg	3	3.0	2
Zinc, mg	8	12.2	12.2
Manganese, μg	134	100	51
Copper, μg	700	2030	1010
Iodine, μg	83	50	200
Sodium, mEq	14	15	13.9
Potassium, mEq	19	27	21
Chloride, mEq	15	19	19.4
Vitamins			
A, μg	800	1658	3030
D, μg	12	31	55
E, IU	15	32	51
K, μg	70	100	65
Thiamine (B_1), μg	800	2030	1620

*No longer produced for use in the United States.
†Nonfat milk and demineralized whey.
‡Nonfat milk, whey protein concentrates.
§Coconut oil, 27%; soy oil, 18%; medium chain triglyceride (MCT) oil, 10%.
‖MCT oil, 50%; soy oil, 30%; coconut oil, 20%.
¶MCT oil, 40%; soy oil, 40%; coconut oil, 20%.
#Includes 17.4 g MCT oils.
**Lactose, 50%; glucose polymers, 50%.
††Glucose polymers, 60%; lactose, 40%.
From American Academy of Pediatrics. *Pediatric Nutrition Handbook.* 4th ed. Elk Grove Village, IL: American Academy of Pediatrics, 1998.

TABLE 11-4

FORMULAS FOR LOW-BIRTH-WEIGHT AND PREMATURELY BORN INFANTS (24 CAL/OZ; 81 CAL/DL) PER LITER—cont'd

	"Preemie"* SMA 24 Liquid (Wyeth, Philadelphia, Pa)	Similac Special Care 24 Liquid (Ross, Columbus, Ohio)	Enfamil Premature 24 Liquid (Mead Johnson, Evansville, Ind)
Riboflavin (B_2), μg	1300	5030	2400
Pyridoxine, μg	500	2030	1220
B_{12}, μg	2	4.5	2
Niacin, mg	6.3	40.6	32
Folic acid, μg	100	300	280
Pantothenic acid, mg	3.6	15.4	9.7
Biotin, μg	18	300	32
C (ascorbic acid), mg	70	300	162
Choline, mg	127	81	97
Inositol, mg	32	45	138

misinterpreted a research study about mixing artificial milk with human milk. The study showed significantly decreased lysozyme activity when equal parts of formula and human milk were mixed.[27] This finding cannot be generalized to "inoculating" a feeding with milk or colostrum.

Water

Glucose Water

A decade or so ago, glucose water was routinely given to healthy full-term newborns either to replace a feeding—typically a night feeding—or to "top off" a breast feeding. Fortunately, most hospitals have given up offering glucose as a prelacteal feed (a feeding prior to initiation of breastfeeding), but this practice still occurs in some hospitals[28] and during the neonatal period.[29] Citing other sources,[30-33] the American Academy of Pediatrics strongly forbids use of glucose water.[1] Glucose water feedings during the first few days of

life may contribute to introduction of artificial milk during the first month of life. In a recent prospective study 80% of newborns who did not receive glucose water continued to be exclusively breastfed during the first month of life, whereas only 65% of those fed glucose water were not receiving any artificial milk at that time.[34]

Several clinical situations were thought to be helped by giving glucose water, including inadequate fluids, jaundice, and hypoglycemia (see Chapter 6 for a discussion of these conditions). Hypoglycemic infants were routinely fed 5% or 10% glucose water on the belief that it would promote normoglycemia, and on the presumption that the newborn could not or would not consume enough human or artificial milk to improve his situation. This reasoning is entirely incorrect. Newborns who are given the glucose water generally experience a "sugar high" and then a "sugar crash" because after absorbing this simple sugar the infant once again becomes hypoglycemic. Nursery protocols should avoid this and instead favor the use of human or artificial milk,[35] which contains protein and

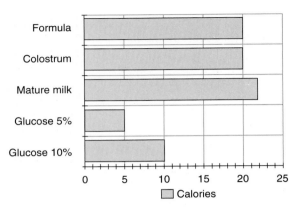

Fig. 11-2 Calories in human milk, artificial milk, and glucose water.

SUMMARY

When direct breastfeeding is not possible, the parents, as well as the health care team, need a thorough understanding of the options. Mother's own fresh milk is always the first choice. Mother's own milk, previously stored, is an excellent choice. Whether given fresh or frozen, mother's own milk may be more beneficial if it is given with fortifiers, or given as hindmilk only to some compromised infants. Donor milk, available from donor milk banks, may have lost some of its goodness because of the high heat required for the pasteurization process, but it is still a good alternative for infants whose mothers are unable to provide their own milk. Artificial milk, in all circumstances, is inferior to human milk.

therefore maintains normoglycemia over a period of time.

Furthermore, if the newborn is a reluctant feeder, he would obtain more calories by consuming human or artificial milk, as shown in Figure 11-2. The explanation for this is simple: 5% glucose water contains 5 kcal per ounce, and 10% glucose water provides 10 kcal per ounce. Human or artificial milk provides about 20 to 24 kcal per ounce, depending on human milk maturity or the commercial formula provided. Therefore, the newborn would need to consume at least twice as much volume to obtain the same amount of calories from the glucose water as from the milk.

Sterile Water

Sterile water was once thought to be appropriate for a first feeding (prelacteal feeding). This idea was based on the fear that if the infant aspirated, it would be more physiological to aspirate sterile water than another substance. However, this practice is no longer used, and there is no evidence-based reason for giving sterile water to any newborn.

References

1. American Academy of Pediatrics Work Group on Breastfeeding. Breastfeeding and the use of human milk. *Pediatrics* 1997;100:1035-1039.
2. Bates CJ, Liu DS, Fuller NJ, Lucas A. Susceptibility of riboflavin and vitamin A in breast milk to photodegradation and its implications for the use of banked breast milk in infant feeding. *Acta Paediatr Scand* 1985;74:40-44.
3. Atkinson SA, Radde IC, Anderson GH. Macromineral balances in premature infants fed their own mothers' milk or formula. *J Pediatr* 1983;102:99-106.
4. Brooke OG, Onubogu O, Heath R, Carter ND. Human milk and preterm formula compared for effects on growth and metabolism. *Arch Dis Child* 1987;62:917-923.
5. DeCurtis M, Brooke OG. Energy and nitrogen balances in very low birthweight infants. *Arch Dis Child* 1987;62:830-832.
6. Cooper PA, Rothberg AD, Pettifor JM, Bolton KD, Devenhuis S. Growth and biochemical response of premature infants fed pooled preterm milk or special formula. *J Pediatr Gastroenterol Nutr* 1984;3:749-754.

7. Atkinson SA, Bryan MH, Anderson GH. Human milk feeding in premature infants: protein, fat, and carbohydrate balances in the first two weeks of life. *J Pediatr* 1981;99:617-624.

8. Davies M. National Childbirth Trust: breastfeeding. *Nurs Times* 1977;73(43):1678-1679.

9. Kashyap S, Schulze KF, Forsyth M, Dell RB, Ramakrishnan R, Heird WC. Growth, nutrient retention, and metabolic response of low-birthweight infants fed supplemented and unsupplemented preterm human milk. *Am J Clin Nutr* 1990;52:254-262.

10. Stein H, Cohen D, Herman AA, et al. Pooled pasteurized breast milk and untreated own mother's milk in the feeding of very low birth weight babies: a randomized controlled trial. *J Pediatr Gastroenterol Nutr* 1986;5:242-247.

11. Gross SJ. Growth and biochemical response of preterm infants fed human milk or modified infant formula. *N Engl J Med* 1983;308:237-241.

12. Schanler RJ, Abrams SA. Postnatal attainment of intrauterine macromineral accretion rates in low birth weight infants fed fortified human milk. *J Pediatr* 1995;126:441-447.

13. Schanler RJ. Fortified human milk: nature's way to feed premature infants. *J Hum Lact* 1998;14:5-11.

14. Lucas A, Fewtrell MS, Morley R, et al. Randomized outcome trial of human milk fortification and developmental outcome in preterm infants. *Am J Clin Nutr* 1996;64:142-151.

15. Valentine CJ, Hurst NM, Schanler RJ. Hindmilk improves weight gain in low-birth-weight infants fed human milk. *J Pediatr Gastroenterol Nutr* 1994;18:474-477.

16. Lucas A, Morley R, Cole TJ, Gore SM. A randomised multicentre study of human milk versus formula and later development in preterm infants. *Arch Dis Child* 1994;70(2 spec no):F141-F146.

17. Sigman M, Burke KI, Swarner OW, Shavlik GW. Effects of microwaving human milk: changes in IgA content and bacterial count. *J Am Diet Assoc* 1989;89:690-692.

18. Ford JE, Marshall VME, Reiter B. Influence of the heat treatment of human milk on some of its protective constituents. *J Pediatr* 1977;90:29-35.

19. Davies DP. Human milk banking. *Arch Dis Child* 1982;57:3-5.

20. Liebhaber M, Lewiston NJ, Asquith MT, Olds Arroyo L, Sunshine P. Alterations of lymphocytes and of antibody content of human milk after processing. *J Pediatr* 1977;91:897-900.

21. Lawrence RA. *Breastfeeding: A Guide for the Medical Profession*. 4th ed. St. Louis: Mosby; 1994.

22. Stocks RJ, Davies DP, Carroll LP, Broderick B, Parker M. A simple method to improve the energy value of bank human milk. *Early Hum Dev* 1983;8:175-178.

23. Gibbs JH, Fisher C, Bhattacharya S, Goddard P, Baum JD. Drip breast milk: its composition, collection and pasteurization. *Early Hum Dev* 1977;1:227-245.

24. Lucas A, Gibbs JA, Baum JD. The biology of human drip breast milk. *Early Hum Dev* 1978;2:351-361.

25. Foman SJ. *Nutrition of Normal Infants*. St. Louis: Mosby; 1993.

26. American Academy of Pediatrics Committee on Nutrition. Soy protein–based formulas: recommendations for use in infant feeding. *Pediatrics* 1998;10:148-153.

27. Quan R, Yang C, Rubinstein S, Lewiston NJ, Stevenson DK, Kerner JA Jr. The effect of nutritional additives on anti-infective factors in human milk. *Clin Pediatr (Phila)* 1994;33:325-328.

28. Zimmerman DR, Bernstein WR. Standing feeding orders in the well-baby nursery: "water, water everywhere . . .". *J Hum Lact* 1996;12:189-192.

29. Scariati PD, Grummer-Strawn LM, Fein SB. Water supplementation of infants in their first month of life. *Arch Pediatr Adolesc Med* 1997;151:830-832.

30. American Academy of Pediatrics and the American College of Obstetrics and Gynecology. *Guidelines for Perinatal Care*. 3rd ed. Elk Grove Village, IL: American Academy of Pediatrics; 1992.

31. Committee on Nutrition American Academy of Pediatrics. *Pediatric Nutrition Handbook*. Elk Grove Village, IL: American Academy of Pediatrics; 1993.

32. Shrago L. Glucose water supplementation of the breastfed infant during the first three days of life. *J Hum Lact* 1987;3:82-86.

33. Goldberg NM, Adams E. Supplementary water for breast-fed babies in a hot and dry climate—not really a necessity. *Arch Dis Child* 1983;58:73-74.

34. Calama JM, Bunuel J, Valero MT, et al. The effect of feeding glucose water to breastfeeding newborns on weight, body temperature, blood glucose, and breastfeeding duration. *J Hum Lact* 1996;13:209-213.

35. World Health Organization. Hypoglycemia of the Newborn: Review of the Literature. Geneva: World Health Organization; 1997.

12

Techniques for Delivering Human and Artificial Milk

*U*nder most circumstances, the healthy infant who has ready access to his mother can usually meet all of his nutritional and fluid needs by suckling her breasts. In cases where the infant does not have ready access to his mother's breasts—for example, the mother and infant are separated as described in Chapter 10—or the infant is not completely well, nourishment will need to be given some other way. While human milk is the preferred nutritional source for all infants, as described in Chapter 11, artificial milk may also be given. When the newborn is not feeding directly at the breast or when supplementation is medically indicated, the question then becomes: How exactly should this nourishment be delivered to the infant?

The aim of this chapter is to describe ways to deliver enteral or oral feedings of human milk or artificial milk. Infants who cannot obtain all of their nourishment at the breast can be viewed as being on a continuum from those who cannot tolerate oral feedings at all to those who vigorously suckle the breast but occasionally obtain their nourishment by some other means. Furthermore, preterm infants can sometimes suckle the breast, then receive the remainder of their feeding by gavage if they become fatigued.

Indirect breastfeeding (consuming human milk through means other than suckling) usually occurs when the infant is too ill to feed directly at the breast, or the mother and infant are well but separated from one another. In either case, it is often assumed that the infant who is not suck-

T A B L E   12-1

EFFECT OF FEEDING OPTIONS ON MOTHER AND CHILD

Feeding Options	Will Promote Goal of Long-Term Breastfeeding?	Is Infant Actually Breastfeeding?	What Is Infant's Energy/Time Expenditure?	Does Infant Receive Human Milk?
Continue frequent breastfeeding	Possibly	Yes	High	Yes
Supplement after breast (bottle, cup, dropper)	No	Yes	High	If uses pumped human milk
Temporarily bottle feed pumped human milk, then resume breastfeeding	Possibly	No	Low	Yes
Bottle feed pumped human milk	No	No	Low	Yes
Feeding tube device with pumped human milk	Yes	Yes	Low	Yes
Feeding tube device with formula	Yes	Yes	Low	Half
Finger feeding by tube/syringe on finger	No	No	High, if slow feeder	If uses pumped human milk
Quit breastfeeding for bottle feeding	No	No	Low	No

Copyright: Kittie Frantz, 1992.

Box 12-1
Priorities for Care During Nonexclusive Breastfeeding

- Determine why indirect breastfeeding and/or artificial milk supplementation has been initiated and proceed with clinical management and counseling as appropriate.
- Build the mother's confidence in herself and her ability to nourish her infant. Avoid any implication that the supplement is just as good as or superior to her own milk.
- Facilitate consumption of human milk, if appropriate.
- If it is not possible for the infant to receive human milk, suggest ways to make the supplements more similar to human milk. "Inoculating" artificial milk with human milk helps the newborn to associate feeding with the smell of human milk. Warm artificial milk so that it is about the same temperature as milk directly from the breast. Suggest other ways to stimulate the breastfeeding experience, including positioning, skin-to-skin contact, and eye contact.
- Identify and correct breastfeeding problems that can be solved by better clinical management. Usually, this means assisting infants who are not latched on correctly.
- Give specific information to parents of infants who are ill or unable to suckle. Emphasize that supplementation is usually a temporary strategy, and estimate how long supplementation is expected to continue. Meanwhile, devise a plan to facilitate full breastfeeding.
- Reassure mothers who wish to (e.g., the employed mother) or need to supplement that supplementation will not "ruin" breastfeeding. Do not try to starve the reluctant nurser into submission. Help the family to choose a supplementation method that works for them.
- Whenever possible, choose a method for delivering milk that is least disruptive to the breastfeeding relationship.
- Show families the technique for the chosen method; require a return demonstration and provide positive and negative feedback to help them master the technique.
- Reinforce the importance of expressing to maintain milk supply.
- Evaluate the infant's weight gain, the family's comfort level, and the mother's lactation status. Do not assume that all is well!

Is Infant Gaining Weight?	Is It Safe for Infant?	What Is Effect on Milk Supply?	What Is Maternal Time Expenditure?
May be poor	Yes, if weight monitored	Decreases	High
Yes	Yes (cup = aspiration danger)	Decreases	High
Yes, if enough milk pumped	Yes	Decreases	Medium
Yes, if enough milk pumped	Yes	Decreases if long term	Medium
Yes, if enough milk pumped	Yes	Good	Medium to high
Yes	Yes	Good	Medium
Not always	Aspiration danger	Decreases	High
Yes	Yes	Gone	Low

ling must have artificial milk, and that is entirely untrue; *what* is given is an issue entirely separate from *how* it is given. Figure 12-1 shows a flowchart[1] that separates issues of what from how. Human milk, as well as artificial milk, may be given by a variety of methods. All methods have distinct advantages and disadvantages for the infant, the mother, or both.[1] Table 12-1 summarizes the advantages and disadvantages of several feeding options.

Like any intervention, supplementation can have a variety of adverse effects. Some are readily apparent; for example, a supplemented infant will demand less, which in turn can reduce the mother's milk supply. Some adverse effects are less obvious; for example, when the mother hears that her newborn needs to be supplemented, the implicit message is that her milk (and therefore she) is inadequate. It is the nurse's responsibility to carry out supplementation in a way that preserves the breastfeeding relationship to the greatest extent possible. Priorities for care when supplementing infants are presented in Box 12-1.

GAVAGE FEEDINGS

If the infant's gastrointestinal tract is completely unable to tolerate food, nourishment is given parenterally (i.e., intravenously). If his gastrointestinal tract can tolerate food, however, he may nonetheless be unable to ingest the food orally, for one of many reasons. Infants are unable to take oral feedings if they have anomalies of the digestive tract (see Chapter 7), an inability to coordinate suck/swallow, severe debilitation, respiratory distress, or unconsciousness.[2] Rather than being fed orally, these infants are fed enterally (i.e., through the stomach or small intestine). A gastrostomy feeding—feeding through a tube passed directly into the stomach from the abdominal wall—is initiated if the infant has an anomaly of the mouth, pharynx, esophagus, or cardiac sphincter of the stomach. More frequently, however, newborns are fed by *gavage* feedings.

Gavage feeding is accomplished by passing a small tube via the nares (nasogastric gavage, or NG) or via the mouth (orogastric gavage, or OG) directly into the stomach. The tube may contain

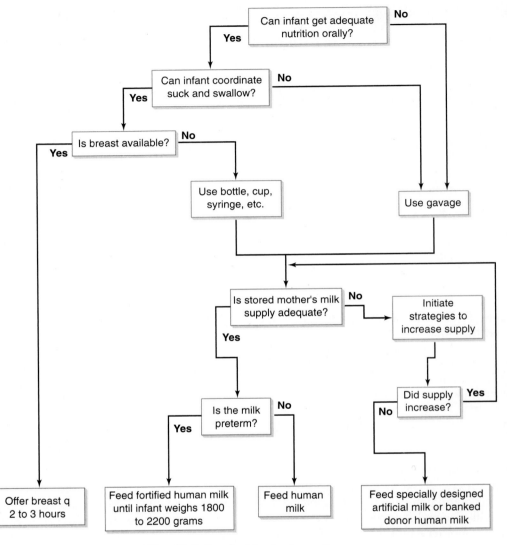

Fig. 12-1 Flowchart for feeding options.

either human or artificial milk, but preterm infants tolerate enteral feeding of human milk sooner than artificial milk.[3] Usually, if only a few gavage feedings are anticipated, the tube is inserted each time. For very ill infants, however, the tube is usually indwelling (i.e., not removed for each feeding). The feeding may be given by bolus (intermittent gavage) or administered continuously (continuous gavage; i.e., the feeding is infused via a pump). The rate of the infusion depends on the infant's general health status. (A complete discussion of how to provide enteral feedings is found in most pediatric textbooks.)

Infants who are very sick or preterm usually have continuous OG or NG feedings, and the human milk or artificial milk is given via an electronic infusion pump, similar to those used to deliver intravenous fluids. Infants who weigh more than 1000 g are more likely to be gavaged by an intermittent bolus, whereas those who weigh less are usually fed by continuous pump.[4] (These data are old, and practice varies regionally, but for the most part this is still true.) Although gavage feedings are always invasive, oxygen desaturation is three times more likely with bottle feedings than with bolus gavage feedings.[5] In the very-low-birth-weight (VLBW) infant, intermittent gavage can lead to respiratory difficulties[6] but growth rate and length of hospitalization does not differ significantly whether the gavage feedings are continuous or intermittent.[7] Continuous slow-infusion feedings of human milk result in loss of calcium and phosphorus[8] and lipids.[9-12] When continuous slow infusions are being used, weight loss may occur because lipids (high in caloric value) may stick to the sides of the tubes. Therefore, it is critical to monitor for weight loss if infants are receiving continuous gavage feedings of human milk.

Administration Responsibilities for Delivering Human Milk via Gavage

Continuous infusion can potentially decrease lipid delivery and increase pathogens. Therefore, several evidence-based clinical implications emerge for the nurse.

- Place the syringe *below* the isolette with the tip pointed upward so that the fat will rise and be pushed through the tube first.[13] The fat that has accumulated during a continuous feeding will rise toward the end of the feeding; a 25- to 40-degree angle is best.[14] This will improve fat delivery to the infant.

- Watch for weight loss. Fat and protein losses occur with continuous gavage,[12] and a slow rate of infusion magnifies the problem.[10] Milk that is fortified with medium-chain triglycerides adheres to the feeding tube.[15] Homogenized milk seems to lower the fat loss during tube feedings.[16]

- Reduce the threat of infection and nutrient loss by infusing the milk over 10 to 20 minutes for an intermittent feeding (depending on what is safe for the newborn) and deliver milk through minibore tubing rather than standard-bore tubing, to better preserve the *creamatocrit*[17]; use short feeding tubes. (Creamatocrit is the percentage of cream in human milk.)

- Ensure adequate fat intake. Advocate for measuring human milk creamatocrit at least once a day[18,19] to estimate the caloric value. Collect the sample from the distal end of the infusion set.

- Change the syringe and tubing at least every 4 hours.[11,20] Less frequent tubing changes may result in excessive bacteria.

Nonnutritive Sucking During Gavage Feeding

In the late 1980s, studies led to the practice of encouraging VLBW infants to suck on a pacifier when being gavage fed. VLBW infants more quickly made the transition from gavage to oral feeding when they sucked on a pacifier, presumably because of an accelerated maturation of the sucking reflex.[21] Whether these infants make better weight gains when they suck on a pacifier during tube feedings is uncertain; some researchers suggest that they do[21,22] while others suggest they do not.[23] Infants who suck on a pacifier during intermittent gavage feedings exhibit less behavioral distress.[24]

In planning care for the gavage-fed newborn, however, there may be a better alternative to sucking on a pacifier. The mother's breast, after being "emptied," gives the infant the benefits of warmth, comfort, and the soothing sound of the mother's heartbeat. Furthermore, sucking on the mother's breast gives the needed stimulation to improve her milk supply and offers the mother an opportunity to actively participate in her infant's care. When newborns are allowed to suck on the mother's breast in this manner, feeding at the breast is the next logical step in the infant's growth and development. Besides the obvious physiological benefits for both mother and infant, those who use this practice are more likely to continue breastfeeding for a longer period than those who do not.[25]

T A B L E 12-2

GUIDELINES FOR INITIATING ORAL FEEDINGS OF HUMAN MILK FOR LBW AND VLBW INFANTS

The suggested guidelines below may be considered for inclusion in hospital protocols, but should not be used without approval from the neonatologist.

Infant's Birth Weight	Begin Feedings	Continue Feedings
750-1000 g	2 ml human milk × 4 feedings 3 ml human milk × 4 feedings 4 ml human milk × 4 feedings 4 ml human milk × 4 feedings	Continue to advance 2 ml every 4 feedings until the newborn is consuming 150 ml/kg/day
1001-1250 g	3 ml human milk × 4 feedings 4 ml human milk × 4 feedings 6 ml human milk × 4 feedings 8 ml human milk × 4 feedings	Continue to advance 2 ml every 4 feedings until the newborn is consuming 150 ml/kg/day
1251-1500 g	6 ml human milk × 4 feedings 8 ml human milk × 4 feedings 10 ml human milk × 4 feedings 12 ml human milk × 4 feedings 14 ml human milk × 4 feedings 16 ml human milk × 4 feedings	Continue to advance 2-3 ml every 4 feedings until the newborn is consuming 150 ml/kg/day
1501-1800 g	6 ml human milk × 4 feedings 9 ml human milk × 4 feedings 12 ml human milk × 4 feedings 15 ml human milk × 4 feedings 18 ml human milk × 4 feedings 21 ml human milk × 4 feedings	Continue to advance 3-4 ml every 4 feedings until the newborn is consuming 150 ml/kg/day
1801-2100 g	10 ml human milk × 4 feedings 15 ml human milk × 4 feedings 20 ml human milk × 4 feedings 25 ml human milk × 4 feedings	Continue to advance 5 ml every 4 feedings until the newborn is consuming 150 ml/kg/day
2101-2500 g	15 ml human milk × 4 feedings 20 ml human milk × 4 feedings 25 ml human milk × 4 feedings 30 ml human milk × 4 feedings	Continue to advance 5-10 ml every 4 feedings until the newborn is consuming 150 ml/kg/day
Over 2500 g	Begin with 25-45 ml human milk (indirect or direct feedings); if tolerated, feed ad lib	If tolerated feed ad lib

Source: University of Rochester Medical Center.

Infants who no longer need to have gavage feedings can make a gradual transition to oral feedings. LBW and VLBW infants are typically unable to consume volumes needed to support their needs for maintenance and growth. The goal is for the infant to consume at least 150 ml/kg/day. Gradually increasing the amount of volume given through indirect feedings, as shown in Table 12-2, helps to achieve this goal. Human milk, however, may also be given directly, requiring test-weighing before and after the feeding. A combination of direct and indirect feedings often works well.

ORAL FEEDINGS

Oral feedings are clearly best, as the biological, psychological, and cultural values associated with feedings are preserved. Oral feedings are not invasive and provide a time for interaction between the infant and caregiver. However, the compromised infant is frequently unable to get all of the nourishment he needs at the breast, and hence the professional or parent must ask: *How* can we best deliver human milk (or artificial milk, if human milk is unavailable) orally? Several alternatives, offering different advantages and disadvantages, are available.

Bottles

Bottles are widely used in the United States to give supplementary nourishment to newborns. The newer angled bottles appear to offer a few physiological advantages,[26] but for the most part bottles are all about the same, and many health care professionals presume them to be harmless. Advocates of breastfeeding clearly discourage bottles. Most of their objections, however, are not really about the bottle but, rather, about artificial nipples.

Any claim that an artificial nipple is "just like mother" is false. Frequently, consumers and health care providers promote the Nuk type of nipple (Figure 12-2) for breastfed infants, but in one expert's words, "The Nuk type . . . is promoted as being similar in shape to the human nipple, but the functional superiority of these nipples is yet to be proved."[27] Frequently, mothers need to experiment a bit to find a nipple that works well for their individual infant. Mothers may perceive that some artificial nipples are better than others, but *different* would be a more appropriate descriptor than *better*.

Although there are several variations, there are three basic styles of artificial nipples: standard, preterm, and Nuk. The styles differ from one another in shape, size, consistency (malleability), distensibility (ability to elongate when sucked), and the size and configuration of the nipple hole. (The nipple hole may be plain or crosscut, and some holes are larger than others.) Most artificial nipples are less compressible than the human nipple.[28] Although one artificial nipple can deliver milk posteriorly to the foramen cecum region of the tongue and can elongate 120% from its resting state, the human nipple elongates 200% from its resting state.[29]

One study examined different nipple units to evaluate the milk flow characteristics of artificial nipples on the market. An apparatus was set up to mimic infant sucking, and two different amounts of negative pressure were tested. Preterm nipple

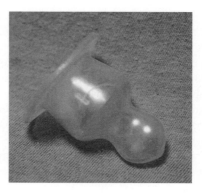

Fig. 12-2 Nuk-style nipple.

units required fewer "sucks" than the standard nipple units to yield the same amount of milk. Nuk nipple units required more "sucks" than the standard nipple units. Larger nipple holes and greater distensibility resulted in greater milk flow rate. However, the nipple unit itself was only one part of the equation in the evaluation of the nipple unit; the amount of negative pressure exerted was the other part of the equation. When the amount of negative pressure was doubled, the number of needed sucks decreased significantly.[30]

Research has shown, however, that there are some clear disadvantages to using bottles to feed healthy, full-term infants as well as for preterm or ill newborns. Recognizing that human milk may be in the bottle, the disadvantages listed here focus only on disadvantages of artificial nipples.

Before the advent of the Baby Friendly™ Hospital Initiative, full-term healthy breastfed newborns were routinely given artificial nipples atop formula bottles when they were supplemented. Nipple confusion, while not a term fully accepted by the medical community, may hinder successful breastfeeding for term or preterm newborns.[31] However, there is evidence that jaw development is hindered by bottle-feeding; masseter muscle activity is significantly reduced in bottle-fed infants who are 2 to 6 months old.[32]

There are several physiological disadvantages to suckling an artificial nipple. In one study, systolic blood pressure changed significantly when healthy, term breast-fed infants between 24 and 92 hours of age were offered a bottle. Bottle-fed infants also had an increase in their basal blood pressure when they began sucking the bottle, but the change was not as dramatic.[33] There is a higher sucking frequency when newborns suckle at the breast compared with when they suck at the bottle,[34] which requires a greater expenditure of energy. Furthermore, when those same newborns were fed human milk from a bottle and artificial milk from a bottle, there was no difference in either sucking frequency or sucking pressure.[34] Therefore, it appears that the act of sucking at

Box 12-2
Behavioral Clues That Indicate Infant Cannot Respond to Faster Flow of Milk From Bottle

- Clenched fists
- Hyperextension of the head, back, and legs
- Elevated shoulders
- Facial grimace
- Milk spilled from the mouth
- Gulping sounds as the infant swallows
- Uneven respirations
- Breath holding, with eventual pauses between swallows to breathe

Source: Weber F, Woolridge MW, Baum JD. An ultrasonographic study of the organization of sucking and swallowing by newborn infants. *Devel Med Child Neurol* 1986;28:19-24.

the bottle—not the fluid that is consumed—determines the suck and breathing patterns of newborns. Box 12-2 lists signs that milk flow from the bottle is too fast for the infant to handle adequately.

The effects of respiratory compromise are perhaps the most significant disadvantage to artificial nippling, especially for preterm infants. The decrease in oxygen saturation for preterm infants while bottle feeding is well documented.[35,36]

It becomes apparent, therefore, that bottles are not the ideal method for delivering oral nutrition to infants, particularly those who are preterm. If direct breastfeeding is not possible, the first step is to develop a plan for moving toward direct breastfeeding, as described in Chapter 7. In the meantime, generate alternative strategies for delivering the feeding.

Alternatives to Bottles

Oral feedings of human milk or artificial milk can be given by a bottle or, preferably, by one of several alternative methods. Such methods have distinct advantages and disadvantages. One factor to

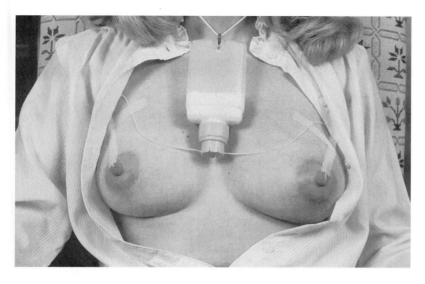

Fig. 12-3 Supplemental Nursing System. *(Courtesy Medela.)*

especially consider is that of personal preference; some methods are considered awkward or undesirable simply because the nurse, mother, or other caregiver simply doesn't like to use them. The priority is to generate alternatives and to choose one that is most practical and least objectionable. When the pediatrician prescribes supplementation he usually does not specify how it should be given, but it is important to muster his support for the method chosen. More frequently, it is the mother who has strong feelings about which method she uses. Ideally, after being presented with multiple options, the mother should choose one method of supplementation and the entire health care team should support that decision. It is counterproductive for several individuals to recommend or teach several methods; the mother is unlikely to choose or use any of them when seemingly conflicting recommendations are given.

Nursing Supplementers

Nursing supplementers are devices with tubes that are placed on the mother's nipple; the infant suckles both the human nipple and the tube. Hence, the infant who has a weak suck or requires extra calories gets more reward for his efforts by using this device, which can be filled with either human milk or artificial milk.

The nursing supplementer may be useful for infants who have poor oral motor functions, such as those with neurological impairments, because the flow of milk helps to organize their suck/swallow reflex. It can also be used successfully for mothers who have a low milk supply, because the infant is suckling the breast, which stimulates better production. This device can also be used for adoptive mothers.

The most popular of these devices are the Supplemental Nursing System™ (Figure 12-3) and the Starter Supplemental Nursing System™ (SNS) by Medela and the Lact-Aid® Nursing Trainer System™ by Lact-Aid International (Figure 12-4). Although these devices are similar, they are not identical. Most notably, the Lact-Aid Training System has a collapsible bag, which is usually positioned so that its bottom is below the infant's chin. (The device may, however, be hung so that gravity assists in milk delivery for special circumstances.) Thus, the infant obtains milk without having to overcome the vacuum created in a rigid container.

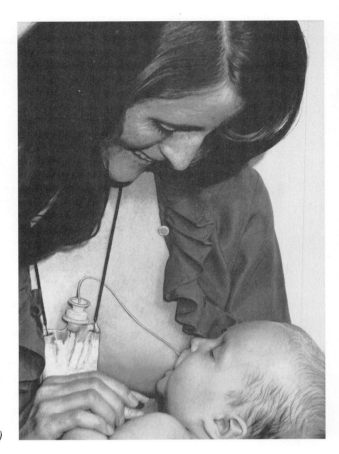

Fig. 12-4 Lact-Aid® Nursing Trainer System.
(Courtesy Jimmie Lynn Avery, Lact-Aid International.)

By using the collapsible bag, pressure is the same as atmospheric pressure. There is one tube coming from the container, and it is available in one size. It does not have to be positioned in the exact center of the infant's lower lip. Instructions are included for adjusting flow to accommodate more viscous artificial milk.

The Supplemental Nursing System uses a rigid container and is hung from the mother's neck. There are two tubes coming from the container: one to the right breast and one to the left. The one not in use is clamped off, while the one going to the infant remains open. Thus, milk flows by the negative pressure exerted by the infant, with assistance from gravity. The device

comes with tubes of three different sizes; the larger tubes better accommodate the thicker viscosity of artificial milk. The tube to the infant should be positioned in the center of his lower lip.

These devices offer many advantages, as outlined in Table 12-1. Most important, the infant receives human milk and the mother's breast receives stimulation. Furthermore, the flow of milk from the device actually stimulates the suck/swallow response. As Chapter 5 explains, swallowing is really a continuation of the sucking reflex. Hence, in situations where the infant is unable to organize this suck/swallow response with the breast only, or only when the mother has a

T A B L E   12-3

POTENTIAL PROBLEMS AND SOLUTIONS WITH SUPPLEMENTAL DEVICES

Possible Problem	Possible Strategies
Infant rejects tube because he has previously been fed with NG tube and responds to the noxious presence of the tube	Try kangaroo care before trying the nursing supplementer; this will give the infant a sense of familiarity with being near the breast, smelling the milk, etc. Pull the tube up slightly so that infant is able to feel the breast first
Difficulty getting milk to drip well	Ask mother to first practice (without the infant) using water in the system Other suggestions include: • Check for any blockage in system • Determine if this is the right size tubing • Adjust the height according to the flow desired
Breast skin breakdown; tape on skin	Lact-Aid generally does not require tape; for SNS, use paper tape (hair-setting tape found in most drugstores also works well and is inexpensive) Applying a warm cloth to the skin after removing the tape may be soothing
Formula too thick to go through tubing	For SNS use largest size tubing For Lact-Aid refer to instructions included with the device Devise a makeshift supplementary system: use a no. 5 feeding tube; tape to mother's nipple and attach other end to syringe; slowly push formula through the tube with the syringe Determine if infant can have human milk for one feeding instead of artificial milk
Infant unable to suck tube successfully (e.g., has cleft palate)	For Lact-Aid see instructions for gravity-assisted flow

milk-ejection response, the nursing supplementer may help to better organize the infant's response.

The major disadvantage is that mothers may consider the device somewhat of a nuisance to get on and off. The Lact-Aid is somewhat less obtrusive, whereas it may be difficult or impossible to camouflage the Supplemental Nurser System under the woman's clothing. Some practical problems can arise in using the supplementer. Potential problems, as well as possible solutions, are listed in Table 12-3. Furthermore, the nursing supplementer should not serve as a substitute for good breastfeeding management.

Cup Feeding

Cup feeding has become popular in the last few years, but its use dates back several decades.[37,38] While earlier papers have described this practice as unsafe,[1] a controlled study at Yale–New Haven Hospital has recently shown it to be safe for well infants who are at least 32 weeks' postconceptional age (see Research Highlight).[39] Furthermore, preterm newborns are more likely to be exclusively breastfeeding at discharge when they have been cup fed rather than bottle fed,[40] and cup feeding has been used safely and effectively with preterm twins.[41] A protocol, based on related research, has been developed for using cup feeding in the neonatal intensive care setting[42]; Table 12-4 suggests appropriate assessments, contraindications, implementation, and evaluation for cup feeding. Cup feeding the newborn is a simple procedure, as shown in Figure 12-5; Appendix B lists resources for the how-to. The key is for the infant, not the caregiver, to control the rate at which the feeding is given.

Syringe

A variety of syringes can be used to give oral feedings. A regular syringe, of any size, can be filled with artificial or human milk, then squirted slowly and gently into the newborn's mouth. Use

---

T A B L E   12-4

SAMPLE PROTOCOL: CUP FEEDING A NEWBORN

Title: Cup Feeding a Newborn
Purpose: To provide human milk or artificial milk (formula) to a newborn who has a weak or inadequate suck or who is separated from his mother
Level: Independent; does not require a physician's order for implementation
Supportive Data: Clinical cases and research studies show that cup feeding improves the likelihood that newborns will be exclusively breastfeeding at time of hospital discharge. This alternative to bottle feeding is noninvasive and while research is ongoing, thus far cup feeding has not been shown to have any adverse effects for either term or preterm infants.

Contents

Key Words	Nursing/Clinical Care
Initial Assessment	***General***
	• Any infant who can tolerate oral feedings is a potential candidate for cup feeding. This includes both breastfed and bottle-fed newborns.
	• A newborn does not necessarily need to "prove himself" by sucking a rubber nipple or suckling a breast before the initiation of cup feeding. Feeding cues are a signal for cup feedings.
	• The infant must have a gag reflex present and tongue movement.
	The Term Infant
	• Any infant whose mother is unavailable for breastfeeding.
	• When infant requires feeding or supplement for medical reasons, as determined by the physician.
	The Preterm Infant
	• Demonstrates coordination of lips/tongue and swallowing, but does not need to coordinate bottle sucking with swallow before cup feeding is initiated. Initiate at nurse's discretion.
	Other Situations
	• Newborns who cannot form an adequate seal, exert adequate suction, or suck effectively (at the breast or with the bottle) may use cup feeding. This may include newborns with clefts or other defects.
Contraindications	• Any newborn who is likely to aspirate is not a candidate for cup feeding. Newborns with a poor gag reflex, those who are lethargic in general, or others who have marked neurologic deficits should be excluded.

From Biancuzzo M. Creating and implementing a protocol for cup feeding. *Mother Baby Journal* 1997;2(3):27-33.

---

an appropriate-sized syringe to accommodate the amount of milk that the newborn is anticipated or required to consume. For example, a very preterm infant may consume only a few milliliters of colostrum, so a 3-ml syringe would work well. A preterm infant who is required to consume at least 18 ml per feeding could be fed with a 20-ml syringe. Similar to the regular syringe found at the nurse's station, an Asepto-type syringe can also be used. It is considerably larger, and therefore more

useful for a full-term infant who is unable to breastfeed but is capable of consuming 50 ml in a feeding. A piece of pediatric catheter tubing attached to the end of any syringe is sometimes helpful. The caregiver is in control of this method of feeding, however, and must be extremely cautious not to overwhelm the infant with too great a volume.

Periodontal syringes, with a curved end (Figure 12-6), improve the "aim" of the caregiver but

T A B L E　12-4	
SAMPLE PROTOCOL: CUP FEEDING A NEWBORN—cont'd	
Key Words	Nursing/Clinical Care
Contraindications—cont'd	• Newborns who are less than 35 weeks' gestation should be evaluated on a case-by-case basis for respiratory and other conditions that may affect safety.
Ongoing Assessment and Implementation	• Cup can contain human milk, human milk with fortifiers, or artificial milk. • Use in conjunction with nasogastric or orogastric feeding, as appropriate. • Wrap infant securely to prevent his hands from interfering with the cup. • Support infant in an upright position. • Tip cup so cup just touches lips. • *Do not pour:* Allow the rim of the cup to touch or rest on lower lip, tip the cup, and wait for the infant to sip. Do not apply pressure to lower lip. Allow infant to set the pace.
Evaluation	• Determine if infant consumes required number of milliliters each feeding (if ordered). • If the infant refuses cup feeding (or is "not interested"), consider gavage.
Documentation	• Record volume consumed "via cup" on infant Kardex.
References	List four or fewer references that you and your colleagues believe best substantiate the protocol you create.

1. _____

2. _____

3. _____

4. _____

Approval/review/revision

Person, title, and/or committee _____ Approval date _____ By _____

Revision date (date last reviewed) _____ Anticipated review date _____

Distribution

Persons receiving copies _____

Location _____

offer no other distinct advantage and are not designed for nutritional purposes. Occasionally, some hospitals require a written physician's order for using the periodontal syringe, although this is often not the case.

Finger Feeding

Finger feeding is a method in which the mother or other caregiver allows the infant to suck on a finger while food is being delivered, as shown in Figure 12-7. It can be accomplished using a periodontal syringe or a feeding tube.

How or if finger feeding is implemented is a matter of personal preference and dexterity. Some clinicians prefer this method because it does offer advantages, including clear sensory signals to the trigeminal nerve via the hard palate.[43] I have never become comfortable with finger feeding because I am unable to simultaneously hold the in-

RESEARCH HIGHLIGHT
The physiological and neurobehavioral effects of a single cup feeding on 10 healthy preterm infants

Citation

Ackerman B, Sabo B, Tillinghast K, Kravitz M. The psychologic and neurobehavioral effects of a single cup feeding on 10 healthy preterm infants: pilot study results. Unpublished data. Yale–New Haven Hospital; 1998.

Cup feeding has been suggested in the literature as an alternative method of providing nutrition by mouth to the preterm infant; however standard practice in Neonatal Intensive Care settings in the United States is to provide oral feedings by breast and by artificial nipple. If cup feeding is a safe alternative to artificial nipple feeding for the preterm infant and if cup feeding contributes to the preterm infant's success at breastfeeding, as suggested in the literature, then cup feeding could be an acceptable alternative to artificial nipple feeding in the neonatal preterm breastfeeding population. The purpose of this observational pilot study was to identify physiological and/or neurobehavioral changes, if any, associated with a single cup feeding on the well-being of healthy preterm infants by monitoring their physiological and neurobehavioral responses prior to, during, and following one cup-feeding session. The study sample consisted of a convenience sample of 10 appropriate-for-gestation (AGA) preterm infants, divided into two groups, five who were 32 weeks postconceptional age and five who were 34 weeks' postconceptional age at study time. This pilot study, using the methods described, suggests a cup feeding does not put the healthy preterm infant at risk.

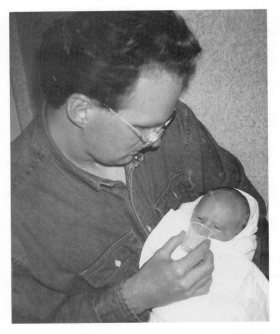

Fig. 12-5 Cup feeding. *(Courtesy Martha Schult.)*

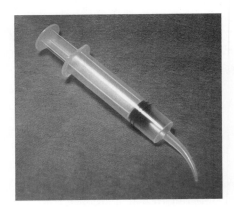

Fig. 12-6 Periodontal syringe.

fant, keep a stiff finger in the infant's mouth, and regulate the syringe.

Perhaps an easy way to accomplish finger feeding is to attach a feeding tube to a finger of the caregiver's dominant hand and instruct her to insert it, pad side up, toward the infant's palate. In this way, the infant can use his tongue in an undulating motion to suck (on a finger) and swallow about every third suck as the caregiver delivers about .5 ml of milk. The infant should not exert suction on the tube; the idea is to have a troughed tongue much like breastfeeding. (If the infant does not first lower and then trough his tongue, apply slight downward pressure on the posterior part of the tongue, then release.) As the infant sucks, the caregiver can gently push about .5 ml of milk from the attached syringe into the infant's mouth about every third suck. The feed-

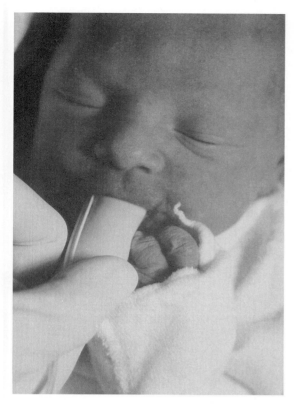

Fig. 12-7 Finger feeding. ©*Debi Bocar, Lactation Consultant Services, Oklahoma City, Oklahoma. Used with permission.*

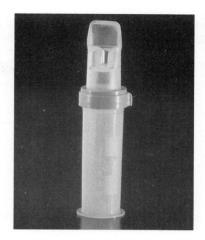

Fig. 12-8 SoftFeeder. *(Courtesy Medela.)*

ing should be unhurried and should continue for about 20 to 30 minutes.

Other Devices

Various other devices have been used for supplementing infants. Medicine droppers work fairly well for newborns. They offer the advantage of easy handling and a way to measure the volume given, and they can be easily sterilized in the autoclave if hospital policy requires them to be sterile. A disadvantage is that they do not provide the infant with much, if any, tactile stimulation to the oral cavity, and they may limit the infant's ability to control the feeding.

Variations of the spoon have also been used. Other versions of the spoon include the Rosti bottle, used in the United Kingdom, and the SoftFeeder (Figure 12-8), manufactured by Medela. Both have a spoonlike device at the end of a handle and are convenient for administering feedings.

THE TRANSITION TO DIRECT AND EXCLUSIVE BREASTFEEDING

All of the techniques for delivering nourishment described in this chapter are inferior to direct breastfeeding. Ideally, then, the situation of indirect breastfeeding or supplementing the infant with artificial milk should be considered temporary. A teaching plan for parents of preterm infants is presented in Chapter 7. A plan for the transition from indirect or supplemental feedings to exclusive direct feeding is found in Table 12-5.

T A B L E 12-5

TRANSITION TO EXCLUSIVE DIRECT BREASTFEEDING

Nursing Responsibility	Clinical Strategy	Rationale
Determine readiness to breastfeed	Introduce breastfeedings before bottle feedings	There is no need for an infant to "prove himself" by sucking a bottle before going to breast. Traditional criteria—arbitrary minimum weights, tolerance of bottle feedings, gestational age, stability of body temperature, or impending discharge—are not supported by scientific research. Ability to coordinate suckling and swallowing with minimal changes in cardiorespiratory response (bradycardia, apnea, hypoxemia) is the current criteria for initiating breastfeeding (until further research-based criteria are identified). Criteria for "breastfeeding" and "bottle feeding" should be restated as ability to tolerate oral feedings.
Prepare infant for first direct breastfeedings	Teach infant to associate mother with feedings (e.g., place mother's breast pad in isolette)	Infant will begin to associate maternal odors with feedings (discourage use of perfume by parents).
	Gavage with nipple in infant's mouth	Sucking improves oxygenation of infant. Infant associates suckling with satiety. Practice may be associated with increased weight gains.[21,44]
	Practice kangaroo care	Increases mother's confidence in holding infant. Increases infant's familiarity with mother's breast and nipple. Nuzzling previously pumped breast prior to planned feedings optimizes experience. Diminishes the "event" atmosphere of first feeding. Reduces mother's anxiety.
	Maximize mother's milk production prior to first feedings	Easier for infant to transfer milk with an abundant milk supply compared with milk trickling from breast. If milk flows too forcefully, pump 2-3 minutes prior to feeding to reduce flow rate.
	Gently stimulate lips and mouth	Stimulating mouth and lips—e.g., having parent perform mouth care—helps infant to become aware of his oral cavity. Avoiding bottle nipples reduces possibility of infant developing confusion between breast and bottle nipples.
Initiate first feedings	Establish reasonable expectations—tolerating the positioning and opening wide may be only expectation for very first feed	Parents almost always have expectations that infant will breastfeed like a champion the very first time. Helping the parent to anticipate small gains encourages rather than disappoints them.
	Provide reassurance and optimal environment	Staying with mother and giving help optimizes feeding interactions. Providing warm, comfortable, private location free from visual and auditory distractions and drafts helps with maternal relaxation (and hence milk ejection) and helps stabilize infants' vital signs and temperature.
	Position the mother; use footstool and pillows as appropriate	Comfortable position that facilitates good alignment, areolar grasp, areolar compression, and audible swallowing, as described in Chapter 5, facilitates milk transfer.

Source: Bocar D. *Breastfeeding Educator Resource Notebook*. Oklahoma City, OK: Lactation Consultant Services; 1998.

T A B L E 12-5

TRANSITION TO EXCLUSIVE DIRECT BREASTFEEDING—cont'd

Nursing Responsibility	Clinical Strategy	Rationale
Initiate first feedings—cont'd	Stimulate infant—use alerting techniques (see Chapter 6)	Helps infant to be in an optimal state for feeding.
	Maintain thermoneutral environment; monitor infant temperature according to unit protocol	Mother's breasts are warmer than the rest of her body. If necessary, supplemental heat (overhead warmer, heat lamp) can be used to increase ambient temperature during the feeding experience.
	Use most optimal position for infant	"Nesting" infant with physical boundaries (pillows, towel rolls, etc.) helps hypotonic infant to maintain postural control and conserve energy. Infants may experience less apnea if positioned prone.[45] Transitional hold allows for good control of infant and good visibility of preterm or hypotonic infant.
	Cue the infant to suckle	Gently touching the lips with the nipple helps the infant to open wide.
	Entice infant to suck • Express milk onto lips • Elicit milk-ejection reflex • Offer breast with easier flow first • Instill a *few* drops of milk in the infant's mouth via feeding tube to elicit suckle-swallow reflex	Gentle perioral stimulation before infant is ready for first feed, as described above, helps infant to become aware of his oral cavity. The suckle-swallow reflex is a chained response. By having the milk readily available and in abundant supply, the infant is more likely to get into the rhythm of the chained suckle-swallow response.
	Monitor infant physiological responses to breastfeeding	Alterations in heart rate, respiratory rate, oxygen saturation, body temperature, color (especially perioral cyanosis) are signs of distress.
	Determine if milk transfer is occurring	Infants can suck without actually obtaining milk. A reassuring sign is when infants have audible swallowing. Perform pre- and postfeeding weight assessments.
	Continue feeding, unless otherwise indicated	Unless the infant shows signs of fatigue or stress cues, the feeding may be continued until he is satiated. Allowing infants to rest can be restorative. Interrupting a feeding on the "first" side may result in cessation of breastfeeding for that session.
Facilitate transition to cue-based feeding	Develop nursery protocols that support cue-based feedings prior to discharge	Research indicates that preterm infants benefit from cue-based feedings rather than scheduled feedings. Term infants consume more milk and grow faster when fed frequently and in response to hunger cues. Preterm infant may be on "modified" cue-based feeding plan at approximately 35-36 weeks' gestational age—setting maximum intervals between feedings (2-3 hours) with one longer sleep-cycle each 24 hours. Cue-based feedings in the hospital help prepare mothers and infants for cue-based feedings at home.

SUMMARY

Ideally, all infants will breastfeed directly and exclusively. In circumstances where they do not, however, alternative methods for delivering nourishment must be explored. Ideally, the nourishment delivered should be human milk, but artificial milk may be given if desired or medically indicated. Multiple devices, each having its own advantages and disadvantages, can be used to give nourishment to the infant who is not exclusively breastfeeding.

References

1. Frantz KB. The slow-gaining breastfeeding infant. *NAACOGS Clin Issu Perinat Womens Health Nurs* 1992;3:647-655.

2. Wong DL. *Whaley and Wong's Nursing Care of Infants and Children*. 5th ed. St. Louis: Mosby; 1995.

3. Simmer K, Metcalf R, Daniels L. The use of breastmilk in a neonatal unit and its relationship to protein and energy intake and growth. *J Paediatr Child Health* 1997;33(1):55-60.

4. Churella HR, Bachhuber WL, MacLean WC Jr. Survey: methods of feeding low-birth-weight infants. *Pediatrics* 1985;76(2):243-249.

5. Poets CF, Langner MU, Bohnhorst B. Effects of bottle feeding and two different methods of gavage feeding on oxygenation and breathing patterns in preterm infants. *Acta Paediatr* 1997;86(4):419-423.

6. Blondheim O, Abbasi S, Fox WW, Bhutani VK. Effect of enteral gavage feeding rate on pulmonary functions of very low birth weight infants. *J Pediatr* 1993;122:751-755.

7. Silvestre MA, Morbach CA, Brans YW, Shankaran S. A prospective randomized trail comparing continuous versus intermittent feeding methods in very low birth weight neonates. *J Pediatr* 1996;128:748-752.

8. Bhatia J, Rassin DK. Human milk supplementation: delivery of energy, calcium, phosphorus, magnesium, copper, and zinc. *Am J Dis Child* 1988;142:445-447.

9. Brooke OG, Barley J. Loss of energy during continuous infusions of breast milk. *Arch Dis Child* 1978;53(4):344-345.

10. Greer FR, McCormick A, Loker J. Changes in fat concentration of human milk during delivery by intermittent bolus and continuous mechanical pump infusion. *J Pediatr* 1984;105:745-749.

11. Lemons PM, Miller K, Eitzen H, Strodtbeck F, Lemons JA. Bacterial growth in human milk during continuous feeding. *Am J Perinatol* 1983;1:76-80.

12. Stocks RJ, Davies DP, Allen F, Sewell D. Loss of breast milk nutrients during tube feeding. *Arch Dis Child* 1985;60:164-166.

13. Arnold LDW, ed. *Recommendations for Collection, Storage, and Handling of a Mother's Milk for Her Own Infant in the Hospital Setting*. West Hartford, CT: Human Milk Banking Association of North America; 1993.

14. Narayanan I, Singh B, Harvey D. Fat loss during feeding of human milk. *Arch Dis Child* 1984; 59:475-477.

15. Mehta NR, Hamosh M, Bitman J, Wood DL. Adherence of medium-chain fatty acids to feeding tubes during gavage feeding of human milk fortified with medium-chain triglycerides. *J Pediatr* 1988;112:474-476.

16. Rayol MR, Martinez FE, Jorge SM, Goncalves AL, Desai ID. Feeding premature infants banked human milk homogenized by ultrasonic treatment. *J Pediatr* 1993;123:985-988.

17. Brennan-Behm M, Carlson GE, Meier P, Engstrom J. Caloric loss from expressed mother's milk during continuous gavage infusion. *Neonatal Netw* 1994;13(2):27-32.

18. Lucas A, Gibbs JA, Lyster RL, Baum JD. Creamatocrit: simple clinical technique for estimating fat concentration and energy value of human milk. *Br Med J* 1978;1:1018-1020.

19. Lemons JA, Schreiner RL, Gresham EL. Simple method for determining the caloric and fat content of human milk. *Pediatrics* 1980;66:626-628.

20. Botsford KB, Weinstein RA, Boyer KM, Nathan C, Carman M, Paton JB. Gram-negative bacilli in human milk feedings: quantitation and clinical consequences for premature infants. *J Pediatr* 1986;109:707-710.

21. Bernbaum JC, Pereira GR, Watkins JB, Peckham GJ. Nonnutritive sucking during gavage feeding enhances growth and maturation in premature infants. *Pediatrics* 1983;71:41-45.

22. Field T, Ignatoff E, String ES, et al. Nonnutritive sucking during tube feedings: effects on preterm neonates in an intensive care unit. *Pediatrics* 1982;70:381-384.

23. Ernst JA, Rickard KA, Neal PR, et al. Lack of improved growth outcome related to non-nutritive sucking in very low birth weight premature infants fed a controlled nutrient intake: a randomized prospective study. *Pediatrics* 1989;83:706-716.

24. DiPietro JA, Cusson RM, Caughy MO, Fox NA. Behavioral and physiologic effects of nonnutritive sucking during gavage feeding in preterm infants. *Pediatr Res* 1994;36:207-214.

25. Narayanan I, Mehta R, Choudhury DK, Jain BK. Sucking on the "emptied" breast: non-nutritive sucking with a difference. *Arch Dis Child* 1991;66:241-244.

26. Farber SD, VanFossen RL, Koontz SW. Quantitative and qualitative video analysis of infant feeding: angled and straight-bottle feeding systems. *J Pediatr* 1995;126:S118-S124.

27. Mathew OP. Science of bottle feeding. *J Pediatr* 1991;114:511-519.

28. Nowak AJ, Smith WL, Erenberg A. Imaging evaluation of artificial nipples during bottle feeding. *Arch Pediatr Adolesc Med* 1994;148:40-42.

29. Nowak AJ, Smith WL, Erenberg A. Imaging evaluation of breast-feeding and bottle-feeding systems. *J Pediatr* 1995;126:S130-S134.

30. Mathew OP. Nipple units for newborn infants: a functional comparison. *Pediatrics* 1988;81:688-691.

31. Neifert M, Lawrence R, Seacat J. Nipple confusion: toward a formal definition. *J Pediatr* 1995;126:S125-S129.

32. Inoue N, Sakashita R, Kamegai T. Reduction in masseter muscle activity in bottle-fed babies. *Early Hum Dev* 1995;42:185-193.

33. Cohen M, Witherspoon M, Brown DR, Myers MM. Blood pressure increases in response to feeding in the term neonate. *Dev Psychobiol* 1992;25:291-298.

34. Mathew OP, Bhatia J. Sucking and breathing patterns during breast- and bottle-feeding in term neonates: effects of nutrient delivery and composition. *Am J Dis Child* 1989;143:588-592.

35. Meier P. Bottle- and breast-feeding: effects on transcutaneous oxygen pressure and temperature in preterm infants. *Nurs Res* 1988;37:36-41.

36. Bier JB, Ferguson AE, Morales Y, et al. Breastfeeding infants who were extremely low birth weight. *Pediatrics* 1997;100. URL: http://www.pediatrics.org/cgi/content/full/100/6/e3.

37. Davis HV, Sears RR, Miller HC, Brodbeck AJ. Effects of cup, bottle and breast feeding on oral activities of newborn infants. *Pediatrics* 1948;2:549-558.

38. Fredeen RC. Cup feeding of newborn infants. *Pediatrics* 1948;2:544-548.

39. Ackerman B, Sabo B, Tillinghast K. The physiologic and neurobehavioral effects of a single cup feeding on 10 healthy preterm infants: pilot study results. Unpublished data. Yale–New Haven Hospital; 1998.

40. Lang S, Lawrence CJ, Orme RL. Cup feeding: an alternative method of infant feeding. *Arch Dis Child* 1994;71:365-369.

41. Biancuzzo M. Breastfeeding preterm twins: a case report. *Birth* 1994;21:96-100.

42. Biancuzzo M. Creating and implementing a protocol for cup feeding. *Mother Baby Journal* 1997;2(3):27-33.

43. Hazelbaker AK. In defense of finger feeding. *Rental Roundup* 1997;2(14):10-11.

44. Gill NE, Behnke M, Conlon M, McNeely JB, Anderson GC. Effect of nonnutritive sucking on behavioral state in preterm infants before feeding. *Nurs Res* 1988;37(6):347-350.

45. Kurlak LO, Ruggins NR, Stephensen TJ. Effect of nursing position on incidence, type, and duration of clinically significant apnoea in preterm infants. *Arch Dis Child* 1994;71:F16-F19.

Appendices

Community Breastfeeding Support

*T*his appendix provides a way to contact organizations that provide products or services that help mothers to initiate or continue breastfeeding. Mothers have direct access to these organizations. Mention of these organizations does not constitute endorsement of their services or products by the author or the publisher. This list is not intended to be all-inclusive. Other local or national organizations may also be helpful to the breastfeeding mother.

A-1 Support Groups for Parents

La Leche League International

La Leche League International (LLLI), started by a group of breastfeeding women in 1957, continues today as an international organization focusing on consumer support and advocacy for breastfeeding. LLLI also provides materials, continuing education, and products for professionals. There are more than 3500 local chapters in about 50 countries throughout the world. To contact local chapters, contact La Leche League International and ask for the chapter in your area.

LA LECHE LEAGUE INTERNATIONAL
PO Box 4079
Schaumburg, IL 60168-4079
(847) 519-7730
(800) LALECHE
FAX: (847) 519-0035
www.lalecheleague.org

Cleft Palate Foundation

The Cleft Palate Foundation (CPF) was founded in 1973 by its parent, the American Cleft Palate–Craniofacial Association (ACPA) to be the public service arm of the professional association. CPF is a non-profit organization that aims to enhance the quality of life for individuals with congenital facial deformities and their families through education, research support, and facilitation of family-centered care. CPF's major activities include the operation of CleftLine and the dissemination of CPF publications. To contact local chapters, call the hotline listed below, and ask for the chapter in your area.

THE CLEFT PALATE FOUNDATION
1829 E. Franklin Street
Suite 1022
Chapel Hill, NC 27514
(919) 933-9044
(800) 24-CLEFT
FAX: (919) 933-9604
www.cleft.com
cleftline@aol.com

National Down Syndrome Society

The National Down Syndrome Society (NDSS) was established in 1979 to increase public awareness about Down Syndrome, to assist families in addressing the needs of children born with this genetic condition, and to sponsor and encourage scientific research. NDSS supports research, sponsors symposia, advocates on behalf of families, provides information and referral services through their toll-free number, and develops and distributes educational materials.

NATIONAL DOWN SYNDROME SOCIETY
666 Broadway, 8th Floor
New York, NY 10012-2317
(212) 460-9330
(800) 221-4602
FAX: (212) 979-2873
www.ndss.org

National Organization of Mothers of Twins Clubs

The National Organization of Mothers of Twins Clubs, Inc. (NOMOTC) was founded in 1960 to promote the special aspects of child development related specifically to multiple-birth children. NOMOTC is a network of about 475 local clubs representing over 21,000 individual parents of multiples. NOMOTC is funded by dues, donations, and grants.

NATIONAL ORGANIZATION OF MOTHERS OF TWINS
  CLUBS INC. (NOMOTC)
PO Box 23188
Albuquerque, NM 87192-1188
(505) 275-0955
(800) 243-2276
www.nomotc.org
NOMOTC@aol.com

Parents of Multiple Births Association of Canada

The Parents of Multiple Births Association (POMBA) of Canada is a non-profit organization of parents of multiples across Canada. The organization provides parent-to-parent support and information for raising twins, triplets, quadruplets, and quintuplets. More than 50 local clubs have been established throughout Canada.

PARENTS OF MULTIPLE BIRTHS ASSOCIATION OF
  CANADA
240 Graff Avenue, Box 22005
Stratford, Ontario CANADA N5A 7V6
(519) 272-2203
FAX: (519) 272-1926
www.pomba.org
office@pomba.org

A-2 Equipment Companies

Many companies in the United States and abroad manufacture breast pumps and related equipment. Companies who provided photos for this book are listed below:

AVENT AMERICA
501 Lively Blvd.
Elk Grove Village, IL 60007
(800) 54AVENT
FAX: (847) 228-6142
www.aventamerica.com

HOLLISTER'S AMEDA/EGNELL
2000 Hollister Drive
Libertyville, IL 60048
(847) 918-5882
(800) 323-4060
FAX: (847) 918-5875
www.hollister.com

LACT-AID INTERNATIONAL
PO Box 1066
Athens, TN 37371-1066
(423) 744-9090
FAX: (423) 744-9116
www.lact-aid.com
info@lact-aid.com

MEDELA
PO Box 660
McHenry, IL 60051-0660
(800) 435-8316
(815) 363-1166
FAX: (800) 995-7867
FAX: (815) 363-1246
www.medela.com

WHITE RIVER CONCEPTS
924 C Calle Negocio
San Clemente, CA 92673
(800) 342-3906
(714) 366-8960
FAX: (714) 366-1664
www.whiteriver.com

A-3 Donor Human Milk Banks in North America

A donor human milk bank is defined by the Human Milk Banking Association of North America as a service established for the purpose of collecting, screening, processing, storing, and distributing donated human milk to meet the specific needs of individuals for whom human milk is prescribed by physicians. (Further information is given in Chapter 10.) Eight donor human milk banks in North America currently meet that criteria; they are listed below. All of these banks are members of the Human Milk Banking Association of North America (HMBANA), 8 Jan Sebastian Way, #13, Sandwich, MA 02563, (508) 888-4041, FAX: (508) 888-8050, milkbank@capecod.net:

BANCO DE LECHE DR. RAFAEL LUCIO
Xalapa, VERACRUZ, MEXICO
52-55-14-45-10, ext. 204
FAX: 52-55-14-45-51

COMMUNITY HUMAN MILK BANK
Georgetown University Hospital
Washington, DC
(202)784-6455

LACTATION SUPPORT SERVICE
British Columbia Children's Hospital
Vancouver, BC CANADA
(604) 875-2345, ext. 7607

MOTHERS' MILK BANK
Columbia P/SL Medical Center
Denver, CO
(303) 869-1888

MOTHERS' MILK BANK
Valley Medical Center
San Jose, CA
(408) 998-4550

REGIONAL MILK BANK
Medical Center of Central Massachusetts
Worcester, MA
(508) 793-6005

TRIANGLE LACTATION CENTER AND MOTHERS'
    MILK BANK
Wake Medical Center
Raleigh, NC
(919) 250-8599

WILMINGTON MOTHERS' MILK BANK
Christiana Care Health System
Wilmington, DE
(302) 733-2340

Parent Education Media

*T*his appendix is designed to identify selected materials for parent education. Materials listed here can be obtained by contacting the respective publishers, producers, and distributors of these materials as listed in Appendix E, or—in the case of paperback books and some other materials—by visiting a bookstore. Many items are available from other vendors than those listed; only vendors in the United States are listed here. The author welcomes suggestions about other places where these materials may be easily obtained. Readers or vendors may send comments to: bookcomments@wmc-worldwide.com.

All materials are in English; additional languages are listed. All videotapes are in NTSC format; additional formats may be avail-able. Materials listed in this appendix do not necessarily constitute endorsement by the author or the publisher, and this list is not intended to be all-inclusive. The author and the publisher have made every attempt to verify the information listed herein. However, availability is subject to change, and prices are approximate and in most cases do not include shipping and handling charges. The author has determined that the resources listed below are aimed primarily at a consumer audience, but acknowledges that some of these materials may be helpful for professionals also.

B-1 Motivating Women to Breastfeed

These audio, visual, and audiovisual materials are designed to motivate women to breastfeed by discussing benefits or debunking myths about breastfeeding. In general, these are most helpful when used during the prenatal period, but it is never too late to provide them.

Key words are attached to help the reader quickly focus on pertinent aspects of the education materials. All media listed are in English; every attempt is made to list other language versions where available. Prices are approximate and are subject to change and in most cases do not include shipping and handling.

Key Word/Target Population	Media	Length	Additional Languages	Author	Date
Advantages	Pamphlet	Multifold		Health Education Associates	Not listed
Advantages	Pamphlet	Multifold		Health Education Associates	Not listed
Advantages	Pamphlet	Multifold		Health Education Associates	Not listed
Advantages	Pamphlet	Multifold	Spanish, Cambodian, Russian, French, Vietnamese	Health Education Associates	Not listed
Advantages	Videotape	9 minutes	Spanish	Texas WIC	1989
Advantages	Videotape	22 minutes		Best Start	Not listed
Advantages, options	Pamphlet	Multifold		Health Education Associates	Not listed
Advantages	Videotape	19 minutes	Spanish	McElaney, L.	1998
African-American	Videotape	14 minutes		Maryland WIC Program, features Anita Baker	1993
African-American	Videotape	14 minutes		Maryland WIC Program	1997
Allergies	Pamphlet	Multifold		Health Education Associates	Not listed
Avoiding problems	Videotape	13 minutes	Spanish	Texas WIC	1989
Cow's milk	Pamphlet	Multifold	Spanish	Health Education Associates	Not listed
Easy to do	Pamphlet	Multifold	Spanish, Vietnamese	Health Education Associates	Not listed
Economically disadvantaged	Videotape	22 minutes	Spanish	Best Start	1989

Title	Publisher	Available From	Price
Breastfeeding: It's NOT Just Food	Health Education Associates	Health Education Associates	$.50 ≤ 24; quantity discounts available
Have You Thought About Breastfeeding?	Health Education Associates	Health Education Associates	$.50 ≤ 24; quantity discounts available
Why Do Mothers Breastfeed?	Health Education Associates	Health Education Associates	$.50 ≤ 24; quantity discounts available
Breastfeeding: Best for Baby and You	Health Education Associates	Health Education Associates	$.50 ≤ 24; quantity discounts available
A Loving Way	Texas WIC	Tele-Print Express	Single copies no charge
Loving Our Children, Loving Ourselves	Best Start	Best Start	$25
Is It Worth It to Breastfeed?	Health Education Associates	Health Education Associates	$.50 ≤ 24; quantity discounts available
Breastfeeding: The Why-to, How-to, Can-do Videos. Part I: Why-to	Vida Health Communications	Vida Health Communications	$195 single/$295 set
Giving You the Best That I've Got, Baby	Maryland Dept. of Health and Mental Hygiene and Johns Hopkins University School of Public Health	Johns Hopkins University	$20
Learning How to Breastfeed Your Baby: Breastfed Is Bestfed	Maryland Dept. of Health and Mental Hygiene and Johns Hopkins University School of Public Health	Johns Hopkins University	Not listed
Breastfeeding Advice for Families With Allergies	Health Education Associates	Health Education Associates	$.50 ≤ 24; quantity discounts available
Yes, You Can Breastfeed	Texas WIC	Tele-Print Express	Not listed
NO Cow's Milk in the First Year	Health Education Associates	Health Education Associates	$.50 ≤ 24; quantity discounts available
Nursing Is Easy When You Know How	Health Education Associates	Health Education Associates	$.50 ≤ 24; quantity discounts available
For All the Right Reasons	Best Start	Best Start	$24

Continued

Key Word/ Target Population	Media	Length	Additional Languages	Author	Date
Family	Pamphlet	Multifold		Health Education Associates	Not listed
Family, sexuality	Pamphlet	Multifold	Spanish	Health Education Associates	Not listed
Fathers	Videotape	5 minutes	Spanish	Vida Health Communications	1998
Fathers	Pamphlet	Multifold		Health Education Associates	Not listed
Lifestyle	Pamphlet	Bifold		Best Start	1997
Options—comic book format	Pamphlet	Multifold		Health Education Associates	Not listed
Support	Pamphlet	Bifold	Spanish	Best Start	1997
Teens	Pamphlet	Multifold		Health Education Associates	Not listed
Teens	Videotape	22 minutes	Spanish	Best Start	1993

Title	Publisher	Available From	Price
If Your Grandchild Is Breastfed	Health Education Associates	Health Education Associates	$.50 ≤ 24; quantity discounts available
Men Ask About Breastfeeding	Health Education Associates	Health Education Associates	$.50 ≤ 24; quantity discounts available
(Title to be determined)	Vida Health Communications	Vida Health Communications	To be determined
Fathers Ask Questions About Breastfeeding	Health Education Associates	Health Education Associates	$.50 ≤ 24; quantity discounts available
Busy Moms	Best Start	Best Start	$0.16 each for ≤ 1000; quantity discounts available
Breastfeeding: Too Good to Miss Out On!	Health Education Associates	Health Education Associates	$.50 ≤ 24; quantity discounts available
Encouragement	Best Start	Best Start	$0.16 each for ≤ 1000; quantity discounts available
Teens Can Breastfeed	Health Education Associates	Health Education Associates	$.50 ≤ 24; quantity discounts available
Nobody Loves Them Like You	Best Start	Best Start	$25

B-2 Managing Breastfeeding In Wellness Situations

These audio, visual, and audiovisual materials are designed to help the clinician manage breastfeeding for well infants and their mothers. One key word has been assigned to help the reader quickly identify pertinent points, but multiple points are usually covered in the media. Prices are approximate and are subject to change, and most do not include shipping and handling.

Key Word	Media	Length	Additional Languages	Author	Date
Attachment	Pamphlet	Multifold		Health Education Associates	Not listed
Attachment, milk supply	Pamphlet	Multifold	Spanish, French, Cambodian, Russian, Vietnamese	Health Education Associates	Not listed
Attachment, positioning	Book	225 pages		Renfrew, M., Fisher, C., & Arms, S.	1990
Attachment, positioning	Pamphlet	Multifold		Health Education Associates	Not listed
Attachment, positioning	Videotape	14 minutes	Spanish	Frantz, K.	1986
Attachment, positioning	Videotape	15 minutes		Frantz, K.	1986
Attachment, positioning	Videotape	15 minutes		Medela	1990
Attachment, positioning	Videotape	20 minutes	Spanish	Smith, L.	1991
Attachment, positioning	Videotape and tear-off tablet	24 minutes	Spanish	Tully, M.R., & Overfield, M.	1991
Avoiding problems	Videotape	13 minutes	Spanish	Texas WIC	1989
Burping	Videotape	18 minutes	Spanish	Frantz, K.	1986
Drugs	Pamphlet	Multifold		Health Education Associates	Not listed
Early discharge	Videotape	30 minutes		Royal College of Midwives/ Fisher, C.	1996
Early discharge	Pamphlet	14 pages		Walker, M.	1998
Early discharge	Videotape	25 minutes		Frantz, K.	1996
Early initiation	Videotape	6 minutes		Righard, L.	1992/ 1995
Easy to do	Pamphlet	Multifold	Spanish, Vietnamese	Health Education Associates	Not listed
Embarrassment	Pamphlet	Multifold		Health Education Associates	Not listed
Expression, hand	Pamphlet	Multifold		Health Education Associates	Not listed
Feeding cues and behavior	Pamphlet	Multifold		Health Education Associates	Not listed

Title	Publisher	Available From	Price
Learning About Breastfeeding	Health Education Associates	Health Education Associates	$.50 ≤ 24; quantity discounts available
How to Nurse Your Baby	Health Education Associates	Health Education Associates	$.50 ≤ 24; quantity discounts available
Bestfeeding: Getting Breastfeeding Right for You	Celestial Arts	Birth and Life Bookstore	$15
An Easy Way to Get Started at Breastfeeding	Health Education Associates	Health Education Associates	$.50 ≤ 24; quantity discounts available
Breastfeeding Techniques That Work! Volume 1: First Attachment	Geddes Productions	Geddes Productions	$39.95
Breastfeeding Techniques That Work! Volume 2: First Attachment in Bed	Geddes Productions	Geddes Productions	$39.95
Breastfeeding Your Baby: Positioning Instructional Video	Medela	Medela	$7.80
A Healthier Baby by Breastfeeding	Television Innovation Company	Childbirth Graphics, LLLI; or Bright Futures	$22
Breastfeeding: A Special Relationship	Eagle Productions	Eagle Productions	$79
Yes, You Can Breastfeed	Texas WIC	Tele-Print Express	Not listed
Breastfeeding Techniques That Work! Volume 4: Burping the Baby	Geddes Productions	Geddes Productions	$39.95
Drugs in Breast Milk	Health Education Associates	Health Education Associates	$.50 ≤ 24; quantity discounts available
Breastfeeding: Coping With the First Week	Royal College of Midwives	Growing With Baby	$80
Everything You Need to Know About Breastfeeding in 24 Hours or Less	Lactation Associates	Lactation Associates	$2.50; quantity discounts available
Breastfeeding Techniques That Work! Volume 8: The First Week	Geddes Productions	Geddes Productions	$39.95
Delivery Self Attachment	Geddes Productions	Geddes Productions, Childbirth Graphics	$14.95
Breastfeeding Is Easy When You Know How	Health Education Associates	Health Education Associates	$.50 ≤ 24; quantity discounts available
How to Nurse Modestly	Health Education Associates	Health Education Associates	$.50 ≤ 24; quantity discounts available
Breast Massage and Hand Expression of Breast Milk	Health Education Associates	Health Education Associates	$.50 ≤ 24; quantity discounts available
Breastfeeding: Those First Weeks at Home	Health Education Associates	Health Education Associates	$.50 ≤ 24; quantity discounts available

Continued

Key Word	Media	Length	Additional Languages	Author	Date
How-to	Videotape	75 minutes	Spanish, Cantonese, Mandarin	Livingstone, V.	1994
How-to	Videotape	24 minutes	Spanish	McElaney, L.	1998
How-to	Book	176 pages		Kitzinger, S.	1998
How-to	Book			Pryor, K.	1991
How-to	Book	62 pages	Spanish, Creole, French	Wiggins, P.	1995
How-to	Book	117 pages	Spanish	Gotsch, G.	1994
How-to	Book	176 pages		Wiggins, P.K.	1996
How-to	Book	180 pages		King. F.S.	1992
How-to	Book	256 pages		Huggins, K. (ed).	1995
How-to	Book	234 pages		Moody, J., Britten, J., & Hogg, K.	1996
How-to	Book	480 pages	Spanish, other	La Leche League International	1991
How-to	Book	105 pages	Spanish	Spangler, A.	1995
How-to	Booklet	32 pages		Stacy, L., & Mizumoto, D.	1993
How-to	Pamphlet	12 pages	Spanish	Danner, S.C.	1998
How-to	Booklet	30 pages		Danner, S.C.	1997
How-to	Videotape	23 minutes			1986
How-to	Videotape	15 minutes		Medela	Not listed
How-to	Videotape	35 minutes	Spanish, French	Nylander, G.	1994
Nutrition	Pamphlet	Multifold		Health Education Associates	Not listed
Nutrition	Pamphlet	Multifold	Spanish, Vietnamese	Health Education Associates	Not listed
Sleep	Audiotape	33 minutes		Woodford, T.	
Sleep	Book	176		Thevenin, T.	1996
Sleep	Pamphlet	Multifold		Health Education Associates	Not listed
Sleep	Pamphlet	Multifold		Health Education Associates	Not listed
Weaning	Pamphlet	Multifold		Health Education Associates	Not listed

Title	Publisher	Available From	Price
The Art of Successful Breast-feeding (4 chapters)	University of British Columbia	Vancouver Breastfeeding Centre	$20 for home use; $130, institutional price
Breastfeeding: The Why-to, How-to, Can-do, Videos. Part 2: How-to	Vida Health Communications	Vida Health Communications	$195 single/$295 set
Breastfeeding Your Baby	Knopf	Birth & Life Bookstore	$20
Nursing Your Baby	Pocket Books	Birth & Life Bookstore	$6
Why Should I Nurse My Baby	L.A. Publishing	L.A. Publishing	$5; bulk rate available
Breastfeeding Pure and Simple	La Leche League International	LLLI, Childbirth Graphics, Birth & Life Bookstore	$10
Breastfeeding: A Mother's Gift	L.A. Publishing	L.A. Publishing	$10; quantity rate available
Helping Mothers to Breastfeed (revised edition)	African Medical and Research Foundation	African Medical and Research Foundation	$12
The Nursing Mothers Companion (3rd edition)	Harvard Common Press	Harvard Common Press	$22 hardcover; $12 softcover
Breastfeeding Your Baby	Natural Childbirth Trust Publishing	HMSO Publications Centre	Not listed
The Womanly Art of Breastfeeding	La Leche League International	LLLI, Childbirth Graphics	$13
Amy Spangler's Breastfeeding: A Parent's Guide (6th ed.)	Amy Spangler	Author, Childbirth Graphics, Birth & Life Bookstore	$6
Breast-feeding: Nature's Best for You and Your Baby	American Dietetic Association	American Dietetic Association	$1.80 nonmembers; $1.50 members
Nursing Your Baby for the First Time	Childbirth Graphics	Childbirth Graphics	$.82 each; quantity discounts available
Nursing Your Baby Beyond the First Days	Childbirth Graphics	Childbirth Graphics	$.82; quantity discounts available
Beginning Breastfeeding	Polymorph Films	Polymorph Films	$295
Breastfeeding Your Baby, A Mother's Guide	Medela	Medela	$9.95
Breast Is Best	Norwegian Film Institute	INFACT Canada	$55
An Easy Diet for Breastfeeding Mothers	Health Education Associates	Health Education Associates	$.50 ≤ 24; quantity discounts available
Nutrition for Breastfeeding Mothers	Health Education Associates	Health Education Associates	$.50 ≤ 24; quantity discounts available
Baby-Go-to-Sleep Tape	Flying Colors	Four Dee Products	$12.95
Family Bed: An Age-Old Concept in Child Rearing	Avery Publishing	Bookstores	$10
Helping Your Baby Sleep Through the Night	Health Education Associates	Health Education Associates	$.50 ≤ 24; quantity discounts available
Sleep Patterns of Breastfed Babies	Health Education Associates	Health Education Associates	$.50 ≤ 24; quantity discounts available
Weaning Your Breastfed Baby	Health Education Associates	Health Education Associates	$.50 ≤ 24; quantity discounts available

B-3 Managing Breastfeeding in Wellness Situations With Special Focus

These audio, visual, and audiovisual materials are designed to help manage or prevent problems for mostly well infants, or to provide advice about feeding the infant when special situations arise, for example, multiple gestation. (As employed mothers deal mostly with issues of separation, employment is listed in the next section.) One key word has been assigned to help the reader quickly identify pertinent points, but multiple points are usually covered in the media. Prices are approximate and subject to change, and most do not include shipping and handling charges.

Key Word/ Target Population	Media	Length	Additional Languages	Author	Date
Adoption	Book	141 pages		Peterson, D.	1995
Allergies	Pamphlet	Multifold		Health Education Associates	Not listed
Cesarean	Videotape	26 minutes		Frantz, K.	1986
Cesarean	Pamphlet	Multifold		Health Education Associates	Not listed
Diabetes	Pamphlet	Multifold		Health Education Associates	Not listed
Employment	Videotape	56 minutes		Frantz, K.	1988
Engorgement	Pamphlet	Multifold (8)		Bocar, D.	1997
How-to	Videotape	75 minutes	Spanish, Cantonese, Mandarin	Livingstone, V.	1994
How-to	Videotape	35 minutes	Spanish, French	Nylander, G.	1994
Insufficient milk	Videotape	10 minutes	Spanish	Texas WIC	1991
Jaundice	Pamphlet	Multifold		Health Education Associates	Not listed
Legal rights	Pamphlet	8 pages		La Leche League International	1991
Legal rights	Packet	Multiple pages		La Leche League International	1991
Multiple gestation	Pamphlet	Multifold		Health Education Associates	1993
Multiple gestation	Book	128 pages		Gromada, K.	1991
Multiple gestation	Book	368 pages		Noble, E.	1991
Multiple gestation	Videotape	30 minutes		Gromada, K.	1998
Problems	Pamphlet	Multifold		Health Education Associates	Not listed
Tandem	Pamphlet	20 pages		Berke, G.	1989

Title	Publisher	Available From	Price
Breastfeeding the Adopted Baby	Corona Publishing	Bookstores	$9
Breastfeeding Advice for Families With Allergies	Health Education Associates	Health Education Associates	$.50 ≤ 24; quantity discounts available
Breastfeeding Techniques That Work! Volume 3: First Attachment After a Cesarean	Geddes Productions	Geddes Productions	$39.95
Breastfeeding After a Cesarean	Health Education Associates	Health Education Associates	$.50 ≤ 24; quantity discounts available
Breastfeeding and the Diabetic Mother	Health Education Associates	Health Education Associates	$.50 ≤ 24; quantity discounts available
Breastfeeding Techniques That Work! Volume 5: Successful Working Mothers	Geddes Productions	Geddes Productions	$39.95
Engorgement	Lactation Consultant Services	Lactation Consultant Services	Special pricing
The Art of Successful Breastfeeding (4 chapters)	University of British Columbia	Vancouver Breastfeeding Centre	$20 for home use; $130 for institutional price
Breast Is Best	Norwegian Health Institute	INFACT Canada	$55
The Missing Milk Caper	Texas WIC	Tele-Print Express	Not listed
Jaundice in Newborn Babies	Health Education Associates	Health Education Associates	$.50 ≤ 24; quantity discounts available
Legal Rights of Breastfeeding Mothers: USA Scene	La Leche League International	La Leche League International	$.75
Breastfeeding Rights Packet	La Leche League International	La Leche League International	$10
Breastfeeding Your Twins	Health Education Associates	Health Education Associates	$.50 ≤ 24; quantity discounts available
Mothering Multiples (3rd ed.).	La Leche League International	LLLI, Childbirth Graphics	$8
Having Twins: A Parent's Guide to Pregnancy, Birth & Early Childhood (2nd ed.)	Houghton Mifflin	Four Dee Products, LLLI, Publisher	$16
Double Duty: The Joys and Challenges of Caring for Newborn Twins	DLF Enterprises	Four Dee Products	Special pricing
Breastfeeding Problems Can Be Avoided	Health Education Associates	Health Education Associates	$.50 ≤ 24; quantity discounts available
Nursing for Two, Is It for You?	La Leche League International	La Leche League International	$2.50

B-4 Preventing or Managing Breastfeeding Problems

These audio, visual, and audiovisual materials are designed to help manage breastfeeding for newborns or mothers who have special problems.

Prices are approximate and are subject to change and in most cases do not include shipping and handling.

Topic	Media	Length	Additional Languages	Author	Date
Cleft	Videotape	16 minutes		Children's Mercy Hospital	1996
Cleft	Videotape	23 minutes	French	Herzog-Isler, C. & Honigmann, K.	1996
Cleft	Pamphlet	Foldover	Spanish	Cleft Palate Foundation	1997
Cleft	Pamphlet	16 pages		Danner, S.C., & Cerutti, E.R.	1996
Cleft	Booklet	31 pages	French	Herzog-Isler, C., & Honigmann, K.	1996
Down syndrome	Pamphlet	12 pages		LLLI	Not listed
Down syndrome	Pamphlet	12 pages		Danner, S.C., & Cerutti, E.R.	1996
Neurologically impaired	Pamphlet	8 pages		Danner, S.C., & Cerutti, E.R.	1996
Preterm	Videotape	14 minutes		Egnell-Ameda (U.K.)	1996
Preterm	Pamphlet	8 pages		Danner, S.C., & Cerutti, E.R.	1996
Preterm	Videotape	23 minutes		Driscoll, J.W., & Lawhon, G.	1986
Preterm	Videotape	16 minutes		Driscoll, J.W., & Lawhon, G.	1986
Preterm	Videotape	17 minutes		Driscoll, J.W., & Lawhon, G.	1986
Preterm	Booklet	28 pages	Spanish	Gotsch, G.	1990
Preterm	Pamphlet	Multifold		Health Education Associates	1992
Preterm	Pamphlet	Multifold		Health Education Associates	Not listed
Preterm	Book	222 pages		Ludington-Hoe, S.M.	1993
Preterm	Videotape	18 minutes		Northwestern Memorial Hospital	1995
Preterm	Pamphlet	16 pages		Walker, M.	1998

Title	Publisher	Available From	Price
The Special Touch Babies Need: Caring for the Infant with Cleft Lip/Palate	Children's Mercy Hospital	Children's Mercy Hospital	$45
Samuel: Breastfed Infants With Cleft Lip and Cleft Palate	Medela	Medela	$46
Feeding an Infant With a Cleft	Cleft Palate Foundation	Cleft Palate Foundation	Not listed
Nursing Your Baby With Cleft Palate or Cleft Lip	Childbirth Graphics	Childbirth Graphics	$2 each; quantity discounts available
Give Us a Little Time	Medela	Medela	$1.50
Breastfeeding the Baby With Down Syndrome	La Leche League International	La Leche League International	$1.50
Breastfeeding Your Baby With Down Syndrome	Childbirth Graphics	Childbirth Graphics	$2 for single copy; quantity discounts available
Nursing Your Neurologically Impaired Baby	Childbirth Graphics	Childbirth Graphics	$2 for single copy; quantity discounts available
Breastfeeding the Preterm Infant: A Positive Approach	Egnell-Ameda (U.K.)	Ameda-Egnell/Hollister	$26.50
Breastfeeding Your Premature Baby	Childbirth Graphics	Childbirth Graphics	$2 for single copy; quantity discounts available
Breastfeeding the Premature Infant: Part I: Initiating and Maintaining Milk Supply	PGG Associates	Care Video Productions	Series of 3; $45 to rent each tape (or $120 to rent series) or purchase one tape for $150 or purchase all three for $350
Breastfeeding the Premature Infant: Part II: Initiating Breastfeeding in the Hospital Nursery	PGG Associates	Care Video Productions	Series of 3; $45 to rent each tape (or $120 to rent series) or purchase one tape for $150 or purchase all three for $350
Breastfeeding the Premature Infant: Part III: Discharge Planning and Breastfeeding at Home	PGG Associates	Care Video Productions	Series of 3; $45 to rent each tape (or $120 to rent series) or purchase one tape for $150 or purchase all three for $350
Breastfeeding Your Premature Baby	La Leche League	LLLI, Birth & Life Bookstore	Not listed
Breastfeeding Your Premie	Health Education Associates	Health Education Associates	$.50 ≤ 24; quantity discounts available
Your Premie Needs You	Health Education Associates	Health Education Associates	$.50 ≤ 24; quantity discounts available
Kangaroo Care: The Best You Can Do to Help Your Preterm Infant	Bantam Publishing Group	Bookstores	$11
Kangaroo Care: A Parent's Touch	Northwestern Memorial Hospital	Northwestern Memorial Hospital	$65
Breastfeeding Your Premature or Special Care Baby	Lactation Associates	Lactation Associates	$5.50; quantity discounts available

B-5 Introducing Supplements and Facilitating Indirect Breastfeeding During Separation Periods

These audio, visual, and audiovisual materials are designed to help mothers successfully breastfeed even in situations where they are separated from their newborns, or where supplementation is required. The word *expression* is listed as a key word, but it includes pumps and pumping. Prices are approximate and subject to change, and most do not include shipping and handling.

Key Word	Media	Length	Additional Languages	Author	Date
Cup feeding	Videotape	10 minutes		Lang, S.	1995
Employment	Book	160 pages		Grams, M.	1985
Employment	Book	256 pages		Mason, D.J., & Ingersoll, D.	1986
Employment	Pamphlet	4 pages		Walker, M.	1994
Employment	Pamphlet	7 pages		La Leche League International	1991
Employment	Pamphlet	8 pages		Bocar, D.	1997
Employment	Pamphlet	13 pages		HMHB Breastfeeding Promotion Committee	1997
Employment	Book (soft cover)	208 pages		Pryor, G.	1997
Employment	Pamphlet	Multifold		Health Education Associates	Not listed
Employment	Pamphlet	Multifold (8)		Bocar, D.	1992
Employment	Videotape	17 minutes	Spanish	Texas WIC	1994
Employment	Videotape	56 minutes		Frantz, K.	1988
Expression	Pamphlet	4 pages	Spanish	Marmet, C.	1988
Expression	Pamphlet	6 pages		Walker, M.	1992
Expression	Pamphlet	12 pages		Bernshaw, N.	1991
Expression	Pamphlet	Multifold		Health Education Associates	Not listed
Expression	Pamphlet	12 pages		Danner, S.C.	1997

Title	Publisher	Available From	Price
The Baby Feeding Cup	Ameda-Egnell	Ameda-Egnell/Hollister	$14.75
Breastfeeding Success for Working Mothers	Achievement Press	Bookstores	$15
Breastfeeding and the Working Mother: The Complete Guide for Today's Nursing Mother	St. Martin's Press	Bookstores	$12
Working and Nursing	Lactation Associates	Lactation Associates	Single copy $0.60; $30 for 100 copies
Practical Hints for Working and Breastfeeding	La Leche League International	La Leche League International	$.75
Combining Breastfeeding and Employment: A Planning Checklist	Lactation Consultant Services	Lactation Consultant Services	Special pricing
Working and Breastfeeding	Healthy Mothers Healthy Babies	Healthy Mothers Healthy Babies and Best Start	Single pamphlet free; 51 cents in bulk
Nursing Mother, Working Mother: The Essential Guide for Breastfeeding and Staying Close to Your Baby After You Return to Work	Harvard Common Press	Bookstores	$10.50
Time Out for Breastfeeding Mothers	Health Education Associates	Health Education Associates	$.50 ≤ 24; quantity discounts available
Engorgement	Lactation Consultant Services	Lactation Consultant Services	Special pricing
Breastfeeding and Working: It's Worth the Effort	Texas WIC	Tele-Print Express	$4
Breastfeeding Techniques That Work! Volume 5: Successful Working Mothers	Geddes Productions	Geddes Productions	$39.95
Manual Expression of Breast Milk: Marmet Technique	Lactation Institute	Lactation Institute	$1
Expressing, Storing, and Transporting Breastmilk	Lactation Associates	Lactation Associates	$35/100 copies
A Mother's Guide to Milk Expression and Breast Pumps	La Leche League International	La Leche League International	$.95
When Your Baby Needs Your Milk	Health Education Associates	Health Education Associates	$.50 ≤ 24; quantity discounts available
Expressing Breastmilk	Childbirth Graphics	Childbirth Graphics	$.82 each; quantity discounts available

Continued

Key Word	Media	Length	Additional Languages	Author	Date
Expression	Videotape	18 minutes	Spanish	Frantz, K.	1988
Expression, pumping	Videotape		Spanish, French	Medela	Not listed
Expression, pumping	Videotape		Spanish, French	Medela	Not listed
Expression, pumping	Videotape	16 minutes	Spanish, French	Medela	Not listed
Options	Pamphlet	Multifold		Health Education Associates	Not listed
Supplemental nurser	Videotape	23 minutes	Spanish	Frantz, K.	1989
Supplementation	Pamphlet	Multifold		Health Education Associates	Not listed

B-6 Other Problems and Related Resources

Media for other problems are listed here.

Topic	Media	Length	Additional Languages	Author	Date
Massage	Videotape	15 minutes		Guyer, E.	1992
Fussy baby	Book	192 pages		Sears, W.	1989
Bonding	Book	272 pages		Klaus P.H., Klaus, M.H., & Kennel, J.H.	1995

Title	Publisher	Available From	Price
Breastfeeding Techniques That Work! Volume 6: Hand Expression	Geddes Productions	Geddes Productions	$39.95
Lactina Instructional Video	Medela	Medela	$7.00
Spring Express Instructional Video	Medela	Medela	$7.00
Classic Instructional Video	Medela	Medela	$7.00
Time Out for Breastfeeding Mothers	Health Education Associates	Health Education Associates	$.50 ≤ 24; quantity discounts available
Breastfeeding Techniques That Work! Volume 7: Supplemental Nursing System	Geddes Productions	Geddes Productions	$39.95
Combining Breast and Bottle Feeding	Health Education Associates	Health Education Associates	$.50 ≤ 24; quantity discounts available

Title	Publisher	Available From	Price
Heart to Heart Baby Massage	Gentle Touch	Gentle Touch	$50
The Fussy Baby	LLLI	LLLI, Bookstores	$5
Bonding: Building the Foundations of Secure Attachment and Independence	Addison Wesley	Bookstores	$22

B-7 Media Critique

It is difficult, if not impossible, to find a video-tape, pamphlet, or book that is ideal for all parents. Furthermore, several people, rather than one individual, usually choose the patient education media to be stocked in the hospital or clinic.

The following template is a useful tool for each member of the interdisciplinary team to note the media's pertinent criteria. If each member of the group looks for each point listed below, a lively discussion afterward can help the group to determine which media should be stocked.

Title

BACKGROUND

Produced by:

Compliments of:

Intended audience:

Length of media:

Content expert:

PURPOSE OF MEDIA:

CONTENT:

CRITIQUE OF MEDIA:

> Rating Scale:
> 0 = totally unacceptable
> 1 = acceptable, but needing modification
> 2 = generally acceptable
> 3 = superb

Purpose fits needs of intended audience

Conservative and realistic

Appropriate for our population: terminology, cultural aspect, etc.

Tone/approach

Pictures

Organization

Content relevant

Content complete

Content accurate

Explanations clear

Overall rating of this media

Is purpose of media evident to clinician?

What is greatest strength of this media?

What is greatest weakness of this media?

Price:

Other comments

APPENDIX C
Professional Development and Support

*T*his appendix seeks to provide a starting point for professionals who wish to find material and human resources to support breastfeeding.

C-1 Organizations and Associations

Listed below are organizations whose main mission is to assist health care professionals. All attempts have been made to provide the latest contact information.

AFRICAN MEDICAL AND RESEARCH FOUNDATION
PO Box 30125
Nairobi, Kenya
(254) 2-501301
FAX: (254) 2-609518
www.amref.org
amrefhq@users.africaonline.co.ke

AMERICAN ACADEMY OF FAMILY PHYSICIANS
8880 Ward Parkway
Kansas City, MO 64114-2797
(816) 333-9700
www.aafp.org
fp@aafp.org

AMERICAN ACADEMY OF PEDIATRICS
141 Northwest Point Boulevard
Elk Grove Village, IL 60007-1098
(847) 228-5005
FAX: (847) 228-5097
www.aap.org
kidsdoc@aap.org

AMERICAN CLEFT PALATE—CRANIOFACIAL
ASSOCIATION
1829 Franklin Street, Suite 1022
Chapel Hill, NC 27514
800-24-CLEFT
(919) 933-9044
FAX: (919) 933-9604
www.cleft.com
cleftline@aol.com

AMERICAN COLLEGE OF NURSE-MIDWIVES
818 Connecticut Avenue NW, Suite 900
Washington, DC 20006
(202) 728-9860
FAX: (202) 728-9897
www.acnm.org
info@acnm.org

AMERICAN COLLEGE OF OBSTETRICIANS AND
GYNECOLOGISTS
409 12th Street SW
PO Box 96920
Washington, DC 20090-6920
(800) 762-2264
(202) 554-3490
FAX: (202) 554-3490
www.acog.org

AMERICAN DIETETIC ASSOCIATION
216 West Jackson Boulevard
Chicago, IL 60606-6995
(800) 745-0775
(312) 899-0040
FAX: (312) 899-1979
www.eatright.org

ASSOCIATION OF WOMEN'S HEALTH, OBSTETRIC
   & NEONATAL NURSES
2000 L Street NW
Suite 740
Washington, DC 20036
(800) 673-8499
(800) 245-0231 (in Canada)
(202) 261-2400
FAX: (202) 728-0575
www.awhonn.org

BEST START SOCIAL MARKETING
3500 East Fletcher Avenue #519
Tampa, FL 33613-4708
(800) 277-4975
(813) 971-2119
FAX: (813) 971-2280
beststart@mindspring.com

BRITISH COLUMBIA BREASTFEEDING SOCIETY
9131 Evancio Crescent
Richmond, BC V7E 5J2 CANADA

BRITISH DIETETIC ASSOCIATION
Elizabeth House
22 Suffolk Street Queensway
Birmingham, B1 1LS ENGLAND
0121-643-5483
FAX: 0121 633 4399
bda@dial.pipex.com
www.vois.org.uk/bda

BRITISH PAEDIATRIC ASSOCIATION
5 St. Andrews Place
Regents Park
London, NW1 4LB
0181-441-2269
www.rcpch.ac.uk/paediatrics

DIETITIANS OF CANADA
480 University Avenue, Suite 604
Toronto, ONTARIO M5G 1V2 CANADA
(416) 596-0857
FAX: (416) 596-0603
www.dietitians.ca

HEALTHY MOTHERS HEALTHY BABIES
121 North Washington Street
Suite 300
Alexandria, VA 22314
(703) 836-6110
FAX: (703) 836-3470
www.hmhb.org
webmaster@hmhb.org

HUMAN MILK BANKING ASSOCIATION OF NORTH
   AMERICA
8 Jan Sebastian Way #13
Sandwich, MA 02563
(508) 888-4141
milkbank@capecod.net

INFACT CANADA
6 Trinity Square
Toronto, CANADA M5G 1B1
(416) 595-9819
FAX: (416) 591-9355
www.infactcanada.ca
infact@ftn.net

INSTITUTE FOR REPRODUCTIVE HEALTH
2115 Wisconsin Avenue NW
Washington, DC 20007
(202) 687-1392
FAX: (202) 687-6846

INTERNATIONAL CHILDBIRTH EDUCATION
   ASSOCIATION
PO Box 20048
Minneapolis, MN 55420
(612) 854-8660
FAX: (612) 854-8772
www.icea.org
info@icea.org

INTERNATIONAL CONFEDERATION OF MIDWIVES
10 Barley Mow Passage
Chiswick
GB-London W4 4PH ENGLAND
+44-181-994-6477
FAX: +44-181-995-1332

INTERNATIONAL FEDERATION OF GYNECOLOGY AND
    OBSTETRICS
27 Sussex Place
Regent's Park
GB-London, NW1 4RG ENGLAND
+44-171-723-2951
FAX: +44-171-258-0737

INTERNATIONAL PEDIATRIC ASSOCIATION
601 Elmwood Avenue
URMC Box 777
Rochester, NY 14642
(716) 275-0225
FAX: (716) 273-1038

INTERNATIONAL LACTATION CONSULTANT
    ASSOCIATION
4101 Lake Boone Trail
Raleigh, NC 27607
(919) 787-5181
FAX: (919) 787-4916
www.ilca.org
ilca@erols.com

INTERNATIONAL SOCIETY FOR RESEARCH ON
    HUMAN MILK AND LACTATION
URMC Box 777
601 Elmwood Avenue
Rochester, NY 14642
(716) 275-4354

LACTATION STUDY CENTER
URMC Box 777
601 Elmwood Avenue
Rochester, NY 14642
(716) 275-0088
FAX: (716) 461-3614

LACTATION SUPPORT SERVICE
British Columbia Children's Hospital
4480 Oak
Vancouver, BC CANADA
(604) 875-2345 ext. 7607

LAMAZE INTERNATIONAL
1200 19th Street NW, Suite 300
Washington, DC 20036-2422
(202) 857-1128
(800) 368-4404
FAX: (202) 223-4579
www.lamaze-childbirth.com
lamaze@dc.sba.com

MARCH OF DIMES BIRTH DEFECTS FOUNDATION
1275 Mamaroneck Avenue
White Plains, NY 10605
800-367-6630
(717) 820-8104
FAX: (717) 825-1987
www.modimes.org
ProfEd@modimes.org

NATIONAL ALLIANCE FOR BREASTFEEDING
    ADVOCACY (NABA)
9684 Oak Hill Drive
Ellicott City, MD 21042-6321
(410) 995-3726
FAX: (410) 992-1977

NATIONAL ALLIANCE FOR BREASTFEEDING
    ADVOCACY RESEARCH EDUCATION AND LEGAL
    FUND (NABA REAL)
254 Conant Road
Weston, MA 02493-1756
(781) 893-3553
FAX: (781) 893-8608

NATIONAL ASSOCIATION OF CHILDBEARING
    CENTERS
3123 Gottschall Road
Perkiomenville, PA 18074
(215) 234-8068
FAX: (215) 234-8829
birthctr@midwives.org

NATIONAL ASSOCIATION OF WIC DIRECTORS
2001 S Street, NW, Suite 580
PO Box 53355
Washington, DC 20009-3355
(202) 232-5492
FAX: (202) 387-5281

NATIONAL DOWN SYNDROME SOCIETY
666 Broadway, 8th Floor
New York, NY 10012-2317
(212) 460-9330
(800) 221-4602
FAX: (212) 979-2873
www.ndss.org

NATIONAL PERINATAL ASSOCIATION
3500 E. Fletcher Avenue, Suite 209
Tampa, FL 33613-4712
(813) 971-1008
FAX: (813) 971-9306
www.nationalperinatal.org
npaonline@aol.com

ROYAL COLLEGE OF MIDWIVES
15 Mansfield Street
London W1M OBE ENGLAND
0171-872-5100
FAX: 0171-872-5101

ROYAL COLLEGE OF OBSTETRICIANS AND
   GYNAECOLOGISTS
27 Sussex Place
Regent's Park
London NW1 4RG ENGLAND
+44 (0) 171-772-6200
FAX: +44 (0) 171-723-0575
www.rcog.org.uk

UNICEF
Nutrition Section, TA 24 A
3 United Nations Plaza
New York, NY 10017
(212) 326-7000
FAX: (212) 888-7465
www.unicef.org
netmaster@unicef.org

UNITED STATES NATIONAL BREASTFEEDING
   COMMITTEE
(no address at press time)
www.wmc-worldwide.com/usnbc
usnbc-info@wmc-worldwide.com

U.S. COMMITTEE FOR UNICEF
333 E. 38th Street
New York, NY 10016
(800) 367-5437
www.unicefusa.org

WELLSTART INTERNATIONAL
4062 First Avenue
San Diego, CA 92103-2045
(619) 295-5192
FAX: (619) 574-8159
inquiry@wellstart.org

WORLD ALLIANCE FOR BREASTFEEDING ADVOCACY
PO Box 1200
10890 Penang MALAYSIA
+60-4-884816
FAX: +604-872655

WORLD HEALTH ORGANIZATION (WHO)
20 Av. Appia
1211 Geneva 27, SWITZERLAND
+41-22 791 21 11
FAX: +41-22 791 0746
www.who.ch
info@who.ch

C-2 Suggested Library for Professionals

References that may be helpful for those involved in breastfeeding management are listed below. This list is not meant to be all-inclusive and is not meant to endorse any product. Rather, it has been compiled to identify media that the author or her colleagues have found helpful in clinical practice. All videotapes are in NTSC format; additional formats may be available. Prices are approximate, and most do not include ship-

Videotapes/Pamphlets/Booklets

Key Word/ Target Population	Media	Length	Additional Languages	Author	Date
Advantages	Videotape	15 minutes		Georgetown University Institute for Reproductive Health	1993
Ankylglossia	Videotape	20 minutes		Jain, E.	1996
Attachment, positioning	Videotape	14 minutes	Spanish	Frantz, K.	1986
Attachment, positioning	Videotape	15 minutes		Frantz, K.	1986
Attachment, positioning	Videotape	20 minutes		Royal College of Midwives/ Fisher, C.	1990
Baby-Friendly	Videotape	33 minutes		U.S. Committee for UNICEF	1994
Burping	Videotape	18 minutes	Spanish	Frantz, K.	1986
Cesarean	Videotape	26 minutes		Frantz, K.	1986
Cleft	Booklet	31 pages	French	Herzog-Isler, C., & Honigmann, K.	1996
Counseling	Videotape	20 minutes		Fisher, C.	1994
Counseling	Videotape/ manual	8 minutes		Best Start	1997
Cup feeding	Videotape	10 minutes		Lang, S.	1995
Early discharge	Videotape	30 minutes		Royal College of Midwives/ Fisher, C.	1996
Early initiation	Videotape	6 minutes		Righard, L.	1992
Employment	Videotape	56 minutes		Frantz, K.	1988

ping and handling charges. Many items are available from other vendors than those listed; only vendors in the United States are listed here. The author welcomes suggestions about other places where these materials may be easily obtained.

Readers or vendors may send comments to bookcomments@wmc-worldwide.com. Contact information for vendors is listed in Appendix E. Prices are approximate and subject to change, and most do not include shipping and handling.

Title	Publisher	Available From	Price
Breastfeeding: Protecting a Natural Resource	Georgetown University Institute for Reproductive Health	Academy for Educational Development	$20
Tongue-Tie: Impact on Breastfeeding		Ameda-Egnell/Hollister	$60
Breastfeeding Techniques That Work! Volume 1: First Attachment	Geddes Productions	Geddes Productions	$39.95
Breastfeeding Techniques That Work! Volume 2: First Attachment in Bed	Geddes Productions	Geddes Productions	$39.95
Helping a Mother Breastfeed: No Finer Investment	London Healthcare	Childbirth Graphics	$46.95
Learning to Be Baby Friendly: One Hospital's Experience	U.S. Committee for UNICEF	Baby-Friendly U.S.A.	$13
Breastfeeding Techniques That Work! Volume 4: Burping the Baby	Geddes Productions	Geddes Productions	$39.95
Breastfeeding Techniques That Work! Volume 3: First Attachment After a Cesarean	Geddes Productions	Geddes Productions	$39.95
Give Us a Little Time	Medela	Medela (U.S. and Switzerland)	$1.50
She Needs You—Chloe Fisher at the Swedish Breastfeeding Institute	Swedish Breastfeeding Institute	Health Education Associates	$39.95 includes shipping
Best Start Training Program (includes What Difference Does It Make) and a new training manual	Best Start	Best Start	$72, includes manual and guide
The Baby Feeding Cup	Ameda-Egnell	Ameda-Egnell/Hollister	$14.75
Breastfeeding: Coping With the First Week	Royal College of Midwives	Growing With Baby	$80
Delivery Self Attachment	Geddes Productions	Geddes Productions, Childbirth Graphics	$14.95
Breastfeeding Techniques That Work! Volume 5: Successful Working Mothers	Geddes Productions	Geddes Productions	$39.95

Continued

Videotapes/Pamphlets/Booklets—cont'd

Key Word/ Target Population	Media	Length	Additional Languages	Author	Date
Employment	Pamphlet	4 pages		HMHB Breastfeeding Promotion Committee	1993
Expression, hand	Videotape	18 minutes	Spanish	Frantz, K.	1988
General	Videotape		Spanish, French	UNICEF	
General	Book	272 pages		Klaus, P.H., Klaus, M.H., Kennel, J.H.	1995
Hospital routines	CAI module	2 hours		Page-Goertz, S., & McCamman, S.	1996
How-to	Videotape	75 minutes	Spanish, Cantonese, Mandarin	Livingstone, V.	1994
How-to	Videotape	25 minutes		Frantz, K.	1996
How-to	Videotape	35 minutes	Spanish, French	Nylander, G.	1994
How-to	Videotape	40 minutes		McElaney, L.	1998
Hyperbilirubinemia	CAI module	90 minutes		Page-Goertz, S., & McCamman, S.	1996
Lactational amenorrhea	Videotape	26 minutes		Georgetown Institute for Reproductive Health	1996
Nipple trauma	CAI module	2 hours		Page-Goertz, S., & McCamman, S.	1996
Preterm	Videotape	14 minutes	Spanish	UNICEF	Not listed
Preterm	Videotape	29 minutes	Spanish, French	UNICEF	Not listed
Sore breasts, nipples	Videotape	24 minutes		Royal College of Midwives/ Fisher, C. & Inch, S.	1997
States of consciousness	Videotape	10 minutes		Danner, S.	1994
States of consciousness	Videotape	25 minutes			1991
Supplemental nurser	Videotape	23 minutes	Spanish	Frantz, K.	1989
Telephone	Booklet	116 pages		Jolley, S.	1996
WIC	Videotape	17 minutes		Texas WIC	1990

Title	Publisher	Available From	Price
What Gives These Companies a Competitive Edge: Worksite Support for Breastfeeding Employees	Healthy Mothers Healthy Babies	Healthy Mothers Healthy Babies	Free
Breastfeeding Techniques That Work! Volume 6: Hand Expression	Geddes Productions	Geddes Productions	$39.95
Breastfeeding: A Global Priority	UNICEF	UNICEF	Special pricing
Bonding: Building the Foundations of Secure Attachment and Independence	Addison Wesley	Bookstores	
Breastfeeding Management Series: Creating Breastfeeding Friendly Environments	Best Beginnings Productions	TENSOR	$200
The Art of Successful Breastfeeding (4 chapters)	University of British Columbia	Vancouver Breastfeeding Centre	$20 for home use; $130 for institutions
Breastfeeding Techniques That Work! Volume 8: The First Week	Geddes Productions	Geddes Productions	$39.95
Breast is Best	Norwegian Health Institute	INFACT Canada	$55
Breastfeeding: The Why-to, How-to, Can-do Videos Part II: How-to	Vida Health Communications	Vida Health Communications	To be determined
Breastfeeding Management Series: Hyperbilirubinemia in the Breastfeeding Infant	Best Beginnings Productions	TENSOR	$125
Taking the First Steps: The Lactational Amenorrhea Method for Family Planning	Georgetown University	Academy for Educational Development	$20
Breastfeeding Management Series: Nipple Trauma	Best Beginnings Productions	TENSOR	$150
Mother Kangaroo, a Light of Hope	UNICEF	UNICEF	Special pricing
Feeding Low Birth Weight Babies	UNICEF	UNICEF	Special pricing
Breastfeeding: Dealing With the Problems	Mark-it Television	Growing With Baby, Childbirth Graphics	$50-60
Baby Talk	State University of NY at Stonybrook	State University of NY at Stonybrook	$20
Early Parent-Infant Relationships	March of Dimes	March of Dimes	Not listed
Breastfeeding Techniques That Work! Volume 7: Supplemental Nursing System	Geddes Productions	Geddes Productions	$39.95
Breastfeeding Triage Tool (3rd edition)	Seattle-King County Department of Public Health	Childbirth Graphics	$10
Breastfeeding: You Can Make the Difference	Texas WIC	Tele-Print Express	

Books and Other Hard Copy

American Academy of Pediatrics and the American College of Obstetricians and Gynecologists. *Guidelines for Perinatal Care*. 4th ed. Elk Grove Village, IL: American Academy of Pediatrics, 1997.

Biancuzzo M. *Breastfeeding the Healthy Newborn: A Nursing Perspective*. White Plains, NY: March of Dimes Birth Defects Foundation; 1994. Revised edition forthcoming.

Briggs GG, Freeman RK, Yaffe SJ. *Drugs in Pregnancy and Lactation*. 5th ed. Baltimore: Williams & Wilkins; 1998.

Committee on Nutrition, American Academy of Pediatrics. *Pediatric Nutrition Handbook*. 4th ed. Elk Grove Village, IL: American Academy of Pediatrics; 1998.

Dowling D, Danner SC, Coffey P. *Breastfeeding the Infant With Special Needs*. White Plains, NY: March of Dimes Birth Defects Foundation; 1997.

Enkin M, Keirse JNC, Renfrew M, Neilson J, eds. *Guide to Effective Care in Pregnancy and Childbirth*. 2nd ed. Cary, NC: Oxford University Press; 1995.

Foman SJ. *Nutrition of Normal Infants*. St. Louis: Mosby; 1993.

Frantz K. *Breastfeeding Product Guide 1994*. Sunland, CA: Geddes Productions; 1993.

Goldman AS, Atkinson SA, Hanson LA. *Human Lactation 3. The Effects of Human Milk on the Recipient Infants*. New York: Plenum Press; 1987.

Hale T. *Medications and Mother's Milk*. 7th ed. Amarillo, TX: Pharmasoft Publishing; 1998.

Hamosh M, Goldman AS. *Human Lactation 2. Maternal and Environmental Factors*. New York: Plenum Press; 1986.

Henschel D. *Breastfeeding: A Guide for Midwives*. Cheshire, England: Books for Midwives Press; 1996. (Available from Butterworth-Heinemann.)

Institute of Medicine. *Nutrition During Lactation*. Washington, DC: National Academy Press; 1991.

Jensen RG, ed. *Handbook of Milk Composition*. San Diego: Academic Press; 1995.

Jensen RG, Neville MC. *Human Lactation: Milk Components and Methodologies*. New York: Plenum Press; 1985.

Labbok M, Cooney C, Coly S. *Guidelines: Breastfeeding, Family Planning and the Lactational Amenorrhea Method—LAM*. Washington, DC: Georgetown University Institute for Reproductive Health; 1994. (Available from Academy for Educational Development.)

La Leche League International. *The Womanly Art of Breastfeeding*. 6th ed. Schaumburg, IL: La Leche League International; 1997.

Lauwers J, Woessner C. *Counseling the Nursing Mother*. 2nd ed. Chalfont, PA: Breastfeeding Support Consultants; 1990.

Lawrence RA, Bryant C, Quint-Adler L. *Breastfeeding Care: Setting the Environment, Supporting the Process*. White Plains, NY: March of Dimes; 1994.

Lawrence RA. The management of lactation as a physiologic process. *Clin Perinatol* 1987;14:1-10. Use library; out of print.

Lawrence RA. *Breastfeeding: A Guide for the Medical Profession*. 5th ed. St. Louis: Mosby; 1999.

Lawrence RA. *A Review of the Medical Benefits and Contraindications to Breastfeeding in the United States (Maternal and Child Health Technical Information Bulletin)*. Arlington, VA: National Center for Education in Maternal and Child Health; 1997. (Available from National Maternal and Child Health Clearinghouse.)

Minchin MK. *Breastfeeding Matters*. Sydney, Australia: Alma Publications; 1989.

Mohrbacher N, Stock J. *The Breastfeeding Answer Book*. 2nd ed. Schaumburg, IL: La Leche League International; 1996.

Neville MC, Neifert MR. *Lactation: Physiology, Nutrition and Breast-feeding*. New York: Plenum Press; 1983.

Newton N. *Newton on Breastfeeding*. Seattle: Birth & Life Bookstore; 1987.

Palmer G. *The Politics of Breastfeeding*. London: Pandora; 1988.

Parenteau-Carreau S, Cooney KA. *Breastfeeding, Lactational Amenorrhea Method and Natural Family Planning Interface: Teaching Guide*. Washington, DC: Georgetown University Institute for Reproductive Health; 1994. (Available from Academy for Educational Development.)

Riordan J, Auerbach K. *Breastfeeding and Human Lactation* 2nd ed. Boston: Jones and Bartlett; 1998.

Savage-King F. *Helping Mothers to Breastfeed*. Nairobi, Kenya: African Medical and Research Foundation; 1992.

Sokol, EJ. *The Code Handbook: A Guide to Implementing the International Code of Marketing of Breastmilk Substitutes*. Penang (Malaysia): IBFAN; 1997

Spisak S, Gross SS. *Second Followup Report: The Surgeon General's Workshop on Breastfeeding and Human Lactation*. Washington, DC: National Center for Education in Maternal and Child Health; 1991. (Available from National Maternal and Child Health Clearinghouse.)

Stuart-Macadam P, Dettwyler KA. *Breastfeeding: Biocultural Perspectives*. Hawthorne, NY: Aldine de Gruyter; 1995.

Tsang RC, Nichols BL. *Nutrition During Infancy*. Philadelphia: Hanley and Belfus; 1988.

United States Department of Health and Human Services. *Report of the Surgeon General's Workshop on Breastfeeding and Human Lactation*. Rockville, MD: Health Resources and Services Administration; 1984. (Available from National Maternal and Child Health Clearinghouse.)

WHO and UNICEF. *Innocenti Declaration: 30 July to 1 Aug, 1990, Florence, Italy*. Geneva: Author; 1990.

UNICEF and WHO. *Breastfeeding Management and Promotion in a Baby-Friendly Hospital: An 18-Hour Course for Maternity Staff*. New York: UNICEF; 1993.

World Health Organization. *International Code of Marketing of Breast-Milk Substitutes*. Geneva: World Health Organization; 1981.

World Health Organization. *A Common Review and Evaluation Framework*. Geneva: World Health Organization; 1996.

World Health Organization. *Hypoglycemia of the Newborn: Review of the Literature*. Geneva: World Health Organization; 1997.

Worthington-Roberts B, Williams SR. *Nutrition in Pregnancy and Lactation*. Madison, WI: Brown Benchmark; 1997. (Available from McGraw-Hill.)

C-3 Sources of Continuing Education for Professionals

Multiple sources exist for continuing education in the United States. Sources listed below are those with which the author has had direct contact, which offer continuing education on a regular basis, and have been offering continuing education to professionals for more than 10 years.

AMERICAN DIETETIC ASSOCIATION
216 West Jackson Boulevard
Chicago, IL 60606-6995
(800) 745-0775
FAX: (312) 899-1979
www.eatright.org

MARIE BIANCUZZO
PO Box 387
Herndon, VA 20172
(703) 758-0092
FAX: (703) 758-0891
www.wmc-worldwide.com
marie@wmc-worldwide.com

BREASTFEEDING SUPPORT CONSULTANTS
228 Park Lane
Chalfont, PA 18914-3135
(215) 822-1281
FAX: (215) 997-7879
www.bsccenter.org
info@bsccenter.org

GEDDES PRODUCTIONS
10546 McVine
Sunland, CA 91040
(818) 951-2809
FAX: (213) 257-7209
www.geddespro.com

HEALTHY CHILDREN PROJECT
8 Jan Sebastian Way #13
Sandwich, MA 02563
(508) 888-8044
FAX: (508) 888-8050
www.aboutus.com/a100/hc2000
hea@capecod.net

INTERNATIONAL BOARD OF LACTATION
    CONSULTANT EXAMINERS
PO Box 2348
Falls Church, VA 22042-0348
(703) 560-7330
FAX: (703) 560-7332
www.iblce.org
iblce@erols.com
(Offers recognition, not courses)

LA LECHE LEAGUE INTERNATIONAL
PO Box 4079
Schaumburg, IL 60168-4079
(847) 519-7730
(800) LALECHE
FAX: (847) 519-0035
www.lalecheleague.org

LACTATION ASSOCIATES
254 Conant Road
Weston, MA 02493-1756
(781) 893-3553
FAX: (781) 893-8608
marshalact@aol.com

LACTATION CONSULTANT SERVICES
11320 Shady Glen Road
Oklahoma City, OK 73162
(405) 722-2163
FAX: (405) 722-2197
dbocar@aol.com

LACTATION EDUCATION RESOURCES
4339 Montgomery Avenue
Bethesda MD 20814
(301) 986-5546
FAX: (301) 986-0441
www.LERon-line.com
vergieh@ix.netcom.com

LACTATION INSTITUTE
16430 Ventura Boulevard
Suite 303
Encino, CA 91436
(818) 995-1913
marmet@beachnet.com

MARCH OF DIMES BIRTH DEFECTS FOUNDATION
1275 Mamaroneck Avenue
White Plains, NY 10605
(800) 367-6630
(717) 820-8104
FAX: (717) 825-1987
www.modimes.org
ProfEd@modimes.org

WELLSTART INTERNATIONAL
4062 First Avenue
San Diego, CA 92103-2045
(619) 295-5192
FAX: (619) 574-8159
inquiry@wellstart.org

Breastfeeding Protection and Promotion

$\mathcal{T}$his appendix gives a broad overview of political, legislative, and regulatory actions that have promoted breastfeeding.

D-1 International Code of Marketing of Breast-Milk Substitutes: Summary of Provisions

The International Code of Marketing was developed in 1981 by the World Health Organization. The United States endorsed the principles of this International Code in 1994 but has not fully embraced the Code; for example, artificial milk companies continue to advertise to U.S. consumers in clear violation of article 5. The Code is an essential part of the Baby-Friendly™ Hospital Initiative and a summary of its provisions follows. The Code in its entirety can be purchased from the World Health Organization (see Appendix C-1 for address).

International Code of Marketing of Breast-Milk Substitutes (1981)

Summary of Provisions

ARTICLE 1: AIM OF THE CODE The aim of this code is to contribute to the provision of safe and adequate nutrition for infants by the protection and promotion of breast-feeding, and by ensuring the proper use of breast-milk substitutes, when these are necessary, on the basis of adequate information and through appropriate marketing and distribution.

ARTICLE 2: SCOPE OF THE CODE The Code applies to the marketing, and practices related thereto, of the following products: breast-milk substitutes, including infant formula, other milk products, food, and beverages, including bottle-fed complementary foods, when marketed or otherwise represented to be suitable, with or without modification, for use as a partial or total replacement of breast-milk, feeding bottles and teats. It also applies to their quality and availability, and to information concerning their use.

ARTICLE 3: DEFINITIONS The Code defines the terms *breast-milk substitute*, *complementary food*, *container*, *distributor*, *health care system*, *health worker*, *infant formula*, *label*, *manufacturer*, *marketing*, *marketing personnel*, *samples*, and *supplies*. The distinction between samples and supplies of infant formula is especially relevant to hospital policies, because the Code recommends that the former not be distributed, whereas the latter may be donated or sold at low-cost to an institution or organization for social purposes (e.g., families in need) if they are not used as a sales inducement. These supplies should be given only to infants who have to be fed a breast-milk substitute, and should be continued for as long as they are medically indicated.

ARTICLE 4: INFORMATION AND EDUCATION FOR THE PURPOSES OF THE CODE Governments should have the responsibility to ensure that objective and consistent information is provided on infant and young child feeding for use by families and those involved in the field of infant and young child nutrition. This responsibility should cover either the planning, provision, design and dissemination of information, or their control.

ARTICLE 5: THE GENERAL PUBLIC AND MOTHERS There should be no advertising or other form of promotion to the general public of products within the scope of this Code. Manufacturers and distributors should not provide, directly or indirectly, to pregnant women, mothers or members of their families, samples of products within the scope of this Code.

ARTICLE 6: HEALTH CARE SYSTEMS No facility of a health care system should be used for the purpose of promoting infant formula or other products within the scope of this Code.

ARTICLE 7: HEALTH WORKERS Health workers should encourage and protect breastfeeding. Information provided by manufacturers and distributors to health professionals regarding products should be restricted to scientific and factual matters. No financial or material inducements to promote products should be offered by manufacturers or distributors to health workers or members of their families, nor should these be accepted by health care workers. Samples of infant formula and other products or of equipment or utensils for their preparation or use should not be provided to health workers except when necessary for the purpose of professional evaluation or research at the institutional level.

ARTICLE 8: PERSONS EMPLOYED BY MANUFACTURERS AND DISTRIBUTORS The volume of sales of products within the scope of this Code should not be included in the calculation of bonuses, nor should quotas be set specifically for sales of these products. Personnel employed in marketing products should not perform educational functions in relation to pregnant women or mothers.

ARTICLE 9: LABELING Labels should be designed to provide the necessary information about the appropriate use of the product, and so as not to discourage breastfeeding.

ARTICLE 10: QUALITY Quality of products is an essential element for the protection of the health of infants and therefore should be of a high recognized standard. Food products should meet applicable standards recommended by the Codex Alimentarius Commission.

ARTICLE 11: IMPLEMENTATION AND MONITORING Governments should take action to give effect to the principles and aim of this Code, as appropriate to their social and legislative framework, including the adoption of national legislation, regulations or other suitable measures. Responsibility for monitoring the application of this Code lies with governments. Manufacturers and distributors and appropriate nongovernmental organizations, professional groups, and consumer organizations should collaborate with governments to this end. Independently of any other measures, manufacturers and distributors should regard themselves as responsible for monitoring their marketing practices according to the principles and aim of this Code, and for taking steps to ensure that their conduct at every level conforms to them. Nongovernmental organizations, professional groups, institutions, and individuals concerned should have the responsibility of drawing the attention of manufacturers or distributors to activities which are incompatible with the principles and aim of this Code. The appropriate governmental authority should also be informed. Manufacturers and distributors should apprise their marketing personnel of the Code and their responsibilities under it. Member States shall communicate annually to the Director-General information on action taken to give effect to the principles and aim of this Code. Director-General shall report in even years to the World Health Assembly on the status of implementation of the Code; and shall provide technical support to Member States in implementation and furtherance of the principles and aim of this Code.

D-2 Baby-Friendly™ Hospital Initiative

The Baby Friendly™ Hospital Initiative is discussed in Chapter 3. Following are documents that are central to the Baby-Friendly™ initiative.

Hospital Self-Appraisal

HOSPITAL DATA   Date _____

If no nursery for normal well newborns exists, write "none" in space provided.

Hospital Name: _____

Address: _____

City, District, or Region: _____ Country: _____

Name of Chief Hospital Administrator: _____ Telephone: _____

Names of senior Nursing Officers (or other personnel in charge):

    For the Facility: _____ Telephone: _____

    For the Maternity Ward: _____ Telephone: _____

    For the Antenatal Service: _____ Telephone: _____

Name of person to be contacted for additional information: _____

Type of Hospital: Government   Private—Not for profit   Private—For profit

                       Mission   Teaching   Other: _____

HOSPITAL CENSUS DATA

Total bed capacity: _____

_____ in labor and delivery area

_____ in the maternity ward

_____ in the normal nursery

_____ in the special care nursery

_____ in other areas for mothers and children

Total deliveries for 12 months ending _____

_____ were by Caesarean   Caesarean rate _____%

_____ were low-birth-weight babies (<2500 g)   Low-birth-weight rate _____%

_____ were in special care   Special care rate _____%

Infant feeding data for deliveries from records or staff reports:

_____ mother/infant pairs discharged in the past month

_____ mother/infant pairs breastfeeding at discharge in the past month   _____ %

_____ mother/infant pairs breastfeeding exclusively from birth to discharge
in the past month   _____ %

_____ infants discharged in the past month who have received at least
one bottlefeed since birth   _____ %

How was the infant feeding data obtained?

_____ From records

_____ Percentages are an estimate, provided by: _____

Name of person(s) filling out this form:

_____

STEP 1. Have a Written Breastfeeding Policy That Is Routinely Communicated to All Health Care Staff.

1.1   Does the health facility have an explicit written policy for protecting, promoting, and supporting breastfeeding that addresses all 10 steps to successful breastfeeding in maternity services?   Yes ❑   No ❑

1.2   Does the policy protect breastfeeding by prohibiting all promotion of and group instruction for using breast-milk substitutes, feeding bottles, and teats?   Yes ❑   No ❑

1.3   Is the breastfeeding policy available so all staff who take care of mothers and babies can refer to it?   Yes ❑   No ❑

1.4   Is the breastfeeding policy posted or displayed in all areas of the health facility that serve mothers, infants, and/or children?   Yes ❑   No ❑

1.5   Is there a mechanism for evaluating the effectiveness of the policy?   Yes ❑   No ❑

STEP 2. Train All Health Care Staff in Skills Necessary to Implement This Policy.

2.1 Are all staff aware of the advantages of breastfeeding and acquainted with the facility's policy and services to protect, promote, and support breastfeeding?   Yes ❑   No ❑

2.2 Are all staff caring for women and infants oriented to the breastfeeding policy of the hospital on their arrival?   Yes ❑   No ❑

2.3 Is training on breastfeeding and lactation management given to all staff caring for women and infants within 6 months of their arrival?   Yes ❑   No ❑

2.4 Does the training cover at least eight of the Ten Steps to Successful Breastfeeding?   Yes ❑   No ❑

2.5 Is the training on breastfeeding and lactation management at least 18 hours in total, including a minimum of 3 hours of supervised clinical experience?   Yes ❑   No ❑

2.6 Has the health care facility arranged for specialized training in lactation management of specific staff members?   Yes ❑   No ❑

STEP 3. Inform All Pregnant Women About the Benefits and Management of Breastfeeding.

3.1 Does the hospital include an antenatal care clinic? Or an antenatal inpatient ward?   Yes ❑   No ❑

3.2 If yes, are most pregnant women attending these antenatal services informed about the benefits and management of breastfeeding?   Yes ❑   No ❑

3.3 Do antenatal records indicate whether breastfeeding has been discussed with the pregnant woman?   Yes ❑   No ❑

3.4 Is a mother's antenatal record available at the time of delivery?   Yes ❑   No ❑

3.5 Are pregnant women protected from oral or written promotion of group instruction for artificial feeding?   Yes ❑   No ❑

3.6 Does the health care facility take into account a woman's intention to breastfeed when deciding on the use of a sedative, an analgesic, or an anesthetic (if any) during labor and delivery?   Yes ❑   No ❑

3.7 Are staff familiar with the effects of such medicaments on breastfeeding?   Yes ❑   No ❑

3.8 Does a woman who has never breastfed or who has previously encountered problems with breastfeeding receive special attention and support from the staff of the health care facility?   Yes ❑   No ❑

STEP 4. Help Mothers Initiate Breastfeeding Within a Half Hour of Birth.

4.1   Are mothers whose deliveries are normal given their babies to hold, with skin contact, within a half hour of completion of the second stage of labor and allowed to remain with them for at least the first hour?   Yes ❏   No ❏

4.2   Are the mothers offered help by a staff member to initiate breastfeeding during this first hour?   Yes ❏   No ❏

4.3   Are mothers who have had cesarean deliveries given their babies to hold, with skin contact, within a half hour after they are able to respond to their babies?   Yes ❏   No ❏

4.4   Do the babies born by cesarean stay with their mothers, with skin contact, at this time for at least 30 minutes?   Yes ❏   No ❏

STEP 5. Show Mothers How to Breastfeed and How to Maintain Lactation, Even If They Should Be Separated From Their Infants.

5.1   Does nursing staff offer all mothers further assistance with breastfeeding within 6 hours of delivery?   Yes ❏   No ❏

5.2   Are most breastfeeding mothers able to demonstrate how to correctly position and attach their babies for breastfeeding?   Yes ❏   No ❏

5.3   Are breastfeeding mothers shown how to express their milk or given information on expression and/or advised of where they can get help should they need it?   Yes ❏   No ❏

5.4   Are staff members or counselors who have specialized training in breastfeeding and lactation management available full-time to advise mothers during their stay in health care facilities and in preparation for discharge?   Yes ❏   No ❏

5.5   Does a woman who has never breastfed or who has previously encountered problems with breastfeeding receive special attention and support from the staff of the health care facility?   Yes ❏   No ❏

5.6   Are mothers of babies in special care helped to establish and maintain lactation by frequent expression of milk?   Yes ❏   No ❏

STEP 6. Give Newborn Infants No Food or Drink Other Than Breast Milk, Unless Medically Indicated.

6.1   Do staff have a clear understanding of what the few acceptable reasons are for prescribing food or drink other than breast milk for breastfeeding babies?   Yes ❏   No ❏

6.2   Do breastfeeding babies receive no other food or drink (than breast milk) unless medically indicated?   Breast milk only   Yes ❏

                                                                       Some other food/drink   No ❏

6.3   Are any breast-milk substitutes, including special formulas which are used in the facility, purchased in the same way as any other foods or medicines?   Yes ❑   No ❑

6.4   Do health facility and health care workers refuse free or low-cost* supplies of breast-milk substitutes, paying close to retail market price for any?   Yes ❑   No ❑

6.5   Is all promotion of infant foods or drinks other than breast milk absent from the facility?   Yes ❑   No ❑

STEP 7. Practice Rooming-in—Allow Mothers and Infants to Remain Together—24 Hours a Day.

7.1   Do mothers and infants remain together (rooming-in or bedding-in) 24 hours a day, except for periods of up to an hour for hospital procedures or if separation is medically indicated?   Yes ❑   No ❑

7.2   Does rooming-in start within an hour of a normal birth?   Yes ❑   No ❑

7.3   Does rooming-in start within an hour of when a cesarean mother can respond to her baby?   Yes ❑   No ❑

STEP 8. Encourage Breastfeeding on Demand.

8.1   By placing no restrictions on the frequency or length of breastfeeds, do staff show they are aware of the importance of breastfeeding on demand?   Yes ❑   No ❑

8.2   Are mothers advised to breastfeed their babies whenever their babies are hungry and as often as their babies want to breastfeed?   Yes ❑   No ❑

STEP 9. Give No Artificial Teats or Pacifiers (Also Called Dummies or Soothers) to Breastfeeding Infants.

9.1   Are babies who have started to breastfeed cared for without any bottle feeds?   Yes ❑   No ❑

9.2   Are babies who have started to breastfeed cared for without using pacifiers?   Yes ❑   No ❑

9.3   Do breastfeeding mothers learn that they should not give any bottles or pacifiers to their babies?   Yes ❑   No ❑

9.4   By accepting no free or low-cost feeding bottles, teats, or pacifiers, do the facility and the health workers demonstrate that these should be avoided?   Yes ❑   No ❑

---

*Low-cost: below 80% open-market retail cost. Breast-milk substitutes intended for experimental use of "professional evaluation" should also be purchased at 80% or more of retail prices.

STEP 10. Foster the Establishment of Breastfeeding Support [Groups] and Refer Mothers to Them On Discharge from the Hospital or Clinic.

10.1 Does the hospital give education to key family members so that they can support the breastfeeding mother at home? Yes ❏ No ❏

10.2 Are breastfeeding mothers referred to breastfeeding support groups, if any are available? Yes ❏ No ❏

10.3 Does the hospital have a system of follow-up support for breastfeeding mothers after they are discharged, such as early postnatal or lactation clinic checkups, home visits, telephone calls? Yes ❏ No ❏

10.4 Does the facility encourage and facilitate the formation of mother-to-mother or health care worker–to-mother support groups? Yes ❏ No ❏

10.5 Does the facility allow breastfeeding counseling by trained mother-support group counselors in its maternity services? Yes ❏ No ❏

Becoming a Baby-Friendly™ Hospital

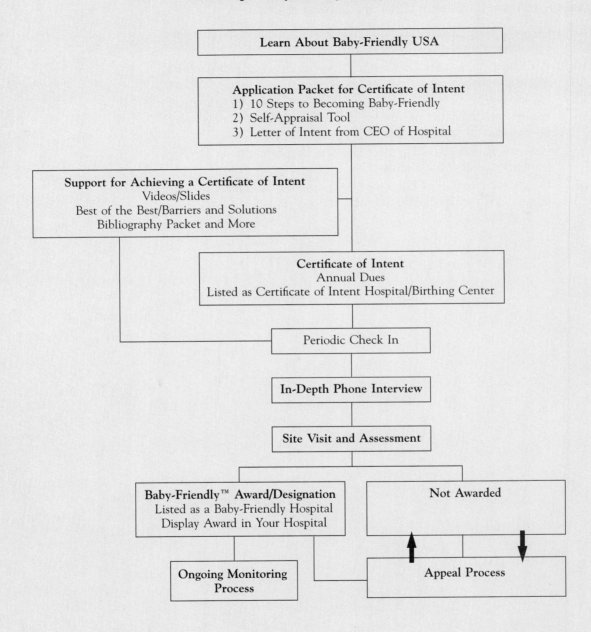

Ten Steps to Successful Breastfeeding

The Baby-Friendly™ Hospital Initiative promotes, protects, and supports breastfeeding through The Ten Steps to Successful Breastfeeding for Hospitals as outlined by UNICEF and WHO. The steps for the United States are:

1. Have a written breastfeeding policy that is routinely communicated to all health care staff.
2. Train all health care staff in skills necessary to implement this policy.
3. Inform all pregnant women about the benefits and management of breastfeeding.
4. Help mothers initiate breastfeeding within an hour of birth.*
5. Show mothers how to breastfeed and how to maintain lactation even if they should be separated from their infants.
6. Give newborn infants no food or drink other than breastmilk, unless medically indicated.
7. Practice 'rooming-in' by allowing mothers and infants to remain together 24 hours a day
8. Encourage breastfeeding on demand.
9. Give no artificial teats, pacifiers, dummies, or soothers to breastfeeding infants.
10. Foster the establishment of breastfeeding support groups and refer mothers to them on discharge from the hospital or birthing center.

D-3 Innocenti Declaration

On the Protection, Promotion and Support of Breastfeeding:

---

*When written in 1989, this step required breastfeeding initiation within the first *half* hour. Research in the 1990s showed that the natural sequence of behavior is for suckling to occur within the first hour. Therefore, this step was modified for United States hospitals.
From Baby-Friendly USA.

Recognising that Breastfeeding is a unique process that:

- provides ideal nutrition for infants and contributes to their healthy growth and development;
- reduces incidence and severity of infectious diseases, thereby lowering infant morbidity and mortality;
- contributes to women's health by reducing the risk of breast and ovarian cancer, and by increasing the spacing between pregnancies;
- provides social and economic benefits to the family and the nation;
- provides most women with a sense of satisfaction when successfully carried out; and that

Recent research has found that:

- these benefits increase with increased exclusiveness[1] of breastfeeding during the first 6 months of life, and thereafter with increased duration of breastfeeding with complementary foods; and
- programme interventions can result in positive changes in breastfeeding behaviour;

We therefore declare that

As a global goal for optimal maternal and child health and nutrition, all women should be enabled to practise exclusive breastfeeding and all infants should be fed exclusively on breast milk from birth to 4-6 months of age. Thereafter, children should continue to be breastfed, while receiving appropriate and adequate complementary foods, for up to 2 years of age or beyond. This child-feeding ideal is to be achieved by creating

---

[1]Exclusive breastfeeding means that no other drink or food is given to the infant; the infant should feed frequently and for unrestricted periods.

an appropriate environment of awareness and support so that women can breastfeed in this manner.

Attainment of the goal requires, in many countries, the reinforcement of a "breastfeeding culture" and its vigorous defence against incursions of a "bottle-feeding culture." This requires commitment and advocacy for social mobilization, utilizing to the full the prestige and authority of acknowledged leaders of society in all walks of life.

Efforts should be made to increase women's confidence in their ability to breastfeed. Such empowerment involves the removal of constraints and influences that manipulate perceptions and behaviour towards breastfeeding, often by subtle and indirect means. This requires sensitivity, continued vigilance, and a responsive and comprehensive communications strategy involving all media and addressed to all levels of society. Furthermore, obstacles to breastfeeding within the health system, the workplace and the community must be eliminated.

Measures should be taken to ensure that women are adequately nourished for their optimal health and that of their families. Furthermore, ensuring that all women also have access to family planning information and services allows them to sustain breastfeeding and avoid shortened birth intervals that may compromise their health and nutritional status, and that of their children.

All governments should develop national breastfeeding policies and set appropriate national targets for the 1990s. They should establish a national system for monitoring the attainment of their targets, and they should develop indicators such as the prevalence of exclusively breastfed infants at discharge from maternity services, and the prevalence of exclusively breastfed infants at 4 months of age.

National authorities are further urged to integrate their breastfeeding policies into their overall health and development policies. In so doing they should reinforce all actions that protect, promote and support breastfeeding within complementary programmes such as prenatal and perinatal care, nutrition, family planning services, and prevention and treatment of common maternal and childhood diseases. All healthcare staff should be trained in the skills necessary to implement these breastfeeding policies.

Operational Targets:

All governments by the year 1995 should have:

- appointed a national breastfeeding coordinator of appropriate authority, and established a multisectoral national breastfeeding committee composed of representatives from relevant government departments, non-governmental organizations, and health professional associations;

- ensured that every facility providing maternity services fully practises all ten of the *Ten Steps to Successful Breastfeeding* set out in the joint WHO/UNICEF statement[2] "Protecting, promoting and supporting breastfeeding: the special role of maternity services";

- taken action to give effect to the principles and aim of all Articles of the International Code of Marketing of Breast-Milk Substitutes and subsequent relevant World Health Assembly resolutions in their entirety; and

- enacted imaginative legislation protecting the breastfeeding rights of working women and established means for its enforcement.

We also call upon international organizations to:

- draw up action strategies for protecting, promoting and supporting breastfeeding, including global monitoring on evaluation of their strategies;

---

[2]World Health Organisation, Geneva, 1989.

- support national situation analyses and surveys and the development of national goals and targets for action; and
- encourage and support national authorities in planning, implementing, monitoring and evaluating their breastfeeding policies.

The Innocenti Declaration was produced and adopted by participants at the WHO/UNICEF policy makers' meeting on "Breastfeeding in the 1990s: A Global Initiative," cosponsored by the United States Agency for International Development (AID) and the Swedish International Development Authority (SIDA), held at the Spedale degli Innocenti, Florence, Italy, on 30 July to 1 August 1990. The Declaration reflects the content of the original background document for the meeting and the views expressed in group and plenary sessions.

D-4 Acceptable Medical Reasons for Supplementation

A few medical indications in a maternity facility may require that individual infants be given fluids or food in addition to, or in place of, breastmilk.

It is assumed that severely ill babies, babies in need of surgery, and very low birth weight infants will be in a special care unit. Their feeding will be individually decided, given their particular nutritional requirements and functional capabilities, although breastmilk is recommended whenever possible. These infants in special care are likely to include:

- Infants with very low birth weight (less than 1500 g) who are born before 32 weeks gestational age

From WHO/UNICEF. Baby-Friendly Hospital Initiative. Part 2: Hospital-Level Implementation, 1992.

- Infants with severe dysmaturity with potentially severe hypoglycemia, or who require therapy for hypoglycemia, and who do not improve through increased breastfeeding or by being given breastmilk

For infants who are well enough to be with their mothers on the maternity ward, there are very few indications for supplements. In order to assess whether a facility is inappropriately using fluids or breast-milk substitutes, any infants receiving additional supplements must have been diagnosed as:

- Infants whose mothers have severe maternal illness (e.g., psychosis, eclampsia, or shock)
- Infants with inborn errors of metabolism (e.g., galactosemia, phenylketonuria, maple syrup urine disease)
- Infants with acute water loss, for example, during phototherapy for jaundice, whenever increased breastfeeding or use of expressed breastmilk cannot provide adequate hydration
- Infants whose mothers require medication which is contraindicated when breastfeeding (e.g., cytotoxic drugs, radioactive drugs, and anti-thyroid drugs other than propylthiouracil)

When breastfeeding has to be temporarily delayed, interrupted, or supplemented, mothers should be helped to establish or maintain lactation, for example, through manual or hand-pump expression of milk, in preparation for the moment when full breastfeeding may be begun or resumed. If the interruption is due to problems with the infant, milk can be expressed, stored if necessary, and provided to the infant as soon as medically advisable. If it is due to a maternal medication or disease which negatively affects the quality of milk, the milk should be pumped and discarded.

D-5 Legislation Related to Breastfeeding

State Legislation Related to Breastfeeding

The following highlights state legislation related to breastfeeding (data derived from La Leche League's Web site). Updates can be found by visiting various Web sites that provide links to state legislation activities, for example, www.multistate.com/weblist.htm.
You may also contact thomas.loc.gov for links to state legislation.

The Right to Breastfeed in Public

Breastfeeding in public is not illegal. However, breastfeeding women have been frequently humiliated or excluded from public places if they are breastfeeding, which has resulted in some states passing a law specifically guaranteeing their right to breastfeed. States that have passed legislation, or have pending legislation on this issue, include:

California, 1997
  (Full text at
  www.leginfo.ca.gov/bilinfo.html)
Connecticut, 1997
Delaware, 1996
Florida, 1993
Illinois, 1995
Michigan, 1994
Nevada, 1995
New Jersey, 1997
New York, 1994
North Carolina, 1993
Texas House, 1995
Utah, 1995
Virginia, 1994
Wisconsin, 1995
Minnesota: Bill introduced March 19, 1998.
  (Updates: See www.revisor.leg.state.mn.us)

Exempting Breastfeeding Mother From Jury Duty

Idaho, 1996
Iowa, 1994

Projects to Determine Support Policies for State Employees

Florida, 1994
Texas, 1995

Breastfeeding Support Incentives for Private Employers

Texas, 1995

Public Health Law: New York State

AVAILABILITY OF HUMAN MILK
STATE OF NEW YORK
An Act to amend the public health law, in relation to the availability of human breast milk for infant consumption.

The people of the State of New York, represented in Senate and Assembly, do enact as follows:

§1. Legislative findings. The legislature hereby finds and declares that human breast milk, the preferred food for all infants, provides a superior, well-tolerated nutritional source because of its unique components. It contains substances, lacking in other forms of infant nutrition, which help control infection and aid in preventing infant disease. For premature infants or those with low birth weight or infants who are allergic to cow's milk and infant formulas, human breast milk is essential.

It shall be the declared policy of the state of New York that any and all infants requiring human breast milk be assured access to sufficient quantities of wholesome human breast milk, donated by concerned lactating mothers on a continual and systematic basis. The availability of such a supply of human breast milk should be made known to the public so that health providers and families of infants with particular need for human breast milk will be aware of its accessibility.

§2. The public health law is amended by adding a new section twenty-five hundred five to read as follows:

§2505. Human breast milk; collection, storage, and distribution; general powers of the commissioner. The commissioner is hereby empowered to:

(a) Adopt regulations and guidelines including, but not limited to donor standards, methods of collection, and standards for storage, and distribution of human breast milk;

(b) Conduct educational activities to inform the public and health care providers of the availability of human breast milk for infants determined to require such milk and to inform potential donors of the opportunities for proper donation;

(c) Establish rules and regulations to effectuate the provisions of this section.

§3 This act shall take effect immediately.

New York State Health Code in Support of Breastfeeding (Added 1984)

CHAPTER V, SUBCHAPTER A, ARTICLE 2, PART 405
Hospitals—minimum standards
(Statutory authority: Public Health law §2803)
405.8 Maternal, child health and newborn services

From Office of Health Systems Management, Bureau of Standards Development, New York State Department of Health, Empire State Plaza, Albany NY, 1984.

(10)(i) The hospital, with the advice of the maternity staff, shall formulate a program of instruction and provide assistance for each maternity patient(s) in the fundamentals of (normal) infant care including infant feeding choice and techniques, post-pregnancy care and family planning.

(ii) The hospital shall provide instruction and assistance to each maternity patient who has chosen to breast-feed and shall provide information on the advantages and disadvantages of breast-feeding to women who are undecided as to the feeding method for their infants. As a minimum:

(a) the hospital shall designate at least one person who is thoroughly trained in breast-feeding physiology and management to be responsible for ensuring the implementation of an effective breast-feeding program; and

(b) policies and procedures shall be developed to assist the mother to breast-feed which shall include, but not be limited to:

(1) prohibition of the application of standing orders for antilactation drugs;

(2) placement of the infant for breast-feeding immediately following delivery, unless contraindicated;

(3) restriction of the infant's supplemental feedings to those indicated by the medical condition of the infant or of the mother;

(4) provision for the infant to be fed on demand; and

(c) assurance that an educational program has been given as soon after admission as possible which shall include but not be limited to:

(1) the nutritional and physiological aspects of human milk;

(2) the normal process for establishing

lactation, including care of breasts, common problems associated with breast-feeding and frequency of feeding;

(3) dietary requirements for breast-feeding;

(4) diseases and medication or other substances which may have an effect on breast-feeding;

(5) sanitary procedures to follow in collecting and storing human milk; and

(6) sources for advice and information available to the mother following discharge.

Federal Legislation Related to Breastfeeding

The following highlights federal legislation related to breastfeeding. Updates to federal legislation can be found by visiting the Government Printing Office's Web site at www.access.gpo.gov and searching for the keyword "breastfeeding."

Special Supplemental Nutrition Program for Women, Infants and Children (WIC)

The Special Supplemental Nutrition Program for Women, Infants and Children (WIC) was legislated by Congress in 1972 as a pilot program and authorized as a permanent program in 1975. For eligible women, infants, and children, WIC provides supplemental foods that are high in protein, iron, vitamins A and C, and calcium. In 1989 the United States Department of Agriculture set aside $8 million for breastfeeding promotion each year, which WIC state agencies were required to spend on breastfeeding promotion and support. Furthermore, each WIC state agency is required to designate a breastfeeding coordinator. A brief description of the history of WIC and its involvement in breastfeeding promotion is found in Chapter 1. Addresses of regional, state, and tribal WIC coordinators are listed below. WIC directors belong to:

NATIONAL ASSOCIATION OF WIC DIRECTORS
2001 S Street, N.W. Suite 580
PO Box 53355
Washington, DC 20009-3355
(202) 232-5492
FAX: (202) 387-5281

MID-ATLANTIC REGIONAL OFFICE
Regional Director
Supplemental Food Programs, Mid-Atlantic
  Regional Office
Food and Consumer Service, USDA
Mercer Corporate Park
300 Corporate Boulevard
Robbinsville, NJ 08691-1598
(609) 259-5163
FAX: MARO (609) 259-5026
FAX: SFP (609) 259-5147

DELAWARE
WIC Nutrition Education Coordinator
Supplemental Food Program
Division of Public Health—WIC Program
Blue Hen Corporate Center
655 Bay Road, Suite 4-B
Dover, DE 19901
(302) 739-3671
FAX: (302) 739-3970

DISTRICT OF COLUMBIA
WIC Nutrition Coordinator
Department of Human Services
Commission of Public Health
2100 Martin Luther King Avenue, SE
Washington, DC 20020
(202) 645-5662
FAX: (202) 645-0516

MARYLAND
WIC Nutrition Services Coordinator
WIC Administration
Maryland Dept. of Health and Mental
    Hygiene
201 West Preston Street, 1st Floor
Baltimore, MD 21201
(410) 767-5244
FAX: (410) 333-5243

NEW JERSEY
State WIC Nutrition Coordinator
Dept. of Health and Senior Services
Family Health Services—WIC
CN 364
Trenton, NJ 08625
(609) 292-9560
FAX: (609) 292-3580

PENNSYLVANIA
State WIC Nutrition Coordinator
Division of Special Food Programs (WIC)
Pennsylvania Dept. of Health
PO Box 90
Harrisburg, PA 17108
(717) 783-1289
FAX: (717) 772-0323

PUERTO RICO
WIC Nutrition Director
Puerto Rico Dept. of Health, WIC Program
#1086 Munoz Rivera Avenue
Rio Piedras, PR 00928-5220
(787) 766-2804
FAX: (787) 765-8817

VIRGIN ISLANDS
Nutrition Coordinator
Virgin Islands Dept. of Health—WIC
Charles Harwood Complex
3500 Estate Richmond
Christiansted
St. Croix, VI 00821
(809) 773-9157
FAX: (809) 773-6495

VIRGINIA
WIC Nutrition Coordinator
State Division of Chronic Disease
Prevention/Nutrition
Virginia Dept. of Health
1500 E. Main Street, Suite 132
PO Box 2448
Richmond, VA 23218
(804) 692-0681
FAX: (804) 371-6162

WEST VIRGINIA
State Nutrition Coordinator
WVA State WIC Program
1411 Virginia Street, East
Charleston, WV 25301-3013
(304) 558-0030
FAX: (304) 558-1541

MIDWEST REGIONAL OFFICE
Regional Director
Special Supplemental Nutrition Programs
Midwest Regional Office
Food and Nutrition Service, USDA
77 West Jackson Boulevard, 20th Floor
Chicago, IL 60604-3507
(312) 353-7710
FAX: (312) 886-1937

ILLINOIS
Nutrition Services Coordinator
Division of Health Assessment and Screening
Illinois Dept. of Public Health
535 W. Jefferson Street
Springfield, IL 62761
(312) 793-8243
FAX: (312) 793-4666

INDIANA
Director, Nutrition and Clinic Services
Division of Nutrition WIC Program
Indiana State Dept. of Health
2 North Meridian Street, Suite 700
Indianapolis, IN 46204
(219) 234-6072
FAX: (219) 234-0331

MICHIGAN
WIC Nutrition Education Coordinator
Western Region, BCS
Michigan Dept. of Public Health
2150 Apollo Drive
PO Box 30195
Lansing, MI 48909
(517) 335-9174
FAX: (517) 335-8835

MINNESOTA
Nutrition Coordinator
Minnesota Dept. of Health
717 SE Delaware Street
PO Box 9441
Minneapolis, MN 55440
(612) 623-5400
FAX: (612) 623-5442

OHIO
Nutrition and Administrative Services
   Supervisor
Bureau of Nutrition Services & WIC Program
Ohio Dept. of Health
246 North High Street
PO Box 118
Columbus, OH 43266-0118
(614) 644-8047
FAX: (614) 644-9850

WISCONSIN
Public Health Nutritionist
Wisconsin WIC Program
Wisconsin Dept. of Health and Social Services
1414 East Washington Avenue, Rm. 96
Madison, WI 53703
(608) 267-3674
FAX: (608) 266-3125

MOUNTAIN PLAINS REGIONAL OFFICE
Regional Director
Nutrition and Technical Services
Supplemental Nutrition Programs
Mountain Plains Regional Office
USDA, Food and Consumer Service
1244 Speer Boulevard, #903
Denver, CO 80204
(303) 844-0308
FAX: (303) 844-6203

COLORADO
Chief Nutritionist
FCHSD-NS-A4
Colorado Dept. of Public Health and
   Environment
4300 Cherry Creek Drive South
Denver, CO 80222-1530
(303) 692-2400
FAX: (303) 756-9926

IOWA
Nutrition Services Coordinator
Bureau of Nutrition and WIC
Iowa Department of Public Health
Lucas Building, 3rd Floor
Des Moines, IA 50319-0075
(515) 281-7769
FAX: (515) 281-4913

KANSAS
Nutrition Services Coordinator
Kansas Department of Health and
    Environment
Bureau of Family Health—WIC Division
Landon State Office Building, 10th Floor
900 SW Jackson
Topeka, KS 66612-1290
(913) 296-1322
FAX: (913) 296-1326

MISSOURI
Associate Chief for Nutrition Services
Missouri Dept. of Health
WIC Program
PO Box 570
Jefferson City, MO 65102
(573) 751-6204
FAX: (573) 526-1470

MONTANA
Nutrition Coordinator
Montana Department of Public Health and
    Human Services
Cogswell Building
Helena, MT 59620
(406) 444-2841
FAX: (406) 444-0239

NEBRASKA
WIC Nutrition Coordinator
Family Health Section
301 Centennial Mall South
PO Box 95007
Lincoln, NE 68509-5007
(402) 471-2781
FAX: (402) 471-7049

NORTH DAKOTA
WIC/MCH Nutrition Services Coordinator
North Dakota Dept. of Health
600 East Boulevard Avenue
Bismarck, ND 58505-0200
(701) 328-2496
FAX: (701) 328-1412

SOUTH DAKOTA
Nutrition Consultant
WIC Program
South Dakota Dept. of Health
445 East Capitol
Pierre, SD 57501-2080
(605) 773-5740
FAX: (605) 773-5509

UTAH
WIC Nutrition Coordinator
Utah WIC Program
288 North 1460 West
Box 144470
Salt Lake City, UT 84114-4470
(801) 538-6960
FAX: (801) 538-6729

WYOMING
WIC Nutrition Coordinator
Wyoming WIC Program
456 Hathaway Building, 4th Floor
Cheyenne, WY 82002-0050
(307) 777-7494
FAX: (307) 777-5643

CHEYENNE RIVER SIOUX TRIBE
WIC Nutrition Education Coordinator
Cheyenne River Sioux Tribe
PO Box 590
Eagle Butte, SD 57625-0590
(605) 964-3947
FAX: (605) 964-4151

NEBRASKA INDIAN INTER-TRIBAL DEVELOPMENT
CORPORATION
WIC Nutritionist
Nebraska Indian Inter-Tribal Development
  Corporation
Rt. 1, Box 66-A
Winnebago, NE 68071
(402) 878-2242
FAX: (402) 878-2504

ROSEBUD SIOUX TRIBE
WIC Nutrition Coordinator
Rosebud Sioux WIC Program
PO Box 99
400 WIC Drive
Rosebud, SD 57570-0099
(605) 747-2617
FAX: (605) 747-2612

SHOSHONE/ARAPAHOE JOINT BUSINESS COUNCIL
Shoshone and Arapahoe WIC Program
PO Box 860
Washakie, WY 82514
Fort Washakie: (307) 332-6733
Fort Arapahoe: (307) 856-8142
FAX: (307) 332-4196

STANDING ROCK SIOUX TRIBE
WIC Nutrition Coordinator
Standing Rock WIC Program
PO Box 437
Fort Yates, ND 58538-0437
(701) 854-7263
FAX: (701) 854-7122

THREE AFFILIATED TRIBES
Nutritionist
Three Affiliated Tribes
WIC Program
HC 3, Box 2
New Town, ND 58763-9401
(701) 627-4777
FAX: (701) 627-3805

UTE MOUNTAIN TRIBE
Nutrition Coordinator
Ute Mountain WIC Program
PO Box II
Towaoc, CO 81334
(970) 565-4441
FAX: (970) 565-7412

NORTHEAST REGIONAL OFFICE
Regional Director
Supplemental Food Programs
Northeast Regional Office
Food and Nutrition Service, USDA
10 Causeway Street
Boston, MA 02222-1066
(617) 565-6444
FAX: (617) 565-6472

CONNECTICUT
WIC Nutrition Coordinator
Dept. of Public Health
410 Capitol Avenue, MS #11WIC
PO Box 340308
Hartford, CT 06134-0308
(860) 509-8055
FAX: (860) 509-7855

MAINE
WIC Nutrition Coordinator
WIC Program
Dept. of Human Services
State House—Station 11
151 Capitol Street
Augusta, ME 04333
(207) 287-5341
FAX: (207) 287-3993

MASSACHUSETTS
Asst. Director, Nutrition Services
Massachusetts Dept. of Public Health
WIC Program
250 Washington Street, 6th Floor
Boston, MA 02108-4619
(617) 624-6100
FAX: (617) 624-6179

NEW HAMPSHIRE
Nutrition Coordinator
Bureau of WIC Nutrition Services
Office of Health Management
Health & Welfare Building
6 Hazen Drive, H+H Bldg.
Concord, NH 03301-6527
(603) 271-4252
FAX: (603) 271-4779

NEW YORK
State WIC Nutrition Coordinator
New York State Dept. of Health
Division of Nutrition
Bureau of Supplemental Food Programs
11 University Place, 2nd Floor
Albany, NY 12203-3399
(518) 458-6840
FAX: (518) 458-5508

RHODE ISLAND
State WIC Nutrition Coordinator
WIC Program
Rhode Island Dept. of Health
Cannon Building
3 Capitol Hill, Room 303
Providence, RI 02908-5097
(401) 277-3940
FAX: (401) 277-1442

VERMONT
State WIC Nutrition Coordinator
Dept. of Health
108 Cherry Street
PO Box 70
Burlington, VT 05402-0070
(802) 863-7333
FAX: (802) 863-7425

PASSAMAQUODDY TRIBE
WIC Program
Indian Township Health Center
One Newell Drive
PO Box 97
Indian Township, ME 04668-0097
(207) 796-2321
FAX: (207) 796-2422

PASSAMAQUODDY TRIBE
WIC Nutritionist
Pleasant Point Health Center
PO Box 351
Perry, ME 04667
(207) 853-0644
FAX: (207) 853-2347

SENECA NATION
WIC Nutritionist
WIC Nutrition Unit
1510 Route 438
Irving, NY 14081
(716) 532-0167
FAX: (716) 532-0110

SOUTHEAST REGIONAL OFFICE
Regional Director
Supplemental Food Programs
Southeast Regional Office
Food and Nutrition Service, USDA
61 Forsyth Street, SW, Room 8T36
Atlanta, GA 30303-3427
(404) 562-7100
FAX: (404) 527-4518

ALABAMA
Nutrition Services Administrator
Division of WIC
Bureau of Family Health Services
Alabama Dept. of Public Health
434 Monroe Street
Montgomery, AL 36130-3017
(334) 242-5673
FAX: (334) 240-3330

FLORIDA
Public Health Nutrition Program
Manager
Florida Dept. of Health, WIC, and Nutrition
    Services
1317 Winewood Boulevard
Tallahassee, FL 32399-0700
(904) 488-8985
FAX: (904) 922-3936

GEORGIA
Director
Office of Nutrition
Georgia Dept. of Human Resources
2 Peachtree Street
Room 8-413
Atlanta, GA 30303-3186
(404) 657-2884
FAX: (404) 657-2886

KENTUCKY
WIC Nutrition Coordinator
Nutrition Branch
Kentucky Cabinet for Health Services
Dept. of Public Health
275 East Main Street
Frankfort, KY 40621
(502) 564-2339
FAX: (502) 564-8389

MISSISSIPPI
WIC Nutrition Coordinator
Bureau of Health Services
Mississippi State Dept. of Health
PO Box 1700
2423 North State Street
Jackson, MS 39215-1700
(601) 987-6732
FAX: (601) 987-6740

NORTH CAROLINA
Head, Clinical Services Branch
Division of Maternal and Child Health
Nutrition Services Section
Department of Environment, Health and
    Natural Resources
PO Box 10008
Raleigh, NC 27605-0008
(919) 715-0645
FAX: (919) 733-1384

SOUTH CAROLINA
WIC Nutrition Coordinator
WIC Division/Maternal and Child Health
South Carolina Dept. of Health and
    Environmental Control
2600 Bull Street
Columbia, SC 29201
(804) 737-3840
FAX: (804) 734-4448

TENNESSEE
WIC Nutrition Coordinator
Community Nutrition Services
Tennessee Dept. of Health
Cordell Hull Building—5th floor
426 Fifth Avenue, North
Nashville, TN 37247-5225
(615) 741-7218
FAX: (615) 532-7189

CHEROKEE
WIC Nutrition Education Coordinator
Eastern Band of Cherokee Indians
PO Box 1145
Cherokee, NC 28719
(704) 497-7297
FAX: (704) 497-4470

CHOCTAW
Director of Nutrition and Dietetics
Mississippi Band of Choctaw Indians
Route 7, Box 21
Philadelphia, MS 39350
(601) 656-2211
FAX: (601) 656-0931

SEMINOLE
Director of Nutrition Services and WIC
Seminole Tribe of Florida
3006 Josie Billie Avenue
Hollywood, FL 33024
(305) 962-2009
FAX: (305) 985-8456

SOUTHWEST REGIONAL OFFICE
Regional Director
Supplemental and Indian Food Programs
Southwest Regional Office
Food and Nutrition Service, USDA
1100 Commerce Street
Dallas, TX 75242
(214) 290-9812
FAX: (214) 767-9599

ARKANSAS
WIC Nutrition Coordinator
Arkansas Dept. of Health
4815 West Markham Street, Slot 43
Little Rock, AR 72205-3867
(501) 661-2473
FAX: (501) 661-2004

LOUISIANA
WIC Nutrition Coordinator
Nutrition Section
Louisiana Dept. of Health and Hospitals
PO Box 60630
New Orleans, LA 70160
(504) 568-5065
FAX: (504) 568-3065

NEW MEXICO
WIC Nutrition Coordinator
New Mexico Dept. of Health
525 Camino Delos Marquez, West Suite
Santa Fe, NM 87501
(505) 476-8522
FAX: (505) 476-8512

OKLAHOMA
Nutrition Division Director
WIC Services
Oklahoma State Dept. of Health
Shepherd Mall
2520 Villa Prom Street
Oklahoma City, OK 73107-2419
(405) 271-4676
FAX: (405) 271-5763

TEXAS
Nutrition Director
Bureau of WIC Nutrition
Texas Dept. of Health
1100 West 49th Street
Austin, TX 78756
(512) 458-7444
FAX: (512) 458-7446

ACL
Nutrition Coordinator
WIC Program
PO Box 310
New Laguna, NM 87038
(505) 552-6068
FAX: (505) 552-6306

CHEROKEE NATION
Nutrition Coordinator
Cherokee Nation WIC Program
PO Box 948
Tahlequah, OK 74465
(918) 456-0671 Ext. 290
FAX: (918) 458-5539

CHICKASAW NATION
WIC Nutrition Coordinator
Chickasaw Nation
PO Box 1548
Ada, OK 74820
(405) 436-7255
FAX: (405) 436-7225

CHOCTAW NATION OF OKLAHOMA
WIC Nutrition Coordinator
Choctaw Nation of Oklahoma
PO Drawer 1210
Durant, OK 74702
(405) 924-8280
FAX: (405) 924-4831

EIGHT NORTHERN INDIAN PUEBLOS
WIC Nutrition Coordinator
Eight Northern Indian Pueblos Council
PO Box 969
San Juan Pueblo, NM 87566
(505) 455-3144
FAX: (505) 455-3055

FIVE SANDOVAL INDIAN PUEBLOS
WIC Nutrition Coordinator
Five Sandoval Indian Pueblos, Inc.
1043 Highway 313
Bernalillo, NM 87004
(505) 867-3351
FAX: (505) 867-3514

INTER-TRIBAL COUNCIL
WIC Nutrition Coordinator
ITC, Incorporated
PO Box 1308
Miami, OK 74355
(918) 542-4486
FAX: (918) 540-2500

MUSCOGEE CREEK NATION
WIC Nutrition Coordinator
1801 East 4th Street
PO Box 2158/OSU Okmulgee
Okmulgee, OK 74447-3901
(918) 758-2722
FAX: (918) 756-4949

OSAGE NATION
WIC Nutrition Coordinator
Osage Nation
627 Grandview
Pawhuska, OK 74056
(918) 287-1040
FAX: (918) 287-1050

OTOE MISSOURIA
WIC Nutrition Coordinator
Route 1, Box 62
Red Rock, OK 74651
(405) 723-4411
FAX: (405) 723-4273

POTAWATOMI INDIANS OF OKLAHOMA
WIC Nutrition Coordinator
Potawatomi Indians of Oklahoma
1901 S. Gordon Cooper Drive
Shawnee, OK 74801
(405) 273-5236
FAX: (405) 878-4052

PUEBLO OF ISLETA
WIC Nutrition Coordinator
PO Box 670
Isleta, NM 87022
(505) 869-2662
FAX: (505) 869-8309

PUEBLO OF SAN FELIPE
WIC Nutrition Coordinator
Pueblo of San Felipe
PO Box 4339
San Felipe Pueblo, NM 87001
(505) 867-2466
FAX: (505) 867-3383

PUEBLO OF ZUNI
WIC Nutrition Coordinator
Pueblo of Zuni
PO Box 339
Zuni, NM 87327
(505) 782-2929
FAX: (505) 782-2700

SAC AND FOX NATION
WIC Nutrition Coordinator
Sac and Fox Nation
Route 2, Box 247
Stroud, OK 74079
(918) 968-9531
FAX: (918) 968-4453

SANTO DOMINGO PUEBLO
WIC Nutrition Coordinator
Santo Domingo Pueblo
PO Box 238
Santo Domingo, NM 87052
(505) 465-2214
FAX: (505) 465-2688

WCD ENTERPRISES
WIC Nutrition Coordinator
WCD Enterprises, Inc.
PO Box 247
Anadarko, OK 73005
(405) 247-2533
FAX: (405) 247-5277

WESTERN REGIONAL OFFICE
Regional Director
Supplemental Nutrition Programs
Western Regional Office
Food and Consumer Service, USDA
550 Kearny Street, Room 400
San Francisco, CA 94108
(415) 705-1313
FAX: (415) 705-1029

ALASKA
WIC Nutritionist
Maternal, Child, and Family Health
Division of Public Health
Dept. of Health and Social Services
1231 Gambell Street
Anchorage, AK 99501-4627
(907) 269-3442
FAX: (907) 269-3414

AMERICAN SAMOA
Certified Nutritionist
American Samoa WIC Program
Agency on Aging and Food and Nutrition
    Services
American Samoa Government
Pago Pago, AS 96799
9-011-684-633-2614
FAX: 9-011-684-633-2618

ARIZONA
WIC Nutrition Education Consultant
Office of Nutrition Services
Dept. of Health Services
1740 West Adams Street, Room 203
Phoenix, AZ 85007
(602) 542-1886
FAX: (602) 542-1890

CALIFORNIA
WIC Nutrition Coordinator
WIC Supplemental Nutrition Branch
Dept. of Health Services
3901 Lennane Drive
Sacramento, CA 95834
(916) 928-8522
FAX: (916) 928-0709

GUAM
WIC Nutrition Coordinator
Nutrition Health Services
Dept. of Public Health and Social Services
Government of Guam
PO Box 2816
Agana, GU 96932
(671) 475-0294
FAX: (671) 477-7945

HAWAII
WIC Nutrition Coordinator
Nutrition Branch
Dept. of Health
PO Box 3378
Honolulu, HI 96801
(808) 586-8070
FAX: (808) 586-8189

IDAHO
WIC Nutrition Coordinator
Dept. of Health and Welfare
(6230-94)
PO Box 83720
Boise, ID 83720-0036
(208) 334-4934
FAX: (208) 332-7362

NEVADA
WIC Nutrition Coordinator
State Health Division
505 East King Street, Room 204
Carson City, NV 89710
(702) 436-0037
FAX: (702) 687-6789

OREGON
WIC Nutrition Consultant
WIC Program
Oregon State Health Division, Suite 865
800 NE Oregon Street, #21
Portland, OR 97232
(503) 731-4125
FAX: (503) 731-3477

WASHINGTON
WIC Nutrition Coordinator
Washington State Dept. of Health
PO Box 47886
Olympia, WA 98504-7886
(360) 586-5062
FAX: (360) 586-3890

INTER-TRIBAL COUNCIL OF ARIZONA
Nutrition Education
Inter-Tribal Council of Arizona, Inc.
4205 North 7th Avenue, Suite 200
Phoenix, AZ 85013
(602) 248-0071
FAX: (602) 248-0080

INTER-TRIBAL COUNCIL OF NEVADA
State WIC Director/Nutritionist
Inter-Tribal Council of Nevada
PO Box 7440
Reno, NV 89510
(702) 355-0600
FAX: (702) 355-0648

Navajo Nation
WIC Nutrition Coordinator
Navajo Nation WIC Program
Division of Health
PO Box 1390
Window Rock, AZ 86515
(520) 327-9951
FAX: (520) 871-6255

Healthy Meals for Healthy Americans Act (1994) Public Law 103-448

Healthy Meals for Healthy Americans Act, passed by Congress in 1994, revised the formula for determining the amount of funds to be spent for WIC breastfeeding promotion and support. The act replaced the $8 million target level with a national maximum for breastfeeding promotion and support expenditures of $21 for each pregnant and breastfeeding woman. The $21 is adjusted annually based on inflation.

Family and Medical Leave Act (FMLA) (1993), 29 CFR Part 825, Public Law 103-3, 107

The FMLA generally requires private-sector employers of 50 or more employees and public agencies to provide up to 12 work weeks of unpaid, job-protected leave to eligible employees for certain specified family and medical reasons; to maintain eligible employees' preexisting group health insurance coverage during period of FMLA leave; and to restore eligible employees to their same or an equivalent position at the conclusion of the FMLA leave. This is WH Publication #1419 and can be obtained by contacting Division of Policy Analysis, Wage and Hour Division, Employment Standards Administration, U.S. Department of Labor, Room S-3506, 200 Constitution Avenue NW, Washington, DC 20210; telephone 202-219-8412.

New Mothers' Breastfeeding Promotion and Protection Act of 1998

This legislation, initiated by Representative Carolyn Maloney of New York, seeks to amend several laws including:

- An amendment to Title VI of the civil rights act of 1964 by inserting the word "breastfeeding," after "childbirth," and by adding at the end the following: "For purposes of this subsection, the term 'breastfeeding' means the feeding of a child directly from the breast or the expression of milk from the breast by a lactating woman."
- Amend Chapter 1 of the Internal Revenue Code of 1986 by adding, "credit for employer expenses incurred to facilitate employed mothers who breastfeed or express milk for their children."
- Amend the Family and Medical Leave Act of 1993 by providing for nursing mothers' breaks and intermittent leave.
- Amend Section 6382 of Title 5, United States Code, by adding statements about leave.
- Amend the Child Nutrition Act of 1966 to increase support for breastfeeding promotion and support activities under the WIC program.

A copy of this bill can be obtained by visiting the congressional web site, thomas.loc.gov.

Helpful Government Web Sites

Department of Health and Human Services
  www.hhs.gov
Agency for Health Care Policy and Research (AHCPR) www.ahcpr.gov

Food and Drug Administration (FDA) www.fda.gov

Health Resources and Services Administration (HRSA) www.hrsa.dhhs.gov

National Institutes for Health www.nih.gov

Health Care Financing Administration (HCFA) www.hcfa.gov

Department of Labor www.dol.gov

Federal Legislation thomas.loc.gov

Government Printing Office www.gpo.gov

Healthy People 2000 Initiative odphp.osophs.dhhs.gov/Pubs/HP2000/

United States Department of Agriculture—WIC- www.usda.gov/FCS/wic.htm

D-6 Statements on Breastfeeding

Listed below are position statements issued by various organizations and associations that pertain to the promotion of breastfeeding. Most of the position papers are found in the organization's official journal as listed below. Unless otherwise noted, the remainder can be obtained by visiting the organization's Web site or by contacting the organization; the organization's address is found in Appendix C-1.

American Academy of Pediatrics Work Group on Breastfeeding. Breastfeeding and the Use of Human Milk. *Pediatrics* 1997;100:1035-1039. Earlier statements were issued in 1980 and 1982.

American Academy of Family Physicians. Academy endorses the 10 steps and criteria of the breast-feeding health initiative. *Am Fam Physician* 1994;50:457-458.

American Academy of Pediatrics and the American College of Obstetrics and Gynecology. *Guidelines for Perinatal Care*. 4th ed. Elk Grove Village, IL: American Academy of Pediatrics; 1997.

American Academy of Family Physicians. *Policy on Breastfeeding and Infant Nutrition*. Kansas City, MO: American Academy of Family Physicians; 1989.

American College of Nurse Midwives. Statement on breast-feeding. *J Nurse Midwifery* 1993;38:4.

American Dietetic Association. Position of the American Dietetic Association: promotion of breast-feeding. *J Am Diet Assoc* 1997;97:662-666.

American Hospital Association. *Something to Think About . . . Promotion of Breastfeeding*. Chicago: American Hospital Association; 1992.

American Medical Association. *AMA Policy Compendium*. Chicago: American Medical Association; 1990.

American Public Health Association. Position paper 8022: Infant feeding in the United States. *Am J Public Health* 1981;71:207-211.

Association of Women's Health, Obstetric and Neonatal Nurses (AWHONN). *Position Statement: Breastfeeding; 1991*. Available from AWHONN. A newer statement is in progress at press time.

British Pediatric Association. Statement of the Standing Committee on Nutrition. *Arch Dis Child* 1994;71:376-380.

Holy Father. Breast-feeding protects against disease and creates bonds of love. *L'Osservatore Romano*. May 1995;21-24.

International Childbirth Education Association. *ICEA Position Paper on Infant Feeding*. 1992.

International Federation of Gynecology and Obstetrics. Recommendations of the International Federation of Gynecology and Obstetrics for action to encourage breastfeeding. *Int J Gynaecol Obstet* 1982;20:171-172.

International Lactation Consultant Association. *Position Paper on Infant Feeding*. Raleigh, NC: International Lactation Consultant Association; 1994.

Lamaze International. *Position Paper on Infant Feeding*. Washington, DC: Lamaze International (formerly ASPO Lamaze); 1995.

National Association of WIC Directors. *Guidelines for Breastfeeding Promotion and Support in the WIC Program*. Washington, DC: National Association of WIC Directors; 1994.

National Association of Pediatric Nurse Associates and Practitioners. NAPNAP policy statement on breastfeeding. *J Pediatr Health Care* 1988;2:314.

Spisak S, Gross SS. *Second Followup Report: The Surgeon General's Workshop on Breastfeeding and Human Lactation.* Washington, DC: National Center for Education in Maternal and Child Health; 1991. Available from National Maternal and Child Health Clearing House.

United States Department of Health and Human Services. *Followup Report: The Surgeon General's Workshop on Breastfeeding and Human Lactation.* Rockville, MD: Health Resources and Services Administration; 1985. Out of print.

United States Department of Health and Human Services. *Healthy People 2000: National Health Promotion and Disease Prevention Objectives.* Washington, DC: Government Printing Office; 1991. Current version available at www.gpo.gov; new version in progress.

United States Department of Health and Human Services. *Report of the Surgeon General's Workshop on Breastfeeding and Human Lactation.* Rockville, MD: Health Resources and Services Administration; 1984. Available from National Maternal and Child Health Clearing House.

WHO and UNICEF. *Innocenti Declaration: 30 July to 1 Aug. 1990, Florence, Italy.* Geneva: Author; 1990. Available from WHO.

WHO and UNICEF. *Protecting, Promoting, and Supporting Breast-Feeding: The Special Role of Maternity Services.* Geneva: World Health Organization; 1989. Available from WHO Publications Center.

World Health Organization. *International Code of Marketing of Breast-Milk Substitutes.* Geneva: World Health Organization; 1981.

APPENDIX E
Publishers/Producers/Distributors

Contact list for publishers, producers, and distributors who carry breastfeeding media listed in other appendices in this book. Every effort has been made to ensure accuracy of the contact information listed below; however, this information changes rapidly. Suggestions from readers or vendors are welcomed; please send comments to bookcomments@wmc-worldwide.com.

ACADEMIC PRESS
(Division of Harcourt Brace)
525 B Street, Suite 1900
San Diego, CA 92101-4495
(800) 321-5068
(407) 345-3800
FAX: (407) 345-4060
www.harcourtbrace.com

ACADEMY FOR EDUCATIONAL DEVELOPMENT
1875 Connecticut Avenue, NW
Washington, DC 20009
(202) 884-8822
FAX: (202) 884-8400
www.aed.org

ADDISON WESLEY LONGMAN
One Jacob Way
Reading, MA 01867-3999
(800) 447-2226
(781) 944-3700
FAX: (800) 367-7198
FAX: (781) 944-3700
www.awl.com

AFRICAN MEDICAL AND RESEARCH FOUNDATION
P.O. Box 30125
Nairobi, Kenya
(254) 2-501301
FAX: (254) 2-609518
www.amref.org
amrefhq@users.africaonline.co.ke

ALDINE DE GRUYTER
200 Saw Mill River Road
Hawthorne, NY 10532
(914) 747-0110
FAX: (914) 747-1326
www.degruyter.de
wdg-info@deGruyter.de

AMEDA-EGNELL
2000 Hollister Drive
Libertyville, IL 60048
(847) 918-5882
(800) 323-4060
FAX: (847) 918-5875
www.hollister.com

AMERICAN ACADEMY OF PEDIATRICS
141 Northwest Point Boulevard
Elk Grove Village, IL 60007-1098
(847) 228-5005
FAX: (847) 228-5097
www.aap.org
kidsdoc@aap.org

AMERICAN DIETETIC ASSOCIATION
216 West Jackson Boulevard
Chicago, IL 60606-6995
(800) 745-0775
(312) 899-0040
FAX: (312) 899-1979
www.eatright.org

AVERY PUBLISHING GROUP
120 Old Broadway
New Hyde Park, NY 11040-5000
(800) 548-5757
(516) 741-2155
FAX: (516) 742-1892
Averypubg@aol.com

BABY-FRIENDLY USA
8 Jan Sebastian Way #13
Sandwich, MA 02563
(508) 888-8044
FAX: (508) 888-8050
www.aboutus.com/a100/bfusa
hea@capecod.net

BEST START SOCIAL MARKETING
3500 East Fletcher Avenue #519
Tampa, FL 33613-4708
(800) 277-4975
(813) 971-2119
FAX: (813) 971-2280
beststart@mindspring.com

BIRTH & LIFE BOOKSTORE
Division of Cascade HealthCare Products
141 Commercial Street NE
Salem, OR 97301
(800) 443-9942
(503) 378-7545
FAX: (503) 371-5395

BREASTFEEDING SUPPORT CONSULTANTS
228 Park Lane
Chalfont, PA 18914-3135
(215) 822-1281
FAX: (215) 997-7879
www.bsccenter.org
info@bsccenter.org

BRIGHT FUTURE LACTATION RESOURCE CENTRE
6540 Cedarview Court
Dayton, OH 45459
(937) 438-9458
FAX: (937) 438-3229
www.bflrc.com

BUTTERWORTH-HEINEMANN
225 Wildwood Ave. #B
Woburn, MA 01801-2041
(617) 928-2500
FAX: (617) 933-6333

CARE VIDEO PRODUCTION
1650-F Crossings Parkway
Westlake, OH 44145
(216) 835-5872

CELESTIAL ARTS PUBLISHING CO
PO Box 7123
Berkeley, CA 94707
(510) 845-8414
(800) 841-BOOK
FAX: (510) 524-1052

CHILDBIRTH GRAPHICS
PO Box 21207
Waco, TX 76702-1207
(800) 299-3366
(254) 776-6461
FAX: (888) 977-7653
FAX: (254) 751-0221
www.wrsgroup.com
sales@wrsgroup.com

CHILDREN'S MERCY HOSPITAL
2401 Gillam Road
Kansas City, MO 64108
(816) 234-1613

CLEFT PALATE FOUNDATION
1829 Franklin Street, Suite 1022
Chapel Hill, NC 27514
(800) 24-CLEFT
(919) 933-9044
FAX: (919) 933-9604
www.cleft.com
cleftline@aol.com

EAGLE PRODUCTIONS
2201 Woodnell Drive
Raleigh, NC 27603-5240
(800) 869-7892
FAX: (919) 779-7284
eaglevid@mindspring.com

FOUR DEE PRODUCTS
13312 Redfish Lane #104
Stafford, TX 77477
(800) 526-2594
(281) 261-2291
FAX: (281) 261-5442
www.fourdee.com
4dee@ghg.net

GEDDES PRODUCTIONS
10546 McVine Avenue
Sunland, CA 91040
(818) 951-2809
FAX: (818) 951-9960
www.geddespro.com

GENTLE TOUCH
1720 Willow Creek Circle, Suite 518
Eugene, OR 97402
(888) 448-9489
(541) 431-6283
FAX: (541) 485-7372

GROWING WITH BABY
1230 Marsh Street
San Luis Obispo, CA 93401
(805) 543-6988
(800) 524-9554
FAX: (805) 543-6692

HANLEY & BELFUS, INC.
210 S 13th Street
Philadelphia, PA 19107
(215) 546-7293
(800) 962-1892
FAX: (215) 790-9330
www.hanleyandbelfus.com

HARVARD COMMON PRESS
535 Albany Street
Boston, MA 02118
(617) 423-5803
(888) 657-3755
FAX: (617) 695-9794

HEALTH EDUCATION ASSOCIATES
8 Jan Sebastian Way #13
Sandwich, MA 02563-2359
(888) 888-8077
(508) 888-8044
FAX: (508) 888-8050
www.aboutus.com/a100/healthed/
hea@capecod.net

HEALTH SCIENCES CENTER FOR EDUCATIONAL
RESOURCES
University of Washington
T252 Health Sciences, Box 357161
Seattle, WA 98195-7161
(206) 685-1156
FAX: (206) 543-8051
cer.hs.washington.edu/hscer/
center@u.washington.edu

HEALTHY MOTHERS HEALTHY BABIES
121 N. Washington St., Suite 300
Alexandria, VA 22314
(703) 836-6110
FAX: (703) 836-3470
www.hmhb.org
webmaster@hmhb.org

HMSO PUBLICATIONS CENTRE
PO Box 276
London, SW8 5DT UK
0171-873-9090
FAX: 0171-873-8200

HOLLISTER'S AMEDA-EGNELL
2000 Hollister Drive
Libertyville, IL 60048
(847) 918-5882
(800) 323-4060
FAX: (847) 918-5875
www.hollister.com

HOUGHTON-MIFFLIN
222 Berkeley Street
Boston, MA 02116
(617) 351-5000
(800) 257-9107
FAX: (617) 351-1125
www.hmco.com

INFACT CANADA
6 Trinity Square
Toronto, CANADA M5G 1B1
(416) 595-9819
FAX: (416) 591-9355
www.infactcanada.ca
infact@ftn.net

INJOY PRODUCTIONS
3970 Broadway Street, Suite B4
Boulder, CO 80304
(303) 447-2082
(800) 326-2082
FAX: (303) 449-8788

INTERNATIONAL CHILDBIRTH EDUCATION
    ASSOCIATION
PO Box 20048
Minneapolis, MN 55420
(612) 854-8660
FAX: (612) 854-8772
www.icea.org
info@icea.org

INTERNATIONAL LACTATION CONSULTANT
    ASSOCIATION
4101 Lake Boone Trail
Raleigh, NC 27607
(919) 787-5181
FAX: (919) 787-4916
www.ilca.org
ilca@erols.com

JOHNS HOPKINS UNIVERSITY
Center for Communications Programs
111 Market Place, Suite 310
Baltimore, MD 21202-4024
(410) 659-6290
FAX: (410) 659-6266
www.jhuccp.org
webadmin@jhuccp.org

JONES AND BARTLETT PUBLISHERS
40 Tall Pine Drive
Sudbury, MA 01776
(978) 443-5000
(800) 832-0034
FAX: (978) 443-8000
www.jbpub.com
custserve@jbpub.com

L.A. PUBLISHING
PO Box 773
Franklin, VA 23851
(800) 397-5833
FAX: (757) 569-1447
lapco@gc.net

LA LECHE LEAGUE INTERNATIONAL
PO Box 4079
Schaumburg, IL 60168-4079
(847) 519-7730
(800) LALECHE
FAX: (847) 519-0035
www.lalecheleague.org

LACTATION ASSOCIATES
254 Conant Road
Weston, MA 02493-1756
(781) 893-3553
FAX: (781) 893-8608
marshalact@aol.com

LACTATION CONSULTANT SERVICES
11320 Shady Glen Road
Oklahoma City, OK 73162
(405) 722-2163
dbocar@aol.com

LACTATION INSTITUTE AND BREASTFEEDING CLINIC
16430 Ventura Boulevard, Suite 303
Encino, CA 91436
(818) 995-1913
marmet@beachnet.com

LAKEVIEW BREASTFEEDING CLINIC
6628 Crowchild Trail SW
Calgary, Alberta, CANADA T3E 5R8
(403) 246-7076

LEARNING CURVE OF WEINGART DESIGN
4614 Prospect Avenue #421
Cleveland, OH 44103-4314
(800) 795-9295
(216) 881-5151
FAX: (216) 881-7177
www.learningcurve1.com
weingartd@aol.com

MARCH OF DIMES
Birth Defects Foundation
1275 Mamaroneck Avenue
White Plains, NY 10605
(800) 367-6630
(717) 820-8104
FAX: (717) 825-1987
www.modimes.org
ProfEd@modimes.org

MARYLAND WIC
201 West Preston Street
Baltimore, MD 21201
(410) 767-6902

McGRAW-HILL COMPANIES
PO Box 182604
Columbus, OH 43272
(800) 262-4729
FAX: (614) 759-3644
www.mhhe.com
customer.service@mcgraw-hill.com

MEDELA
PO Box 660
McHenry, IL 60051-0660
(800) 435-8316
(815) 363-1166
FAX: (800) 995-7867
FAX: (815) 363-1246
www.medela.com

MOSBY
11830 Westline Industrial Drive
St. Louis, MO 63146
(800) 426-4545
(314) 872-8370
FAX: (314) 432-1380
www.mosby.com

NATIONAL ACADEMY PRESS
2101 Constitution Avenue NW
Lockbox 285
Washington, DC 20055
(800) 624-6242
(202) 334-3313
FAX: (202) 334-2451
www.nap.edu
amerchan@nas.edu

NATIONAL MATERNAL AND CHILD HEALTH
 CLEARING HOUSE
2070 Chain Bridge Road, Suite 450
Vienna, VA 22182-2536
(703) 356-1964
FAX: (703) 821-2098
www.circsol.com/mch/
nmchc@circsol.com

NEW YORK STATE DEPARTMENT OF HEALTH
 BUREAU OF CHILD AND ADOLESCENT HEALTH
890 Corning Tower Building
Albany, NY 12237
(518) 474-2084
www.health.state.ny.us

NORTHWESTERN MEMORIAL HOSPITAL
250 E. Superior Street
Chicago, IL 60611-2950
(312) 908-7398
www.nmh.org

OXFORD UNIVERSITY PRESS
2001 Evans Road
Cary, NC 27513
(800) 451-7556
(919) 677-0977
FAX: (919) 677-1303
www.oup-usa.org

PHARMASOFT PUBLISHING
21 Tascocita Circle
Amarillo, TX 79124
(800) 378-1317
(806) 358-8138
FAX: (806) 356-9480
calx.ama.ttuhsc.edu

PLENUM PUBLISHING CORP.
233 Spring Street
New York, NY 10013-1578
(800) 221-9369
FAX: (212) 647-1898
www.plenum.com
info@plenum.com

POLYMORPH FILMS
118 South Street
Boston, MA 02111
(800) 223-5107
(617) 965-9335
FAX: (617) 542-4957
www.pfilms.com

SPANGLER, AMY
PO Box 501046
Atlanta, GA 31150-1046
(770) 913-9331
FAX: (770) 913-0822
akspangler@aol.com

SUNY STONYBROOK
School of Nursing HSC
Stonybrook, NY 11794-8240
(516) 444-3200
FAX: (516) 444-3136
www.umc.sunysb.edu/nursing/

TELE-PRINT EXPRESS VIDEO COPY CENTER
220 W Martin Luther King Jr Boulevard
Austin, TX 78701
(512) 480-8080

TENSOR
12008 W. 87th Street Parkway #303
Lenexa, KS 66215-2888
(913) 894-8885

UNICEF
Nutrition Section, TA 24 A
3 United Nations Plaza
New York, NY 10017
(212) 326-7000
FAX: (212) 888-7465
www.unicef.org
netmaster@unicef.org

VANCOUVER BREASTFEEDING CENTRE
611 West 11th Avenue
Vancouver, BC V5Z 1M1
(604) 875-4678
FAX: (604) 875-5017
mypage.direct.ca/m/millerb/
millerb@direct.ca

VIDA HEALTH COMMUNICATIONS
6 Bigelow Street
Cambridge, MA 02139
(617) 864-4334
FAX: (617) 864-7862
vidahealth@aol.com

WELLSTART INTERNATIONAL
4062 First Avenue
San Diego, CA 92103-2045
(619) 295-5192
FAX: (619) 574-8159
inquiry@wellstart.org

WHO PUBLICATIONS CENTER
49 Sheridan Avenue
Albany, NY 12210
(518) 436-9686
FAX: (518) 436-7433

WILLIAMS AND WILKINS
351 West Camden Street
Baltimore, MD 21201-2436
(410) 528-4223
(800) 638-0672
FAX: (800) 447-8438
FAX: (410) 528-8550
www.wwilkins.com
custserv@wwilkins.com

WORLD HEALTH ORGANIZATION (WHO)
20 Av. Appia
1211 Geneva 27, SWITZERLAND
+41-22 791 21 11
FAX: +41-22 791 0746
www.who.ch
info@who.ch